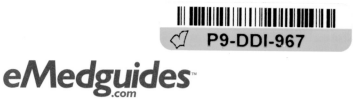

eMedguides™
.com

online and in-print Internet directories in medicine

Cardiology

AN INTERNET RESOURCE GUIDE

December 2001 — November 2002

Consulting Editor

Stephen C. Achuff, M.D.

The David J. Carver Professor of Medicine,
Division of Cardiovascular Medicine,
The Johns Hopkins University School of Medicine

Visit **Cardiology**
at www.eMedguides.com

Access code: **0216**

eMedguides.com, Inc., a Thomson Healthcare company, Princeton, New Jersey

For electronic browsing of this book, see
http://www.eMedguides.com/cardiology

The publisher offers discounts on the eMedguides
series of books. For more information, contact:

Sales Department
eMedguides.com, Inc.
15 Roszel Road
Princeton, NJ 08540
tel   800-230-1481 x16
fax   609-520-2023
e-mail   sales@eMedguides.com
web   http://www.eMedguides.com/books

This book is set in Avenir, BaseNine, Gill Sans, and
Sabon typefaces and was printed and bound in the
United States of America.

10 9 8 7 6 5 4 3 2 1

ISBN 0-9676811-5-4

eMedguides™
.com

Cardiology
AN INTERNET RESOURCE GUIDE

Stephen C. Achuff, M.D., *Consulting Editor*
The David J. Carver Professor of Medicine,
Division of Cardiovascular Medicine,
The Johns Hopkins University School of Medicine

Karen M. Albert, MLS,
Consulting Medical Librarian
Director of Library Services, Fox Chase Cancer Center

Daniel R. Goldenson, *Publisher*

Alysa M. Wilson, *Editor-in-Chief*

Karen B. Schwartz, *Managing Editor*

Ravpreet S. Syalee, *Production Editor*

Barbara Morrison, *Manuscript Editor*

Joyce Milione, *Production Assistant*

Sue Bannon, *Graphic Designer*

eMedguides.com, Inc.,
a Thomson Healthcare company
15 Roszel Road, Princeton, NJ 08540

Daniel R. Goldenson
General Manager

Amy Ma, Ph.D,
Coordinator, Publication Development

Kim Seok,
Coordinator, Finance Administration

Book Orders & Feedback
Book orders • http://www.eMedguides.com/books
Phone orders • 800.230.1481 x16
Facsimile • 609.520.2023
E-mail • cardiology@eMedguides.com
Web • http://www.eMedguides.com/cardiology

2001–2002
Annual Editions

Allergy & Immunology
Anesthesiology & Pain Management
Arthritis & Rheumatology
Cardiology
Dental Medicine
Dermatology
Diet & Nutrition
Emergency Medicine
Endocrinology & Metabolism
Family Medicine
Gastroenterology
General Surgery
Infectious Diseases & Immunology
Internal Medicine
Neurology & Neuroscience
Nurse Practitioners
Obstetrics & Gynecology
Oncology & Hematology
Ophthalmology
Orthopedics & Sports Medicine
Osteopathic Medicine
Otolaryngology
Pathology & Laboratory Medicine
Pediatrics & Neonatology
Physical Medicine & Rehabilitation
Psychiatry
Radiology
Respiratory & Pulmonary Medicine
Urology & Nephrology
Veterinary Medicine

Disclaimer

eMedguides.com, Inc., hereafter referred to as the "publisher," has developed this book for informational purposes only, and not as a source of medical advice. The publisher does not guarantee the accuracy, adequacy, timeliness, or completeness of any information in this book and is not responsible for any errors or omissions or any consequences arising from the use of the information contained in this book. The material provided is general in nature and is in summary form. The content of this book is not intended in any way to be a substitute for professional medical advice. One should always seek the advice of a physician or other qualified healthcare provider. Further, one should never disregard medical advice or delay in seeking it because of information found through an Internet Web site included in this book. The use of the eMedguides.com, Inc. book is at the reader's own risk.

All information contained in this book is subject to change. Mention of a specific product, company, organization, Web site URL address, treatment, therapy, or any other topic does not imply a recommendation or endorsement by the publisher.

Non-liability

The publisher does not assume any liability for the contents of this book or the contents of any material provided at the Internet sites, companies, and organizations reviewed in this book. Moreover, the publisher assumes no liability or responsibility for damage or injury to persons or property arising from the publication and use of this book; the use of those products, services, information, ideas, or instructions contained in the material provided at the third-party Internet Web sites, companies, and organizations listed in this book; or any loss of profit or commercial damage including but not limited to special, incidental, consequential, or any other damages in connection with or arising out of the publication and use of this book. Use of third-party Web sites is subject to the Terms and Conditions of use for such sites.

Copyright Protection

Information available over the Internet and other online locations may be subject to copyright and other rights owned by third parties. Online availability of text and images does not imply that they may be reused without the permission of rights holders. Care should be taken to ensure that all necessary rights are cleared prior to reusing material distributed over the Internet and other online locations.

Trademark Protection

The words in this book for which we have reason to believe trademark, service mark, or other proprietary rights may exist have been designated as such by use of initial capitalization. However, no attempt has been made to designate as trademarks or service marks all personal computer words or terms in which proprietary rights might exist. The inclusion, exclusion, or definition of a word or term is not intended to affect, or to express any judgment on, the validity or legal status of any proprietary right that may be claimed in that word or term.

EMEDGUIDES.COM ONLINE

Instant access to every Web site in this book at www.eMedguides.com!

This volume, *in its entirety*, can be browsed online at eMedguides.com. Simply point and click to surf to the latest Web sites in your specialty! eMedguides.com is continually updated with URL and content changes, as well as new sites in each specialty. Start your search for medical information, in any specialty, with the trusted assistance of eMedguides.com.

THREE WAYS TO SURF WITH AN EMEDGUIDE:

FAST Drill down at eMedguides.com to the Web information you seek.

FASTER Find a site in the print edition and type the URL into your browser.

FASTEST Find a site in the print edition and type in the e-Link code instead of the URL (for example, go to site G-1234 by typing: www.eMedguides.com/G-1234).

GENERAL MEDICINE REFERENCE
Part Two of every book (General Medical Web Resources) is always available in the sidebar.

E-LINK WITH THE URL
Type in the e-Link code (found next to each entry in this book) after www.eMedguides.com/. You will go directly to the site you seek, even if the URL has changed.

TELL US ABOUT A SITE
When you find a terrific site, tell us about it. Fill out a simple form and we may add your site immediately to eMedguides.com, and we may include it in our next print edition too.

BUY MORE BOOKS
Quickly order books in any of our available specialties, including patient guides, from our online store.

FREE JOURNALS & ASSOCIATIONS
Hundreds of links to journals and associations in each of over 20 specialties are provided.

BROWSE THE TABLE OF CONTENTS
You can quickly find every topic using the full table of contents.

FULL PRINT EDITION, ONLINE
Click to view the sites in a topic. An access code is required; you can find it on the title page of this book.

E-LINK OR SEARCH
Enter an e-Link code (found next to each site in this book) or enter a text string to search the entire specialty.

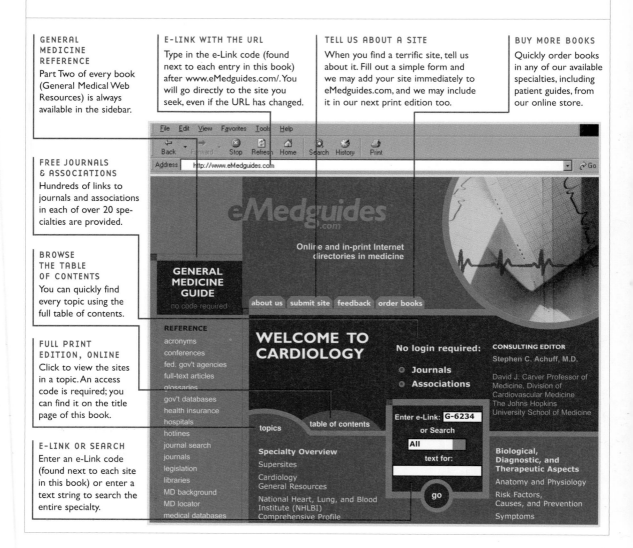

PRAVACHOL®
pravastatin sodium 40 mg tablets

Please see full prescribing information
in appendix A at the end of this book.

TABLE OF CONTENTS

New NCEP* guidelines† identify
more patients than ever in the **CV RISK ZONE**

Help bring your patients to the

PRAVACHOL
PROTECTION
ZONE:

Aggressive cardioprotection. Proven safety.

Now the CV Risk Zone includes patients with†:

**Borderline-high LDL-C
(LDL-C 130-159 mg/dL)**

2+ risk factors

**≥10% ten-year risk for
major CHD events**

**Diabetes — now a
CHD risk equivalent**

LDL-C ≥100 mg/dL

**>20% ten-year risk for
major CHD events**

* NCEP = National Cholesterol Education Program
† Executive Summary of the Third Report of the National Cholesterol Education Program (NCEP)
Expert Panel on Detection, Evaluation, and Treatment of High Blood Cholesterol in Adults (Adults
Treatment Panel III). *JAMA*. 2001L285:2486-2497.

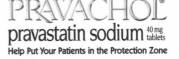

PRAVACHOL lowers CV risk — NOW with reduced recommendations for LFT monitoring*

Aggressive cardioprotection

In addition to diet, when diet and exercise are not enough in patients with elevated cholesterol or CHD

- PRAVACHOL is the only statin proven to reduce the risk of both first and recurrent MI, as well as stroke[1-4]

- Reduce the risk of total mortality by reducing coronary death[1,4]

* Proven safety

- It is recommended that liver function tests be performed prior to initiating therapy, prior to increasing the dose, and when otherwise clinically indicated

- If a patient develops increased transaminase levels, or signs and symptoms of liver disease, more frequent monitoring may be required

- Reduced potential for CYP450 3A4 drug interactions

Important Safety Information:

- Pravachol is contraindicated for patients who are pregnant or nursing and in the presence of active liver disease or unexplained persistent transaminase elevations.

- Myopathy should be considered in any patient with diffuse myalgias, muscle tenderness or weakness, and/or marked elevation of creatine phosphokinase (CPK). Patients should be advised to report promptly unexplained muscle pain, tenderness, or weakness, particularly if accompanied by malaise or fever. The risk of myopathy during treatment with another HMG-CoA reductase inhibitor is increased with concurrent therapy with erythromycin, cyclosporin, niacin or fibrates. The combined use of Pravachol and fibrates should be avoided unless the benefit of further alterations in lipid levels is likely to outweigh the increased risk of this drug combination.

- Pravachol is well tolerated. The most common adverse events are rash, fatigue, headache, and dizziness.

1. Pravachol product labeling, Bristol-Myers Squibb Company.
2. Shepherd J. Cobbe SM, Ford I, et al. Prevention of coronary heart disease with pravastatin in men with hypercholesterolemia. N Engl J Med. 1995;333:1301-1307.
3. Sacks FM, Pfeffer MA, Moye LA, et al. The effect of pravastatin on coronary events after myocardial infarction in patients with average cholesterol levels. N Engl J Med. 1996;335:1001-1007.
4. The Long-Term intervention with Pravastatin in Ischaemic Disease (LIPID) Study Group. Prevention of cardiovascular events and death with pravastatin in patients with coronary heart disease and a broad range of initial cholesterol levels. N Eng J Med. 1998;339:1349-1357

Please see full prescribing information in appendix A at the end of this book.

PRAVACHOL®
pravastatin sodium 40 mg tablets
Help Put Your Patients in the Protection Zone

PART TWO   General Medical Web Resources

10. REFERENCE INFORMATION AND NEWS SOURCES 361

11. PROFESSIONAL TOPICS AND CLINICAL PRACTICE 415

PREFACE

The American Medical Association has estimated that more than half of America's physicians use the Internet, and the trend-line is rising. Although much use may be attributed to e-mail and personal research, the clinical uses of the World Wide Web cannot be ignored. The Internet facilitates communication among professionals, ease of examination of numerous medical journals, focused topical research, and patient education. And in the very near future, if not already, we will do our clinical transactions over the Internet.

The second annual edition of *Cardiology: An Internet Resource Guide* is now one in a series of more than ten similar volumes that cover the various fields of medicine in great depth. Designed for clinicians, researchers, medical students, and allied healthcare professionals, the books put the user in touch with extensive resources on the Internet, with a format somewhat like a medical textbook.

For cardiologists and their staffs, there are daily news sites, conference schedules, clinical trials information, and new drug data appearing in a section called Quick Reference. More than one hundred journals are available where article abstracts for current issues may be consulted at any time. Newly published books and resources on CME add to some of the educational features of this compendium.

In the clinical sections, dozens of diagnostic tests, surgical procedures, and therapeutics are referenced, with links to applicable Web sites, followed by an exploration into more than twenty diverse clinical and educational topics.

A long chapter is devoted to hundreds of diseases and disorders, categorized extensively for the reader's convenience.

The last section of the book is devoted to general medical information resources covering a wide range of topics, from general reference to insurance and patient planning.

I am pleased to invite physicians and healthcare professionals to delve into the Internet and use this volume as a starting point for research explorations and as a source for patient education.

Daniel R. Goldenson
Publisher

INTRODUCTION

1.1 WELCOME TO eMEDGUIDES

Welcome to eMedguides and to the second edition of *Cardiology: An Internet Resource Guide*. As a user of this book, you have a gateway to an extraordinary amount of information, now much expanded, to help you find every useful resource in your field, from electronic journals to selected Web sites on dozens of common and uncommon diseases and disorders.

Over the past year, eMedguides have reached hundreds of thousands of physicians, healthcare professionals, researchers, and medical students. We have published guides to cardiology, dermatology, endocrinology and metabolism, infectious diseases and immunology, neurology and neuroscience, psychiatry, oncology and hematology, urology and nephrology, internal medicine, and respiratory and pulmonary medicine. Several additional important specialties are on the way.

This second edition is built upon a comprehensive table of contents in order to provide a broad overview of topics and issues in the field. We have added hundreds of additional Web sites, revising every category to meet the demanding information requirements of our sophisticated audience.

We would like to thank our Consulting Medical Editor, Stephen C. Achuff, M.D., The David J. Carver Professor of Medicine, Division of Cardiovascular Medicine, The Johns Hopkins University School of Medicine, for his continued contribution to the preparation of this volume. In addition, we appreciate the assistance and guidance from our Consulting Medical Librarian, Karen M. Albert, Director of Library Services for the Fox Chase Cancer Center.

How to Benefit Most from this Book

The most efficient method for finding information in this volume is to scan the table of contents. Our aim has been to organize the material logically, topic by topic, giving descriptions of Web sites that we feel our readers will want to visit. Part One focuses just on the fields of cardiology, including biological, diagnostic, and therapeutic aspects, as well as recent books, CME sites, disorder resources, journal access, organization sites, and other topical information. Part Two concentrates on the broad fields of medicine reference, clinical practice, and patient education. This includes online databases, sources of current news and legislation, library access sites, government agencies, pharmaceutical data, student resources, and patient planning information.

A very extensive index is also included, covering all included topics and Web site titles, to make the fact-finding mission as efficient as possible.

Physicians and researchers will find that a wide array of material exists in the field. In addition to "supersites," many individual diseases, diagnoses, and therapies have dedicated Web sites intended for professional audiences. We have provided a comprehensive list of journal Web sites which provide access to thousands of articles and abstracts every month. A further exploration can lead to content-rich government sites, hospital and school departments, clinical research centers, recent drug trial results, and sites that provide quick updates on news, CME, and upcoming conferences.

Although much of the material in this book is intended for a professional medical audience, key patient Web resources are also provided. Physicians may wish to refer patients to these sites. Many patient sites include up-to-date news and research and clear descriptions of diseases and their treatments.

Finding a Site

We provide the full URL for each site in this volume, which can be typed into the address bar of your Internet browser. With our second edition, we also provide an identification number called an "e-Link," which will quickly take you to a specific Web site. Simply type in the eMedguides address, followed by a forward slash (/), followed by the e-Link number (found in the box next to each Web site in this book). For example, to reach the National Institutes of Health, enter www.eMedguides.com/g-0050. The e-Link number is associated with a Web site address in our database. Since we update Web addresses continually, you will always be directed to the appropriate address. This is especially important for medical Web site addresses, which change quite often as new information is added to bring sites up to date.

All of the content in this volume can also be accessed at our Web site, www.eMedguides.com, using the entry code found on the title page of this book. At our site you can explore the field by simply clicking on Web sites, as with a traditional Web directory. General medical sites are located in the sidebar, while specialty-specific information can be reached from the Cardiology section (use www.eMedguides.com/cardiology as a shortcut).

The Benefits of Both Print and Online Editions

We feel that both the print and online editions of eMedguides play an important role in the information gathering process. The print edition is a "hands-on" tool, enabling the reader to thumb through a comprehensive directory, finding Web information and topical sources that are totally new and unexpected. Each page can provide discoveries of resources previously unknown to the reader that may never have been the subject of an online search. Without knowing what to expect, the reader can be introduced to useful Web site information just by glancing at the book, looking through the detailed table of contents, or examining the extensive index. This type of browsing is difficult to achieve online.

The online edition serves a different purpose. It provides direct links to each Web site so the user can visit the destination instantaneously, without having to type the Web address or our new e-Link identification code into a browser. In addition, there are search features in this edition that can be used to find specific information quickly, and then the user can print out only what he or she wishes to use.

The online edition also represents the most up-to-date information about our selected Web sites. We update our database throughout the year, adding new resources as they become available, and editing those that change. The eMedguides Web site also provides a platform for communication with our Submit a Site feature, which lets you share your online discoveries with us and, hence, other readers in a future update.

We hope you will find the print and online versions of this volume to be useful Internet companions, always on hand to consult.

1.2 RATINGS AND SITE SELECTION

Site Selection Criteria

Our medical research staff has carefully chosen the sites for this guide. We perform extensive searches for all of the topics listed in our table of contents and then select only the sites that meet carefully established criteria. The pertinence and depth of content, timeliness of the material, presentation, and usefulness of the site for physician and advisory purposes are taken into account.

The selection of sites in this physician guide includes detailed reference material, news, clinical data, and current research articles. We also include and appropriately identify numerous sites that may be useful for patient reference. The large majority of our Web sites are maintained by reputable academic, government-sponsored, or professional and research organizations. Additional material is derived from online textbooks or scholarly, referenced journals in the field. Sites operated by private individuals or corporations are only included if they are content-rich and useful to the physician. In these cases, we clearly identify the operator in the title or description of the site.

In addition, if a site requires a fee, some fees, or a free registration/disclosure of personal information, we indicate this information at the end of the site description.

Ratings Guide

Those sites that are identified based on the selection criteria are subsequently rated on a scale of one apple (🍎) to three apples (🍎🍎🍎). Scholarly material, aimed at a professional audience, and authoritative educational materials that are useful to both students and healthcare consumers are eligible for inclusion. The three-apple designation denotes a site that is a comprehensive source of relevant information derived from a major educational institution, government-sponsored organization, noteworthy professional or research group, or authoritative publication. The timeliness and accuracy of the material, its usefulness to users, and its depth of content are considered to be high. A one-apple site contains accurate, relevant information in a more succinct format.

Abbreviations

See "Medical Abbreviations and Acronyms" under "Reference Information and News Sources" in Part Two for Web sites that provide acronym translation. Below are a few acronyms you will find throughout this volume:

ACC	American College of Cardiology
AHA	American Heart Association
AMA	American Medical Association
CME	Continuing Medical Education
FAQ	Frequently Asked Questions
NHLBI	National Heart, Lung, and Blood Institute
NIH	National Institutes of Health
PDQ	Physician Data Query
URL	Uniform Resource Locator (the address of a Web site on the Internet)

1.3 GETTING ONLINE

The Internet is growing at a rapid pace, but many individuals are not yet online. What is preventing people from jumping on the "information highway"? There are many factors, but the most common issues are a general confusion about what the Internet is, how it works, and how to access it.

The following few pages are designed to clear up any confusion for readers who have not yet accessed the Internet. We will look at the process of getting onto and using the Internet, step by step.

It is also helpful to consult other resources, such as the technical support department of the manufacturer or retailer where you purchased your computer. Although assistance varies widely, most organizations provide startup assistance for new users and are experienced with guiding individuals onto the Internet. Books can also be of great assistance, as they provide a simple and clear view of how computers and the Internet work, and can be studied at your own pace.

What is the Internet?

The Internet is a large network of computers that are all connected to one another. A good analogy is to envision a neighborhood, with houses and storefronts, all connected to one another by streets and highways. Often the Internet is referred to as the "information super-highway" because of the vastness of this neighborhood.

The Internet was initially developed to allow people to share computers. That is, share part of their "house" with others. The ability to connect to so many other computers quickly and easily made this feasible. As computers proliferated and increased in computational power, people started using the Internet for sending information quickly from one computer to another.

For example, the most popular feature of the Internet is electronic mail (e-mail). Each computer has a mailbox, and an electronic letter can be sent instantly. People also use the Internet to post bulletins, or other information, for others to see. The process of sending e-mail or viewing this information is simple. A computer and a connection to the Internet are all you need to begin.

How is an Internet connection provided?
The Internet is accessed either through a "direct" connection, which is found in businesses and educational institutions, or through a phone line. Phone line connections are the most common access method for users at home, although direct connections are becoming available for home use. There are many complex options in this area. However, for the new user it is simplest to use an existing phone line to experience the Internet for the first time. A dual telephone jack can be purchased at many retail stores. Connect the computer to the phone jack, and then use the provided software to connect to the Internet. Your computer will dial the number of an Internet provider and ask you for a user name and password. Keep in mind that while you are using the Internet, your phone line is tied up and callers will hear a busy signal. Additionally, call waiting can sometimes interrupt an Internet connection and disconnect you from the Internet.

Who provides an Internet connection?
Several Internet providers exists at both the local and national levels. One of the easiest ways to get online is with America Online (AOL). They provide software and a user-friendly environment through which to access the Internet. Because AOL manages both this environment and the actual connection, they can be of great assistance when you are starting out. America Online takes you to a menu of choices when you log in, and while using their software you can read and send e-mail, view Web pages, and chat with others.

Many other similar services exist, and most of them also provide an environment using Microsoft or Netscape products. These companies, such as the Microsoft Network (MSN) and Earthlink, also provide simple, easy-to-use access to the Internet. Their environment is more standard and not limited to the choices America Online provides.

Internet connections generally run from $10-$30 per month (depending on the length of commitment) in addition to telephone costs. Most national providers have local phone numbers all over the country that should eliminate any telephone charges. The monthly provider fee is the only direct charge for accessing the Internet.

How do I get on the Internet?
Once you've signed up with an Internet provider and installed their software (often only a matter of answering basic questions), your computer will be set up to access the Internet. By simply double-clicking on an icon, your computer will dial the phone number, log you in, and present you with a Web page (a "home" page).

What are some of the Internet's features?
From the initial Web page there are almost limitless possibilities of where you can go. The address at the top of the screen (identified by an "http://" in front) tells you where you are. You can also type the address of where you would like to go next. When typing a new address, you do not need to add the "http://". The computer adds this prefix automatically after you type in an address and press return. Once you press return, the Web site will appear in the browser window.

You can also navigate the Web by "surfing" from one site to another using links on a page. A Web page might say, "Click here for weather." If you move the mouse pointer to this underlined phrase and click the mouse button, you will be taken to a different address, where weather information is provided.

The Internet has several other useful features. E-mail is an extremely popular and important service. It is free and messages are delivered instantly. Although you can access e-mail through a Web browser (AOL has this feature), many Internet services provide a separate e-mail program for reading, writing, and organizing your correspondence. These programs send and retrieve messages from the Internet.

Another area of the Internet offers chat rooms where users can hold roundtable discussions. In a chat room you can type messages and see the replies of other users around the world. There are chat rooms on virtually every topic, although the dialog certainly varies in this free-for-all forum. There are also newsgroups on the Internet, some of which we list in this book. A newsgroup is similar to a chat room but each message is a separate item and can be viewed in sequence at any time. For example, a user might post a question about Lyme disease. In the newsgroup you can read the question and then read the answers that others have provided. You can also post your own comments. This forum is usually not managed or edited, particularly in the medical field. Do not take the advice of a chat room or newsgroup source without first consulting your physician.

How can I find things on the Internet?

Surfing the Internet, from site to site, is a popular activity, but if you have a focused mission, you will want to use a search engine. A search engine can scan lists of Web sites to look for a particular site. We provide a long list of medical search engines in this book.

Because the Internet is so large and unregulated, sites are often hard to find. In the physical world it is difficult to find good services, but you can turn to the yellow pages or other resources to get a comprehensive list. Physical proximity is also a major factor. On the Internet, the whole world is at your doorstep. Finding a reliable site takes time and patience, and can require sifting through hundreds of similar, yet irrelevant, sites.

The most common way to find information on the Internet is to use a search engine. When you go to the Web page of a search engine, you will be presented with two distinct methods of searching: using links to topics or using a keyword search. The links often represent the Web site staff's best effort to find quality sites. This method of searching is the core of the Yahoo! search engine (http://www.yahoo.com). By clicking on Healthcare, then Disorders, then Lung Cancer, you are provided with a list of sites the staff has found on the topic.

The keyword approach is definitely more daring. By typing in search terms, the engine looks through its list of Web sites for a match and returns the results. These engines typically only cover 15 percent of the Internet, so it is not a comprehensive process. They also usually return far too many choices. Typing "lung cancer" into a search engine box will return thousands of sites, including one entry for every site where someone used the words lung cancer on a personal Web page.

Where do eMedguides come in?

eMedguides are organized listings of Web sites in each major medical specialty. Our team of editors continually scours the Net, searching for quality Web sites that relate to specific specialties, disorders, and research topics. More importantly, of the sites we find, we only include those that provide professional and useful content. eMedguides fill a critical gap in the Internet research process. Each guide provides more than 1,000 Web sites that focus on every aspect of a single medical discipline.

Other Internet search engines rely on teams of "surfers" who can only cover a subject on its surface because they survey the entire Internet. Search engines, even medical search engines, return far too many choices, requiring hours of time and patience to sift through. eMedguides, on the other hand, focus on medical and physician sites in a specialty. With an eMedguide in hand, you can quickly identify the sites worth visiting on the Internet and jump right to them. At our site, http://www.eMedguides.com, you can access the same listings as in this book and can simply click on a site to go directly to it. In addition, we provide continual updates to the book through the online site and annually in print. Our editors do the surfing for you and do it professionally, making your Internet experience efficient and fulfilling.

Our new e-Link identification code provides a method of instantly accessing selected sites without having to type in lengthy and cumbersome Web addresses.

Taking medical action must involve a physician

As interesting as the Internet is, the information that you will find is both objective and subjective. Our goal is to expose our readers to Web sites on hundreds of topics for informational purposes only. If you are not a physician and become interested in the ideas, guidelines, recommendations, or experiences discussed online, bring these findings to a physician for personal evaluation. Medical needs vary considerably, and a medical approach or therapy for one individual could be entirely misguided for another. Final medical advice and a plan of action must come only from a physician.

CARDIOLOGY
WEB RESOURCES

QUICK REFERENCE

2.1 DISORDER PROFILES

The following Web sites provide resources on a large number of disorders for quick reference purposes. A far more extensive treatment of individual diseases and disorders appears in a later section of the volume.

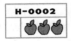

American Heart Association (AHA): Heart and Stroke Encyclopedia An A-to-Z guide is found at this site, which provides comprehensive access to AHA consumer publications. Consumer brochures address a wide variety of cardiovascular and stroke-related illnesses, with each document offering an introduction to the selected condition's symptoms, diagnosis, and management options. http://216.185.112.5/presenter.jhtml?identifier=10000056

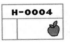

Karolinska Institutet: Cardiovascular Diseases A virtual library of heart disease information is contained at this reference of the Karolinska Institutet. Hundreds of fact sheets and other patient information, as well as a wide selection of professional resources, are available. Guidelines for assessment, diagnosis, and management of disorders are presented, including resources for arrhythmias, angina pectoris, congestive heart failure, myocardial infarction, and dozens of additional cardiovascular conditions.
http://micf.mic.ki.se/Diseases/c14.html

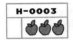

Medical College of Wisconsin: Cardiovascular System Offering physicians a quick reference guide, this site lists a large number of cardiovascular disorders and provides a short clinical description of each of them. Included in many citations are links to related articles in the Medical College of Wisconsin HealthLink.
http://chorus.rad.mcw.edu/index/2.html

Merck Manual of Diagnosis and Therapy: Cardiovascular Disorders Section 16 of the online *Merck Manual of Diagnosis and Therapy* offers 17 searchable chapters on diseases of the cardiovascular system, including arrhythmias, endocarditis, and pericardial disease. By accessing a specific chapter, visitors arrive at a comprehensive overview of included disorders, accompanied by several additional connections to specific disorders within the classification and details regarding pathophysiology, diagnosis, and treatment.
http://www.merck.com/pubs/mmanual/section16/sec16.htm

2.2 Glossaries

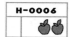

Society of Thoracic Surgeons: Glossary of Heart Surgery Terms
Created by the Society of Thoracic Surgeons, this glossary provides patients with an alphabetical list and definitions of terms associated with heart surgery. Within the text, there are links to other organizations and hyperlinks to other terms in the glossary.
http://www.sts.org/doc/3564

Texas Heart Institute: Glossary of Cardiovascular Terminology
This glossary of cardiovascular terminology is provided by the Texas Heart Institute Heart Information Service. In addition to the large number of entries, a link to anatomy of the heart is provided for diagrammatic clarification.
http://www.tmc.edu/thi/glossary.html

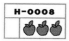

ThromboSite: ThromboGlossary
The ThromboGlossary provides definitions of terms related to the pathophysiology, pharmacology, and clinical aspects of thrombosis, thrombotic disorders, and hemostasis. Definitions are intended for use by medical professionals.
http://www.thrombosite.com/thrombo_glos.html

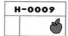

University of Michigan: Cardiology Terminology Glossary
Definitions of medical terms that patients may commonly hear or read about are provided at this online glossary, as a service of the Patient Information Center/Heart Care Program. http://www.med.umich.edu/hcp/pa_info/glossary.htm

2.3 Conferences in Cardiology

A number of key Web sites that offer event calendars along with details of conference programs and locations are provided here. Although an extensive conference calendar is provided by the PSL Group's *Doctor's Guide,* the other listed sites have valuable additional listings. Taken together, this group provides an overall source of conference scheduling information for the year.

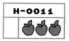

American Heart Association (AHA): Scientific Conferences and Meetings
A listing of professional meetings and development seminars is found at this AHA site, including dates, program details, and links to in-depth information on educational objectives and curriculum, sponsored by the AHA and associated councils. Cosponsored conferences are also included.
http://www.americanheart.org/presenter.jhtml?identifier=1200035

Doctor's Guide: Medical Conferences and Meetings
This extensive listing of conferences and meetings in cardiology offers dates, locations, and other meeting details. The information is updated frequently. The reader can click on any conference listing to additional information such as travel arrangements and local weather. http://www.pslgroup.com/dg/cardio.htm

Health On the Net (HON) Foundation: Conferences and Events A search for "cardiology" events results in this listing of CME activities and national and international professional activities. Details on meeting coverage and location are found, with links available to specific conference URLs. A mailbox option delivers updates to the list electronically.
http://www.hon.ch/cgi-bin/confevent?theme+alp+C+G02.403.776.409.163

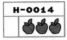

MedicalConferences.com MedicalConferences.com is a comprehensive resource for information on forthcoming conferences and meetings. Visitors can enter specific search terms into the site's search engine to receive a lengthy listing of conferences to be held over the next 12 months or longer. Each conference is an active link in itself, providing access to further information about the event. http://www.medicalconferences.com/

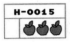

MediConf Online: Cardiology and Cardiovascular Meetings MediConf Online provides a directory of upcoming meetings and conferences in every major medical specialty. This site, specific to cardiology and cardiovascular meetings, provides a listing of events, complete with contact information and a link to the city, through which the visitor can learn about accommodations, weather, and community information. Web sites specific to the courses and conferences offer program and scientific details, as well as registration opportunities. http://www.mediconf.com/

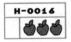

Medscape: Cardiology Conference Coverage Requiring a free registration, this Medscape site offers reviews of conference coverage, authored by leading authorities in the field of cardiology. Selected session summaries are available, as well as printable versions of the activities. Many of the programs are valid for CME, including those of the North American Society of Pacing and Electrophysiology and the American College of Cardiology. (free registration)
http://cardiology.medscape.com/Home/Topics/
cardiology/directories/dir-CARD.ConfSummaries.html

2.4 TOPICAL SEARCH TOOLS

American College of Cardiology (ACC): Search Engine By entering keywords at the ACC search engine, visitors are returned an assortment of documents, including ACC news, highlights in cardiovascular medicine, journal excerpts, and minutes from Scientific Sessions. The entire site may searched as well as clinical statements across a variety of subspecialties.
http://www.acc.org/

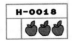

American Heart Association (AHA): Search Engine The search engine of the AHA allows users to search the Web by selecting from a series of menus or by entering specific topics. Also available are the Heart and Stroke A-to-Z Guide, which provides direct links to commonly requested information, and the Scientific Statements search for quick access to professional management resources. http://www.americanheart.org/presenter.jhtml?identifier=1200000

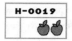

AtCardiology.com AtCardiology.com offers visitors the opportunity to locate information quickly on commonly searched cardiology terminology or to perform an individualized cardiology Internet search. By clicking on any one of the frequently searched topics, users are returned a listing of journal articles, scientific statements, and practice guidelines in the area. Alternatively, a keyword search of Internet documents pertaining to the field of cardiovascular medicine may be performed.

http://www.atcardiology.com/cardiology

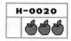

CardioGuide.com CardioGuide.com allows for efficient Internet searching in the field of cardiology, including both the cardiology-specific MEDLINE search and the keyword cardiology Internet search. Visitors are returned a listing of either article abstracts within the chosen topic or an assortment of case studies, clinical trials, scientific statements, and visualizations. Quick patient information reference guides are available at the page, and premier cardiology disorder, educational, and organizational sites are recommended and accessible.

http://www.mymedline.com/cardio

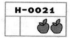

Cardiothoracic Surgery Network (CTSNet) Using keywords, this useful tool allows visitors to locate desired articles from the CTSNet Document Library and Image Library. These resources offer online archives of scholarly publications related to cardiothoracic practice, as well as figures, photographs, illustrations, and tables from the *Annals of Thoracic Surgery* and the Internet pages of Cardiothoracic Surgery Network.

http://www.ctsnet.org/search

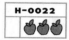

Global Cardiology Network This user-friendly resource for cardiology professionals, patients, and others with an interest in the specialty provides access to a wealth of information in the subject area. Documents available from member organizations' Web sites include journal articles, practice guidelines, clinical trials, CME, meetings and conferences, grants and fellowships, patient information, and organization home pages in cardiology.

http://www.globalcardiology.org/search/search.asp

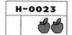

National Heart, Lung, and Blood Institute (NHLBI): Site Search Engine An extensive collection of cardiovascular health resources may be found using the NHLBI's powerful search engine, allowing visitors access to an assortment of publications, statistics, and clinical guidelines and trials. Access to the laboratories of the NHLBI, specialty divisions and health initiative information, educational programs of the organization, NIH news releases, and a multitude of additional cardiovascular health documents may be found.

http://www.nhlbi.nih.gov/search/index.htm

2.5 CARDIOLOGY NEWS

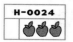

American College of Cardiology (ACC): Media, Journal, & News
Research headlines are the focus of this site of the ACC, presented by WebMD

and Cardiosource. Additional news departments of the organization can be accessed from the page and include ACC News and News Releases and Annual Scientific Session Media. A related patient education department is offered, as well as Web editorials.

http://www.acc.org/media/media_journals.htm

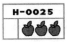

Cardiology Today: Current News in Cardiovascular Disease Front page headlines, editorials, and access to back issues are found at this page, provided by Slack, Inc. A free e-mail newswire service is available following a simple registration, and additional features, such as clinical trial scorecards, online articles in practice management, and upcoming events, are included.

(free registration) http://www.cardiologytoday.com/

CTSNet Newswire This site contains the latest headlines from Reuters Health Information, as a courtesy of the Cardiothoracic Surgery Network. Headlines are listed by date and are accessible for 10 days, with articles on new pharmacotherapeutic agents, related governmental spending, statistical reports, and new surgical techniques and treatments.

http://www.ctsnet.org/reuters

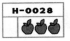

Doctor's Guide: Cardiology Daily News Updated daily, this site provides links to the latest information in the field of cardiology and pharmacotherapeutics, with access to press releases and news reports regarding new treatments and other interesting summaries of clinical study. Full articles may be accessed, and source information is provided. Archived articles are available for up to one year prior to the current date. Visitors are also offered the opportunity to subscribe to a free Internet newsletter.

http://www.pslgroup.com/dg/cardionews.htm

Heart Information Network Containing original content and cardiovascular news, this site provides the latest information in the field of cardiology. The articles may be viewed by topic or in chronological order, beginning with the most recent. Angina, congenital heart defects, diet, health insurance, and artificial valves are a small selection of the topics covered. Links to other resources of the Heart Information Network are also available.

http://www.heartinfo.org

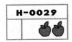

Heart Surgery Network News This site, created by the Heart Surgery Forum, provides summaries of recent articles and books written about heart surgery practice. Also found are reviews of new Web sites and industry press releases. The site offers Heart Surgery Forum announcements, awards, and a LISTSERV. http://www.hsforum.com/frameset1.asp?loc=/default1.asp

HeartLinx.com: Cardiovascular News HeartLinx.com is an indispensable professional resource that provides daily searches of the Internet for relevant articles and clinical reports in the field of cardiology. Visitors to this comprehensive site will find headlines related to cardiovascular medicine, links to corresponding abstracts and news releases, registration details for a free e-mail news-

letter, and access to news archive sources. A medical query search tool is provided, and headlines under relevant subtopics, including arrhythmias, cardiac surgery, congenital heart diseases, and related diagnostics, can be retrieved.
http://www.heartlinx.com

Medscape: Cardiology News   Maintained by Medscape, this site offers today's cardiology news and headlines, with additional links to conference summaries, upcoming conference schedules, and the CBS health information channel. Online reviews of new therapies via CME links, a library of current clinical management news, and highlights of related medical journals are found, courtesy of Journal Scan, MEDLINE, and additional sources. A current review of the global economic burden of cardiovascular disease is provided.
(free registration) http://cardiology.medscape.com/Home/Topics/cardiology/cardiology.html

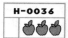

National Heart, Lung, and Blood Institute (NHLBI): News and Press Releases   Alerts, news, and press releases from the NHLBI are listed by month at this Web site. Headlines link to full-text versions of each item, including clinical advisories, statements of the National Institutes of Health (NIH), NHLBI clinical trial review, and new health initiatives of this NIH division.
http://www.nhlbi.nih.gov/new/index.htm

2.6 STATISTICS

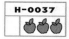

American Heart Association (AHA): Statistics   The statistics Web site of the AHA offers specific statistical information through the *2001 Heart and Stroke Statistical Update,* which is available online as a PDF file. Several biostatistical fact sheets are found, demonstrating the effects of heart disease across various populations. General information on how to interpret statistical information can also be accessed.
http://www.americanheart.org/presenter.jhtml?identifier=1200026

National Center for Health Statistics   The National Center for Health Statistics (NCHS) is a key professional tool for monitoring the nation's health. Access to FEDSTATS provides information from more than 70 U.S. governmental agencies, and "FASTATS A-to-Z" offers an assortment of statistical information in heart disease and across related medical specialties and disorders. Comprehensive data download opportunities exist, and access to several governmental survey and data collection systems, such as the National Health and Nutrition Examination Survey (NHANES), is found.
http://www.cdc.gov/nchs

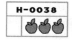

National Center for Health Statistics: Heart Disease   Focusing exclusively on statistics for cardiovascular disease, this page connects viewers to general information on mortality and heart disease as a cause of death by age, race, and sex. Heart disease prevalence documents, which consider occurrence rates by family income and geographic region, are viewable or downloadable in PDF format. http://www.cdc.gov/nchs/fastats/heart.htm

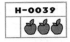

Society of Thoracic Surgeons: National Cardiac Surgery Database

This site features the data analyses of the STS National Cardiac Surgery Database. Visitors can view table summaries of all cardiac procedures in the United States from 1970-1998, as well as a section on annual trends and summaries of procedure volume, age, gender, status, valve type, and preoperative and postoperative length of stay. Other sections cover mortality by procedure, operative mortality summaries, incidence of complications and operative morbidity summaries, and key procedure data by predicted risk group.

http://www.sts.org/doc/2986

2.7 CLINICAL STUDIES AND TRIALS

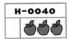

CenterWatch: Listings of Studies at the National Institutes of Health

CenterWatch provides this comprehensive resource for information on clinical trials conducted by the various NIH divisions at the Warren Grant Magnuson Clinical Center in Bethesda, Maryland. By accessing the cardiovascular/vascular diseases section, visitors are returned a listing of over 40 clinical trials in the treatment, evaluation, and prevention of heart diseases. Participating research divisions include the National Heart, Lung, and Blood Institute (NHLBI), the National Institute of Allergy and Infectious Diseases (NIAID), and the National Institute of Diabetes and Digestive and Kidney Diseases (NIDDK). Concise protocol abstracts offer summaries of research goals, a sponsoring institute listing, and recruitment details.

http://www.centerwatch.com/patient/nih/nih_index.html

CenterWatch: Trial Listings by Medical Specialty

An excellent tool for patient referral and professional reference, CenterWatch features a listing of cardiology/vascular disease clinical trials by state in over 30 cardiology disease subcategories, including angina, atherosclerosis, atrial fibrillation, cardiac surgery, heart failure, and peripheral vascular disease. Each categorical listing provides links to the participating clinical research center, a summary of the clinical trial, and research coordinator contact information.

http://www.centerwatch.com/studies/listing.htm#Section1

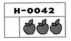

ClinicalTrials.gov

This page, a service of the National Institutes of Health, provides a variety of methods for searching for clinical trial information. A focused search by disease, location, treatment, or sponsor may be performed by entering appropriate terms, or a keyword search of all clinical trials can be conducted. Users of the site can also browse trials by specific disease or view a list of studies listed by funding organization. Additional patient resources are available, including information on the clinical trial process.

http://www.clinicaltrials.gov

National Heart, Lung, and Blood Institute (NHLBI): Clinical Trials Database

By selecting a disease or condition of interest, study titles and objectives of research are returned. Principal investigator and contact details are provided for those interested in learning more about or enrolling in the chosen clinical trial. Links at the top of the pages offer connection to additional information on study background, subjects, design, and current status of research. The site can also be searched by entering an age group for subjects or selecting a current trial stage.

http://apps.nhlbi.nih.gov/clinicaltrials/

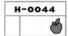

University of Medicine and Dentistry of New Jersey: Clinical Trials in Cardiology An alphabetical listing of clinical trials in cardiology is found at this address, maintained by Dr. Olga Shindler. Study titles, citations for published results, and some details of research objectives are included.

http://www2.umdnj.edu/~shindler/trials.html

2.8 Drug Pipeline: Approved and Developmental Drugs

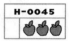

CenterWatch: Drugs Approved by the FDA By accessing any specific approval year and specialty, visitors are returned a listing of products approved by the FDA during that time period. General information, clinical results, side effects, and mechanism of action are reviewed for each new therapy.

http://www.centerwatch.com/patient/drugs/druglsal.html

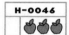

CenterWatch: Drugs in Clinical Trials Database This online resource offers professional and consumer viewers information on over 1,300 new therapies in phase II and III clinical trials. Details about each new treatment, brand and generic names, sponsoring research company, and contacts for research centers are provided. Visitors are returned results by selecting from the large variety of medical conditions listed.

http://www.centerwatch.com/patient/cwpipeline/default.asp

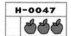

Food and Drug Administration (FDA): Center for Drug Evaluation and Research In addition to an alphabetical listing of all prescription drugs approved during the 1998-2001 time period, visitors will find links to a regularly updated, reverse chronological listing; several resources for prescription drug information; and the online *Orange Book,* which lists all FDA-approved prescription drugs and their generic equivalents. Major drug information pages on individual products and the Consumer Drug Information Page, which lists basic label information and provides complete package inserts, are found.

http://www.fda.gov/cder/drug/default.htm

2.9 Online Texts and Tutorials

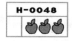

Family Practice Notebook.com: Cardiovascular Medicine A variety of book chapters can be accessed from the cardiovascular medicine index of this family medicine resource. Presented in outline form, chapters include review of arrhythmias, coronary artery disease, congestive heart failure, examination and

diagnostic testing, hypertension, management procedures, and symptom evaluations. Information is also provided on diseases of the eye as they relate to cardiovascular disease, infectious diseases of the heart, pulmonology, cardiovascular pharmacology, diagnostic imaging, and surgical interventions.
http://www.fpnotebook.com/CV.htm

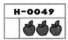

Merck Manual of Diagnosis and Therapy: Cardiovascular Disorders
Section 16 of this online reference from Merck includes chapters on patient evaluation and diagnostic cardiovascular procedures, as well as several disease-specific sections. Visitors to the site will also find general disease information, classification and etiology, pathophysiology, symptoms, diagnosis, and treatment details. Links to related chapters, subtopics, tables, and figures are provided throughout this searchable publication.
http://www.merck.com/pubs/mmanual/section16/sec16.htm

Virtual Hospital: Cardiology
Externally peer reviewed by Mosby, this site offers review of ischemic heart disease, cardiac arrhythmias, congestive heart failure, acute pulmonary edema, and a variety of additional cardiac disorder topics. Each chapter offers a disease definition, diagnostic findings and information, and therapeutic measures in a concise, encyclopedic format.
http://www.vh.org/Providers/ClinRef/FPHandbook/02.html

Journals, Articles, and Latest Books

3.1 Abstract, Citation, and Full-Text Search Tools

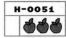

CliniWeb International: Heart Diseases Maintained by the Oregon Health and Science University, CliniWeb provides extensive listings of cardiology literature, courtesy of several preeminent academic and professional institutions. Preformatted query links to PubMed are available for a large variety of cardiology disorders and topics, including review, therapeutic, and diagnostic searches, ranging from arrhythmia to ventricular outflow obstruction.
http://www.ohsu.edu/cliniweb/C14/C14.280.html

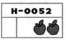

Heart Surgery Forum: Literature Searches The site features large collections of abstracts dealing with topics such as coronary artery bypass grafting, valve disorders, aortic diseases, congenital heart disease, transplantation, myocardial preservation, cardiopulmonary bypass, pharmacology, and tumors. The listings of references returned are representative of sample articles related to the topic requested. Keywords searched are listed, and abstracts from the National Library of Medicine are viewable.
http://www.hsforum.com/search

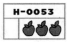

MEDLINE/PubMed at the National Library of Medicine (NLM) PubMed is a free MEDLINE search service providing access to 11 million citations with links to the full text of articles of participating journals. Probably the most heavily used and reputable free MEDLINE site, PubMed permits advanced searching by subject, author, journal title, and many other fields. It includes an easy-to-use "citation matcher" for completing and identifying references, and its PreMEDLINE database provides journal citations before they are indexed, making this version of MEDLINE more up-to-date than most.
http://www.ncbi.nlm.nih.gov/PubMed

MedNets: Cardiology Journals The MedNets professional online community offers a listing of over 50 of the top cardiology journals, with a search feature that allows retrieval of specific research inquiries from these publications and additional abstracts and articles. By entering keywords, visitors are returned the beginning of journal abstracts, access to journal-specific entries, and, in most cases, the opportunity to obtain full-text articles.
http://www.internets.com/mednets/cvsweb.htm

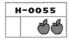

MyMedline.com: Cardiology This search engine, provided as a service of AtCardiology.com, browses the most commonly searched cardiology and cardiology-related journals. Visitors may enter keywords, choose journals to be searched, and add a date of publication. Other variables for limiting document return are provided.
http://www.atlife.com/medline/cardiology.php3

3.2 ARTICLES AND REVIEWS

MCP Hahnemann University Libraries: Cardiology Health Reviews Full-text review articles related to cardiovascular disease are available through this directory, provided for use by primary care physicians. Articles are listed under sub topic headings, including hypertension, atherosclerosis and coronary disease, myocardial disease, congestive heart failure, valvular heart disease, arrhythmias, and vascular disease. Links are also available to other sources for cardiology information.
http://library.mcphu.edu/resources/reviews/card.htm

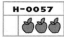

Medical Journals: WebMedLitPlus Presented by WebMedLit, this site offers an extensive listing of recent articles on cardiology from medical journals around the world. Listings provide source information, authors, and an abstract. For each article abstract, there is a link to the publisher's abstract site with, in most cases, the opportunity to download the complete text.
http://webmedlit.silverplatter.com/topics/cardio.html

3.3 JOURNALS ON THE INTERNET: CARDIOLOGY

INDIVIDUAL JOURNAL WEB SITES

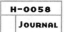

Acta Haematologica
Publisher: Karger **Free:** Table of Contents, Abstracts **Pay:** Articles
http://www.karger.ch/journals/aha/aha_jh.htm

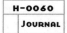

American Heart Journal
Publisher: Mosby **Free:** Table of Contents, Abstracts **Pay:** Articles
http://www1.mosby.com/mosbyscripts/mosby.dll?action=searchDB&searchDBfor=current&id=hj

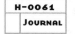

American Journal of Cardiology
Publisher: Elsevier Science **Free:** Table of Contents, Abstracts **Pay:** Articles
http://www.elsevier.com/inca/publications/store/5/2/5/0/4/8

American Journal of Hematology
Publisher: John Wiley & Sons, Inc. **Free:** Table of Contents, Abstracts **Pay:** Articles
http://www.interscience.wiley.com/jpages/0361-8609

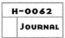

American Journal of Hypertension

Publisher: American Society of Hypertension **Free:** Table of Contents, Abstracts, Articles
Pay: None http://www-east.elsevier.com/ajh/index.html

American Journal of Physiology: Heart and Circulatory Physiology

Publisher: American Physiological Society **Free:** Table of Contents, Abstracts **Pay:** Articles
http://ajpcon.physiology.org/

Angiogenesis

Publisher: Kluwer Academic Publishers **Free:** Table of Contents **Pay:** Abstracts, Articles
http://www.wkap.nl/prod/j/0969-6970

Annals of Emergency Medicine

Publisher: Mosby **Free:** Table of Contents, Abstracts **Pay:** Articles
http://www1.mosby.com/scripts/om.dll/serve?
action=searchDB&searchDBfor=home&id=EM

Annals of Hematology

Publisher: Springer-Verlag **Free:** Table of Contents, Abstracts **Pay:** Articles
http://link.springer.de/link/service/journals/00277/index.htm

Annals of Noninvasive Electrocardiography

Publisher: Futura Publishing Company, Inc. **Free:** Table of Contents **Pay:** Articles
http://www.futuraco.com/ane.htm

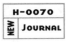

Annals of Thoracic Surgery

Publisher: Elsevier Science **Free:** Table of Contents **Pay:** Abstracts, Articles
http://www.elsevier.nl/inca/publications/store/5/0/5/7/4/7/

Annals of Vascular Surgery

Publisher: Springer-Verlag **Free:** Table of Contents, Abstracts **Pay:** Articles
http://link.springer.de/link/service/journals/10016/

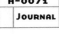

Applied Cardiopulmonary Pathophysiology

Publisher: Pabst Science Publishers **Free:** Table of Contents, Abstracts **Pay:** Articles
http://www.pabst-publishers.de/Medizin/med%20Zeitschriften/acp/

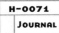

Arteriosclerosis, Thrombosis, and Vascular Biology

Publisher: Lippincott Williams & Wilkins **Free:** Table of Contents, Abstracts **Pay:** Articles
http://atvb.ahajournals.org

Artificial Cells, Blood Substitutes and Immobilization Biotechnology

Publisher: Marcel Dekker **Free:** Table of Contents, Abstracts **Pay:** Articles
http://www.dekker.com/servlet/product/productid/BIO

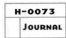

Atherosclerosis

Publisher: Elsevier Science **Free:** Table of Contents **Pay:** Abstracts, Articles
http://www.elsevier.com/inca/publications/store/5/2/2/7/9/0

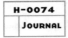

Basic Research in Cardiology
Publisher: Steinkopff Verlag **Free:** Table of Contents, Abstracts **Pay:** Articles
http://link.springer.de/link/service/journals/00395/index.htm

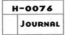

British Medical Journal
Publisher: BMJ Publishing Group **Free:** Table of Contents, Abstracts, Articles **Pay:** None
http://www.bmj.com/

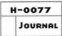

Canadian Journal of Cardiology
Publisher: Pulsus Group Inc. **Free:** Table of Contents, Abstracts **Pay:** Articles
http://www.pulsus.com/CARDIOL/home.htm

Cardiac and Vascular Regeneration
Publisher: Futura Publishing Company, Inc. **Free:** Table of Contents **Pay:** Abstracts, Articles http://futuraco.com/cvr.htm

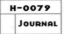

Cardiac Consult
Publisher: Cleveland Clinic Heart Center **Free:** Table of Contents, Articles **Pay:** None
http://www.clevelandclinic.org/heartcenter/pub/professionals/cardiacconsult/

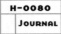

Cardiac Electrophysiology Review
Publisher: Kluwer Academic Publishers **Free:** Table of Contents **Pay:** Abstracts, Articles
http://www.wkap.nl/journalhome.htm/1385-2264

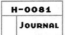

CardioConsult Reviews
Publisher: PharmInfoNet **Free:** Table of Contents **Pay:** Articles
http://www.cardioconsult.org/news.html#ccr

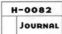

Cardiology
Publisher: Karger **Free:** Table of Contents, Abstracts **Pay:** Articles
http://www.karger.com/journals/crd

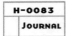

Cardiology Clinics
Publisher: W. B. Saunders **Free:** Table of Contents **Pay:** Abstracts, Articles
http://www.harcourthealth.com/scripts/om.dll/serve?action=searchDB&searchDBfor=home&id=ccar

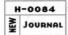

Cardiology in Review
Publisher: Lippincott Williams & Wilkins **Free:** Table of Contents **Pay:** Articles
http://www.cardiologyinreview.com

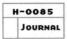

Cardiology in the Young
Publisher: Greenwich Medical Media Ltd. **Free:** Table of Contents, Abstracts **Pay:** Articles
http://www.greenwich-medical.co.uk/detail.asp?catalogid=136

Cardiology Today
Publisher: Slack Inc. **Free:** Table of Contents, Abstracts, Articles **Pay:** None
http://www.cardiologytoday.com/default.asp?article=cthome.asp

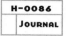

Cardiovascular and Interventional Radiology
Publisher: Springer-Verlag **Free:** Table of Contents, Abstracts **Pay:** Articles
http://link.springer.de/link/service/journals/00270/index.html

| H-0087 | JOURNAL |

Cardiovascular Disease Management
Publisher: COR Healthcare Resources **Free:** Table of Contents **Pay:** Articles
http://www.corhealth.com/cdm/CDMHome4.asp

| H-0088 | NEW JOURNAL |

Cardiovascular Diseases and Cardiovascular Surgery
Publisher: Elsevier Science **Free:** Table of Contents **Pay:** Abstracts, Articles
http://www.elsevier.nl/inca/publications/store/5/0/5/9/8/7/

| H-0089 | JOURNAL |

Cardiovascular Drug Reviews
Publisher: Neva Press, Inc. **Free:** Table of Contents **Pay:** Abstracts, Articles
http://www.nevapress.com/cdr/home.html

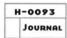

Cardiovascular Drugs and Therapy
Publisher: Kluwer Academic Publishers **Free:** Table of Contents **Pay:** Articles
http://www.wkap.nl/journalhome.htm/0920-3206

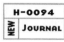

Cardiovascular Engineering
Publisher: Kluwer Academic Publishers **Free:** None **Pay:** Table of Contents, Abstracts, Articles http://kapis.www.wkap.nl/journalhome.htm/1567-8822

| H-0092 | JOURNAL |

Cardiovascular Pathology
Publisher: Elsevier Science **Free:** Table of Contents, Abstracts **Pay:** Articles
http://www.elsevier.com/inca/publications/store/5/2/2/7/5/0

| H-0093 | JOURNAL |

Cardiovascular Pharmacology and Therapeutics
Publisher: W. B. Saunders **Free:** Table of Contents **Pay:** Articles
http://www.harcourthealth.com/fcgi-bin/displaypage.pl?isbn=10742484

| H-0094 | NEW JOURNAL |

Cardiovascular Radiation Medicine
Publisher: Elsevier Science **Free:** Table of Contents **Pay:** Abstracts, Articles
http://www.elsevier.nl/inca/publications/store/6/2/0/0/4/2/

| H-0095 | JOURNAL |

Cardiovascular Radiation Therapy
Publisher: Cardiovascular Research Institute **Free:** Table of Contents, Abstracts, Articles **Pay:** None http://www.radiationonline.com

| H-0096 | JOURNAL |

Cardiovascular Research
Publisher: Elsevier Science **Free:** Table of Contents, Abstracts, Articles **Pay:** None
http://www.elsevier.nl/homepage/sab/cardio

| H-0097 | JOURNAL |

Cardiovascular Surgery
Publisher: Elsevier Science **Free:** Table of Contents **Pay:** Abstracts, Articles
http://www.elsevier.com/inca/publications/store/3/0/3/9/5

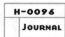

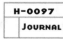

Catheterization and Cardiovascular Diagnosis
Publisher: Wiley-Liss, Inc. **Free:** Table of Contents, Abstracts **Pay:** Articles
http://www3.interscience.wiley.com/cgi-bin/jtoc?ID=32535

Catheterization and Cardiovascular Interventions
Publisher: Wiley-Liss, Inc. **Free:** Table of Contents, Abstracts **Pay:** Articles
http://www3.interscience.wiley.com/cgi-bin/jtoc?ID=10005205

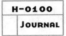

Cerebrovascular Diseases
Publisher: Karger **Free:** Table of Contents, Abstracts **Pay:** Articles
http://www.karger.ch/journals/ced/ced_jh.htm

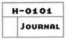

Chest
Publisher: American College of Chest Physicians **Free:** Table of Contents, Abstracts **Pay:** Articles http://www.chestjournal.org

Chest Medicine On-Line
Publisher: Priory Lodge Education Ltd. **Free:** Table of Contents **Pay:** Articles
http://www.priory.com/chest.htm

Circulation
Publisher: American Heart Association **Free:** Table of Contents, Abstracts **Pay:** Articles
http://circ.ahajournals.org

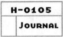

Circulation Research
Publisher: American Heart Association **Free:** Table of Contents, Abstracts **Pay:** Articles
http://circres.ahajournals.org

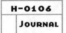

Clinical and Applied Thrombosis/Hemostasis
Publisher: Lippincott Williams & Wilkins **Free:** Table of Contents **Pay:** Articles
http://www.thrombosis-hemostasis.com

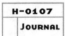

Clinical and Experimental Hypertension
Publisher: Marcel Dekker **Free:** Table of Contents, Abstracts **Pay:** Articles
http://www.dekker.com/servlet/product/productid/CEH

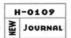

Clinical and Laboratory Haematology
Publisher: Blackwell Science **Free:** Table of Contents, Abstracts **Pay:** Articles
http://www.blackwell-science.com/~cgilib/jnlpage.bin?Journal=clh&File=clh&Page=aims

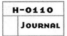

Clinical Cardiology
Publisher: Foundation for Advances in Medicine and Science **Free:** Table of Contents, Abstracts **Pay:** Articles http://www.clinical-cardiology.org

Clinical Radiology
Publisher: Harcourt International **Free:** Table of Contents, Abstracts **Pay:** Articles
http://www.harcourt-international.com/journals/crad/default.cfm

Don't type in long URLs – add the site number to the eMedguides URL: www.eMedguides.com/**G-1234**.

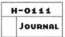

Clinical Transplantation
Publisher: Munksgaard **Free:** Table of Contents **Pay:** Articles
http://www.blackwellmunksgaard.com/clinicaltransplantation

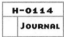

Clinics in Chest Medicine
Publisher: W. B. Saunders **Free:** Table of Contents **Pay:** Articles
http://www.harcourthealth.com/fcgi-bin/displaypage.pl?isbn=02725231

Core Journals in Cardiology
Publisher: Elsevier Science **Free:** None **Pay:** Table of Contents, Abstracts, Articles
http://www.elsevier.com/locate/corecard

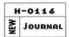

Coronary Artery Disease
Publisher: Lippincott Williams & Wilkins **Free:** Table of Contents **Pay:** Articles
http://www.coronary-artery.com

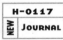

Coronary Health Care
Publisher: Harcourt International **Free:** Table of Contents **Pay:** Articles
http://www.harcourt-international.com/journals/chec

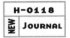

Current Atherosclerosis Reports
Publisher: Current Science Inc. **Free:** Table of Contents **Pay:** Abstracts, Articles
http://current-reports.com/cr_jrnl_home.cfm?JournalID=AT

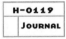

Current Cardiology Reports
Publisher: Current Science Inc. **Free:** Table of Contents **Pay:** Abstracts, Articles
http://www.current-reports.com/cr_jrnl_home.cfm?JournalID=CR

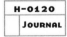

Current Hypertension Reports
Publisher: Current Science Inc. **Free:** Table of Contents **Pay:** Abstracts, Articles
http://current-reports.com/cr_jrnl_home.cfm?JournalID=HR

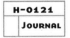

Current Opinion in Cardiology
Publisher: Lippincott Williams & Wilkins **Free:** Table of Contents, Abstracts **Pay:** Articles
http://www.biomednet.com/gateways/car

Current Opinion in Hematology
Publisher: Lippincott Williams & Wilkins **Free:** Table of Contents **Pay:** Articles
http://www.lww.com/cgi-bin/wwonline.storefront/1373204986/Product/View/1065-6251

Current Opinion in Nephrology and Hypertension
Publisher: Lippincott Williams & Wilkins **Free:** Table of Contents, Abstracts **Pay:** Articles
http://www.co-neph-htn.com/

Current Opinion in Organ Transplantation
Publisher: Lippincott Williams & Wilkins **Free:** Table of Contents **Pay:** Articles
http://www.lww.com/cgi-bin/wwonline.storefront/93005394/Product/View/1087-2418

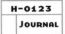

Current Problems in Cardiology
Publisher: Mosby **Free:** Table of Contents, Abstracts **Pay:** Articles
http://www1.mosby.com/mosbyscripts/mosby.dll?action=searchDB&searchDBfor=home&id=cd

Echocardiography Journal
Publisher: University of Medicine and Dentistry of New Jersey **Free:** Table of Contents
Pay: Articles http://www2.umdnj.edu/~shindler/echo.html

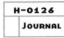

Europace
Publisher: Harcourt International **Free:** Table of Contents, Abstracts **Pay:** Articles
http://www.harcourt-international.com/journals/eupc/default.cfm

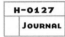

European Heart Journal
Publisher: Harcourt International **Free:** Table of Contents **Pay:** Abstracts, Articles
http://www.harcourt-international.com/journals/euhj

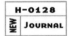

European Journal of Cardio-thoracic Surgery
Publisher: Elsevier Science **Free:** Table of Contents **Pay:** Articles
http://www.elsevier.com/inca/publications/store/6/0/0/1/2/7

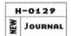

European Journal of Echocardiography
Publisher: Harcourt International **Free:** Table of Contents, Abstracts **Pay:** Articles
http://www.harcourt-international.com/journals/euje/

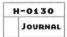

European Journal of Heart Failure
Publisher: Elsevier Science **Free:** Table of Contents **Pay:** Abstracts, Articles
http://www.elsevier.com/locate/ejheart

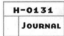

European Journal of Vascular and Endovascular Surgery
Publisher: W. B. Saunders **Free:** Table of Contents, Abstracts **Pay:** Articles
http://journals.harcourt-international.com/wbs/ejv

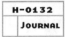

Evidence-Based Cardiovascular Medicine
Publisher: Harcourt International **Free:** Table of Contents **Pay:** Abstracts, Articles
http://www.harcourt-international.com/journals/ebcm/default.cfm

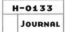

Experimental and Clinical Cardiology
Publisher: Pulsus Group Inc. **Free:** Table of Contents, Abstracts **Pay:** Articles
http://www.pulsus.com/europe/home.htm

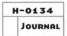

Fibrinolysis and Proteolysis
Publisher: Harcourt International **Free:** Table of Contents, Abstracts **Pay:** Articles
http://www.harcourt-international.com/journals/fipr

Haemostasis
Publisher: Karger **Free:** Table of Contents, Abstracts **Pay:** Articles
http://www.karger.ch/journals/hae/hae_jh.htm

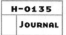

Harvard Heart Letter

Publisher: Harvard Health Publications **Free:** Table of Contents **Pay:** Articles
http://www.health.harvard.edu/aboutheart.shtml

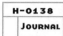

Heart

Publisher: BMJ Publishing Group **Free:** Table of Contents, Abstracts, Articles **Pay:** None
http://heart.bmjjournals.com

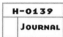

Heart and Lung

Publisher: Mosby **Free:** Table of Contents, Abstracts, Articles **Pay:** None
http://www1.mosby.com/mosbyscripts/mosby.dll?action=searchDB&searchDBfor=home&id=hl

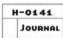

Heart and Vessels

Publisher: Springer-Verlag **Free:** Table of Contents **Pay:** Articles
http://link.springer.de/link/service/journals/00380/index.htm

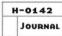

Heart Disease

Publisher: Lippincott Williams & Wilkins **Free:** Table of Contents **Pay:** Articles
http://www.heartdiseasej.com

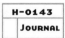

Heart Failure Reviews

Publisher: Kluwer Academic Publishers **Free:** Table of Contents **Pay:** Abstracts, Articles
http://www.wkap.nl/journalhome.htm/1382-4147

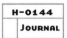

Heart Information Network

Publisher: Center for Cardiovascular Education **Free:** Table of Contents, Abstracts, Articles
Pay: None http://www.heartinfo.org/hrtnews.htm

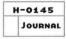

Heart Surgery Forum

Publisher: Heart Surgery Forum **Free:** Table of Contents, Abstracts, Articles **Pay:** None
http://www.hsforum.com

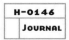

HeartDrug

Publisher: Karger **Free:** Table of Contents **Pay:** Abstracts, Articles
http://www.karger.ch/journals/hed/hed_jh.htm

HeartWeb

Publisher: Amadeus Multimedia Technologies, Ltd. **Free:** Table of Contents
Pay: Abstracts, Articles http://www.heartweb.org/heartweb/index.htm

Hematology and Cell Therapy

Publisher: Springer-Verlag **Free:** Table of Contents, Abstracts **Pay:** Articles
http://link.springer.de/link/service/journals/00282/index.htm

Hypertension

Publisher: American Heart Association **Free:** Table of Contents, Abstracts **Pay:** Articles
http://hyper.ahajournals.org

Don't type in long URLs – add the site number to the eMedguides URL: www.eMedguides.com/**G-1234**.

H-0147 JOURNAL	**Hypertension in Pregnancy** **Publisher:** Marcel Dekker **Free:** Table of Contents, Abstracts **Pay:** Articles http://www.dekker.com/servlet/product/productid/PRG
H-0148 JOURNAL	**International Journal of Angiology** **Publisher:** Springer-Verlag **Free:** Table of Contents, Abstracts **Pay:** Articles http://link.springer.de/link/service/journals/00547/index.htm
H-0149 JOURNAL	**International Journal of Cardiology** **Publisher:** Elsevier Science **Free:** Table of Contents **Pay:** Articles http://www.elsevier.com/inca/publications/store/5/0/6/0/4/1
H-0150 JOURNAL	**International Journal of Cardiovascular Imaging** **Publisher:** Kluwer Academic Publishers **Free:** Table of Contents **Pay:** Articles http://www.wkap.nl/journalhome.htm/0167-9899
H-0151 NEW JOURNAL	**International Journal of Cardiovascular Interventions** **Publisher:** Taylor & Francis Group **Free:** Table of Contents **Pay:** None http://www.tandf.co.uk/journals/md/14628848.html
H-0152 JOURNAL	**International Journal of Hematology** **Publisher:** Carden Jennings Publishing Co., Ltd. **Free:** Table of Contents **Pay:** Articles http://www.cjp.com/stories/storyReader$16
H-0153 JOURNAL	**Internet Journal of Thoracic and Cardiovascular Surgery** **Publisher:** Internet Scientific Publications **Free:** Table of Contents, Abstracts **Pay:** Articles http://www.ispub.com/journals/ijtcvs.htm
H-0154 NEW JOURNAL	**Japanese Heart Journal** **Publisher:** Kluwer Academic Publishers **Free:** None **Pay:** Table of Contents, Abstracts, Articles http://www.baltzer.nl/journalhome.htm/0021-4868
H-0155 JOURNAL	**Journal of Cardiac Failure** **Publisher:** Harcout Health Sciences **Free:** Table of Contents **Pay:** Articles http://www.harcourthealth.com/fcgi-bin/displaypage.pl?isbn=10719164
H-0156 JOURNAL	**Journal of Cardiac Surgery** **Publisher:** Futura Publishing Company, Inc. **Free:** Table of Contents, Abstracts **Pay:** Articles http://www.futuraco.com/jcs.htm
H-0157 JOURNAL	**Journal of Cardiopulmonary Rehabilitation** **Publisher:** Lippincott Williams & Wilkins **Free:** Table of Contents **Pay:** Articles http://www.lww.com/productdetailresults/1,2265,33811462,00.html
H-0158 JOURNAL	**Journal of Cardiothoracic and Vascular Anesthesia** **Publisher:** W. B. Saunders **Free:** Table of Contents, Abstracts **Pay:** Articles http://www.jcardioanesthesia.com

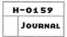

Journal of Cardiovascular Electrophysiology

Publisher: Futura Publishing Company, Inc. **Free:** Table of Contents, Abstracts **Pay:** Articles http://futuraco.com/jce.htm

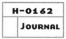

Journal of Cardiovascular Magnetic Resonance

Publisher: Marcel Dekker **Free:** Table of Contents, Abstracts **Pay:** Articles http://www.dekker.com/servlet/product/productid/JCMR

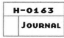

Journal of Cardiovascular Pharmacology

Publisher: Lippincott Williams & Wilkins **Free:** Table of Contents **Pay:** Articles http://www.cardiovascularpharm.com

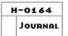

Journal of Cardiovascular Pharmacology and Therapeutics

Publisher: Westminster Publications **Free:** Table of Contents, Abstracts **Pay:** Articles http://www.westminsterpublications.com/therapeutics.htm

Journal of Cardiovascular Risk

Publisher: Lippincott Williams & Wilkins **Free:** Table of Contents **Pay:** Articles http://www.lww.com/cgi-bin/wwonline.storefront/815216653/Product/View/1350-6277

Journal of Cerebral Blood Flow and Metabolism

Publisher: Lippincott Williams & Wilkins **Free:** Table of Contents **Pay:** Articles http://www.jcbfm.com

Journal of Clinical Apheresis

Publisher: John Wiley & Sons, Inc. **Free:** Table of Contents **Pay:** Articles http://www.interscience.wiley.com/jpages/0733-2459

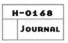

Journal of Electrocardiology

Publisher: W. B. Saunders **Free:** Table of Contents **Pay:** Articles http://www.harcourthealth.com/scripts/om.dll/serve?action=searchDB&searchDBfor=home&id=jelc

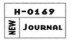

Journal of Endovascular Therapy

Publisher: International Society of Endovascular Specialists **Free:** Table of Contents, Abstracts, Articles **Pay:** None http://www.jevsurg.org/

Journal of Heart and Lung Transplantation

Publisher: Elsevier Science **Free:** Table of Contents **Pay:** Articles http://www.elsevier.com/inca/publications/store/6/0/1/5/3/8

Journal of Heart Valve Disease

Publisher: ICR Publishers Ltd. **Free:** Table of Contents, Abstracts **Pay:** Articles http://www.icr-heart.com/journal/index.htm

Journal of Human Hypertension

Publisher: Nature Publishing Group **Free:** Table of Contents **Pay:** Abstracts, Articles http://www.naturesj.com/jhh/index.html

Journal of Hypertension

Publisher: Lippincott Williams & Wilkins **Free:** Table of Contents, Abstracts, Articles **Pay:** None http://www.jhypertension.com/

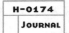

Journal of Interventional Cardiac Electrophysiology

Publisher: Kluwer Academic Publishers **Free:** Table of Contents **Pay:** Abstracts, Articles http://www.wkap.nl/journalhome.htm/1383-875X

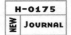

Journal of Interventional Cardiology

Publisher: Futura Publishing Company, Inc. **Free:** Table of Contents, Abstracts **Pay:** Articles http://futuraco.com/jic.htm

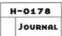

Journal of Invasive Cardiology

Publisher: Medscape **Free:** Table of Contents **Pay:** Abstracts, Articles http://cardiology.medscape.com/HMP/JIC/public/JIC-journal.html

Journal of Long-Term Effects of Medical Implants

Publisher: Begell House, Inc. **Free:** Table of Contents **Pay:** Abstracts, Articles http://www.begellhouse.com/jltemi/jltemi.html

Journal of Molecular and Cellular Cardiology

Publisher: Academic Press **Free:** Table of Contents, Abstracts **Pay:** Articles http://www.academicpress.com/jmcc

Journal of Nuclear Cardiology

Publisher: Mosby **Free:** Table of Contents, Abstracts **Pay:** Articles http://www1.mosby.com/mosbyscripts/mosby.dll?action=searchDB&searchDBfor=home&id=nc

Journal of Stroke and Cerebrovascular Diseases

Publisher: Harcourt Health Sciences **Free:** Table of Contents **Pay:** Articles http://www.harcourthealth.com/fcgi-bin/displaypage.pl?isbn=10523057

Journal of the American College of Cardiology

Publisher: American College of Cardiology **Free:** Table of Contents, Abstracts, Articles **Pay:** None http://www.cardiosource.com/config/jacc/default.htm

Journal of the American Society of Echocardiography

Publisher: Mosby **Free:** Table of Contents, Abstracts, Articles **Pay:** None http://www1.mosby.com/scripts/om.dll/serve?action=searchDB&searchDBfor=home&id=JE

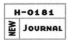

Journal of the Hong Kong College of Cardiology

Publisher: Medcom Limited **Free:** Table of Contents, Abstracts **Pay:** Articles http://medicine.org.hk/hkcc/journal/home.htm

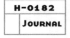

Journal of Thoracic and Cardiovascular Surgery

Publisher: Mosby **Free:** Table of Contents **Pay:** Articles http://www1.mosby.com/scripts/om.dll/serve?action=searchDB&searchDBfor=home&id=TC

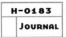

Journal of Thoracic Imaging
Publisher: Lippincott Williams & Wilkins **Free:** Table of Contents **Pay:** Articles
http://www.thoracicimaging.com

H-0184 | JOURNAL

Journal of Thrombosis and Thrombolysis
Publisher: Kluwer Academic Publishing **Free:** Table of Contents **Pay:** Abstracts, Articles
http://www.wkap.nl/journalhome.htm/0929-5305

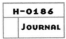

Journal of Vascular and Interventional Radiology
Publisher: Lippincott Williams & Wilkins **Free:** Table of Contents, Abstracts **Pay:** Articles
http://www.jvir.org/

H-0186 | JOURNAL

Journal of Vascular Investigation
Publisher: W. B. Saunders **Free:** Table of Contents **Pay:** Abstracts, Articles
http://www.churchillmed.com/Journals/JVI/jhome.html

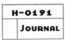

Journal of Vascular Research
Publisher: Karger **Free:** Table of Contents, Abstracts **Pay:** Articles
http://www.karger.ch/journals/jvr/jvr_jh.htm

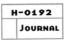

Journal of Vascular Surgery
Publisher: Mosby **Free:** Table of Contents, Abstracts **Pay:** Articles
http://www1.mosby.com/mosbyscripts/mosby.dll?action=searchDB&searchDBfor=home&id=vs

---

Journal Watch Cardiology
Publisher: Massachusetts Medical Society **Free:** Table of Contents **Pay:** Abstracts, Articles
http://www.jwatch.org/card/

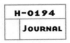

Kidney and Blood Pressure Research
Publisher: Karger **Free:** Table of Contents, Abstracts **Pay:** Articles
http://www.karger.ch/journals/kbr/kbr_jh.htm

H-0191 | JOURNAL

Microcirculation
Publisher: Nature Publishing Group **Free:** Table of Contents **Pay:** Articles
http://www.naturesj.com/mn/index.html

H-0192 | JOURNAL

Microvascular Research
Publisher: Academic Press **Free:** Table of Contents **Pay:** Articles
http://www.apnet.com/www/journal/mr.htm

H-0193 | NEW | JOURNAL

New England Journal of Medicine
Publisher: Massachusetts Medical Society **Free:** Table of Contents, Abstracts **Pay:** Articles
http://content.nejm.org/

H-0194 | JOURNAL

Online Journal of Cardiology
Publisher: McGill University **Free:** Table of Contents **Pay:** Articles
http://www.mmi.mcgill.ca/heart/index.html

Operative Techniques in Thoracic and Cardiovascular Surgery
Publisher: W. B. Saunders **Free:** Table of Contents **Pay:** Articles
http://www.harcourthealth.com/scripts/om.dll/serve?ac-
tion=searchDB&searchDBfor=home&id=otct

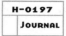

Pacing and Clinical Electrophysiology
Publisher: Futura Publishing Company **Free:** Table of Contents **Pay:** Articles
http://futuraco.com/pace.htm

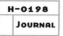

Pediatric Cardiology
Publisher: Springer-Verlag **Free:** Table of Contents, Abstracts **Pay:** Articles
http://link.springer.de/link/service/journals/00246/

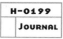

Pediatric Transplantation
Publisher: Munksgaard **Free:** Table of Contents **Pay:** Articles
http://www.blackwellmunksgaard.com/pediatrictransplantation

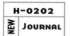

Progress in Cardiovascular Diseases
Publisher: Harcourt Health Sciences **Free:** Table of Contents **Pay:** Articles
http://www.harcourthealth.com/fcgi-bin/displaypage.pl?isbn=00330620

Progress in Pediatric Cardiology
Publisher: Elsevier Science **Free:** Table of Contents **Pay:** Articles
http://www.elsevier.com/inca/publications/store/5/2/5/0/1/8

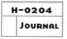

Prostaglandins and Other Lipid Mediators
Publisher: Elsevier Science **Free:** Table of Contents, Abstracts **Pay:** Articles
http://www.elsevier.nl/inca/publications/store/5/2/5/0/1/9/

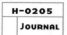

Resuscitation
Publisher: Elsevier Science **Free:** Table of Contents, Abstracts **Pay:** Articles
http://www.elsevier.nl/inca/publications/store/5/0/5/9/5/9/

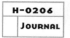

Scandinavian Cardiovascular Journal
Publisher: Taylor & Francis Group **Free:** Table of Contents **Pay:** Articles
http://www.tandf.co.uk/journals/tfs/14017431.html

Seminars in Cardiothoracic and Vascular Anesthesia
Publisher: Harcourt Health Sciences **Free:** Table of Contents **Pay:** Articles
http://www.harcourthealth.com/fcgi-bin/displaypage.pl?isbn=10892532

Seminars in Hematology
Publisher: Harcourt Health Sciences **Free:** Table of Contents **Pay:** Articles
http://www.harcourthealth.com/fcgi-bin/displaypage.pl?isbn=00371963

Seminars in Interventional Cardiology
Publisher: W. B. Saunders **Free:** Table of Contents, Abstracts **Pay:** Articles
http://journals.harcourt-international.com/wbs/sic

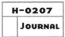

Seminars in Thoracic and Cardiovascular Surgery
Publisher: W. B. Saunders **Free:** Table of Contents **Pay:** Articles
http://www.harcourthealth.com/fcgi-bin/displaypage.pl?isbn=10430679

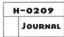

Seminars in Vascular Surgery
Publisher: W. B. Saunders **Free:** Table of Contents **Pay:** Articles
http://www.harcourthealth.com/fcgi-bin/displaypage.pl?isbn=08957967

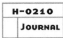

Stroke
Publisher: Lippincott Williams & Wilkins **Free:** Table of Contents **Pay:** Articles
http://stroke.ahajournals.org

Techniques in Vascular and Interventional Radiology
Publisher: W. B. Saunders **Free:** Table of Contents **Pay:** Articles
http://www.harcourthealth.com/fcgi-bin/displaypage.pl?isbn=10892516

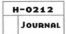

Texas Heart Institute Journal
Publisher: Texas Heart Institute **Free:** Table of Contents, Abstracts **Pay:** Articles
http://www.texasheartinstitute.org/journal.html

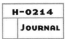

Thrombosis and Haemostasis
Publisher: Schattauer **Free:** Table of Contents **Pay:** Articles
http://www.schattauer.de/zs/startz.asp?load=/zs/thromb/main.asp

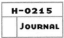

Thrombosis Research
Publisher: Elsevier Science **Free:** Table of Contents **Pay:** Articles
http://www.elsevier.com/inca/publications/store/3/6/9

Transfusion
Publisher: American Association of Blood Banks **Free:** Table of Contents **Pay:** Articles
http://www.transfusion.org

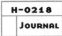

Transfusion Medicine
Publisher: Blackwell Science **Free:** Table of Contents **Pay:** Articles
http://www.blackwell-science.com/products/journals/trans.htm

Transplant International
Publisher: Springer-Verlag **Free:** Table of Contents, Abstracts **Pay:** Articles
http://link.springer.de/link/service/journals/00147/index.htm

Transplantation
Publisher: Lippincott Williams & Wilkins **Free:** Table of Contents **Pay:** Articles
http://www.transplantjournal.com

Transplantation Proceedings
Publisher: Elsevier Science **Free:** Table of Contents **Pay:** Abstracts, Articles
http://www.elsevier.com/inca/publications/store/6/0/0/1/1/4

Don't type in long URLs – add the site number to the eMedguides URL: www.eMedguides.com/**G-1234**.

Transplantation Reviews

Publisher: Harcourt Health Sciences   **Free:** None   **Pay:** Table of Contents, Abstracts, Articles   http://www.harcourthealth.com/fcgi-bin/displaypage.pl?isbn=0955470X

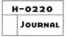

Trends in Cardiovascular Medicine

Publisher: Elsevier Science   **Free:** Table of Contents   **Pay:** Articles
http://www.elsevier.com/inca/publications/store/5/0/5/7/8/2

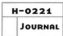

Vascular Medicine

Publisher: Arnold Publishers   **Free:** Table of Contents   **Pay:** Articles
http://www.arnoldpublishers.com/Journals/Journpages/1358863x.htm

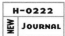

Venous Digest

Publisher: Venous Digest Publications   **Free:** Table of Contents, Abstracts, Articles   **Pay:** None   http://www.venousdigest.com/

Xenotransplantation

Publisher: Munksgaard   **Free:** Table of Contents, Abstracts   **Pay:** Articles
http://www.blackwell-synergy.com/Journals/issuelist.asp?journal=xen

3.4 BOOKS ON CARDIOLOGY PUBLISHED IN 2000/2001

The following listing contains books published during the past 12 months in the field of cardiology. We have categorized the books under major topics, although many of the books contain material that extends beyond the highlighted subject. All of these books may be purchased through Amazon at http://www.amazon.com.

General
Acute Cardiology
Alcohol and Cardiac Disease
Anatomy and Physiology
Angina
Antioxidants
Arrhythmias and
   Dysrhythmias
Artificial Hearts
Atherogenesis
Atherosclerosis
Blood Pressure
Carbon Monoxide
Cardiac Anesthesia
Cardiac Imaging
Cardiac Nursing
Cardiac Surgery

Cardiopulmonary
   Rehabilitation
Cardiovascular Pathology
Cardiovascular Toxicology
Clinical Management
Coding
Computers in Cardiology
Conference Proceedings
Congenital Heart Disease
Coronary Artery Disease
Critical Care Cardiology
Diabetes
Diagnostics and Imaging
Drug-Induced Disorders
Education
Emergency Cardiology
End-Stage Renal Failure

Evidence-Based Cardiology
Exercise
Fetal Cardiology
Genetics
Geriatric Cardiology
Heart Disease
Heart Failure
History
Hypertension
Infection
Interventional Cardiology
Mitral Valve Disease
Myocardial Infarction
Nuclear Cardiology
Nutrition
Pacing and Defibrillation
Pediatric Cardiology

Prevention

Procedures

Sleep Apnea

Terminology

Therapeutics/Pharmacology

Thromboembolism

Transplantation

Vascular Disease

GENERAL

100 Questions in Cardiology, Anthony Palmieri, ACPE, Martin Schiavenato, Denise Tucker, Bandido Books, Diana Holdright, Hugh Montgomery. BMJ Books, ISBN: 1582120382.

Atlas of Heart Disease, Eugene Braunwald, Douglas P. Zipes, Peter Libby. W. B. Saunders Co., ISBN: 0721685544.

Atlas of Heart Disease: Hypertension: Mechanisms and Therapy (CD-ROM), Eugene Braunwald (Editor), Norman K. Hollenberg (Editor). Current Medicine, ISBN: 157340165X.

Atlas of Heart Disease (2-Volume Set CD-ROM Package), Eugene Braunwald, Douglas P. Zipes, Peter Libby. W. B. Saunders Co., ISBN: 0721685560.

Cardiology, Michael H. Crawford, John P. Dimarco. Mosby, Inc., ISBN: 0723431388.

Cardiology for the MRCP, Adam Debelder, Derek Chin. Greenwich Medical Media, ISBN: 1841100102.

Cardiology for the Primary Care Physician, Third Edition, Joseph S. Alpert. Current Medicine, ISBN: 1573401552.

Cardiology for the Primary Care Physician, Vetrovec. Current Medicine, ISBN: 0721665195.

Cardiology in Primary Care, William T. Branch (Editor), R. Wayne Alexander (Editor), Robert C. Schlant (Editor). McGraw-Hill Professional Publishing, ISBN: 0070071624.

Cardiology Pearls, Blase A. Carabello, M.D., Peter C. Gazes, M.D. Hanley & Belfus, ISBN: 1560534036.

Cardiology Secrets, Olivia Vynn Adair. Hanley & Belfus, ISBN: 1560534206.

Cardiology: Patient Pictures, J. Colin Forfar, R. S. Kirby, S. Holmes, C. Carson, Sally C. Pitman. Health Press, ISBN: 1903734045.

Cardiovascular Medicine, James T. Willerson, M.D., Jay N. Cohn, M.D. Churchill Livingstone, ISBN: 0443070008.

CD-ROM for Heart Disease - A Textbook of Cardiovascular Medicine, Zipes Braunwald, Eugene Braunwald, Douglas P. Zipes, Peter Libby. W. B. Saunders Co., ISBN: 0721685528.

Churchill's Pocketbook of Cardiology, Neil R. Grubb, David E. Newby. Churchill Livingstone, ISBN: 0443062218.

Current Pocket Reference, 2000, Cardiology, Larry Shepherd, Thomas Whalen, Mary Ann Riley, Hopkins, Watkins, J. M. Kiel, Mackersie, Kolev, Karl Lennert, A.C. Feller. Springer-Verlag, ISBN: 0964219360.

Essential Atlas of Heart Diseases, Eugene Braunwald, M.D. McGraw-Hill Professional Publishing, ISBN: 0071376453.

Essential Cardiology: Principles and Practice, Clive Rosendorff (Editor). W. B. Saunders Co., ISBN: 0721681441.

Essential Interventional Cardiology, M. S. Norell, John Perrins. W. B. Saunders Co., ISBN: 0702024805.

Hurst's The Heart, Valentin Fuster (Editor), R. Wayne Alexander (Editor), Robert A. O'Rourke, Hein J. J. Wellens. McGraw-Hill Professional Publishing, ISBN: 0071356940.

Hurst's The Heart: Manual of Cardiology, Robert A. O'Rourke (Editor), Valentin Fuster (Editor), R. Wayne Alexander, Spencer B. King, III, Hein J. J. Wellens. McGraw-Hill Professional Publishing, ISBN: 0071354158.

Manual of Cardiovascular Medicine, Steven P. Marso (Editor), Brian P. Griffin (Editor), Eric J. Topol (Editor). Lippincott, Williams & Wilkins, ISBN: 0683306855.

Mayo Clinic Heart Book, Bernard J. Gersh, M.D. (Editor), Michael B. Wood. William Morrow & Co., ISBN: 0688176429.

On Call Cardiology, M. Gabriel Khan, M.D. W. B. Saunders Co., ISBN: 0721692222.

Saint-Frances Guide to Cardiology, Andrew D. Michaels, Craig Frances. Lippincott Williams & Wilkins Publishers, ISBN: 068330660X.

State Of The Heart, Larry W. Stephenson, M.D. Jeffrey L. Rodengen (Contributor), C. Everett Koop (Contributor). Write Stuff Syndicate, ISBN: 0945903634.

Stedman's Cardiology & Pulmonary Words: Includes Respiratory, Lippincott Williams & Wilkins Publishers, ISBN: 0781730562.

The Cardiology Rotation, George J. Taylor, M.D. Blackwell Science Inc., ISBN: 0632043520.

The Cleveland Clinic Heart Book: The Definitive Guide for the Entire Family

from the Nation's Leading Heart Center, Eric J. Topol (Editor), Michael D. Eisner. Hyperion, ISBN: 0786864958.

ACUTE CARDIOLOGY

Acute Coronary Syndromes, Eric J. Topol (Editor). Marcel Dekker, ISBN: 0824704169.

Challenges in Acute Coronary Syndromes, D. P. De Bono (Editor), Burton E. Sobel, David Debono. Blackwell Science Inc, ISBN: 0632055790.

Emergency Medicine Questions Pearls of Wisdom, American College of Cardiology, ACPE, Martin Schiavenato, Denise Tucker, Bandido Books, Stephanie Thibeault, Jarrell, Beckinham, Evans, Finlay, British Medical Association, Mills, Fay, Dollinger, Rebecca Schmidt, Warren Sanger, Thomas Vallombroso, Ken Metcalf, Duane Eichler, William Schwer, Wanda Cloet, Maureen Duncan, Steven Yun, Felix Chew, Steven Greer, William Beachley, Eric Scholar, Joshi Shantaram, Jesse A. Cole, Scott H. Plantz, Lance W. Kreplick, John Trestrail, Elaine St. Johns, Mary T. Dorn, Michael Greenberg. Boston Medical Pub. Inc., ISBN: 1583970436.

ALCOHOL & CARDIAC DISEASE

Moderate Alcohol Consumption and Cardiovascular Disease (Medical Science Symposia Series, Vol. 15) Mitral Valve, Rodolfo Paoletti, A. L. Klatsky, S. Zakhari, A. Poli. Kluwer Academic Publishers, ISBN: 0792365720.

Anatomy and Physiology

Cardiopulmonary Anatomy & Physiology, Desjardins, Terry R. Des Jardins. Delmar Publishers, ISBN: 0766825337.

Cardiopulmonary Anatomy and Physiology, George H. Hicks. W. B. Saunders Co., ISBN: 0721651992.

Cardiovascular Physiology, Robert M. Berne, M.D., Matthew N. Levy, M.D. Mosby, Inc., ISBN: 0323011276.

Cardiovascular Solid Mechanics: Cells, Tissues, and Organs, Jay D. Humphrey. Springer Verlag, ISBN: 0387951687.

Potassium Channels in Cardiovascular Biology, Stephen L. Archer (Editor), Nancy J. Rusch (Editor). Plenum Pub. Corp., ISBN: 0306464020.

The Arterial Circulation: Physical Principles and Clinical Applications, John K-J Li (Editor). Humana Press, ISBN: 0896036332.

The Nervous System and the Heart, Gert J. Ter Horst (Editor), Humana Press, ISBN: 0896036936.

Tumor Angiogenesis and Microcirculation, Emile E. Voest, Patricia A. D'Amore. Marcel Dekker, ISBN: 0824702646.

Angina

Angina, Jackson. Dunitz Martin Ltd, ISBN: 1853176265.

Antioxidants

Antioxidants and Cardiovascular Disease, Jean-Claude Tardif, Martial G. Bourassa. Kluwer Academic Publishers, ISBN: 079236564X.

Arrhythmias and Dysrhythmias

Arrhythmias and Sudden Death in Athletes (Developments in Cardiovascular Medicine, 232), Antonio Bayes De Luna (Editor), F. Furlanello (Editor), B. J. Maron (Editor). Kluwer Academic Publishers, ISBN: 079236337X.

Basic Dysrhythmias: Interpretation & Management, Third Edition, Robert J. Huszar, M.D. Mosby, Inc., ISBN: 0323012442.

Cardiac Arrhythmia: Mechanisms, Diagnosis, and Management, Philip J. Podrid (Editor). Lippincott Williams & Wilkins Publishers, ISBN: 0781724864.

Cardiac Arrhythmias and Device Therapy: Results and Perspectives for the New Century, I. Eli Ovsyshcher, M.D., Ph.D., F.A.C.C. (Editor). Futura Pub. Co., ISBN: 0879934557.

Cardiac Arrhythmias in Children and Young Adults With Congenital Heart Disease, Edward P. Walsh, J. Philip Saul, John K. Triedman. Lippincott Williams & Wilkins Publishers, ISBN: 0397587449.

Cardiac Arrhythmias, 1999, Volume 1: Proceedings of the 6th International Workshop on Cardiac Arrhythmias (Venice, October 5-8, 1999), Antonio Raviele, Springer Verlag, ISBN: 8847000718.

Electrocardiography of Clinical Arrhythmias, Charles Fisch, M.D. (Editor), Suzanne B. Knoebel. Futura Pub. Co., ISBN: 0879934468.

Emergency Dysrhythmias and ECG Injury Patterns, Kevin R. Brown. Delmar Publishers, ISBN: 0766819884.

Foundations of Cardiac Arrhythmias: Basic Concepts and Clinical Approaches (Fundamental and Clinical Cardiology), Peter M. Spooner (Editor), Michael R. Rosen (Editor). Marcel Dekker, ISBN: 0824702662.

Fundamental Approaches to the Management of Cardiac Arrhythmias, Michael R. Lauer, M.D., Ruey J. Sung, M.D. Kluwer Academic Publishers, ISBN: 0792365593.

Irregular Heartbeats: To Control, Reduce and Eliminate Potentially Debilitating and Life Threatening Arrhythmias, Joseph Hessen. 1stBooks Library, ISBN: 1587216906.

Optical Mapping of Cardiac Excitation and Arrhythmias, David S. Rosenbaum (Editor), Jose Jalife (Editor). Futura Pub. Co., ISBN: 0879934816.

Pocket Guide to Basic Dysrhythmias, Robert J. Huszar, Robert J. Huszar M. D. Mosby, Inc., ISBN: 0323012434.

QT Dispersion (Clinical Approaches to Tachyarrhythmias, Vol. 12), Marek Malik, Velislav Batchvarov. Futura Pub. Co., ISBN: 0879934565.

ARTIFICIAL HEARTS

The Mechanization of the Heart: Harvey and Descartes (Rochester Studies in Medical History, 1), Thomas Fuchs, Marjorie Grene (Translator). Univ. of Rochester Press, ISBN: 1580460771.

ATHEROGENESIS

Lipoprotein Metabolism and Atherogenesis, T. Kita (Editor), M. Yokode (Editor). Springer-Verlag, ISBN: 443170261X.

ATHEROSCLEROSIS

Atherosclerosis: Gene Expression, Cell Interactions, and Oxidation, Roger T. Dean (Editor), David T. Kelly (Editor). Oxford University Press, ISBN: 0198506376.

Atherosclerosis: Experimental Methods and Protocols, Angela F. Drew (Editor). Humana Press, ISBN: 0896037517.

Inflammatory and Infectious Basis of Atherosclerosis (Pir-Progress in Inflammation Research), Jay L. Mehta (Editor). Birkhauser, ISBN: 3764361549.

BLOOD PRESSURE

Blood Pressure Monitoring in Cardiovascular Medicine and Therapeutics, William B., Md. White (Editor). Humana Press, ISBN: 0896038408.

Coronary Pressure (Developments in Cardiovascular Medicine Volume 227), Nico H.J. Pijls, Bernard De Bruyne. Kluwer Academic Publishers, ISBN: 0792361709.

The Blood Pressure Book: How to Get It Down and Keep It Down, Stephen P. Fortmann, M.D. Prudence E. Breitrose. Bull Pub. Co., ISBN: 0923521607.

The High Blood Pressure Solution: A Scientifically Proven Program for Preventing Strokes and Heart Disease, Richard D. Moore M.D. Ph.D. Inner Traditions Intl. Ltd, ISBN: 0892819758.

What You Really Need To Know About High Blood Pressure, Robert Buckman, John Cleese (Introduction), Rob Buckman. Lebhar-Friedman Books, ISBN: 0867307951.

CARBON MONOXIDE

Carbon Monoxide and Cardiovascular Functions, Rui Wang (Editor). CRC Press, ISBN: 0849310415.

CARDIAC ANESTHESIA

Cardiac Anesthesia: Principles and Clinical Practice, Second Edition, Fawzy G. Estafanous, M.D. (Editor), Paul G. Barash, M.D. (Editor), J. G. Reves, M.D. Lippincott Williams & Wilkins Publishers, ISBN: 0781721954.

Cardiac, Vascular, and Thoracic Anesthesia, John A. Youngberg (Editor), Carol L. Lake (Editor), Michael F. Roizen. Churchill Livingstone, ISBN: 0443089205.

Transoesophageal Echocardiography in Anaesthesia, Jan Poelaert (Editor), Karl Skarvan (Editor). B M J Books, ISBN: 072791278X.

CARDIAC IMAGING

Cardiac SPECT Imaging, E. Gordon Depuey, M.D. (Editor), Ernest V. Garcia, Ph.D. (Editor), Dani Berman. Lippincott Williams & Wilkins Publishers, ISBN: 0781720079.

Chest and Cardiovascular Imaging, Philippe Grenier, Charles B. Higgins. Isis Medical Media, ISBN: 1901865088.

Imaging in Cardiovascular Disease, Gerald M. Pohost, M.D. (Editor), Robert A. O'Rourke, M.D. (Editor), Daniel S. Berman. Lippincott Williams & Wilkins Publishers, ISBN: 039751591X.

CARDIAC NURSING

Cardiothoracic Surgical Nursing, Betsy A. Finkelmeier. Lippincott, Williams & Wilkins, ISBN: 0781717132.

Springhouse Nurse's Drug Guide (Book with CD-ROM for Windows), Stanley Jablonski, Springhouse, Naina Chohan, Kevin D. Dodds. Lippincott Williams & Wilkins Publishers, ISBN: 1560534877.

CARDIAC SURGERY

Atlas of Cardiac Surgery, William A. Baumgartner, R. Scott Stuart, Vincent L. Gott, Leon Schlossberg. Hanley & Belfus, ISBN: 1560533102.

Beating Heart Coronary Artery Surgery, Tomas A. Salerno (Editor). Futura Pub. Co., ISBN: 0879934735.

Cardiac Surgery Secrets, Paulo R. Soltoski, M.D., Kratch L. Karamanoukian, M.D., Tom Salerno. Hanley & Belfus, ISBN: 1560533617.

Cardio-Aortic and Aortic Surgery (Keio University Symposia for Life Science and Medicine, 7), S. Kawada (Editor), T. Ueda (Editor), H. Shimizu (Editor). Springer-Verlag, ISBN: 4431702911.

Congenital Cardiac Surgery, Bruce A. Reitz. Appleton & Lange, ISBN: 0838515428.

Heart Surgery: What to Expect, How to Handle It, Doug Carter. Xlibris Corporation, ISBN: 0738841188.

Intraoperative Graft Patency Verification in Cardiac and Vascular Surgery, Giuseppe D'Ancona, M.D. (Editor), Hratch L. Karamanoukian, M.D. (Editor). Futura Pub. Co., ISBN: 0879934883.

Operative Atlas of Endoluminal Aneurysm Surgery, S. W. Yusuf (Editor), M. L. Marin (Editor), K. Ivancev (Editor), B. R. Hopkinson. Isis Medical Media, ISBN: 1899066993.

Passing on Bypass Using External Counter Pulsation: An FDA Cleared Alternative to Treat Heart Disease Without Surgery, Drugs or Angioplasty, George J. Jueter-sonke. Pikes Peak Press, Inc, ISBN: 096781281X.

Pediatric Cardiac Surgery, Landes Bioscience, ISBN: 1570595763.

Surgery of the Aorta and Its Branches, Bruce L. Gewertz (Editor), Lewis B. Schwartz (Editor). W. B. Saunders Co., ISBN: 0721677517.

Surgical Remodeling in Heart Failure: Alternative to Transplantation, W. Brett (Editor), A. Todorov (Editor), M. Pfisterer (Editor), H. Zerkowski. Dr. Verlag Steinkipff Dietrich, ISBN: 379851223X.

CARDIOPULMONARY REHABILITATION

Advances in Cardiopulmonary Rehabilitation, Jean-Louis Jobin (Editor), Francois Maltais (Editor), Pierre Leblanc. Human Kinetics Pub, ISBN: 0736003126.

CARDIOVASCULAR PATHOLOGY

Cardiovascular Pathology, Malcolm D. Silver, Avrum I. Gotlieb, Frederick J. Schoen. Churchill Livingstone, ISBN: 0443065357.

Cardiovascular Pathology, Renu Virmani, M.D., James B. Atkinson, M.D., Allen Burke, M.D., Andrew Farb. W. B. Saunders Co., ISBN: 0721681654.

Heart Physiology and Pathophysiology, Nick Sperelakis (Editor), Yoshihisa Kurachi (Editor), Andre Terzic (Editor), Nicholas Sperelakis (Editor), Michael Cohen. Academic Press, ISBN: 0126569754.

CARDIOVASCULAR TOXICOLOGY

Cardiovascular Toxicology, Daniel Acosta (Editor). Taylor & Francis, ISBN: 0415248698.

CLINICAL MANAGEMENT

Handbook of Coronary Care, Joseph S. Alpert, Gary S. Francis. Lippincott Williams & Wilkins Publishers, ISBN: 0781719585.

Homocysteine in Health and Disease, Ralph Carmel, Donald W. Jacobsen. Cambridge Univ. Press (Short), ISBN: 0521653193.

Management and Prevention of Thrombosis in Primary Care, John Spandorfer (Editor), Barbara A. Konkle (Editor), Geno J. Merli (Editor). Edward Arnold, ISBN: 0340761253.

Management of Acute Coronary Syndromes, Peter M. Schofield, Dunitz Martin Ltd., ISBN: 1853177199.

Management of Cardiac Arrhythmias (Contemporary Cardiology), Leonard I. Ganz (Editor). Humana Press, ISBN: 0896038467.

Management of Peripheral Arterial Disease: Medical, Surgical and Interven-

tional Aspects, Mark Creager (Editor). Remedica Pub. Ltd., ISBN: 1901346145.

Manual of Clinical Problems in Cardiology: With Annotated Key References, L. David Hillis. Lippincott Williams & Wilkins Publishers, ISBN: 0781723817.

Mechanisms and Clinical Management of Cardiac Arrhythmias, Clifford Garrett. Login Brothers Book Company, ISBN: 0727911945.

Metabolic Support of the Stunned Myocardium: An Experimental Study on the Influence of Lipid Emulsions on Myocardial Performance (Acta Biomedica Lovaniensia, 213), Marc Van De Velde Leuven University Press, ISBN: 9058670309.

Primary Care Management of Heart Disease, George Jesse Taylor (Editor), S. Charleston. Mosby-Year Book, ISBN: 0323002560.

Primary Care Provider's Guide to Cardiology, Glenn N. Levine (Editor), Douglas L. Mann (Editor). Lippincott Williams & Wilkins Publishers, ISBN: 068330688X.

Recovering From Heart Disease in Body & Mind: Medical and Psychological Strategies for Living with Coronary Artery Disease, Brian Baker, M.B., Paul Dorian, M.D., Bretta Maloff McGraw Hill - NTC, ISBN: 0737303603.

The AHA Clinical Cardiac Consult, Joseph S. Alpert, M.D. (Editor), Gerard P. Aurigemma, M.D. (Editor). Lippincott Williams & Wilkins Publishers, ISBN: 0781724201.

The Hypertrophied Heart, Nobuakira Takeda, M.D. (Editor), Makoto Nagano, M.D. (Editor), Naranja Dhalla. Kluwer Academic Publishers, ISBN: 0792377419.

CODING

Coding Companion for Cardiology - Cardiothoracic Surgery - Vascular Surgery, 2002, St. Anthony. St Anthony Publishing, ISBN: 1563374056.

Coding Companion for Cardiology, 2001 St. Anthony Publishing, ISBN: 1563297175.

ICD-9 CM Easy Coder: Cardiology, 2001, Paul K. Tanaka. Unicor Medical, Inc., ISBN: 1567814336.

ICD-9 CM Easy Coder: Cardiology, 2002, Paul K. Tanaka. Unicor Medical, Inc., ISBN: 1567814344.

COMPUTERS IN CARDIOLOGY

Clinical Application of Computational Mechanics to the Cardiovascular System, T. Yamaguchi (Editor). Springer-Verlag, ISBN: 4431702881.

Computers in Cardiology, 2000, IEEE Engineering in Medicine and Biology Society. Amer. Inst. of Chemical Engineers, ISBN: 0780365593.

Medical Applications of Computer Modeling: Cardiovascular and Ocular Systems (Advances in Computational Bioengineering), T. B. Martonen (Editor). Wit Pr/Computational Mechanics, ISBN: 1853126136.

CONFERENCE PROCEEDINGS

16th International Congress on Thrombosis: Porto, Portugal, May 5-8, 2000 (Haemostasis), M. Campos (Editor), L. M. Cunha-Ribeiro (Editor). S. Karger Publishing, ISBN: 3805570821.

2000 Computers in Cardiology: September 24-27, 2000 Cambridge, Massachusetts, USA (Computers in Cardiology, 2000), IEEE, ISBN: 0780365577.

Harrisons Advances in Cardiology, Eugene Braunwald. McGraw Hill Text, ISBN: 0071370889.

CONGENITAL HEART DISEASE

Congenital Diseases of the Heart: Clinical-Physiological Considerations, Abraham M. Rudolph. Futura Pub. Co., ISBN: 0879934719.

Congenital Heart Diseases in Adults, W. Gersony. McGraw Hill Text, ISBN: 0070329095.

Congenital Heart Malformations in Mammals: An Illustrated Text, Magnus Michaelsson (Editor), Siew Yen Ho (Editor). Imperial College Press, ISBN: 1860941583.

Etiology and Morphogenesis of Congenital Heart Disease: Twenty Years of Progress in Genetics and Developmental Biology, Edward B. Clark (Editor), Makoto Nakazawa (Editor), Atsuyoshi Takao (Editor). Futura Pub. Co., ISBN: 0879934476.

Jesse E. Edwards' Synopsis of Congenital Heart Disease, Brooks S. Edwards, M.D., Jesse E. Edwards, M.D. Futura Pub. Co., ISBN: 0879934530.

The Left Heart in Congenital Heart Disease, Robert H. Anderson. Greenwich Medical Media, ISBN: 1841100560.

CORONARY ARTERY DISEASE

Coronary Artery Disease: An Incredibly Easy! Miniguide, Springhouse Pub. Co., ISBN: 1582550131.

CRITICAL CARE CARDIOLOGY

Critical Care Cardiology in the Perioperative Period, J. L. Atlee (Editor), J. L. Vincent (Editor), Antonino Gullo (Editor) Springer-Verlag, ISBN: 8847001331.

Critical Care Focus 6: Cardiology, Galley, Woolf, Marinker, Scully, Connelly, Charles, Cooklin, Silagy, Haines, Knotterus, Hall, Dawson, Tylee, Rowbotham, Trowell, Fell, Malik, Advanced Life Support Group, McCluskey, Stewart, Taylor, Nunn, Lask, Fay, Dollinger, Sharon Krieger, Rebecca Schmidt, Thomas Vallombroso, Warren Sanger, William Beachley, Donald Kushner, Guy Haskell, Steven Yun, William Schwer, Mary T. Dorn, John Trestrail, Lance W. Kreplick, Scott H. Plantz, Jesse A. Cole. Boston Medical Pub. Inc., ISBN: 0727915436.

Critical Pathways in Cardiology, Christopher P. Cannon (Editor), Patrick T. O'Gara (Editor). Lippincott Williams & Wilkins Publishers, ISBN: 0781726212.

DIABETES

Diabetes and Cardiovascular Disease (Contemporary Cardiology), Michael T. Johnstone, M.D. (Editor), Aristidis Veves, M.D. (Editor). Humana Press, ISBN: 089603755X.

DIAGNOSTICS & IMAGING

A Practical Guide to the Use of the High-Resolution Electrocardiogram, Edward J. Berbari, Jonathan S. Steinberg. Futura Pub. Co., ISBN: 087993445X.

Advances in Non-Invasive Electrocardiographic Monitoring (Developments in Cardiovascular Medicine Volume 229), Hans H. Osterhues (Editor), Vinzenz Hombach (Editor), Arthur J. Moss (Editor). Kluwer Academic Publishers, ISBN: 0792362144.

An Atlas of Contrast-Enhanced Angiography (The Encyclopedia of Visual Medicine Series), R. Mohiaddin. CRC Press-Parthenon Publishers, ISBN: 1842140817.

An Atlas of Heart Rhythms, Roy Pittman. Roy Pittman Publishing, ISBN: 0971051607.

An Introduction to Cardiac Electrophysiology, Antonio Zara (Editor), Michael R. Rose (Editor). Gordon & Breach Science Pub. ISBN: 9057024578.

Chou's Electrocardiography in Clinical Practice: Adult and Pediatric, Borys Surawicz, Timothy Knilans. W. B. Saunders Co., ISBN: 0721686974.

Clinical Electrocardiographic Diagnosis: A Problem-Based Approach, Noble O. Fowler. Lippincott, Williams & Wilkins, ISBN: 0781719577.

Concepts in Echocardiography, Chase. CRC Press-Parthenon Publishers, ISBN: 185070080X.

Coronary Angioscopy, Yasumi Uchida, M.D. Futura Pub. Co., ISBN: 0879934786.

Coronary Arteriography, King-Douglas. McGraw Hill Text, ISBN: 0071343849.

Coronary Magnetic Resonance Angiography, Andre J. Duerinckx (Editor). Springer- Verlag, ISBN: 0387949593.

CT Angiography of the Chest, Lee-Chiong (Editor). Lippincott Williams & Wilkins Publishers, ISBN: 0781727316.

Current Medical Diagnosis & Treatment 2001 CD-ROM (For Windows & Macintosh), Stephen J. McPhee (Editor), Maxine A. AAdakis (Editor), Ralph Gonzales, Papadakis. McGraw-Hill Professional Publishing, ISBN: 0838515592.

Duplex Scanning in Vascular Disorders, D. Eugene Strandness, M. D., Jr. Lippincott Williams & Wilkins Publishers, ISBN: 078172631X.

Dynamic Practical Electrocardiography: A Virtual Clinic and Classroom, Galen S. Wagner, William T. Lawson, Jr., Robert A. Waugh. Lippincott, Williams & Wilkins, ISBN: 0683305883.

ECG Cards, Springhouse Pub Co (Short), ISBN: 1582550085.

ECG's Made Easy Package Book and Pocket Guide, Barbara Aehlert, R.N. Mosby, Inc., ISBN: 0323014321.

ECG's Made Easy Pocket Guide, Barbara Aehlert. Mosby, Inc., ISBN: 032301433X.

Echocardiography, Mosby-Year Book, ISBN: 0815151454.

Echocardiography for the Neonatologist, Jonathan Skinner (Editor), Stewart Hunter, Dale Clark Alverson. Churchill Livingstone, ISBN: 0443054800.

Echo-Morphologic Correlates (Echoardiographic Diagnosis of Congenital Heart Disease), S. Brecker, R. H. Anderson. World Scientific Publishing Co., Inc., ISBN: 1860942407.

Electrocardiograph, Gareth Mallon. Unknown, ISBN: 1873413041.

EZ ECG Video and Booklet, American Safety Video Publishers Staff, Mosby, Goldman, Robert J. Huszar, Stuart N. Chale, Edward R. Stapleton. Mosby, Inc., ISBN: 0323013309.

Guide to ECG Analysis, Joseph T. Catalano. Lippincott Williams & Wilkins Publishers, ISBN: 0781729300.

Handbook of Contrast Echocardiography: Left Ventricular Function and Myocardial Perfusion, Harold Becher, Peter N. Burns. Springer-Verlag, ISBN: 3540670831.

Handbook of Non-Invasive Cardiac Testing, A. Iain McGhie (Editor). Edward Arnold, ISBN: 0340742127.

Interpreting Electrocardiograms: Using Basic Principles and Vector Concepts (Fundamental and Clinical Cardiology, Number 42), J. Willis Hurst. Marcel Dekker, ISBN: 0824705130.

Listening to the Heart: A Comprehensive Collection of Heart Sounds and Murmurs (3 CD-ROMs/Booklet), Daniel Mason. F. A. Davis Co., ISBN: 0803606966.

Magnetic Resonance of the Heart and Great Vessels: Clinical Applications (Medical Radiology), J. Bogaert (Editor), A. J. Duerinckx (Editor), F. E. Rademakers (Editor). Springer- Verlag, ISBN: 3540672176.

Markers in Cardiology: Current and Future Clinical Applications (American Heart Association Monograph Series), Jesse E. Adams, Fred S. Apple, Ph.D. (Editor), Allan S. Jaffe, M. D. Futura Pub. Co., ISBN: 0879934727.

Marridott's Practical Electrocardiography, Galen S. Wagner, Henry J. L. Marriott. Lippincott, Williams & Wilkins, ISBN: 0683307460.

Mastering Auscultation: An Audio Tour to Cardiac Diagnosis (Cardiophonetic CD-ROM), T. Anthony Don Michael. McGraw Hill Text, ISBN: 0078642922.

Noninvasive Electrocardiology in Clinical Practice, Wojciech Zareba (Editor), Emanuela Locati, M.D. (Editor), P. Maison-Blanche. Futura Pub. Co., ISBN: 0879934670.

Pocket Reference to Sensible Analysis of the ECG, Kathryn Monica Lewis, Kathleen A. Handal. Delmar Publishers, ISBN: 0766805220.

Pocket Guide to ECG Diagnosis, Edward K. Chung. Blackwell Science Inc., ISBN: 0865425892.

Pulmonary Differential Diagnosis, Zackon. W. B. Saunders Co., ISBN: 0702025771.

Quick and Accurate 12-Lead ECG Interpretation, Dale Davis. Lippincott Williams & Wilkins Publishers, ISBN: 0781723272.

Rapid Analysis of Electrocardiograms: A Self-Study Program, Emanuel Stein, Thomas Xenakis (Illustrator). Lippincott Williams & Wilkins Publishers, ISBN: 0683306561.

Rapid Interpretation of EKG's, Dale Dubin. Cover Pub Co, ISBN: 0912912065.

Real-World Nursing Survival Guide ECG's and the Heart, Cynthia C. Chernecky (Editor), Christine Alichnie, Ph.D., Beverly George-Gay, Cynthia Terry, Kitty Garrett, Rebecca K Hodges. W. B. Saunders Co., ISBN: 072169036X.

Sensible Analysis of the 12-Lead ECG, Kathryn Monica Lewis, Kathleen A.

Handal. Delmar Publishers, ISBN: 0766805247.

Spiral CT of the Chest, M. Remy Jardin (Editor), J. Remy (Editor), A.L. Baert (Editor), K. Sartor Springer-Verlag, ISBN: 3540411763.

Synopsis of Cardiac Physical Diagnosis, Jonathan Abrams. Butterworth-Heinemann, ISBN: 0750673389.

The Guide to EKG Interpretation (White Coat Pocket Guide Series), John A. Brose (Editor), John C. Auseon, Daniel Waksman, Michael J. Jarosick. Ohio Univ. Press (Txt), ISBN: 0821413287.

Understanding 12 Lead EKGs: A Practical Approach, Michael C. West, Brenda M. Beasley Prentice Hall, ISBN: 0130272817.

Understanding Heart Sounds & Murmurs with an Introduction to Lung Sounds, Ara G. Tilkian, Mary Boudreau Conover. W. B. Saunders Co., ISBN: 072167643X.

DRUG-INDUCED DISORDERS

Heparin-Induced Thrombocytopenia, Theodore E. Warkentin (Editor), Andreas Greinacher. Marcel Dekker, ISBN: 0824702719.

EDUCATION

Basic Electrocardiography in Ten Days, David R. Ferry, M.D., Robert A. O'Rourke. McGraw-Hill Professional Publishing, ISBN: 0071352929.

Lecture Notes on Cardiology (Lecture Notes), Keith D. Dawkins (Contributor), John M. Morgan, Huon Gray, Iain A. Simpson (Contributor). Blackwell Science Inc., ISBN: 0865428646.

Lecture Notes on Molecular Medicine, John Sutherland, M.D., Debbie Durham, William H. Faulkner, M. Rutter, Jeremy Hawker, Norman Begg, E. Taylor, Carolyn Kaut Roth, David W. Hay, Robert T. Smith, Julius Weinberg, John Bradley. Blackwell Science Inc., ISBN: 0632044756.

Todd's CV Review CD, J. Wesley Todd. Cardiac Self Assessment, ISBN: 0965356892.

EMERGENCY CARDIOLOGY

First Aid and CPR for Infants and Children, National Safety Council. Jones & Bartlett Pub. ISBN: 0763713228.

Handbook of Cardiac Emergencies, McConachie, Roberts, Ian McConachie (Editor), David Roberts. Greenwich Medical Media, ISBN: 1841100412.

Handbook of Cardiovascular Emergencies, James W. Hoekstra, M.D. (Editor). Lippincott Williams & Wilkins Publishers, ISBN: 0781724902.

END-STAGE RENAL FAILURE

Cardiovascular Disease in End-Stage Renal Failure, Joseph Loscalzo (Editor), Gerard M. London (Editor). Oxford University Press, ISBN: 0192629875.

EVIDENCE-BASED CARDIOLOGY

Evidence-Based Cardiology, Peter J. Sharis, Christopher P. Cannon. Lippincott Williams & Wilkins Publishers, ISBN: 0781716136.

Evidence-Based Management of the Acute Coronary Syndrome, Roque Pifarre

(Editor), Patrick J. Scanlon, M.D. (Editor). Lippincott Williams & Wilkins Publishers, ISBN: 1560534583.

Evidence-Based Manual of Coronary Care Management, Mark Connaughton. Churchill Livingstone, ISBN: 0443064156.

EXERCISE

Exercise and Circulation in Health and Disease, Bengt Saltin (Editor), Robert Boushel (Editor), Niels Secher (Editor). Human Kinetics Pub., ISBN: 0880116323.

Exercise and Sports Cardiology, Paul D. Thompson (Editor). McGraw-Hill Professional Publishing, ISBN: 0071347739.

FETAL CARDIOLOGY

Fetal Electrocardiography (Series in Cardiopulmonary Medicine), E. Malcolm Symonds, Daljit Sahota, Allan Chang. Imperial College Press, ISBN: 1860941710.

Fetal Origins of Cardiovascular and Lung Disease, David J. P. Barker (Editor). Marcel Dekker, ISBN: 082470391X.

Textbook of Fetal Cardiology, Lindsey Allan, M.D. (Editor), Lisa Hornberger, M.D. (Editor), Gurleen K. Sharland. Greenwich Medical Media, ISBN: 1900151634.

The Fetal and Neonatal Pulmonary Circulations, E. Kenneth Weir (Editor), Stephen L. Archer (Editor), John T. Reeves. Futura Pub. Co., ISBN: 0879934395.

GENETICS

Genetics for Cardiologists: The Molecular Genetic Basis of Cardiovascular Disorders, Ali J. Marian. Remedica Pub. Ltd., ISBN: 1901346099.

GERIATRIC CARDIOLOGY

Cardiac Disease in the Elderly: Interventions, Ethics, Economics, M. Preiss (Editor), M. Grapow (Editor), P. Buser (Editor), H. R. Zerkowski. Dr. Verlag Steinkipff Dietrich, ISBN: 3798512868.

HEART DISEASE

Chest Pain, Richard C. Becker. Butterworth-Heinemann, ISBN: 0750671416.

Heart Disease -- A Textbook of Cardiovascular Medicine, Single volume, Eugene Braunwald, M.D. (Editor), Douglas P. Zipes, M.D. (Editor), Peter Libby. W. B. Saunders Co., ISBN: 0721685498.

Heart Disease (Perspectives on Disease and Illness), Susan R. Gregson. Lifematters Press, ISBN: 0736807497.

Heart Disease (Understanding Illness (Mankato, Minn.), Sue Vander Hook. Smart Apple Media, ISBN: 1583400265.

Heart Disease: A Textbook of Cardiovascular Medicine (2 volume set), Eugene Braunwald (Editor), Douglas P. Zipes (Editor), Peter Lib (Editor). W. B. Saunders Co., ISBN: 0721685617.

Heart Disease: Environment, Stress, and Gender, G. Weidner. IOS Press, ISBN: 1586030825.

Heart Diseases and Disorders Sourcebook: Basic Consumer Health Information About Heart Attacks, Angina, Rhythm Disorders, Heart Failure, Valve Disease, Karen Bellenir (Editor). Omnigraphics, Inc., ISBN: 0780802381.

The ABC's of Coronary Heart Disease, James J. MacIejko. Sleeping Bear Press, ISBN: 1886947996.

Why Me?: Approaching Coronary Heart Disease, Cardiac Catheterization, and Treatment Options from a Position of Strength, Scott M. Nordlicht, M.D., Alan N. Weiss, M.D., Philip A. Ludbrock. Northern Lights Inc., ISBN: 0965761118.

HEART FAILURE

ABC of Heart Failure, Christopher R. Gibbs (Editor), Michael K. Davies (Editor), Gregory Y. H. Lip. B M J Books, ISBN: 072791457X.

An Atlas of Heart Failure (The Encyclopedia of Visual Medicine Series), J. Cleland, M. Davis. CRC Press-Parthenon Publishers, ISBN: 1850700419.

Basics of Heart Failure: A Problem Solving Approach, Brian E. Jaski, M.D. Kluwer Academic Publishers, ISBN: 0792377869.

Choose Health Over Heart Failure, Michael E. McIvor. McGraw-Hill Primis Custom Publishing, ISBN: 0072491841.

Clinical Management of Heart Failure, James Young, Roger Mills. Professional Communications, ISBN: 188473555X.

Fighting Sudden Cardiac Death: A Worldwide Challenge, Etienne Aliot (Editor), Jacques Clementy (Editor), Eric N. Prystowsky. Futura Pub. Co., ISBN: 0879934603.

Heart Failure: Diagnosis and Management, John McMurray. Dunitz Martin Ltd., ISBN: 1853177172.

Heart Failure: Frontiers in Cardiology, Akira Kitabatake (Editor), Shigetake Sasayama (Editor), Gary S. Francis. Springer-Verlag, ISBN: 4431702393.

Heart Failure: An Incredibly Easy! Miniguide, Springhouse Pub. Co., ISBN: 1582550115.

HISTORY

British Cardiology in the 20th Century, Peter Fleming, Arthur Hollman, Desmond Julian, Mark E. Silverman, Peter R. Fleming. Springer-Verlag, ISBN: 185233312X.

Dates in Cardiology, H. S. J. Lee (Editor), J. Wright. CRC Press-Parthenon Publishers, ISBN: 1850704988.

Professor Hein J. J. Wellens: 33 Years of Cardiology and Arrhythmology, J. L. R. M. Smeets (Editor), Pieter A. Doevendans (Editor), M.E. Josephson. Kluwer Academic Publishers, ISBN: 0792362098.

The History of Cardiology, Louis J. Acierno, M.D. CRC Press-Parthenon Publishers, ISBN: 1850700494.

HYPERTENSION

100 Questions and Answers About Hypertension, William M. Manger, M. D., Ray W. Gifford, Jr. Blackwell Science Inc., ISBN: 0632044810.

ABC of Hypertension (ABC Series), Gareth Beevers, Gregory Y. H. Lip, Eoin O'Brien. B M J Books, ISBN: 0727915223.

Clinical Trials in Hypertension, Henry R. Black (Editor). Marcel Dekker, ISBN: 0824702700.

Epidemiology of Hypertension, C. J. Bulpitt (Editor). Elsevier Science Ltd., ISBN: 044482779X.

Hypertension, Lennart Hansen, M.D. (Editor), Jose Rodicio, M.D. (Editor), Albert Zanchetti, M.D. (Editor), Stevo Julius (Editor). McGraw-Hill, ISBN: 0077095235.

Hypertension and Co-Existing Disease, Francisco Leyva, Andrew J. S. Coats, Francisco Leyva-Leon. Blackwell Science Inc., ISBN: 063205073X.

Hypertension in Focus. Unknown, ISBN: 0853694567.

Hypertension Medicine, Michael A. Weber, M.D. (Editor). Humana Press, ISBN: 0896037886.

Hypertension Therapy Annual, Norman M. Kaplin (Editor). Dunitz Martin Ltd., ISBN: 1853177288.

Hypertensive Disorders in Women, Baha M. Sibai, M. D. (Editor). W. B. Saunders Co., ISBN: 0721673740.

Illustrated Pocketbook of Hypertension, P. F. Semple. CRC Press-Parthenon Publishers, ISBN: 1842140574.

Pharmacological Profiles in Hypertension: ACE Inhibitors, V. R. Preedy (Editor), H. Why (Editor). Greenwich Medical Media, ISBN: 1841100315.

The Hypertension Sourcebook, Mary P. McGowan, M.D., Jo McGowan-Chopra. McGraw Hill - NTC, ISBN: 0737305398.

INFECTION

Staphylococci in Cardio-Thoracic Surgery: Epidemiological and Clinical Studies (Comprehensive Summaries of Uppsala Dissertations from the Faculty of), Ann Tammelin Brandemark. Uppsala Universitet, ISBN: 9155450059.

INTERVENTIONAL CARDIOLOGY

Interventional Cardiology: Self-Assessment and Review, Volumes 1 & 2 (in one volume), Martin B. Leon, Robert D. Safian, Mark Freed. Physicians Press, ISBN: 1890114308.

Interventional Cardiovascular Medicine Principles and Practice, Stack, Roubin, O'Neill. Churchill Livingstone, ISBN: 044307979X.

Interventional Electrophysiology, Igor Singer (Editor). Lippincott Williams & Wilkins Publishers, ISBN: 0781723337.

Interventional Radiology Secrets, Murphy. Hanley & Belfus, ISBN: 156053415X.

Interventional Radiology: A Survival Guide, David Kessel, Iain Robertson. Churchill Livingstone, ISBN: 0443062897.

Invasive Cardiology: Manual for Cath. Lab Personnel, Sandy Watson, Bernhard Meier. Physicians Press, ISBN: 1890114316.

Practical Handbook of Advanced Interventional Cardiology, Thach N. Nguyen, M.D. (Editor), Shigeru Saito, M.D. (Editor), Dayi Hu, M.D. Futura Pub. Co., ISBN: 0879934697.

The New Manual of Interventional Cardiology, Mark Freed, Cindy Grines,

Robert D. Safian. Physicians Press, ISBN: 1890114294.

INTERVENTIONAL RADIOLOGY

Handbook of Interventional Radiologic Procedures, Krishna Kandarpa. Lippincott Williams & Wilkins Publishers, ISBN: 0781723582.

MITRAL VALVE DISEASE

Mitral Valve: Floppy Mitral Valve, Mitral Valve Prolapse, Mitral Valvular Regurgitation, Harisios Boudoulas M.D., Ph.D., Charles Wooley, M.D. Futura Pub. Co., ISBN: 0879934484.

MYOCARDIAL INFARCTION

Myocardial Infarction: An Incredibly Easy! Miniguide, Springhouse Pub. Co. ISBN: 1582550093.

Myocardial Viability: A Clinical and Scientific Treatise, Vasken Dilsizian, M.D. (Editor). Futura Pub. Co., ISBN: 0879934379.

Myocardium at Risk and Viable Myocardium: Evaluation by Spet (Developments in Cardiovascular Medicine, 234), Jaume Candell-Riera (Editor), Joan Castell-Conesa (Editor), Aguade-Bruix. Kluwer Academic Publishers, ISBN: 0792367243.

Silent Myocardial Ischemia and Infarction, Peter F. Cohn. Marcel Dekker, ISBN: 0824703545.

NUCLEAR CARDIOLOGY

Nuclear Cardiology (Speedy, V. 1), Kathleen Murphy (Editor). Society of Nuclear Medicine, ISBN: 0932004768.

NUTRITION

The Cholesterol Myths: Exposing the Fallacy that Saturated Fat and Cholesterol Cause Heart Disease, Uffe Ravnskov. NewTrends Publishing, Inc., ISBN: 0967089700.

What You Should Know About Triglycerides: The Missing Link in Heart Disease, Dennis Sprecher, M.D. Wholecare, ISBN: 0380809400.

PACING AND DEFIBRILLATION

A Practical Guide to Cardiac Pacing, H. Weston Moses, Kriegh P. Moulton, Brain D. Miller. Lippincott, Williams & Wilkins, ISBN: 0781719569.

AED: Automated External Defibrillation, Jones & Bartlett Pub. ISBN: 0763716324.

Cardiac Assist Devices, Daniel J. Goldstein (Editor), Mehmet Oz (Editor. Futura Pub. Co., ISBN: 0879934492.

Cardiac Electrophysiology: From Cell to Bedside, Douglas P. Zipes (Editor), Jose Jalife (Editor), Richard Zorab (Editor). W. B. Saunders Co., ISBN: 0721678114.

Cardiac Pacing, Kenneth A. Ellenbogen (Editor), Mark Wood. Blackwell Science Inc, ISBN: 0865425868.

Cardiac Pacing and Defibrillation: A Clinical Approach, David L. Hayes, M.D., Margaret A. Lloyd, M.D., Paul A.

Friedman, M.D. Futura Pub. Co., ISBN: 087993462X.

Cardiac Pacing for the Clinician, Fred M. Kusumoto, M.D. (Editor), Nora F. Goldschlager, M.D. (Editor). Lippincott Williams & Wilkins Publishers, ISBN: 0683307045.

Clinical Cardiac Electrophysiology: Techniques and Interpretations, Adis, ISBN: 0683306936.

Implantable Cardioverter-Defibrillator: A Practical Manual, L. Bing Liem. Kluwer Academic Publishers, ISBN: 079236743X.

Machines in Our Hearts: The Cardiac Pacemaker, the Implantable Defibrillator, and American Health Care, Kirk Jeffrey. Johns Hopkins Univ. Press, ISBN: 0801865794.

Mechanical Support for Cardiac and Respiratory Failure in Pediatric Patients, Brian W. Duncan (Editor). Marcel Dekker, ISBN: 0824702751.

Ventricular Fibrillation: A Pediatric Problem, Linda Quan, M.D. (Editor), Wayne H. Franklin, M.D. (Editor). Futura Pub. Co., ISBN: 0879934522.

Pediatric Cardiology

Moss and Adams' Heart Disease in Infants, Children, and Adolescents: Including the Fetus and Young Adult (2 Volume Set), Hugh D. Allen (Editor), Howard P. Gutgesell (Editor), Edward B. Clark. Lippincott Williams & Wilkins Publishers, ISBN: 0683307428.

Neonatal Cardiology, Michael Artman, David F. Teitel, Lynn Mahony. McGraw Hill Text, ISBN: 0070070989.

Paediatric Cardiology, 2-Volume Set, Robert H. Anderson, Edward J. Baker, Fergus J. McCartney, Michael L. Rigby, Elliot A. Shinebourne, Michael Tynan. Churchill Livingstone, ISBN: 0443079900.

Pediatric Cardiology, Karol Lozasadi, Vilmos Kornyei. Akademiai Kiado, ISBN: 963057702X.

Pediatric Cardiology, Alexander S. Nadas. W. B. Saunders Co., ISBN: 0721666523.

Pediatric Cardiology (Core Handbooks in Pediatrics), Walter H. Johnson, M.D., Jr., James H. Moller, M.D. Lippincott Williams & Wilkins Publishers, ISBN: 0781728789.

Pediatric Cardiovascular Medicine, James H. Moller, Julien I. E. Hoffman. Churchill Livingstone, ISBN: 0443076774.

Practical Pediatric Echocardiography, David T. Linker. Churchill Livingstone, ISBN: 0443076405.

The Heart of a Child: What Families Need to Know About Heart Disorders in Children (Johns Hopkins Press Health Book), Edward B. Clark (Editor), Carleen Clark (Editor), Catherine A. Neill (Editor). Johns Hopkins Univ. Press, ISBN: 0801866367.

Thromboembolic Complications During Infancy and Childhood (With CD-ROM for Windows & Macintosh), Maureen Andrew, M.D., Paul T. Monagle, Luanne Brooker, BC Decker Inc, ISBN: 1550090364.

Prevention

50 Ways Women Can Prevent Heart Disease, M. Sara Rosenthal, Laura Purdy. McGraw Hill - NTC, ISBN: 0737305029.

Every Heart Attack is Preventable, Michael Mogadam, M.D. Lifeline Press, ISBN: 089526207X.

Heal Your Heart: How You Can Prevent or Reverse Heart Disease, K. Lance Gould, M.D. Rutgers Univ. Press, ISBN: 0813528968.

Healthy Heart: Keep Your Cardiovascular System Healthy and Fit at Any Age, Patricia Bragg, Paul C. Bragg. Health Science, ISBN: 0877900965.

Heart Health for Black Women: A Natural Approach to Healing and Preventing Heart Disease, Beverly Yates. Marlowe & Co., ISBN: 156924619X.

Prevention of Disease Progression Throughout the Cardiovascular Continuum: The Role of Adrenergic B-Blockade, Lars E. Ryden (Editor) Springer-Verlag, ISBN: 3540415033.

Preventive Cardiology: Strategies for the Prevention and Treatment of Coronary Artery Disease, Joanne Micale Foody, M.D. (Editor), Eugene Braunwald. Humana Press, ISBN: 0896038114.

Role of Potassium in Preventive Cardiovascular Medicine (Basic Science for the Cardiologist, Volume 8), David B. Young. Kluwer Academic Publishers, ISBN: 0792373766.

The 8-Week Cholesterol Cure: How to Lower Your Blood Cholesterol by Up to 40 Percent Without Drugs or Deprivation [Large Print], Robert E. Kowalski, Albert A. Kattus, M.D. HarperCollins (paper), ISBN: 0060955740.

You Can Beat Heart Disease: Prevention and Treatment, Lester R. Sauvage, M.D. Carol P. Garzona (Foreword), Kathryn D. Barker, Warren Berry, Jerry Gladstone. Better Life Press, ISBN: 0966378822.

PROCEDURES

Atlas of Coronary Stenting, Rothman. Dunitz Martin Ltd. ISBN: 1853177180.

Cardiopulmonary Bypass: Principles and Practice, Glenn P. Gravlee (Editor), Richard F. Davis (Editor), Mark Kurusz (Editor). Lippincott, Williams & Wilkins, ISBN: 0683304763.

Coronary Artery Stenting (Contemporary Cardiology), Sheldon Goldberg (Editor), Igor F. Palacios (Editor). Humana Press, ISBN: 0896038572.

Current Status of Carotid Bifurcation Angioplasty and Stenting, Frank J. Veith (Editor), Max Amor (Editor). Marcel Dekker, ISBN: 0824704959.

Dispersion of Ventricular Repolarization: State of the Art, S. Bertil Olsson, M.D., Ph.D. (Editor), Jan P. Amlie, M.D., Ph.D. (Editor). Futura Pub. Co., ISBN: 0879934581.

Grossman's Cardiac Catheterization, Angiography, and Intervention, Donald S. Baim (Editor), William Grossman, M.D. (Editor). Lippincott Williams & Wilkins Publishers, ISBN: 068330741X.

Handbook of Coronary Stents, Patrick W. Serruys, M.D., Ph.D., Michael J. B. Kutryk, M.D., Ph.D. Dunitz Martin Ltd. ISBN: 1853178020.

Handbook of Noninvasive Cardiovascular Procedures, A. I. McGhie. Lippincott Williams & Wilkins Publishers, ISBN: 0412112914.

Lasers for Ischemic Heart Disease: Update on Alternatives for the Treatment of Diffuse Coronary Artery Disease, Xavier M. Mueller (Editor). Springer-Verlag, ISBN: 3540676546.

Rotary Blood Pumps: New Developments and Current Applications, H. Matsuda (Editor). Springer-Verlag, ISBN: 4431702806.

Stent-Grafts: Current Clinical Practice, Bart L. Dolmatch, M.D. (Editor), Ulrich Blum, M.D. (Editor) Thieme Medical Pub. ISBN: 0865778930.

Sleep Apnea

Sleep Apnea: Implications in Cardiovascular and Cerebrovascular Disease, T. Douglas Bradley (Editor), John S. Floras (Editor). Marcel Dekker, ISBN: 0824702999.

Terminology

Cardiology Words and Phrases, Health Professions Institute. Prentice Hall, ISBN: 013094081X.

Dorland's Cardiology Word Book for Medical Transcriptionists, Sharon B. Rhodes (Editor), Mary David (Editor). W. B. Saunders Co., ISBN: 072169151X.

Illustrated Dictionary of Cardiology, M. Melloni, B. J. Melloni. CRC Press-Parthenon Publishers, ISBN: 1850707111.

Therapeutics/
Pharmacology

120 Years of Nitrate Therapy Prepared for the Next Millennium, J. F. Holubarsch (Editor), T. F. Luscher. Walter De Gruyter, ISBN: 3110168480.

A Textbook on EDTA Chelation Therapy, Elmer M. Cranton (Editor), Linus Pauling. Hampton Roads Pub. Co. ISBN: 1571742530.

Angiotensin II Receptor Antagonists, Murray Epstein, M.D. Hanley & Belfus, ISBN: 1560534532.

Cardio Cures, Gary Bushkin, Estitta Bushkin. McGraw-Hill Professional Publishing, ISBN: 0658015311.

Cardiovascular Therapeutics a Companion to Braunwald's Heart Disease, Antman. W. B. Saunders Co., ISBN: 0721687334.

Cox-2 Inhibitors, Howard A. Bird. Dunitz Martin Ltd, ISBN: 1853177954.

Disease-Modifying Therapy in Vasculitides (Pir-Progress in Inflammation Research), Cornelis Gijsbertus Maria Kallenberg (Editor), J. W. Cohen Tervaert. Birkhauser (Architectural), ISBN: 3764361476.

Drugs for the Heart, Lionel H. Opie, M.D. (Editor), Bernard J. Gersh (Editor), Eugene Braunwald. W. B. Saunders Co. ISBN: 0721687571.

Essentials of Cardiopulmonary Physical Therapy, Ellen A. Hillegass (Editor), H. Steven Sadowsky (Editor). W. B. Saunders Co. ISBN: 0721672884.

Fibrinolytic and Antithrombotic Therapy: Theory, Practice, and Management, Richard C. Becker. Oxford University Press, ISBN: 019512331X.

Fibrinolytics and Antifibrinolytics, F. Bachmann (Editor). Springer-Verlag, ISBN: 3540661263.

Gene Therapy Protocols, Michael D'Ambra. Humana Press, ISBN: 0896037231.

Growth Hormone and the Heart (Endocrine Updates Volume 9), Andrea Giustina (Editor), Filippo Manelli (Editor). Kluwer Academic Publishers, ISBN: 0792372123.

Hormone Replacement Therapy and Cardiovascular Disease (Controversial Issues in Climacteric Medicine, Volume 1), Andrea R. Genazzani (Editor). CRC Press-Parthenon Publishers, ISBN: 1842140388.

Intravascular Brachytherapy: From Theory to Practice, Prabhakar Tripuraneni (Editor). Remedica Pub. Ltd, ISBN: 1901346307.

Molecular Approaches to Heart Failure Therapy, G. Hasenfub (Editor), E. Marban (Editor). Dr. Verlag Steinkipff Dietrich, ISBN: 3798512361.

Natural Treatments for High Cholesterol (The Natural Pharmacist), Darin Ingels. Prima Publishing, ISBN: 0761524673.

Nitric Oxide and the Cardiovascular System (Contemporary Cardiology), Joseph Loscalzo (Editor), Joseph A. Vita (Editor). Humana Press, ISBN: 0896036200.

Optimizing Antiplatelet Therapy in Atherothrombotic Patients: Satellite Symposium to the 9th European Stroke Conference, Vienna, May 2000, J. Boeousslavsky, J. D. Easton (Editor). S. Karger Publishing, ISBN: 3805572352.

Pocket Guide to Injectable Drugs: Companion to Handbook on Injectable Drugs (11th edition), Lawrence A. Trissel, American College of Cardiology, Anna B. Reisman, Janice Ryden, Pamela Charney, Karen Calhoun, American College of Physicians, American Medical Association, Barry Grumbiner, James S. Tan, Paul Blumenthal, David Stevens. American Medical Association, ISBN: 1585280232.

The ABCs of Antihypertensive Therapy, Franz H. Messerli (Editor). Lippincott, Williams & Wilkins, ISBN: 1881063070.

THROMBOEMBOLISM

Thromboembolism: New Insights & Future Prospects: 7th International Symposium on Thromboembolic Diseases, Palma De Mallorca, June 2000: Proceedings), S. Haas, V. J. Marder, M. M. Samama. S. Karger Publishing, ISBN: 3805571771.

Thrombosis and Thromboembolism (Fundamental and Clinical Cardiology), Goldhaber, Ridker. Marcel Dekker, ISBN: 0824706463.

TRANSPLANTATION

Heart & Lung Transplantation, Landes Bioscience, ISBN: 1570596344.

VASCULAR DISEASE

Encyclopedic Reference of Vascular Biology & Pathology, A. Bikfalvi. Springer-Verlag, ISBN: 3540652892.

Inflammatory Diseases of Blood Vessels, Gary Hoffman, Cornelia M. Weyland. Marcel Dekker, ISBN: 0824702697.

Minimal Access Therapy for Vascular Disease, Leahy, Bell, Katzen. Isis Medical Media, ISBN: 1901865274.

Oxidative Stress and Vascular Disease, John F. Keaney, Jr. (Editor). Kluwer Academic Publishers, ISBN: 0792386787.

Pathological Diagnosis of Vascular Disease, B. Austin. Springer-Verlag, ISBN: 2287596607.

Peripheral Arterial Disease Handbook, William R. Hiatt (Editor), Judith Regensteiner (Editor), Alan t Hirsch. CRC Press, ISBN: 0849384133.

Ultrasonography in Vascular Diseases: A Practical Approach to Clinical Problems, Edward I. Bluth (Editor). Thieme Medical Pub. ISBN: 1588900509.

Vascular Anaesthesia: A Practical Handbook, Lawrence Caldicott, M. B. , Andrew B. Lumb, M. B. Butterworth Architecture, ISBN: 0750650001.

Vascular and Endovascular Opportunities, R. M. Greenhalgh (Editor), J. T. Powell (Editor), W. W. Mitchell (Editor). W. B. Saunders Co. ISBN: 0702026107.

Vascular and Endovascular Surgical Techniques: An Atlas, Roger M. Greenhalgh (Editor). W. B. Saunders Co., ISBN: 0702026433.

Vascular and Interventional Radiology: Principles and Practices, Curtis W. Bakal. Thieme Medical Pub. ISBN: 0865776784.

Vascular Brachytherapy, Ron Waksman (Editor). Futura Pub. Co. ISBN: 0879934891.

Vascular Disease and Injury: Preclinical Research (Contemporary Cardiology), Daniel I. Simon, M.D. (Editor), Campbell Rogers, M.D. (Editor), Victor J. Dzau. Humana Press, ISBN: 0896037533.

Vascular Endothelium: Source and Target of Inflammatory Mediators, J. D. Catravas (Editor). IOS Press, ISBN: 1586030922.

Vascular Manifestations of Systemic Auto-Immune Diseases, Ronald A. Asherson (Editor), Ricard Cervera, M.D. (Editor), Steven Abramson. CRC Press, ISBN: 084931335X.

Venous Interventional Radiology with Clinical Perspectives, Scott J. Savander, M.D. (Editor), Scott O. Trerotola, M.D. (Editor). Thieme Medical Pub. ISBN: 0865778949.

Continuing Medical Education (CME)

4.1 CME Resources: Cardiology

American College of Cardiology (ACC): Continuing Education The ACC offers a variety of CME programs in the field and provides registration opportunity at the site for several upcoming titles and dates. Featured online programs, including those on the diabetic patient with heart disease, are available for viewing. Electrocardiogram, echocardiogram, and nuclear cardiology cases of the month are presented free of charge.

(some features fee-based) http://www.acc.org/education/education.htm

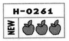

American Heart Association (AHA): Professional Education The opportunities accessible from this site of the AHA include daily summaries of the AHA Scientific Sessions online, a satellite broadcast replay on coronary artery disease in women, issues in arrhythmia management, and additional opportunities for learning in coronary artery disease and revascularization. Late-breaking clinical trial CME, a hypertension primer, Scientific Statements, conference and meeting schedules, and a variety of additional professional publications are found.

http://www.americanheart.org/presenter.jhtml?identifier=1722

American Society of Nuclear Cardiology: Calendar of CME Events Continuously updated, this calendar of CME events from the American Society of Nuclear Cardiology lists conferences, workshops, and symposia held around the world. Details about previous, current, and upcoming events are listed monthly. http://www.asnc.org/cgi-bin/calendar/calendar.cgi

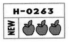

Medscape: Cardiology: CME Center Free, continuously updated CME activities are available at this site from Medscape, including activities for credit and cardiology programs in clinical management. Summaries of important medical conferences are available, as well as reports from conference workshops, authored by experts in the field. Industry-sponsored CME events are also available and are certified by accredited CME providers. A "CME Locator" feature offers a method of viewing all CME activities in the database or searching for programs by keyword entries.

http://www.medscape.com/Home/Topics/cardiology/directories/dir-CARD.CMECenter.html

Medsite CME: Interactive Grand Rounds in Cardiology Created by physicians for physicians, this site offers original, CME-certified cardiovascular medicine resources, with all content authored by nationally recognized leaders in the field. New cases are introduced monthly, and visitors may choose either to access new cases or to resume work in a previously accessed case study. A variety of clinical topics are provided, including arrhythmias, dyslipidemias, hypertension, and immunosuppressive therapy in heart/lung transplantation. Each activity is composed of both a clinical management section and a review article associated with some component of the case. Registration for CME credit is available once both portions have been completed, with no fee required for participation. http://cme.medsite.com

4.2 CME RESOURCES

Accreditation Council for Continuing Medical Education (ACCME) The ACCME offers voluntary accreditation to providers of continuing medical education who are interested in being recognized further for their high standards and quality. At the ACCME Web site, visitors will find information regarding all aspects of the accreditation process, as well as the current activities of the organization regarding communications and quality control protocols. http://www.accme.org

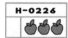

American Medical Association (AMA): CME Locator The American Medical Association CME locator provides access to over 2,000 activities sponsored by CME providers that are either accredited by the Accreditation Council for Continuing Medical Education (ACCME) or approved by the American Medical Association. CME selections of U.S., Canadian, and international conferences, seminars, workshops, and home study courses are contained in the database. By customizing a search through the selection of a specialty, location, and date, visitors are returned a locator result set, which provides access to course objectives, registration information, and related Web address, where applicable. http://www.ama-assn.org/iwcf/iwcfmgr206/cme

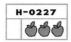

CME Unlimited This division of the nonprofit Audio-Digest Foundation specializes in providing CME programs to physicians and allied healthcare professionals on a subscription basis. It maintains a high-quality selection of over 6,000 CME products from medical associations, institutions, and societies in a variety of formats, including audio, video, and CD-ROM. The offerings at this Web site include 13 specialty series and two jointly sponsored activities, with audio materials of medical symposia, review courses, and specialty meetings available. Each course listing includes its description, sponsor, target audience, accreditation, objectives, and faculty, along with a list of currently available formats. http://www.landesslezak.com/cgi-bin/start.cgi/cmeu/index.htm

CME Web Sites An alphabetical listing of CME sites, collected by Bernard Sklar, M.D., offers information on accredited programs across a variety of

medical specialties. Links are provided to over 200 online CME sites, including those of the American Academy of Family Physicians, FamilyPractice.com, the American College of Cardiology's case-based interactive courses and clinical decision making programs, and Baylor College of Medicine's Online CME courses. Additional sources include the American College of Physicians-American Society of Internal Medicine (ACP-ASIM) and the AMA archives. Registration and participation requirements vary from site to site, with many free and fee-based offerings included.

(some features fee-based) http://www.netcantina.com/bernardsklar/cmelist.html

H-0228

CMEWeb CMEWeb is an online resource for participation in electronic CME courses. It is provided by American Health Consultants, a commercial group accredited by the Accreditation Council for Continuing Medical Education (ACCME). CME resources are only available to registered members of the site, and registration requires a fee.

(fee-based) http://www.cmeweb.com/#pdr

H-0230

Cyberounds Cyberounds is an online, interactive forum moderated by distinguished professionals. It is available for use only by physicians, medical students, and other healthcare professionals. A free registration is required. CME opportunities, an online bookstore, links to quality sites relevant to a variety of specialties, and additional educational resources are available.

http://www.cyberounds.com/links/home.html

H-0231

Ed Credits Ed Credits offers opportunities for CME credits for medical and other professionals. Registration is available for an annual fee, and any number of courses can be taken within this time. Material for the courses is available for free on the Web site, but registration is necessary to take the tests and to receive certificates. (some features fee-based) http://www.edcredits.com

H-0232

Medical Computing Today: CME Sites Medical Computing Today provides this comprehensive, alphabetical listing of currently available category I CME credit offerings accredited by the Accreditation Council for Continuing Medical Education (ACCME). Principal areas of specialty covered at each of 85 sites are listed. Programs are categorized according to whether they cover multiple specialties, or primary care resources, with a listing for cardiology that provides information on CME programs from the ACC, the AHA, the American Venous Forum, Cardiology Today and Tomorrow, selected medical schools and Controversies in Cardiology. CME descriptions, credits, and associated costs are included in the entries, and registration for CME credit may be completed online. (some features fee-based) http://www.medicalcomputingtoday.com/0listcme.html

H-0233

Medical Matrix: CME Courses Online Medical Matrix's CME Courses Online is a resource containing nearly 40 CME credit listing sites. General learning modules are available via the Virtual Lecture Hall Health Professionals CME, and Medscape's Online Articles for CME Reviews. The Cleveland Clinic Foundation, the National Institutes of Health, and Virtual Hospital Online all provide opportunities to access Internet-based CME courses, often with immediate feedback on performance. A multitude of top-rated CME modules and interesting feature sites are available, including the "Interactive Patient," which provides users with the opportunity to view a simulated online patient, request history, perform exams, and review diagnostic data. Credit fees vary by organization site. (some features fee-based) http://www.medmatrix.org

National Institutes of Health (NIH): Continuing Education This CME site, sponsored by the NIH and the Foundation for Advanced Education in the Sciences, invites users to participate in an online experiment in distance learning. Visitors can access consensus statements, details of the CME course, and a CME exam on a variety of health topics.
http://consensus.nih.gov/cme/cme.htm

4.3 Selected Medical School CME Programs

Baylor College of Medicine: Online Continuing Medical Education
Registered visitors to this site can access online CME lectures. Features available in the presentation modules include audio accompaniments to each slide, an index of slide topics, a search tool, access to PubMed for literature searches, a discussion forum organized by topic, and a concluding CME test. Answers to common technical questions about the online lectures are also available.
(free registration) http://www.baylorcme.org

Case Western Reserve University: Continuing Medical Education
Many features are available at this CME page, including grand rounds, activity brochures, and an interactive search for activities by date or specialty. Listings of self-paced learning activities and online programs are available, and visitors can register directly at the site for participation. Special topics on medical practice enhancement and planning CME events are also included.
(some features fee-based) http://cme.cwru.edu/default.htm

Columbia University: Center for Continuing Education in the Health Sciences   Resources for professionals interested in CME programs through Columbia Presbyterian Medical Center are available at this site. Visitors will find a calendar of events and a brochure request form, a general description of CME activities, a mission statement, information about Columbia University and New York City, details of hotel and travel arrangements, and e-mail contact details. http://cpmcnet.columbia.edu/dept/cme

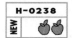

Cornell University Weill Medical College: Office of Continuing Medical Education   The Office of Continuing Medical Education at Cornell University offers listings of weekly departmental grand rounds at both New York Presbyterian Hospital and the Hospital for Special Surgery. Contact details, weekly dates, and weekly times are posted for each department offering rounds. http://www.med.cornell.edu/cme/index.html

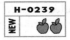

Duke University: Office of Continuing Medical Education A list of CME activities sponsored by Duke University is provided at this site, including listings by specialty/medical topic and date. Brochures for CME activities are available, and a search engine offers direction to specific course details in a number of medical specialties. Several opportunities to participate in CME Cybersessions are available.

(free registration) http://www2.mc.duke.edu/depts/som/docme/

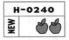

Emory University School of Medicine: Office of Continuing Medical Education Course listings by date and specialty are offered at this page, as well as information on mini-fellowships, grand rounds, and details for course participants. A site index arranges all courses by specialty and topic, and a download page offers course schedule and approval forms, travel expense documents, and other utilities for participation.

http://www.emory.edu/WHSC/MED/CME/index.html

Harvard Medical School: Department of Continuing Education Resources provided by the Harvard Medical School Department of Continuing Education include a list of hospitals, medical groups, and health centers offering CME programs; travel and housing details; and directories of specific CME programs. Visitors can search the directory of courses by topic, specialty, or date. Online registration forms are available. Information and on home study programs, available on CD-ROM, audiocassette, or videocassette, is also found at the site. http://www.med.harvard.edu/conted

Johns Hopkins Medicine: Continuing Medical Education Visitors to this address will find comprehensive resources related to CME programs at Johns Hopkins University. The site offers a calendar of events, a site search engine for locating relevant CME programs, a listing of special programs available by appointment only, information on graduate certificate programs, notices and a registration form for upcoming Franklin Covey CME courses, and contact details for the CME office. Information on distance education, video programs on CD-ROM, and Webcast courses is also available. Readers of these newsletters can receive CME credit through completion of a test at the conclusion of the newsletter. http://www.med.jhu.edu/cme

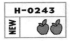

Mayo Medical School: Mayo School of CME The Mayo schedule for CME courses is found at this site, arranged by both month and medical specialty. Some listings offer online information brochures and course information in HTML and PDF formats; brochures can also be sent to a fax machine via the "Fax-On-Demand" service available from the Web site. A course synopsis is found for each program, as well as course location and sponsor.

http://www.mayo.edu/cme/schedule.html

Mount Sinai School of Medicine: Continuing Medical Education A schedule of CME courses can be accessed from this page, providing departmental information, date, and location details. Speaker's Bureau listings offered by Mount Sinai faculty are found, and a calendar of medical events at the Mount Sinai Medical Center is presented. In addition to regularly scheduled

Sinai Medical Center is presented. In addition to regularly scheduled departmental activities, the site also provides access to MSSM-TV, an interactive medical education tool containing live broadcast events and video archives. Many free CME opportunities are available.

(some features fee-based) http://www.mssm.edu/forfaculty/cme.shtml

New York University: Continuing Medical Education Current, past, and in-house conference event listings can be accessed from the menu at this site, which also offers information on accommodations in New York and other general information. Courses can be browsed by subject or month, with each listing offering information on target audience and educational objectives. Printable registration forms for each event are available.

http://www.med.nyu.edu/cme/

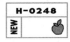

Northwestern University: Continuing Medical Education The CME calendar from Northwestern University provides dates, locations, and contact information for each event. By clicking on the titles of various programs, event description and admission cost are displayed. The site is regularly updated and contains listings of the most current events.

http://www.nums.northwestern.edu/cme/

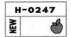

Stanford School of Medicine: Continuing Medical Education With courses accredited by the Accreditation Council for Continuing Medical Education (ACCME), the Office of Postgraduate Medical Education and Stanford University offer quality programs across a variety of medical specialties. Traditional lectures, workshops, and online CME are all available, and the calendar of events can be searched by Stanford department, month, or weekday.

http://www.med.stanford.edu/osa/cme/

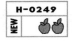

University of California Los Angeles (UCLA): Office of Continuing Medical Education Dates, titles, and locations for a variety of CME programs are offered at this UCLA listing. Some course brochures are available in PDF format. Viewers are encouraged to get up-to-date CME information by submitting an online information form.

http://www.medsch.ucla.edu/CME/

University of California San Diego (UCSD): Continuing Medical Education Offering listings of conferences by date, conferences by specialty, mini-fellowships, and home-study program details, this Web site provides a variety of postgraduate educational opportunities. Event registration forms can be obtained online, and information on instructors, program details, and included workshops are found. Location, cost, and online registration opportunities are available. http://cme.ucsd.edu/

University of California San Francisco (UCSF): Continuing Medical Education Providing over 200 courses each year across a variety of medical specialties, UCSF offers course catalogs at the site for its Department of Medi-

cine, School of Medicine, and Department of Radiology. Downloadable registration forms are available.
http://www.som.ucsf.edu/som/education/cme/

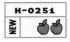

University of Chicago: Center for Continuing Medical Education

The Center for Continuing Medical Education offers this calendar of conferences, seminars, and other opportunities for CME credit through the University of Chicago. Titles, dates, and location details are provided.
http://www.uchicago.edu/bsd/cme

University of Michigan Ann Arbor: Continuing Medical Education

This site of the University of Michigan Medical School provides printable brochures, registration forms, and registration and online payment for most course offerings. Program details are accessible by date or specialty. Additional CME information, such as a staff directory and CME credit approval details, are included. http://cme.med.umich.edu/events/

University of North Carolina at Chapel Hill: Continuing Medical Education

The University of North Carolina School of Medicine offers this connection to CME programs and services, which contains a variety of one-time activities, serial presentations, and enduring materials. Program details include titles, locations, and coordinator contacts. Grand rounds listings from various departments are found, and many brochures of conferences and individual registration forms can be downloaded.
http://www.med.unc.edu/cme/

University of Pennsylvania Health System: Continuing Medical Education

CME resources offered through the University of Pennsylvania Health System are listed at this site. A calendar of events lists current conferences, seminars, grand rounds, mini-fellowships, and ongoing lecture series. Online CME programs are also available from the site.
http://www.med.upenn.edu/cme

University of Pittsburgh: Center for Continuing Education in the Health Sciences

Original features of this CME Web site include a credit transcript link and an interactive program connection for instant CME opportunities. Automatic grading and credit are available, and all online programs are available free of charge. Additionally, current course offerings certified by the Center for Continuing Education in the Health Sciences can be viewed and include online registration opportunities and details on series courses, formal CME, self-study programs, and visiting fellowships. The University of Pennsylvania also offers telemedicine video conferencing services to current faculty and faculty of the University of Pittsburgh. The "Rounds on Tape" series is formatted specifically for CME credit and is available at no cost, provided materials are returned within two weeks of receipt.
http://www.upmc.edu/ccehs/

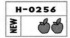

University of Texas Southwestern Medical Center at Dallas: Continuing Education   Specific programs can be located by clicking on a selected month or accessing the "find" feature of one's Web browser. Internet, audiotape, videotape, and CD-ROM distance learning opportunities are available, as well as the calendar for additional North Texas educational programs, including grand rounds and conference program details.
http://www3.utsouthwestern.edu/cme/cemain.html

University of Washington: Continuing Medical Education   A series of downloadable course brochures for on-site CME programs is available at this page. The site provides access to online CME programs following registration and purchase of a password. Additional offerings through the School of Medicine include medical history and ethics courses, radiology teaching files, and rehabilitation medicine. Medical grand rounds links are available to several departments where specific schedules can be accessed.
(some features fee-based) http://www.dom.washington.edu/cme/index.html

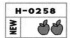

Washington University in St. Louis: Continuing Medical Education
Information on CME programs at Washington University in St. Louis is available from this site. Visitors can search a directory of seminars by specialty and date. Information on program logistics and travel arrangements is available, as well as links to related programs throughout the university.
http://cme.wustl.edu

Yale University School of Medicine: Office of Postgraduate and Continuing Medical Education   Professionals interested in CME at Yale University School of Medicine will find a mission statement; a current schedule of CME courses; accreditation details; a Yale-New Haven Medical Center weekly schedule of events; and subscription details for *The Medical Letter/Yale School of Medicine CME Program,* a publication providing two annual exams for CME credit based on the previous six months' issues of *The Medical Letter on Drugs and Therapeutics.*
http://info.med.yale.edu/CME

CARDIOLOGY OVERVIEW SITES

5.1 SUPERSITES

About.com: Heart Disease/Cardiology This categorical listing of heart disease links includes an introduction to the specialty and information about diagnostics for heart disease, congenital heart disease, coronary artery diseases, heart valve diseases, heart failure, heart alternatives, rhythm disturbances, risk factors, and prevention and rehabilitation. Each category contains links to news, treatment advances, fact sheets, and articles relating to the topic. Connections to additional online heart disease resources, including journals and publications, forums and discussion groups, and major cardiology societies and organizations, are provided at this cardiology health portal.
http://heartdisease.miningco.com/health/heartdisease/mlibrary.htm

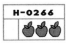

American College of Cardiology (ACC) A professional society with over 26,000 members from around the world, the ACC provides rigorous criteria to improve the quality of care delivered by its members. The college actively participates in healthcare policy debate, and users may access information about its position on specific issues at this site. Visitors will also find a large database of ACC professional publications, programs, and products. Links are available to clinical information, conferences, information on advocacy, career and training opportunities, and patient education.
(free registration) http://www.acc.org

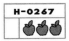

American Heart Association (AHA) The AHA is devoted to providing the public with authoritative information on the prevention and treatment of heart disease and stroke. Resources available from this address include interactive risk assessment tools, fact sheets on a wide range of diseases, drug therapy and prevention information, biostatistical topics, and details regarding AHA educational programs. Local AHA chapter information, public advocacy activities, and other AHA endeavors are explained at the site, and professional resources, such as AHA journal access, scientific statements and guidelines, conference and meeting details, and information on AHA research programs and funding, are provided. Details regarding the AHA Pharmaceutical Roundtable, professional education opportunities, clinical health news, and a comprehensive links section are offered.
http://www.americanheart.org/presenter.jhtml?identifier=1200000

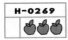

Cardio Info Innovations: Links to Cardiac Anatomy and Disease This online directory offers links to valuable resources related to cardiac anatomy and cardiac disease, with links to case studies, disease atlases, clinical trials, and an online exploration of the heart included. General sites are listed, as well as those related to specific valve disorders, myopathies, structural defects, heart failure, and peripheral disease. Visitors may find this site a useful starting point for the vast array of cardiovascular clinical information on the World Wide Web.
http://www.cardio-info.com/linkanat.htm

Global Cardiology Network The Global Cardiology Network provides a search engine for cardiology professionals and others interested in the field. Search categories include journals, practice guidelines, clinical trials, CME, meetings and conferences, grants and fellowships, patient information, member organizations, and cardiac links. There are direct links to member organizations, including the American College of Cardiology, the American Heart Association, the European Society of Cardiology, the Inter American Society of Cardiology, and the World Heart Federation.
http://www.globalcardiology.org

Hardin MD: Cardiology and Heart Diseases From Hardin MD, this site provides comprehensive listings of links to reliable sources of cardiology information. Sites are categorized by size and include 15 large lists, such as MedMark, MEDLINEplus, and Healthfinder, and several medium-sized lists, including HealthWeb and HealthLinks. The Hardin Meta Directory also offers "Focus Pages," which provide links to lists on specialized topics.
http://www.lib.uiowa.edu/hardin/md/cardio.html

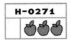

HealthWeb: Cardiology From HealthWeb, this site divides resources into three categories, with links to pages of interest to consumers, healthcare professionals, and students and educators. Professional resources include associations and agencies, such as the American Heart Association and the American Association of Cardiovascular and Pulmonary Medicine. Links to journals, headlines, and discussion groups; consumer information, including the Congenital Heart Disease Resource Page and the Harvard Heart Letter; and resources for students and educators, such as cardiology atlases and the Cardiovascular Pathology Index, are provided.
http://bones.med.ohio-state.edu/hw/cardiology/index.html

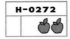

Heart Information Network The Heart Information Network provides continuously updated news and details from landmark studies in the field of cardiology. Patient guides to hypertension, diabetes, heart attack, and stroke are offered, as well as general drug information answers to FAQ's about heart disease, and an online cardiology dictionary. Additional guides within the site include those on cardiology and women's health, nutrition, and fitness.
http://208.133.254.45/

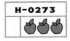

InteliHealth: Heart and Circulatory Index InteliHealth's heart health area provides a wide variety of topical resources, as well as highlights of current issues in cardiology. News stories on such topics as vitamins to reduce heart defects and detection of heart disease risk are found, in addition to a selection of interactive features for patient self-assessments. Anatomy and physiology basics, expert commentary on nutrition and heart disease, and search tools for diseases and drug therapy are provided.

http://www.intelihealth.com/IH/ihtlH/WSIHW000/8059/8059.html?k=zonex408x8059

Karolinska Institutet: Cardiovascular Diseases Cardiovascular disease information is comprehensively covered at the page's assortment of fact sheets, clinical articles, and pathology case studies of major cardiac disorders. The site offers introductory review sites of anatomy and physiology, links to general resources in cardiology, topical links in the field, and online diagnostic imaging.

http://www.mic.ki.se/Diseases/c14.html

Martindale's Health Science Guide: Cardiology and Pulmonary Center This comprehensive site provides links to medical dictionaries and glossaries, metabolic pathways and genetic maps, and literature searches, as well as to doctors and hospitals around the world. There are links to interactive anatomy browsers, pathology case studies, and online medical journals. Links are available to heart and cardiovascular development and function sites, as well as to courses and tutorials, teaching files, cardiology databases, and information regarding artificial hearts, valves, and pulse generators. Connections to virtual examples of cardiology sounds and images are found.

http://www-sci.lib.uci.edu/~martindale/MedicalCardio.html

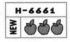

Medem: Healthcare Information Founded by the nation's leading medical societies, such as the American Medical Association, the American Academy of Pediatrics, and the American College of Obstetricians and Gynecologists, this site offers a comprehensive medical library featuring patient education materials on life stages, diseases and conditions, and therapies. Other features of the site include a "Site Builder" that allows physicians to develop their own Web site with links to online physician finders and health plan provider directories, as well as secure messaging for communicating with patients. A physician directory is also featured on the site for patients.

(some features fee-based) http://www.medem.com

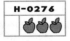

Medical Matrix: Cardiology The cardiology page of the Medical Matrix supersite offers visitors access to Internet cardiology search engines, news in the field of cardiovascular medicine, full-text journals and CME modules online, and multimedia learning opportunities. Diagnostic and therapeutic procedural pages, practice guidelines in cardiology, and pathology case studies are available from one of the top medical supersites on the World Wide Web. The site search engine offers advanced searching options, in addition to a convenient medical spell checker.

(free registration) http://www.medmatrix.org/_SPages/Cardiology.asp

MedMark: Cardiology MedMark offers a comprehensive directory of cardiology resources available on the Internet, including general professional resources, medical schools and hospitals, professional societies, navigational guides, journals, and current news sources. Connections for patients and consumers, pediatric cardiology coverage, emergency information, cardiology equipment and service suppliers, and relevant nonmedical resources are provided. Sites are listed that offer information on basic science, computers and telemedicine technologies, clinical diagnosis and therapy, diseases and disorders, invasive techniques and surgery, and rehabilitation and prevention. This valuable consumer and professional resource is frequently updated, and visitors can search the site by keyword.

http://www.medmark.org/car

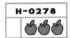

MedNets: Cardiology Databases This MedNets-sponsored site offers access to many online cardiology journals, medical atlases, clinical trials in cardiology, and organizational links in the specialty. The search engine of the National Heart, Lung, and Blood Institute (NHLBI) is found at the Web page and will return users hundreds of documents related to the cardiology topic of one's choosing. Connections available from the site include audible systolic and diastolic murmur pages, several cardiology network search sites, AHA Scientific statements, and pacemaker databases and reports.

http://www.mednets.com/scardiac.htm

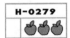

Medscape: Cardiology News, treatment updates, practice guidelines, conference summaries, journal reviews, clinical case studies, patient resources, articles addressing issues in managed care, and links to related sites are available from this comprehensive cardiology resource.

(free registration) http://cardiology.medscape.com/Home/Topics/cardiology/cardiology.html

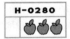

MedWeb: Cardiology Emory University's Health Sciences Center Library contains resources in over 80 topical areas of cardiology (also listed in the "Cardiology" link underneath the "Specialties" category), with each subject link providing an assortment of articles, images, fact sheets, cardiology programs, and late-breaking medical research. Alphabetized topic selections range from academic departments to vascular medicine, with concentrations included in the areas of evidence-based medicine and research design.

http://www.medweb.emory.edu/MedWeb

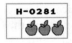

SciCentral: Best Cardiology Online Resources SciCentral's cardiology resources offer a listing of some of the most comprehensive directories in cardiovascular medicine, as well as specialized resources from the AHA and Cardio.net. Research news from MedWeb and Medscape cardiology and articles on current developments in cardiovascular disease prevention, techniques, and computer modeling are found, courtesy of major teaching institutions, organizations, and professional medical journals.

http://www.scicentral.com/H-cardio.html

World Wide Web Cardiology Links This index of links, provided as a service of the European Society of Cardiology, contains more than 300 connections to Web sites in nearly a dozen cardiology categories. Major associations,

public administrations, hospitals and research centers, and cardiology search engines are accessible from the site. Guidelines and clinical trial links, journal listings, and physician and patient-oriented educational materials are available.
http://www.escardio.org/navigation/www_cardio_links.htm

5.2 GENERAL RESOURCES FOR CARDIOLOGY

Cardiology Compass Supported by South County Cardiology Associates, Inc., this site offers a useful Web navigation tool. The site contains hundreds of cardiology links, including research centers, clinician education pages, consumer information, online cases, professional meeting information, and practice guidelines in the field. Additional departments include professional organization listings, telemedicine, and general medical resources.
http://www.cardiologycompass.com/

Cardiology Home Page Serving as a general informational resource to both consumers and providers of healthcare, this extensive site includes a broad scope of topics related to the functions and disorders of the heart and circulation. Links to CME programs and articles on a number of conditions, including hypertension, cardiac arrhythmias, and uremic pericarditis, are found. Information about diagnostics and treatments, an image library, a drug library, and a list of cardiology links are also provided.
http://home.hkstar.com/~shwan/index.html

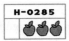

Cardiology Internet Directory The SLACK Cardiology Internet Directory provides visitors with access to a large selection of cardiac medical resources on the Internet. Access to *Cardiology Today* is provided from the site, with current, archived, and breaking news bulletin supplements. Additional resources include links to preeminent cardiothoracic associations, cardiology Internet directories, and related e-mail lists and newsgroups.
http://www.slackinc.com/idirectories/heartnet-x.htm

Cardiosource A wide range of information related to the field of cardiology is accessible from this Web address. The site provides access to more than 10 online journals, including the *American Journal of Hypertension,* the *Annals of Thoracic Surgery,* and the *Journal of the American College of Cardiology.* Other resources include a clinical trials database and search engine. Links to clinical practice guidelines and information pertaining to upcoming meetings, job postings, and current news in the field of cardiology are offered. A free registration is required.
(free registration) http://www.cardiosource.com

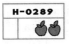

Med Nexus: Cardiology Sites Major cardiology teaching institutions; educational resources, such as a computer simulation and visualization of the cardiovascular system; and an electronic journal are included among the resources found at this directory of medical links from Med Nexus. Visitors have

the opportunity to suggest the medical resource of their choosing and add it to this database by filling out a form at the site.
http://www.mednexus.com/public/mnlinkc.html

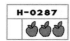

Medem Medical Library: Heart Disease/Stroke   Provided by leading medical societies, including the AMA, the Medem Medical Library offers this Web portal to general resources in the field of cardiology. Guides to a variety of common disorders are presented by the AMA, as well as fact sheets, articles, and professional literature regarding treatment and surgical procedures in the specialty. Medical news and online atlases of the circulatory system are included.   http://www.medem.com/MedLB/sub_detaillb.cfm?parent_id=68&act=disp

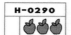

MEDLINEplus Health Information: Heart and Circulation Sites   From aneurysms to Wegener's granulomatosis, this collection of links leads users to comprehensive collections of Web sites on selected disorders. Compiled by the National Library of Medicine, entries for more than 40 diseases provide connections to general overviews of the condition, the latest news concerning disease discoveries and treatment, information on clinical trials, and reviews of prevention, diagnostic tests, treatment, rehabilitation, and specific disease aspects. Sites are selected from a variety of private professional organizations and government divisions and include fact sheets, brochures, and interactive tutorials.
http://www.nlm.nih.gov/medlineplus/heartandcirculation.html

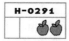

New York Online Access to Health (NOAH): Heart Disease and Stroke   From City University of New York (CUNY), this site contains a comprehensive list of links to information about heart disease and stroke. Categories of information include heart disease and stroke, care and treatment, and general resources. Under each topic heading several subtopics are listed. An alphabetical disease index, discussions regarding nutrition and diet, and information about prevention, clinical trials, medication, tests, and surgical procedures are available.
http://www.noah-health.org/english/illness/heart_disease/heartdisease.html

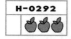

WebDoctor: Cardiology   This clinically oriented Web site offers nearly 10 categories of information in the field of cardiology, including associations, clinical practice guidelines, and multimedia teaching files. By accessing any one of the Web page divisions of the WebDoctor resource, visitors will be taken to an assortment of professional materials, including several sources of clinical diagnostic and management reviews, general references in pediatric cardiology, journal links and articles, and audio teaching files, courtesy of Synapse Publishing.   http://gretmar.com/webdoctor/cardiology.html

Yale Library: Cardiovascular Medicine   Selected Internet resources in cardiovascular medicine are provided by the Cushing/Whitney Medical Library of Yale University. Clinical guidelines in the specialty, online medical textbooks, cardiology associations, and references to disease, statistical, and patient education information are accessible from the site. The online *Yale University School* *of Medicine Heart Book* covers the entire range of cardiovascular diseases, and a link to the *Internist and Cardiology* edition of the *Medical Tribune* is found. http://www.med.yale.edu/library/sir/select.php3? prof_subject=Medicine~Cardiovascular+Medicine

5.3 AWARDS AND HONORS

Public recognition of important contributions in medicine is achieved through awards and honors from major educational, scientific, nonprofit, and corporate organizations. We have included many such awards in this section. Awards and honors are subject to change at any time, however, and some awards may not be granted every year. Organizations periodically discontinue awards, change their terms and qualifications, or add new awards and honors. For these reasons, the reader should visit these Web sites directly to obtain the latest information on current awards and honors.

AWARDS FOR SERVICE

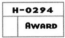

Society for Vascular Surgery: Distinguished Service Award   Individuals who have made original or significant contributions to the clinical practice of vascular surgery or the basic sciences underlying the specialty may be nominated for this award by members of the Society for Vascular Surgery. http://www.vascsurg.org/doc/852.html

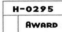

Thoracic Surgery Residents Association: Socrates Award   Given by the Thoracic Surgery Residents Association, the Socrates Award is a monthly and annual award that recognizes outstanding faculty members in cardiothoracic surgery with a strong commitment to resident education and mentorship. Recipients are nominated by cardiothoracic surgery residents in North America. Annual winners are selected from the group of monthly winners. http://ctsnet.org/doc/3812

INVESTIGATOR AND RESEARCH AWARDS

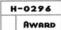

American College of Phlebology: Research Award   These awards, presented by the American College of Phlebology, are presented to recognize and stimulate research in the field of venous disease. Included are the Beiersdorf-Jobst Research Program for Phlebology, intended to stimulate research in the field of phlebology, and the VNUS Medical Technologies Award, intended to promote research on treatment methods for patients with venous disease. Further details and a list of past recipients are found at the site. http://www.phlebology.org/research.htm

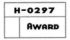

American Heart Association (AHA): Bugher Foundation Awards for the Investigation of Stroke   This monetary award of $100,000 per year (including up to 10 percent indirect) for a maximum of four years is intended to

encourage investigations leading to the development of better stroke preventive measures and stroke interventions. Available to both basic and clinical studies, the focus of applications should involve any aspect of stroke-related brain vascular function. Candidates must have an M.D., Ph.D., D.O., or equivalent doctoral degree. Award distribution began on January 1, 2000, and will end on December 31, 2003.

http://216.185.112.5/presenter.jhtml?identifier=137

H-0298

AWARD

American Heart Association (AHA): Established Investigator Grant

This award supports the career development of promising scientists who have recently achieved independent status and who are involved in research related to cardiovascular function and disease, stroke, or related clinical, basic science, and public health problems. This award is for full-time faculty/staff members holding an M.D., Ph.D., D.O., or equivalent degree. The applicant's first full-time faculty/staff position should have elapsed more than four years but not more than nine years at the time of award activation. For a maximum total award of $300,000 over a four-year period, the grant will not exceed $75,000 per year for salary, fringe benefits, indirect costs, and project costs.

http://216.185.112.5/presenter.jhtml?identifier=2230

H-0299

AWARD

American Heart Association (AHA): Grant-in-Aid

To stimulate and encourage independent investigators undertaking innovative and groundbreaking research programs, this award aims to support projects involving cardiovascular function and disease, stroke, or related clinical, basic science, and public health problems. Candidates must have an M.D., Ph.D., D.O., or equivalent doctoral degree and should be a full-time faculty/staff member. Awarded for a maximum of three years, the grant will not surpass $71,500 per year, including 10 percent indirect costs and up to $15,000 for principal investigator salary and fringe benefits.

http://216.185.112.5/presenter.jhtml?identifier=2275

H-0300

AWARD

American Heart Association (AHA): Scientist Development Award

This award is to support promising new investigators involved in research in cardiovascular function and disease, stroke, or related clinical, basic science, and public health problems. Applicants should be full-time faculty/staff members holding an M.D., Ph.D., D.O., or equivalent doctoral degree. The applicant's first full-time faculty/staff appointment must not have been more than four years at the time of award activation. For a maximum total of $260,000 over a four-year period, the award will not exceed $65,000 per year for salary, fringe benefits, indirect costs, and project costs.

http://216.185.112.5/presenter.jhtml?identifier=2350

H-0301

AWARD

American Roentgen Ray Society: Roentgen Fund

The Roentgen Fund of the American Roentgen Ray Society (ARRS) provides support for the educational, scientific, and research needs of the radiology community. Funded programs include the Figley Fellowships, the Armed Forces Institute of Pathology

(AFIP) Distinguished Scientist support, the ARRS Visiting Scientist at the AFIP, and Radiology Journalism Awards. http://www.arrs.org/scholarships

American Society of Echocardiography: Research Award The American Society of Echocardiography offers two fellowship awards of $25,000 each to support research activities related to echocardiography and meritorious research evaluating the effects of the utilization of echocardiography on patient outcomes, or the cost effectiveness of echocardiography in clinical practice. http://www.asecho.org/Research_2000/2001/body_2001.html

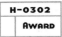

American Society of Transplantation: Faculty Development Award The AST Faculty Development Award is intended to serve as initial funding for a new investigator. This funding will permit the new investigator to acquire research results that will be the basis for an individual research award from another source. The one-time award is $25,000. http://www.a-s-t.org/index.htm

American Society of Transplantation: Fujisawa Fellowship in Transplantation This one-year fellowship of $25,000 is designed to attract promising investigators to clinical research careers in transplantation medicine. Applicants must be sponsored by an active member of the American Society of Transplantation. Applications will be evaluated on the relative strengths of the research and training plan, the environment for training provided by the mentor, and the potential for the applicant's career development if awarded the fellowship. The award recipient is required to submit a final report at the end of the award period. http://www.a-s-t.org/index.htm

American Society of Transplantation: Novartis Fellowship in Transplantation This two-year $50,000 fellowship with $25,000 paid annually is designed to attract investigators to basic science research careers in transplantation medicine/immunology. All applicants must be sponsored by an active AST member in good standing. Funding in the second year is contingent upon the submission of a brief summary of progress written by the mentor. http://www.a-s-t.org/index.htm

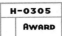

American Society of Transplantation: Roche Investigator Award This award is designed to attract young investigators and is not intended for established senior investigators. It is intended to serve as transitional funding to enable the investigator to acquire research results that will be the basis for future research grant applications. The two-year award of $50,000 will be paid in two annual installments. http://www.a-s-t.org/index.htm

Bracco Diagnostics Inc./Society for Cardiac Angiography and Interventions Fellowship Program By clicking on the "Research Awards" link, viewers will find information on one-year fellowships that are awarded to physicians who have demonstrated medical excellence to support their research in the advancement of cardiovascular imaging and invasive cardiology. Submis-

sions will be judged on four criteria: scientific value, potential for significant imaging advances, potential for improvements in patient care, and potential for successful completion of objectives in one year. Award amounts vary up to a maximum of $25,000 based on research proposals submitted.
http://www.scai.org/main.htm

| H-0308 |
| AWARD |

George H. A. Clowes, Jr., M.D., F.A.C.S.: Memorial Research Career Development Award This award, offered by the American College of Surgeons, is intended to provide five years of support for the research of a promising surgical investigator. The award is $40,000 for each of five years and is not renewable. The award is restricted to a surgeon who has completed specialty training in a residency or an accredited fellowship in general surgery or a surgical specialty within the preceding five years.
http://www.facs.org/about_college/acsdept/fellow_dept/research.html#3

| H-0309 |
| AWARD |

National Heart, Lung, and Blood Institute (NHLBI): Minority Institutional Faculty Mentored Research Scientist Development Award
The program provides support to faculty members at minority institutions who have the potential to conduct quality research in the areas of pulmonary, hematologic, cardiovascular, or sleep disorders. This, in turn, provides hands-on research opportunities for minority students at those institutions. The award supports two students each academic year and summer for up to five years.
http://www.nhlbi.nih.gov/funding/training/redbook/newrek01.htm

| H-0310 |
| AWARD |

National Institutes of Health (NIH): Independent Scientist Award
The Independent Scientist Award provides up to five years of support for newly independent scientists who demonstrate the need for a period of intensive research to improve their careers. This award is intended to aid in the development of excellent scientists and help them expand their potential to make substantial contributions to their field of research.
http://grants.nih.gov/grants/guide/pa-files/PA-00-020.html

| H-0311 |
| AWARD |

National Stroke Association: Research Fellowships in Cerebrovascular Disease Intended to provide opportunities for promising investigators to develop their research interests, this fellowship supports efforts on the causes, mechanisms, and treatment of cerebrovascular disease. A goal of this project is to increase the number of clinical and basic scientists devoted to the field of stroke. Up to four fellowships are granted annually. Each fellowship is in the amount of $30,000 annually for one or two years. Applicants must be sponsored by an established institution in the United States.
http://www.stroke.org/pages/pro_fellow.cfm

| H-0312 |
| AWARD |

Rosanna Degani Young Investigator Award The Rosanna Degani Young Investigator Award is presented by Computers in Cardiology to young investigators in the field of cardiology. The program is designed to encourage young investigators to present their work to the international scientific community. Four finalists are awarded $750. The winner receives a plaque and $1,250. Finalists,

winners, and other applicants present their work at the annual Computers in Cardiology Conference.
http://www.cinc.org/cicyi.htm

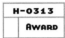

Society of Cardiovascular Anesthesiologists: IREF-Research Mid-Career Grant This award of no more than $20,000 per year for a maximum of two years is intended to support the expenditures of related research projects. Applicants must hold an M.D. or Ph.D. degree and rank of Assistant or Associate Professor. The candidate must also be a member of the Society of Cardiovascular Anesthesiologists.
http://www.scahq.org/sca3/newsletters/mid-career.shtml

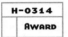

Society of Cardiovascular Anesthesiologists: IREF-Research Starter Grant An award of no more than $10,000 is available to support the project expenditures of new investigators. Candidates must have an M.D. or Ph.D. degree, rank of Assistant Professor or lower, and five years or less of post residency training. The candidate must also be a member of the Society of Cardiovascular Anesthesiologists.
http://www.scahq.org/sca3/newsletters/starter.shtml

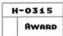

Society of Thoracic Radiology: Seed Grant The Society of Thoracic Radiology is offering seed grant support for young investigators to pursue research in thoracic imaging. The award ranges from $8,000 to $15,000 for one year. Proposals will be evaluated on the basis of originality, scientific merit, and significance. http://www.thoracicrad.org/seed_grant_guide.htm

Scholarship Awards

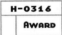

American College of Surgeons: International Guest Scholarship This scholarship is offered to young surgeons who have demonstrated strong interests in teaching and research. The award for $10,000 may be used to participate in clinical, teaching, and research activities in North America and to attend and participate in the educational opportunities and activities of the American College of Surgeons' Clinical Congress.
http://www.facs.org/about_college/acsdept/fellow_dept/research.html#5

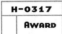

American Roentgen Ray Society: Annual Scholarship The American Roentgen Ray Society Annual Scholarship Program supports study in a field selected by the recipient. The funds, up to $120,000 for one year, are given to departments of radiology for the support of the scholar in his or her program of study. Funds may be used in part as a salary or to support study or travel, or in another way that will contribute to the scholar's advancement as a member of the faculty. http://www.arrs.org/scholarships

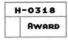

American Roentgen Ray Society: Residents in Radiology Awards Given by the American Roentgen Ray Society, these awards are given for papers produced by residents in radiology and radiological sciences. Papers are eligible

for the President's Award of $2,000 and the Executive Council Awards of $1,000 each. http://www.arrs.org/scholarships

5.4 National Heart, Lung, and Blood Institute (NHLBI) Profile

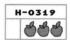

National Heart, Lung, and Blood Institute (NHLBI) This component of the National Institutes of Health conducts and supports basic research, clinical investigations and trials, observational studies, and demonstration and education projects related to diseases of the heart, blood vessels, lungs, and blood. Site resources include informational fact sheets for consumers, patients, and professionals; other NHLBI publications; research resources; information on grants and funding sources; news and press releases; events calendars; and the NHLBI clinical guidelines. A clinical trials database, links to home pages of various large studies, links to individual NHLBI laboratory home pages, and various materials concerning technology transfer within the institute are found. Highlighted resources offered throughout this site include the NHLBI Strategic Plan, clinical guidelines on overweight and obese patients, and interactive patient education resources on cholesterol management and weight loss.
http://www.nhlbi.nih.gov

Departments and Services

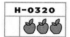

NHLBI: Clinical Guidelines A number of major resource files may be downloaded from this site, including public blood cholesterol screening recommendations; the second report from the Expert Panel on Detection, Evaluation, and Treatment of High Blood Cholesterol in Adults; the *Sixth Report of the Joint National Committee on Prevention, Detection, Evaluation, and Treatment of High Blood Pressure* (JNC VI); and clinical guidelines on overweight and obesity. http://www.nhlbi.nih.gov/guidelines/index.htm

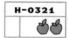

NHLBI: Committees, Meetings, and Events An NHLBI calendar of events and links to additional information about specific meetings, conferences, and other events are available at this site. Links to institute advisory committees and peer-reviewed resources are also provided.
http://www.nhlbi.nih.gov/meetings/index.htm

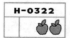

NHLBI: News and Press Releases News alerts from NHLBI are listed by month at this site, and archived news articles are available. NHLBI study results, updates on treatment guidelines, findings on cardiovascular disease risk, and upcoming NIH study summaries are discussed.
http://www.nhlbi.nih.gov/new/index.htm

NHLBI: Office of Technology Transfer and Development The NHLBI Office of Technology Transfer and Development interacts with industry to ap-

ply research findings from the institute to commercial products in an effort to benefit public health. Goals are achieved through Cooperative Research and Development Agreements (CRADAs), Clinical Trial Agreements, Material Transfer Agreements (MTAs), and licensing arrangements. Information is available at this address on NHLBI technologies, including medical reagents, gene therapy, devices, research tools, clinical trials, "technology hotspots," and CRADA opportunities. A staff directory is provided.
http://www.nhlbi.nih.gov/tt/index.htm

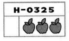

NHLBI: Scientific Resources   Resources for investigators and other professionals include a database of MEDLINE article citations relating to genetically altered animal models of diseases or conditions relevant to NHLBI research, genetics databases, information on the NHLBI Blood Specimen Repository, links to important research studies, information on NHLBI professional courses, and connections to other genetics and animal model resources. Scientific documents and links to major NHLBI research divisions, including the Division of Heart and Vascular Diseases, are also found at this address.
http://www.nhlbi.nih.gov/resources/index.htm

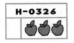

NHLBI: Studies Seeking Patients   Visitors can access the NHLBI Clinical Trials Database from this site. Resources are available concerning specific clinical trials such as the Prevention of Recurrent Thromboembolism Trial (PREVENT), the Magnesium in Coronaries (MAGIC) Trial, and the National Emphysema Treatment Trial (NETT).
http://www.nhlbi.nih.gov/studies/index.htm

EXTRAMURAL FUNDING OPPORTUNITIES

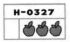

NHLBI: Research Funding   Visitors interested in extramural research funding through NHLBI will find requests for applications (RFAs), requests for proposals (RFPs), and program announcements (PAs) at this address. Training and career development opportunities, resources related to the NHLBI Small Business Innovation Research Program (SBIR), general funding information and policies, and communications from the director of NHLBI are also available.
http://www.nhlbi.nih.gov/funding/index.htm

RESEARCH

H-0327

NHLBI: Cardiology Branch   Three major areas of research are summarized at this address: vascular biology, cardiomyopathy research, and innovative imaging technologies. Diagnostic technologies investigated by this NHLBI branch include stress testing, two-dimensional and three-dimensional echocardiography, nuclear imaging, electrophysiology testing, pacemaker management, and cardiac catheterization. News stories, employment opportunities, resources for patient referral to clinical screening trials, links to current clinical research studies

open to enrollment, connections to specific research sections, and access to related Web pages are provided at the site.
http://www.nhlbi.nih.gov/labs/cardiology/index.htm

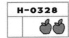

NHLBI: Division of Heart and Vascular Diseases NHLBI research programs investigating the causes, diagnosis, treatment, and prevention of heart and vascular diseases are summarized at this address. Clinical and fundamental research in cardiology is conducted through the Heart Research Program, and research activities in atherosclerosis, cardiovascular homeostasis and bionutrition, and molecular genetics are supported through the Vascular Research Program. http://www.nhlbi.nih.gov/about/dhvd/index.htm

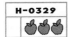

NHLBI: Division of Intramural Research The NHLBI Division of Intramural Research conducts basic research in molecular and cellular biology, genetics, biochemistry, and physiology, as well as clinical research in disease of the heart, blood, and lungs. Research emphasizes an early and rapid transition from basic research findings to human therapies. Arteriosclerosis, vascular biology, cardiac imaging, and the molecular genetics of cardiovascular disease are among the division's major areas of concentration. This address provides a description of the division, links to nearly 20 laboratories and research branches, and a link to NHLBI technology transfer resources.
http://www.nhlbi.nih.gov/labs/index.htm

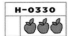

NHLBI: Laboratory of Cardiac Energetics Connections are available through this Web address to the four major research sections within the Laboratory of Cardiac Engineering: Imaging Physics, Cardiovascular Imaging, Medical Imaging, and Integrative Physiology. The laboratory uses noninvasive technologies to study the physiological processes of the cardiovascular system, and a clinical program through the laboratory evaluates the use of magnetic resonance imaging in the diagnosis of cardiovascular disease. The site provides news, recent publications, information on training and employment opportunities, a staff directory, images, and links to related sites.
http://zeus.nhlbi.nih.gov

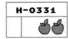

NHLBI: Laboratory of Molecular Cardiology Investigation into the "regulation, expression and function of contractile proteins in vertebrate muscle and nonmuscle cells, and in the role of mutations in cardiac myosin from patients with familial hypertrophic cardiomyopathy as well as the embryonic development of muscle and neuronal tissues" is provided at this NHLBI laboratory. An overview of research topics currently studied through this research group is provided. http://www.nhlbi.nih.gov/labs/molecularcardiology/index.htm

NHLBI: Vascular Biology Branch A brief summary of the Vascular Biology Branch, devoted to research into the pathophysiology of vascular diseases and the development of novel therapeutics, is available from this address.
http://www.nhlbi.nih.gov/labs/vascularbiology/index.htm

6

BIOLOGICAL, DIAGNOSTIC, AND THERAPEUTIC ASPECTS

6.1 ANATOMY AND PHYSIOLOGY

GENERAL RESOURCES

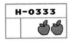

Access Excellence: The Heart and the Circulatory System Access Excellence offers review of the pulmonary and systemic circuits, with discussion of cardiac function, illustrated and labeled diagrams of the circuits, and the depiction of proper stethoscope placement. An overview of blood vessel anatomy, a close-up of the capillary bed, and discussion of circulatory degenerative disease, valvular dysfunction, systemic veins, and capillary bed problems are found. http://www.accessexcellence.org/AE/AEC/CC/heart_anatomy.html

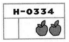

Cardiothoracic Surgery Notes: Cardiac Anatomy General anatomical information on major cardiac features is available from this resource, with labeled illustrations of important structures. Cardiac features listed include cardiac chambers, right atrium, left atrium, right ventricle, left ventricle, the conduction system, cardiac valves, the left ventricular outflow tract, and coronary arteries. http://www.ctsnet.org/residents/ctsn/archives/not02.html

Global Classroom: The Circulatory System General information on the circulatory system, a labeled anatomical diagram of the heart, description of the aorta and arterial system, and basic review of the venous system are provided at this Global Classroom information page.
http://www.globalclassroom.org/hemo.html

Gross Physiology of the Cardiovascular System Authored by Robert M. Anderson, M.D., this site offers a tutorial on the physiology of the cardiovascular system. An introduction and chapters on unique characteristics of the cardiovascular system, normal circulation, pathological circulation, open heart surgery with passive filling mechanical pumps, animal experiments with passive filling heart replacement pumps, and a hydraulic model of the cardiovascular system are presented. A summary and appendix are included.
http://cardiovascular.cx

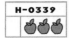

Virtual Hospital: Illustrated Encyclopedia of Human Anatomic Variation in the Cardiovascular System Components of the cardiovascular system are listed alphabetically and by region at this Virtual Hospital site, with clinical descriptions of the arteries, veins, heart, and lymphatics. A glossary of terms, a list of referenced journals, and terminology for the cardiovascular system derived from older English, French, and German literature related to current usage are provided.
http://www.vh.org/Providers/Textbooks/AnatomicVariants/Cardiovascular/Introduction.html

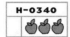

World Federation of Society of Anaesthesiologists: Cardiovascular Physiology Dr. James Rogers of Frenchay Hospital, Bristol, in the United Kingdom, offers a complete online guide to cardiovascular physiology at this address, including a tutorial on the heart, electrophysiology, components of the cardiac cycle, the coronary circulation, cardiac output, and systemic circulation. The formula for the relationship between blood flow and driving pressure is presented, as well as autonomic control of the systemic circulation.
http://www.nda.ox.ac.uk/wfsa/html/u10/u1002_01.htm

CARDIOVASCULAR EMBRYOLOGY

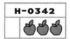

Gray's Anatomy: Development of the Vascular System This page of Henry Gray's *Anatomy of the Human Body* offers a detailed, illustrated record of cardiovascular embryology including the first appearance of blood vessels, the primitive heart, and subsequent cardiovascular development. Also available at the site are enlargeable, labeled images of various developmental stages, illustrating the development of the visceral, umbilical, and parietal veins, as well as the inferior vena cava and venous sinuses of the dura matter. A series of profile images of the dural veins is presented. http://www.bartleby.com/107/135.html

Loyola University: Heart Development This site offers a tutorial on the development of the human heart with lessons on such topics as the formation of the heart tube, partitioning of the atria, atrioventricular canals, and formation of the ventricles. Also found is information on congenital heart defects, such as atrial septal defect, persistent atrioventricular canal, and tetralogy of Fallot. Explanatory diagrams are offered that follow the week-by-week fetal development stages, and a timetable of events is available that may be kept open while processing the tutorial.
http://www.meddean.luc.edu/lumen/MedEd/
GrossAnatomy/thorax0/Heart_Development/HeartIndex.html

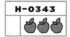

Rush Children's Heart Center: Cardiovascular Embryology A technical discussion of cardiovascular embryology is available for medical students and researchers at this address, complete with summaries of each section for nonprofessional readers. Two- and three-dimensional images and animations accompany the text, with a table outlining gestational age and corresponding cardiovascular development. Specific development topics include embryonic folding, heart looping, systemic veins, pulmonary veins, aortic

bryonic folding, heart looping, systemic veins, pulmonary veins, aortic arches, and the pericardial sac. Known etiological factors in congenital heart diseases are listed, and reference citations are provided.
http://www.rchc.rush.edu/embryology/embryology.htm

THE HEART

Franklin Institute Online: The Heart A virtual tour of the heart and multimedia tutorial provide comprehensive information about the heart, heart development topics, blood vessels, the pulmonary system, and heart monitoring, along with a multitude of interactive educational opportunities, at this page. Examples of echocardiography, information on blood pressure measurement, and a series of videos that address healthy heart issues are found. The site's table of contents provides access to information on a wide variety of additional topics related to the heart.
http://sln.fi.edu/biosci/biosci.html

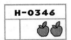

Gray's Anatomy: The Heart Part of a complete online publication, this excerpt from *Anatomy of the Human Body* offers details about components of the heart, enlargeable related images, and a large variety of labeled diagrams. Cardiac muscular tissue, the Purkinje fibers, vessel and nerve supplies, and the cardiac cycle are discussed.
http://www.bartleby.com/107/138.html

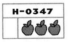

NOVA Online: Map of the Human Heart Originally appearing on the NOVA Web site, "Cut to the Heart," this page offers an illustrated introduction to heart anatomy and physiology. Links provide access to additional information on topics such as heart transplants, the artificial heart, and bioengineering, as well as to related resources.
http://www.pbs.org/wgbh/nova/eheart/human.html

Yale University School of Medicine Heart Book: The Heart and Circulation Provided in PDF format, this document introduces heart chambers, valves, the endocardium and pericardium, and review of the conduction system, cardiac cycle, heart rate and cardiac output, and stroke volume. Related chapters on the circulation, blood components, and control of cardiovascular function are available.
http://info.med.yale.edu/library/heartbk/1.pdf

CONDUCTION SYSTEM

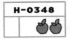

Cardiac Action Potentials, the Cardiac Cycle, and Cardiac Output A discussion of the cardiac cycle from a cellular perspective, including the action potential in cardiac muscle cells and cardiac contractions, is found at this address. Characteristics of cells other than those of the myocardium and rates of spontaneous depolarization in the SA and AV nodes are presented. Terms related to cardiodynamics are defined, and factors controlling the stroke volume are introduced. Additional information includes concepts behind Starling's principle and a discussion of contractility, including both positive and negative inotropic actions.

http://virtual.yosemite.cc.ca.us/dward/physo101/lab_2cardio.htm

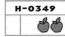

Conduction System   The anatomy of the heart's conduction system is reviewed at this site, authored by a graduate student at Ohio University. Information is provided on the sinoatrial node, the atrioventricular node, and the atrioventricular bundle and is accompanied by a detailed, labeled diagram that can be accessed from various points throughout the text. The physiology of the heart's conduction system is reviewed, including mechanism of sinus nodal rhythmicity, internodal pathways and transmission of the cardiac impulse through the atria, and transmission in the Purkinje system.

http://oak.cats.ohiou.edu/~jr888793/conduction.html

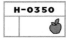

Heart Anatomy and Intrinsic Conduction System   Provided by Modesto Junior College, this site reviews the basic conduction circuit of the heart, describing contractile cells, structural and functional differences between cardiac and skeletal muscle, and automaticity of the conduction system. Discussion questions are listed.

http://virtual.yosemite.cc.ca.us/dward/physo101/lab_1cardio.htm

CARDIAC CYCLE

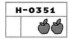

King's College London: Stroke Volume, Cardiac Output, and Coronary Circulation   Key components of the regulation of stroke volume and cardiac output are discussed at this site of the United Medical and Dental Schools of Guy's and St. Thomas' Hospitals. Starling's law, inotropic responses, and causes of cardiac failure are reviewed, in addition to ways of measuring the cardiac output.

http://www.umds.ac.uk/physiology/BDS1B/1B10.htm

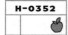

Queen's University: The Cardiac Cycle   Queen's University in Ontario provides an outline of the systole and diastole cycles, including review of ventricular filling, atrial systole, isovolumetric ventricular contraction, ventricular systole, and isovolumetric relaxation. Key points of each and information on related heart sound production are found.

http://meds.queensu.ca/medicine/physiol/undergrad/baer/cardiac/heart4.htm

ELECTROPHYSIOLOGY

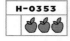

Cardiac Electrophysiology   The basic electrical behavior of the heart is reviewed at this site of the University of Vermont Department of Physiology. The site offers information on cardiac electrophysiology, including a general overview and sections on cellular excitation and electrical control. Subtopics include cellular anatomy, electrical control of the heart, abnormal electrical activity, and adjusting contraction. This detailed, illustrated presentation covers topics ranging from the basics of electrical behavior to issues concerning abnormal electrical activity.

http://physioweb.med.uvm.edu/cardiacep

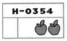

Electrophysiology   The study of the heart's electrical system, including electrophysiological studies, supraventricular tachycardia, automatic defibrillators, and additional management techniques, is reviewed in this document, authored by an expert in the field. Cardiac pacemaker implantation and clinical assessment and follow-up of functioning are discussed.

http://www.heart24.com/electro.html

North American Society of Pacing and Electrophysiology   Dedicated to the study and management of cardiac arrhythmias, this organization offers both patient and professional information, as well as information about the society at this Web site. Professional information includes news and policies, case studies, a calendar of events, scientific studies, educational products, clinical trials, and a list of medical links. The patient portion of the site contains an overview of the function of the heart and a glossary.

http://www.naspe.org

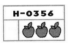

Postgraduate Medicine: Clinical Cardiac Electrophysiology   *Postgraduate Medicine* offers a review of clinical cardiac electrophysiology in this four-part article series, which addresses current treatment, catheter ablation, implantable cardioverter-defibrillators, and the head-upright tilt-table test. Each article provides information regarding advances in the field, examples of abnormal electrophysiology, and clinical management practices.

http://www.postgradmed.com/issues/1998/01_98/symp_int.htm

THE BLOOD

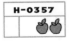

Columbia University: The Blood and Its Components   The *Columbia University College of Physicians and Surgeons Complete Home Medical Guide* offers an online introduction to blood function and components at this page. Formed cells and plasma, ratio of red blood cells in the circulating blood to white blood cells, and additional blood cell types are discussed.

http://cpmcnet.columbia.edu/texts/guide/hmg23_0001.html

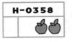

Franklin Institute Online: Lifeblood   An introductory tutorial on components of the blood is found at this site, intended for a consumer audience. Links throughout the text take viewers to further information on the composition of the blood and purpose of red blood cells, white blood cells, plasma, and platelets. Additional pages on blood types and Rh factor, autologous blood, and blood donation are provided.

http://sln.fi.edu/biosci/blood/blood.html

THE CIRCULATION

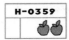

A Better Way: The Circulatory System   This tutorial on the circulatory system includes sections on heart sounds, coronary circulation, the heartbeat, pulmonary circulation, systemic circulation, the lymphatic system, the blood, and heart disease. Heart disease prevention strategies are outlined, and colorful diagrams and illustrations accompany the text.
http://www.A-Better-Way.com/systems/8_1.html

Circulatory System   The anatomy of the circulatory system is described for patients and consumers in this fact sheet, accompanied by simple diagrams and links to resources on the heart; coronary circulation; pulmonary circulation; systemic circulation; the lymphatic system; blood; and the arteries, veins, and vessels. A glossary of terms and a review quiz are provided.
http://prism.troyst.edu/~tiemeyep/circulat.htm

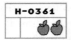

Franklin Institute Online: The Circle of Blood   Intended for a consumer audience, this site provides a collection of pages covering all phases of the circulatory system. Information on blood vessels, the pulmonary circulation, coronary circulation, and systemic circulation is provided, with a related illustration accompanying each page.
http://sln.fi.edu/biosci/systems/circulation.html

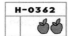

World Federation of Society of Anaesthesiologists: The Coronary Circulation   An overview of coronary circulation is found at this article from *Cardiovascular Physiology,* with definitions related to cardiac output and contractility presented. Information on the systemic circulation, including blood flow, autonomic control, and control of arterial pressure, is found.
http://www.nda.ox.ac.uk/wfsa/html/u10/u1002_02.htm#coro

BLOOD FLOW AND PRESSURE

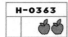

Altruis Biomedical Network: Blood Pressure   A discussion of blood pressure and its maintenance is found at this page, which emphasizes the dependence of blood pressure on cardiac output and peripheral resistance. The kidney's function in regulating blood volume and notes on central blood pressure control, hormonal influences, and impulses generated by cardiopulmonary baroreceptors and chemoreceptors are examined.
http://www.e-cardiovascular.net/bp.html

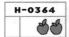

King's College London: Blood Flow   The physics of blood flow is the focus of this site, provided by King's College London. Distinctions between flow and velocity, types of flow, vessel pressure, peripheral resistance, and cardiac output are among the topics addressed.
http://www.umds.ac.uk/physiology/rbm/physbloo.htm

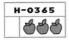

Temple University: Hemodynamics Terms related to the physics of blood flow in the circulation and outlines of static fluid mechanics, dynamic fluid mechanics, and venous pressure and waveforms are found at this site. Illustrations accompany the outline, which also contains sections on stenosis and regurgitation of the aortic valve, pressure measurements, and cardiac output measurement. http://blue.temple.edu/~pathphys/cardiology/hemodynamics2.html

Arterial System

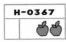

Iowa State University: Arterial System Online lecture notes provide information on components of the arterial system, including how the arterial system provides continuous blood flow to the capillary system, properties of the arterial wall and advantages of compliant arterial walls. Decrease in elasticity with increasing age is discussed, as well as physiological determinants of mean arterial pressure.
http://www.biology.iastate.edu/Courses/Zool%20355/Lecture%2020

Scientific American Online: Coronary Arterial System This site supplies an overview of coronary artery anatomy, providing a descriptive tour of the arterial branches and their courses. A labeled illustration of the arteries, ventricular branch, septal branches, circumflex artery, and marginal and diagonal branches is presented.
http://www.samonline.com/F100134.htm

Venous System

Gray's Anatomy: The Veins Information on the pulmonary, systemic, and portal veins is contained at this online reference of Henry Gray's *Anatomy of the Human Body.* By advancing through this well-illustrated chapter, readers will find thorough coverage of the veins of the heart, head and neck, upper extremities and thorax, lower extremities, abdomen, and pelvis.
http://www.bartleby.com/107/164.html

McGill Medical Informatics: Venous System Development Development of the adult venous system is described and illustrated at this site of McGill University, authored by a medical student and intended to supplement medical curriculum and provide a resource for medical professionals and educators. The complex detailed diagrams are presented, and an accessible table correlates embryonic structures with adult equivalents.
http://sprojects.mmi.mcgill.ca/embryology/cvs/venous.html

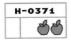

Venous Anatomy and Physiology Anatomy and physiology of the peripheral venous system are reviewed at this site of the American College of Phlebology, accompanied by a description of vein composition, correct venous functioning and its requirements, and the Web-like network of the superficial

venous system. Some examples of venous pathology, such as primary muscle pump failure and deep obstruction, are mentioned.
http://www.phlebology.org/syllabus1.htm

LYMPHATICS

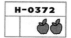

Altruis Biomedical Network: Lymphaticsnet   The composition of lymph and components of the lymphatic system are described at this site, which discusses the removal and return of extracellular fluid from the blood. Connection to further information on the capillaries and an overview of lymphatic capillaries, movement of lymph, and abnormalities of the system's function are provided.   http://www.lymphatics.net/

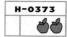

Lymphatic System   Important functions of the lymphatic system in maintaining fluid balance and its specialized role as a component of the circulatory system are discussed at this outline, sponsored by Cayuga Community College. The distribution of the lymphatic vessels is described, and their relationship to blood capillaries is illustrated. An additional figure at the site further illustrates the relationship between the lymphatic and cardiovascular systems.
http://www.cayuga-cc.edu/about/facultypages/greer/biol204/lymphatic1/lymphatic1.html

CONTROL OF CARDIOVASCULAR FUNCTION

University of Illinois at Urbana-Champaign: Autonomic Control of the Cardiovascular System   An assortment of slides can be viewed at this site, addressing autonomic control of the cardiovascular system. Cardiovascular system variables, receptors involved in control of blood pressure, regulation of heart rate and myocardial contractibility, and autonomic pharmacology of the heart are among the topics presented.
http://mipwww.life.uiuc.edu/304%20Labs/
Lab%20%23%20%207%20Autonomic%20CV/AutoCVSlidesWeb30499/index.htm

World Federation of Societies of Anaesthesiologists: Control of Arterial Pressure   A discussion of heart innervation and the conduction system of the heart is found at this online article. Physiological mechanisms responsible for regulation of blood flow, including autonomic nervous system responses, capillary shift mechanisms, hormonal responses, and kidney and fluid balance mechanisms are reviewed. Included figures illustrate pressure increases with advancing age and hormonal blood pressure maintenance.
http://www.nda.ox.ac.uk/wfsa/html/u01/u01_008.htm

6.2 RISK FACTORS AND CAUSES

GENERAL RESOURCES

American Heart Association (AHA): Risk Factors and Coronary Artery Disease An AHA scientific position document is found at this address, which discusses extensive clinical and statistical research identifying heart disease risk factors. Modifiable and nonmodifiable risk factors are reviewed, and links are provided to related information on exercise, diet, cholesterol, and hypertension. A large variety of related AHA publication titles are listed at the site and can be accessed by using the site's search engine.
http://216.185.112.5/presenter.jhtml?identifier=4726

Cardiovascular Risk Assessment: Heart Disease Risk Factors Major and contributing risk factors to heart disease from the American Heart Association are listed at this address. A risk self-assessment test is included.
http://www.heartfriendly.com/risk.html

Heart Disease Risk Factors Recently recognized risk factors in heart disease, including elevated blood homocysteine levels, elevated blood triglycerides, elevated blood fibrinogen levels, infectious agents, and nonspecific inflammatory and blood factors, are presented in this article, provided by Internal Medicine Specialists. Examples of lifestyle modification goals and potential benefits of dietary supplements are reviewed.
http://www.imsdocs.com/Heart%20disease%20risk%20factors.htm

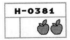

Kansas State University: The Heart Disease Page A guided tour around the Internet is found at this page, providing statistics about heart disease and information on modifiable risk factors. Resources available include those of American Heart Association, the Centers for Disease Control and Prevention, and academic centers.
http://www.kines.uiuc.edu/heart/3.html

Medical College of Wisconsin: Online Clinical Calculator A coronary heart disease risk calculator is found at this page, evaluating for age; sex; smoking; and diabetic, cholesterol, and hypertension status. Points and relative risk are calculated from user input and a low, average, or high risk percentile is assigned. Information for calculation is derived from the Framingham Heart Study, and score sheets for men and women are taken directly from *Circulation*.
http://www.intmed.mcw.edu/clincalc/heartrisk.html

New York Online Access to Health (NOAH): Causes of Heart Disease This index from the New York Online Access to Health provides links to articles and information about the causes of various heart diseases. Conditions listed include atherosclerosis, high cholesterol, and hypertension. Resources related to smoking, smoking cessation, and stress are included, along with resources for information on diabetes, hypertension, and serum cholesterol levels. http://www.noah-health.org/english/illness/heart_disease/heartdisease.html#CAUSES

AGE

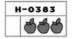

Clinical Geriatrics: Cardiovascular Risk Factors in the Elderly Published by MultiMedia Health Care, this article discusses significant predictors of coronary artery disease and offers information on the benefits of risk factor interventions. The evaluation of blood cholesterol levels, recommendations of the Adult Treatment Panel and the National Cholesterol Education Program, and guidelines for the management of hypercholesterolemia are examined. Traditional risk factors in the elderly, such as hypertension, smoking, and diabetes mellitus, are discussed, as well as appropriate disease prevention strategies. http://www.mmhc.com/cg/articles/CG9911/foody.html

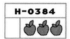

National Institute on Aging (NIA): Hearts and Arteries Age as a major risk factor for cardiovascular disease is the focus of this presentation, introduced by Richard J. Hodes, M.D. Aging, lifestyle, and disease are discussed, and interdependent factors that influence cardiac output are introduced. Studies describing age changes in the heart, blood vessels and the aging process, and cellular components of atherosclerosis are examined. The publication provides a review of heart dynamics and the aging process and how exercise and gene therapy may slow the aging process. http://www.nih.gov/nia/health/pubs/hearts-arteries/p1.htm

ATHEROSCLEROSIS

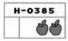

American Heart Association (AHA): Atherosclerosis From the American Heart Association, this fact sheet offers an explanation of atherosclerosis and the risk factors involved in its development. Details regarding current research related to the condition are provided. http://216.185.112.5/presenter.jhtml?identifier=228

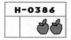

Virtual Hospital: Understanding Your Atherosclerosis and Living with It Treatment of atherosclerosis and prevention of heart attack, stroke, and other conditions are reviewed at this Virtual Hospital article. The discussion contains background information on atherosclerosis, including potential complications, diagnosis, and symptoms, as well as lifestyle modification. http://www.vh.org/Patients/IHB/IntMed/Cardio/Athero/Atherosclerosis.html

BALDNESS

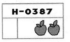

Hair Loss and Heart Disease A commercial publication devoted to hair loss offers this chapter on the link between hair loss and heart disease. Heart attack, atherosclerosis, and cholesterol information is presented, with a thorough discussion on the connection between dihydrotestosterone, hair loss, and heart disease emphasized. Risk factors are discussed, and a glossary of terms is available at the article, authored by Nasser Razack, M.D.
http://www.raztec.com/chapter12.html

PersonalMD.com: Baldness in Men Reflects Higher Heart Disease Risk Research from the Physicians' Health Study, reviewing a possible link between male pattern baldness and heart disease, is the focus of this Reuters Health Information page. Drawn from an article published in the *Archives of Internal Medicine,* the discussion introduces a possible explanation for the connection. An even higher risk of heart disease when combined with other risk factors is noted.
http://www.personalmd.com/news/n0124072050.shtml

C-REACTIVE PROTEIN

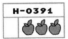

C-Reactive Protein, High Sensitivity An introduction to C-reactive protein and its clinical significance is found at this page, which describes its indications for examining risk of atherosclerosis. Testing methodology and appropriate test application are reviewed, and a table at the site provides a reference interval and interpretive data. Additionally, this address features access to a large collection of recent abstracts and full-text articles that propose the use of C-reactive protein in cardiovascular risk assessment.
http://labmed.hallym.ac.kr/chemistry/hs-CRP.htm

Harvard University Gazette: Protein Predicts Risk of First Heart Attack, Stroke A news story found at this site examines the role of C-reactive protein in the prediction of heart disease risk. Information from the Physicians Health Study, the possibility of the substance being an independent risk factor for heart disease, and other implications of the research are presented. http://www.heartinfo.com/news99/c-react010799.htm

COAGULATION FACTORS

American Heart Association: "Thick" Blood May Increase Stroke Risk The American Heart Association introduces results of research implicating von Willebrand factor, factor VIIIc, and fibrinogen as predictors of ischemic stroke. The previously studied association of these coagulation factors with coronary heart disease and details on the Atherosclerosis Risk in Communities Study are presented. http://www.americanheart.org/presenter.jhtml?identifier=3294

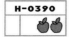

University of California San Francisco (UCSF): Fibrinogen is a Candidate Measure of Allostatic Load   Authored by Eric Brunner and Michael Marmot in collaboration with the Allostatic Load Working Group, this article discusses fibrinogen as a risk factor for cardiovascular disease. Determinants of fibrinogen level, psychosocial factors involved, the relationship between socioeconomic status and fibrinogen level, and other markers of allostatic load are considered.
http://www.macses.ucsf.edu/Research/Allostatic/notebook/fibrogen.html

CULTURE, RACE, AND ETHNICITY

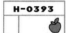

Association of Black Cardiologists: Cardiovascular Disease in the Black Population   A slide presentation at this site outlines age-adjusted death rates due to cardiovascular disease and stroke by race and sex. Graphs illustrate death rates for coronary artery disease and stroke in the African American population, as well as modifiable and nonmodifiable risk factors.
http://www.abcardio.org/NHLBI/module_1/

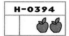

Hispanic-American Cardiovascular Risk Factors   Authored by Stanley L. Bassin, Ed.D., of California State University, this article presents cultural and epidemiological issues related to cardiovascular disease. With a specific focus on Hispanic cultures and lifestyle, the paper addresses risk factors of these groups, including obesity linked to diet and physical inactivity.
http://www.csupomona.edu/~slbassin/html/cardiorisk.html

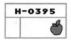

JAMA: Ethnic and Socioeconomic Differences in Cardiovascular Disease Risk Factors   Authors of this *Journal of the American Medical Association* article analyze whether differences in cardiovascular disease risk factors by ethnicity can be attributed to variations in socioeconomic status. Study description, outcome measures, and conclusions of the research are outlined at this abstract, with the full text of the article available for purchase.
(some features fee-based) http://jama.ama-assn.org/issues/v280n4/abs/joc72047.html

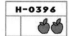

Morbidity and Mortality Weekly Report: Prevalence of Selected Cardiovascular Disease Risk Factors Among American Indians and Alaska Natives   Documenting the prevalence of selected cardiovascular disease risk factors among American Indians and Alaskan natives, this article cites findings that indicate that risk factors and mortality rates are not uniformly distributed across these populations. The importance of prevention activities and the need for population-specific assessments of behavioral risk factors are discussed.   http://www.cdc.gov/epo/mmwr/preview/mmwrhtml/mm4921a1.htm

DIABETES

American Family Physician: Attenuating Cardiovascular Risk Factors in Patients with Type 2 Diabetes   Presented by the American Academy of

Family Physicians, this Web site includes a professionally oriented article, as well as a related patient information handout. Both papers, authored by Alan Garber, M.D., Ph.D., stress connections between hyperglycemia and atherosclerosis. The pathogenesis of atherosclerosis and tables outlining components of atherogenic dyslipidemia and metabolic syndrome are included at the professional resource. Modifiable and predisposing risk factors for cardiovascular disease in diabetics and the need for coronary artery disease prevention measures in the population are emphasized.

http://www.aafp.org/afp/20001215/2633.html

Diabetes, Heart Disease, and Stroke   Diabetes and its role in heart attack and stroke are discussed in this online fact sheet, including information on the mechanisms of increased risk, therapeutic strategies for diabetes control, and optimal blood sugar ranges. Links are available to information on additional risks associated with heart disease and stroke, provided as a service of Health Education Associates.

http://well-net.com/cardiov/hadm.html

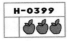

Postgraduate Medicine: Reducing Cardiovascular Risk in Diabetes   Authored by Robert G. Spanheimer, M.D., this portion of a diabetes symposium offers information on the prevalence of cardiovascular disease in type 2 diabetes, major cardiovascular risk factors in diabetes, and details on treatment of hypertension, hyperlipidemia, and hyperglycemia in this population. The importance of risk factor modifications is emphasized, with a table outlining interventions for more than 10 specific risk factors.

http://www.postgradmed.com/issues/2001/04_01/spanheimer.htm

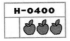

University of Newcastle upon Tyne: Strategy for Arterial Risk Management in Type 2 (Non-Insulin-Dependent) Diabetes Mellitus   Initially published in *Diabetes Medicine,* this article summarizes selected arterial risk factors in diabetes and provides a systematic determination of arterial risk and appropriate management. The significance of dyslipidemia, predictions from serum lipid measurements, interpretation of blood pressure values, and analysis of blood glucose concentration are analyzed. Body mass index, insulin insensitivity, raised albumin excretion rate, and the significance of particular population risks are discussed.

http://www.staff.newcastle.ac.uk/philip.home/ar1998.html

GENDER-SPECIFIC RISK FACTORS

Heart Information Network: Symptoms of Heart Disease: The Difference Between Men and Women   Contributing factors for heart disease in both men and women are examined at this online table, reprinted with permission from Washington Hospital Center. The "ABCs" of heart disease in women, as well as men's symptoms, representative of the textbook clinical picture, are listed.   http://208.133.254.45/search/display.asp?Id=253&caller=455

National Center for Chronic Disease Prevention and Health Promotion: Heart Disease Mortality Among Men   An online atlas, entitled *Men and Heart Disease,* was developed by the Office for Social Environment and Health Research at West Virginia University. Part of the Centers for Disease Control and Prevention database, this site connects users to interactive state maps, fact sheets, and methodological notes. The complete atlas is downloadable in PDF format and emphasizes geographic, racial, and ethnic inequalities in heart disease mortality among men. The related *Women and Heart Disease* publication can be accessed from the site.
http://www.cdc.gov/nccdphp/cvd/mensatlas/

GENETICS

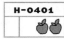

WebMDHealth: Genetics of Coronary Heart Disease   The role of genes in the development of coronary heart disease is the focus of this WebMD article, which introduces the genetic versus environmental debate. Examples of both genetic and environmental factors are reviewed at an online table, and a 1994 study on coronary disease in twins is examined. Genes proposed to be involved in coronary artery disease are discussed, with comments on particular gene regions and related research.
http://my.webmd.com/condition_center_content/cvd/article/1675.50290

HOMOCYSTEINE

American Heart Association (AHA): Homocysteine, Folic Acid, and Cardiovascular Disease   This fact sheet introduces homocysteine and its relationship to cardiovascular risk. The use of folic acid to potentially decrease risk, laboratory testing and risk assessment, and total diet risk profile are considered. http://216.185.112.5/presenter.jhtml?identifier=535

Bandolier: Homocysteine and Heart Disease   Offered as part of Bandolier's evidence-based healthcare collection, this page describes homocysteine's association with heart disease. A discussion of homocysteine's effects on the arteries is provided, along with normal values and research demonstrating the relationship between higher serum levels of homocysteine and cardiovascular disease mortality. Related topics, including homocysteine concentrations and plasma vitamin concentration, as well as therapeutic implications and recommendations, are reviewed.
http://www.jr2.ox.ac.uk/bandolier/band57/b57-3.html

HYPERCHOLESTEROLEMIA

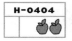

Cholesterol   Produced by the Delaware Cooperative Extension, this site contains patient information regarding cholesterol level interpretation. The site

provides information on "good" and "bad" cholesterol, controlling HDL and LDL levels, effects of cholesterol in the body, dietary fat, and modification of dietary fat intake.
http://bluehen.ags.udel.edu/deces/fnf/fnf-18.htm

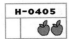

MedicineNet.com: Cholesterol and the Heart This fact sheet provides a list of FAQs for quick reference to information about cholesterol. A general overview of cholesterol and its role in causing heart disease, additional risk factors for coronary heart disease, treatment review, and current research on cholesterol and the heart are provided.
http://www.medicinenet.com/Script/Main/Art.asp?ArticleKey=320

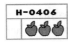

National Cholesterol Education Program Coordinated by the National Heart, Lung, and Blood Institute (NHLBI), the National Cholesterol Education Program is described at an Executive Summary found at this site's links. A discussion of blood cholesterol level and increased risk for coronary heart disease, as well as the use of risk status as a guide to therapy implementation is presented. Cholesterol management, primary prevention, and issues and risks in young adults, in women, and according to age are included. Clinical management, dietary therapy, drug treatment, physical activity, and a variety of related issues are addressed.
http://dragon.labmed.umn.edu/~relson/atp_home.html

HYPERINSULINEMIA

Archives of Internal Medicine: Hyperinsulinemia and the Risk of Cardiovascular Death and Acute Coronary and Cerebrovascular Events in Men An original investigation is discussed at this page, examining whether hyperinsulinemia alone is associated with an increase in cardiovascular morbidity and mortality. An explanation of the relationship found and weaker associations with risk of acute coronary events and stroke are addressed. The option to view the full text of articles on a pay-per-view basis is available.
(some features fee-based) http://archinte.ama-assn.org/issues/v160n8/abs/ioi90166.html

HYPERTENSION

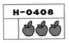

American Family Physician: Hypertension Treatment and the Prevention of Coronary Heart Disease in the Elderly The American Academy of Family Physicians offers this clinical opinion paper, authored by Marvin Moser, M.D., of Yale University School of Medicine. The discussion targets management of systolic and systolic/diastolic hypertension with lifestyle and pharmacologic interventions. The efficacy of various agents and discussion of trials on hypertension in the elderly are analyzed. An algorithm for treatment of elderly patients with hypertension is provided.
http://www.aafp.org/afp/990301ap/1248.html

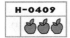

National Heart, Lung, and Blood Institute (NHLBI): High Blood Pressure   Health information for the public is offered at this page, which contains an assortment of articles related to hypertension and heart disease risk. Several publications on lowering blood pressure, facts about the DASH diet, and a link to the National High Blood Pressure Education Program of the NHLBI are available. Publications for several additional risk factor categories for heart disease are included in this extensive collection of publications.
http://www.nhlbi.nih.gov/health/public/heart/

HYPOMAGNESEMIA

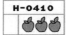

Cardiovascular Risk Factors and Magnesium: Relationships to Atherosclerosis, Ischemic Heart Disease, and Hypertension   Drawn from *Magnesium and Trace Elements,* this article addresses deficits in magnesium intake and low intake as a risk factor for hypertension, cardiac arrhythmias, ischemic heart disease, atherogenesis, and sudden cardiac death. Those at greatest risk for low intake of magnesium and the multiple cellular and molecular effects on cardiac and vascular smooth muscle are examined. Etiology of hypertension, incidence of hypomagnesemia in hospitalized populations, and history of low magnesium intake related to a variety of clinical pictures are addressed.   http://www.execpc.com/~magnesum/alturacv.html

LIPOPROTEIN (a)

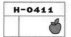

Associated Press: Lipoprotein Ups Heart Attack Risk   Information on lipoprotein(a), the cholesterol risk factor, and research suggesting its association with an increased risk of heart disease are presented at this news release. These findings, originally published in *Circulation,* address the genetic components of lipoprotein(a) and the number of heart attacks occurring in those with higher serum levels compared with those with lower serum concentrations of the substance.   http://www.internetwks.com/pauling/lpa090400.html

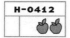

Lipoprotein(a) and Coronary Heart Disease   Summaries of several studies addressing the significance of lipoprotein(a) as compared with established cardiac risk factors, such as elevated total cholesterol and reduced high-density lipoprotein, are presented at this page, courtesy of the Hospital Authority of Hong Kong. The characterization of the lipoprotein(a) particle and a discussion of a genetic disease basis are included.
http://www.ha.org.hk/tmh/medicine/yip5.html

OBESITY AND OVERWEIGHT

American Heart Association (AHA): Obesity in Heart Disease   Provided by the American Heart Association, the article at this site offers information about the relationship of obesity to coronary heart disease and congestive heart failure. Therapeutic approaches for obesity treatment are recommended. http://216.185.112.5/presenter.jhtml?identifier=1751

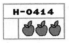

American Heart Association (AHA): Overweight The association between overweight or obesity and heart disease is the focus of this site, which presents a variety of links to weight management information, diet planning, lifestyle interventions, and body composition test details. Details on nutrition labeling, several diet types, and other information related to this modifiable risk factor are available.
http://216.185.112.5/presenter.jhtml?identifier=497

PHYSICAL INACTIVITY/SEDENTARISM

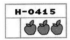

National Institutes of Health (NIH): Physical Activity and Cardiovascular Disease The health burden and prevalence of physical inactivity among various demographic groups are described at this statement, published by the National Institutes of Health as part of its Consensus Development Conference Statement. A review of the indexed literature provides information on the significant health benefits of exercise, evidence indicating physical inactivity as a risk factor for cardiovascular disease, and recommendations regarding daily physical activity requirements.
http://text.nlm.nih.gov/nih/cdc/www/101txt.html#Head3

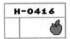

Physical Inactivity and Cardiovascular Disease Provided by the New York State Department of Health, this page provides a definition of physical inactivity, with recommendations for minimum levels of activity supplied. Consequences of physical inactivity, estimates of coronary heart disease mortality due to physical inactivity, and details on reported levels of inactivity in various segments of the population are included.
http://www.health.state.ny.us/nysdoh/chronic/cvd.htm

PHYTOCHEMICALS

American Heart Association (AHA): Phytochemicals and Cardiovascular Disease Recommendations from the *AHA Heart and Stroke Guide* regarding research directions in nutrition are presented at this site. Consumer information about phytochemicals and cardiovascular disease is provided, with sections reviewing the current state of knowledge with regard to flavanoids, plant sterols, and other compounds that may be associated with decreased heart disease risk. http://216.185.112.5/presenter.jhtml?identifier=4722

SEX HORMONES

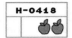

American Heart Association (AHA): Estrogen and Cardiovascular Diseases in Women   This site describes the relationship of estrogen to heart disease risk and the controversy that exists concerning hormone replacement therapy. Facts about both estrogen and combined hormone replacement therapy are presented, including findings from observational studies and other research.
http://216.185.112.5/presenter.jhtml?identifier=4536

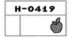

Archives of Internal Medicine: Testosterone and Cardiovascular Risk Factors   Discussion of a variety of opinions regarding the correlation of testosterone with coronary artery disease is found at this editor's correspondence page. One commentary cites major reasons for the continuing controversy and discusses evidence implicating elevated androgens in aspects of atherogenesis. Studies documenting an enhanced tendency toward thrombosis in those receiving exogenous androgens and discussing the possibility that hormones other than androgens are involved are reviewed.
http://archinte.ama-assn.org/issues/v160n13/ffull/ilt0710-4.html

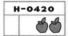

Journal of Gender–Specific Medicine: Estrogens for Heart Disease
This report from the Annual Session of the American College of Cardiology, authored by physicians of Loyola University Medical Center, summarizes research addressing the possible cardioprotective effects of estrogens in postmenopausal women. Comments on retrospective studies, combination hormone replacement therapy, the NIH Women's Health Initiative, selective estrogen receptor modulators, and several other reports and findings noted during the American College of Cardiology's 49th Annual Session are presented.
http://www.mmhc.com/jgsm/articles/JGSM0006/wehrmacher.htm

SMOKING

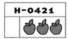

AHA Medical/Scientific Statement: Cigarette Smoking, Cardiovascular Disease, and Stroke   This statement from the American Heart Association offers details concerning the association of cigarette smoking with cardiovascular disease and stroke. Topics discussed include effectiveness of physician intervention, physician training, smoking cessation pharmacotherapy, and multi-component programs.
http://216.185.112.5/presenter.jhtml?identifier=1737

American Heart Association (AHA): Cigarette Smoking and Cardiovascular Diseases   Information on cigarette smoking and cardiovascular disease from the AHA *Heart and Stroke Guide* is provided at this site, in addition to a scientific position statement by the AHA and discussions of risk factors for heart attack and stroke.
http://216.185.112.5/presenter.jhtml?identifier=4545

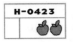 **Dalhousie University Medical Informatics: Smoking and Coronary Heart Disease** This fact sheet offers valuable information on smoking and coronary heart disease, answering commonly asked questions and providing information on harmful substances in cigarettes, the effects of nicotine and carbon monoxide on the body, and secondhand smoke. Techniques for smoking cessation are also listed.
http://www.chebucto.ns.ca/Health/CPRC/smoking.html

Stress

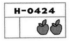 **American Heart Association (AHA): Stress and Heart Disease** From the *Heart and Stroke Guide* of the American Heart Association, this site offers information on the possible link between cardiovascular disease and environmental and psychosocial risk factors. The review provides discussion relating to current research on psychosocial therapies, with an emphasis on the need for more data regarding specific mechanisms by which stress may contribute to heart disease risk.
http://216.185.112.5/presenter.jhtml?identifier=4750

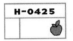 **Johns Hopkins Medicine: Strong Response to Mental Stress Could Indicate Heart Disease** Results of a study published in *Circulation* are reviewed at this press release, emphasizing the possible relationship between stress and heart disease. Results of the study, supported by the National Institutes of Health, indicate that blood flow to the heart decreases in those who have strong responses to stressful events. Additional information on the research is summarized. http://www.hopkinsmedicine.org/press/1997/DECEMBER/199705.htm

Substance Abuse

 WebMDHealth: Pot Impacts Heart, Study Shows Possible increased heart attack risk with marijuana use is the focus of this online story, a result of research initiated in reponse to a report recommendation of the Institute of Medicine. Significant information derived from the research is stated.
http://my.webmd.com/content/article/1728.55387

Triglycerides/Trans Fatty Acids

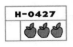 **American Heart Association (AHA): Trans Fatty Acids** Consumers will find a useful discussion of dietary fats, particularly trans fatty acids, in this fact sheet. AHA recommendations on the use of dietary fats are presented, followed by a thorough summary of fatty acids, including different types, food sources, and healthy choices. A description of trans fatty acids includes the hydrogenation process and an explanation of why these fats are unhealthy.
http://216.185.112.5/presenter.jhtml?identifier=4776

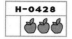

American Heart Association (AHA): Triglycerides Triglycerides are defined and discussed in this fact sheet, which provides information regarding the mechanism of triglyceride creation in the body, reasons why an excess of triglycerides is harmful, and dietary treatment goals in patients diagnosed with hypertriglycerides. Normal, borderline-high, high, and very high triglyceride ranges, as defined by the Second Expert Panel on the Detection, Evaluation, and Treatment of High Blood Cholesterol in Adults, are listed.
http://216.185.112.5/presenter.jhtml?identifier=4778

6.3 SCREENING AND PREVENTION

GENERAL RESOURCES

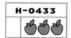

AHA Medical/Scientific Statement: Guide to Primary Prevention of Cardiovascular Disease The contribution physicians can make to primary prevention of coronary heart disease is the focus of this statement, from the AHA Task Force on Risk Reduction. Assessing patients for established risk factors, successful implementation of recommendations regarding the clinical approach to detection, and education regarding healthy lifestyle habits are discussed. A summary of the paper is available, as well as a table outlining risk interventions. http://216.185.112.5/presenter.jhtml?identifier=1788

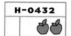

AHA Medical/Scientific Statement: Preventing Heart Attack and Death in Patients with Coronary Disease This statement, excerpted from *Circulation,* offers a comprehensive risk reduction formula for patients with coronary and other vascular disease. Risk interventions and recommendations are listed in table format, and a downloadable print-ready version is available. A guide to primary prevention is found at the site.
http://216.185.112.5/presenter.jhtml?identifier=1316

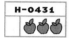

AHA Medical/Scientific Statement: Primary Prevention of Coronary Heart Disease A statement for healthcare professionals is available at this site, addressing contributions of the Framingham Heart Study to the understanding of cardiovascular disease development. Risk factor definitions, as developed by the research; limitations of Framingham risk scores; the possible role of insulin resistance; and suggestions for further research are included. Issues concerning relative versus absolute risk, primary versus secondary prevention, and potential uses of Framingham risk charts are discussed. Additional information on age, smoking, hypertension, serum cholesterol levels, and diabetes mellitus, as well as other potent risk factors is available.
http://216.185.112.5/presenter.jhtml?identifier=1807

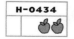

American Family Physician: Heart Disease—How to Reduce Your Risk Information on a variety of factors to consider in reducing one's risk of heart disease is presented at this consumer-oriented brochure. Basic information

on diet and exercise, as well as the detrimental effects of smoking, high blood pressure, hypercholesterolemia, and uncontrolled diabetes, is explained in easy-to-understand terms.
http://familydoctor.org/healthfacts/358/

American Heart Association (AHA): Risk Factors That Can Be Changed   A discussion of both modifiable and nonmodifiable risk factors for heart disease is found at this address, which contains links to collections of documents on five significant and manageable risks. Several documents on one of the most preventable risk factors, cigarette smoking, are provided, and collections of information from the AHA on physical inactivity and exercise, high blood cholesterol, high blood pressure, and overweight are included.
http://216.185.112.5/presenter.jhtml?identifier=494

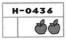

Cardiac HealthWeb: Preventing Heart Disease   Produced by Blacksburg Electronic Village Health Center, this site provides a selection of patient information concerning heart disease prevention. Information includes a risk assessment section, with links to the American Heart Association and the Center for Science in the Public Interest. A section about lifestyle modification includes links to information regarding diet, exercise, and stress management.
http://www.bev.net/health/cardiac/prevention.html

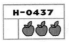

Comprehensive Cardiologic Program   Developed to provide basic knowledge regarding cardiologic preventative care, this program offers a discussion of several risk factors that contribute to cardiac disease, including smoking, diabetes, hypertension, a sedentary lifestyle, high cholesterol, and obesity. A coronary risk test assesses risk of coronary heart disease based on weight, smoking, cholesterol level, blood glucose, heredity, age, gender, physical activity level, and blood pressure. The site contains links to medical sites, including the American College of Cardiology, the American Heart Association, and the World Health Organization.
http://www.geocities.com/HotSprings/1288/index2.htm

National Center for Chronic Disease Prevention and Health Promotion: Cardiovascular Health   A division of the Centers for Disease Control and Prevention, this program promotes epidemiologic surveillance and research, prevention initiatives, and public health education for cardiovascular disease. Activities of this section can be accessed by going directly to one of its several division branches, including the Cardiovascular Health Branch, the Division of Nutrition and Physical Activity, the Office on Smoking and Health, the Division of Diabetes Translation, and the Division of Adolescent and School Health, for which relevant branch publications, recommendations, and press releases can be found. State program activities and research and intervention project information are available.
http://www.cdc.gov/nccdphp/cvd/aboutprogram.htm

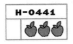

National Heart, Lung, and Blood Institute (NHLBI): Cardiovascular Information for Health Care Professionals   The latest reports by the Na-

tional Heart, Lung, and Blood Institute on high blood pressure, cholesterol, obesity, and heart attacks may be accessed at this site. Some publications must be downloaded, and some require a small fee. The site also contains information on the JumpSTART program, developed by the NHLBI in conjunction with Scholastic, Inc., which promotes the cardiovascular health of children in elementary school through recognition of risk factors and prevention.
(some features fee-based) http://www.nhlbi.nih.gov/health/prof/heart/index.htm

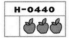

National Heart, Lung, and Blood Institute (NHLBI): Office of Prevention, Education, and Control (OPEC) This office disseminates summaries of research findings and scientific publications to health professionals and the public. Health education programs and initiatives focus on high blood pressure, high blood cholesterol, early warning signs of heart attack, asthma, obesity, and sleep disorders. A description and background information on the office is available from this address, as well as links to information on its national education programs. Links are also available to relevant NHLBI fact sheets and prevention practice guidelines.
http://www.nhlbi.nih.gov/about/opec/index.htm

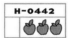

University of California Irvine: Heart Disease Prevention Program
The heart disease prevention program described at this site offers information on clinical research programs, published research on cardiovascular epidemiology, and individualized and community prevention programs. The site features a coronary calcium slide show, a guide to healthy shopping, and recommendations on preventing heart disease, along with clinical studies and heart disease - related links.
http://www.heart.uci.edu

ALCOHOL AND HEART DISEASE

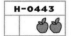

AHA Medical/Scientific Statement: Alcohol From the American Heart Association's *Circulation* publication, this site contains an article exploring the protective effects of alcohol against congestive heart disease, mechanisms for cardio-protective effects of alcohol consumption, and recommendations. References are included. http://216.185.112.5/presenter.jhtml?identifier=1874

ANTIOXIDANT CONSUMPTION

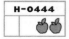

AHA Science Advisory: Antioxidant Consumption and Risk of Coronary Heart Disease As a courtesy of the American Heart Association, this site provides an article on antioxidant consumption and coronary heart disease risk reduction, with an emphasis on vitamin C, vitamin E, and beta-carotene. Topics discussed in this *Circulation* article include the influence of oxidants and antioxidants on the development of atherosclerosis, investigations

of the effects of antioxidants, and overall review of dietary antioxidant potentials for improved clinical outcomes. A PDF reprint version is available.
http://circ.ahajournals.org/cgi/content/full/99/4/591

ASPIRIN

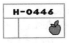

American Heart Association (AHA): Aspirin in Heart Attack and Stroke Prevention   This site provides recommendations for the use of aspirin in secondary prevention of myocardial infarction, unstable angina, ischemic stroke, and transient ischemic attacks. Included are cautions, risks, and information about primary prevention.
http://216.185.112.5/presenter.jhtml?identifier=4456

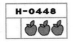

InteliHealth: Daily Aspirin Therapy   Harvard University and InteliHealth have collaborated to bring this introduction to aspirin therapy following a heart attack and in the primary prevention of a first incident. Controversy over the appropriate aspirin dose and risks to be aware of are introduced.
http://www.intelihealth.com/IH/ihtIH/WSIHW000/8124/23697/152228.html?d=dmtContent

BLOOD PRESSURE SCREENING

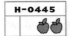

American Heart Association (AHA): Blood Pressure Testing and Measurement   A description of blood pressure measurement and its usefulness as a screening tool are discussed at this page of the AHA. Several related publications are available, including those on factors contributing to high blood pressure and a hypertension primer.
http://216.185.112.5/presenter.jhtml?identifier=4470

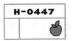

National Institutes of Health (NIH): Screening for Hypertension   Part of the National Institutes of Health's Guide to Clinical Preventive Services, this document examines the prevalence of uncontrolled hypertension and provides information on accurate methods of screening. Errors in blood pressure measurement and factors affecting accuracy are examined, as well as the effectiveness of early detection. Review of the indexed literature, the efficacy of antihypertensive regimens, and recommendations of other groups regarding blood pressure screening and control are presented.
http://text.nlm.nih.gov/cps/www/cps.9.html#CH03

CHOLESTEROL SCREENING AND REDUCTION

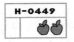

American Heart Association (AHA): Cholesterol Screening   Information on cholesterol screening and its usefulness in raising public awareness of blood cholesterol as a risk factor for heart disease are introduced in this article from the AHA. The potential hazards of poorly conducted community screen-

ing programs, selected screening recommendations, and guidelines for tests, as directed by the National Cholesterol Education Program and the AHA, are addressed. Information on prevention-oriented publications is provided.
http://216.185.112.5/presenter.jhtml?identifier=4504

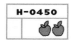

Bandolier: Cholesterol Screening and Treatment An effectiveness review is provided at this site, examining cholesterol as a risk factor and measurement of risk. The accuracy of cholesterol assays, the effectiveness of cholesterol-lowering regimens, and the cost implications associated with treatment, as well as the overall implications in healthcare management, are summarized.
http://www.jr2.ox.ac.uk/bandolier/band5/b5-2.html

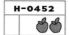

National Heart, Lung, and Blood Institute (NHLBI): Recommendations Regarding Public Screening for Measuring Blood Cholesterol Provided by the American Heart Association, these guidelines are the updated version of a document created in 1989 for cholesterol screening outside of the physician's office. Measurement of LDL lipoprotein cholesterol as a part of the initial evaluation and more aggressive assessment and management are detailed. The document can be viewed online in PDF format or ordered from the site.
http://www.nhlbi.nih.gov/guidelines/cholesterol/chol_scr.htm

DIETARY INTERVENTION

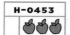

AHA Medical/Scientific Statement: Guidelines for Weight Management Programs for Healthy Adults Guidelines for the development and evaluation of nonpharmacologic and nonsurgical weight control programs are presented at this AHA site. Essential components of an effective management protocol, information to be provided to participants, and the roles of professional personnel in supervising weight loss management are discussed. Recommendations with regard to goals, diet and nutrition, exercise, and ongoing program assessment are included.
http://216.185.112.5/presenter.jhtml?identifier=1226

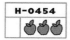

Clinical Cardiology: DASH Diet: A Clinical Success Story in Hypertension Control This supplement to the peer-reviewed *Clinical Cardiology* journal contains four articles, downloadable in PDF format, that review clinical dietary approaches to reduce hypertension. Review of the Dietary Approaches to Stop Hypertension (DASH) study and additional clinical practice experiences are presented, and text abstracts are accessible.
http://www.clinical-cardiology.org/supplements/CC22S3/CC22-3.mainpage.html

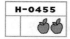

International Task Force for Prevention of Coronary Heart Disease: Olive Oil and the Mediterranean Diet A consensus statement regarding the advantages of the Mediterranean diet is reviewed at this site, along with the mechanisms by which its components are believed to reduce cardiovascular risk factors. A working definition of the diet; evidence of its benefits, specifically in

regard to oleic acid; and heart study reviews corroborating theories of prevention are provided.
http://www.chd-taskforce.com/oliveoil

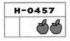

National Institutes of Health (NIH): Counseling to Promote a Health Diet Part of the National Institutes of Health's Guide to Clinical Preventive Services, this recommendation includes limitations of dietary fat intake, caloric balance in the diet, and inclusion of fiber in the diet. Evidence regarding other dietary components is summarized, with specific advice on nutritional counseling by physicians, dieticians, and community intervention programs. Nutritional factors linked to heart disease, the efficacy of risk reduction methods, and dietary interventions in special patient populations are considered.
http://text.nlm.nih.gov/cps/www/cps.62.html#CH56

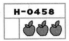

University of Michigan: Preventive Cardiology Guide for Healthy Eating Daily recommendations on food intake shown to reduce cardiovascular disease risk are outlined in this preventive care guide. Recommendations for food groups and portions are provided, as well as links to related topics, courtesy of the University of Michigan Health System.
http://www.med.umich.edu/1libr/primry/prevnt08.htm

EXERCISE/PHYSICAL ACTIVITY

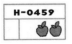

AHA Medical/Scientific Statement: How to Implement Physical Activity in Primary and Secondary Prevention Developed for the Task Force on Risk Reduction, this clinical statement offers practical recommendations for implementing physical activity in primary and secondary prevention of cardiovascular disease. Types of activity, intensity, duration, and frequency are covered. The importance of customizing a fitness regimen to the individual is emphasized. Secondary prevention regimens in the presence or absence of ischemia or significant arrhythmias are also discussed.
http://216.185.112.5/presenter.jhtml?identifier=1687

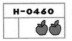

American Heart Association (AHA): Exercise/Physical Activity This informational brochure reviews the scientific position of the AHA regarding the importance of physical activity for the reduction of heart disease. Lifestyle risk factors and exercise recommendations are offered.
http://216.185.112.5/presenter.jhtml?identifier=4563

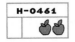

American Heart Association (AHA): National Coalition for Promoting Physical Activity This endeavor of the AHA is discussed at this site in terms of its background, mission, and collaborative efforts in encouraging education, regulatory policies, and outreach efforts for the promotion of physical activity. http://216.185.112.5/presenter.jhtml?identifier=4664

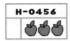

McGill Medical Informatics: Heart Disease and Exercise: Prevention of Disease A lecture review, provided as part of a McGill University lecture series, encourages physicians to advise patients regarding the benefits of exercise. The variety of mechanisms by which physical activity affords protective effects to the heart and cardiovascular system, with positive changes directly related to the intensity of exercise, are stressed, including management of diabetes mellitus through exercise, decreasing blood pressure, reducing weight, and increasing levels of HDL cholesterol. Professional exercise guidance recommendations and projected benefits are outlined.

http://www.mmip.mcgill.ca/heart/welex9701.html

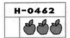

National Institutes of Health (NIH): Counseling to Promote Physical Activity   Risk reduction through the promotion of physical activity is the focus of this chapter of the NIH's Guide to Clinical Preventive Services. Efficacy of risk reduction strategies toward the prevention of coronary heart disease, obesity, hypertension, and non-insulin-dependent diabetes mellitus is discussed in the statement, and information on appropriate quantity and intensity of physical exercise necessary to promote cardiovascular fitness is presented. Additionally, recommendations of the NIH and other groups concerning the benefits of counseling in this area are stated.

http://text.nlm.nih.gov/cps/www/cps.61.html#CH55

GENDER-SPECIFIC RISK FACTOR MANAGEMENT

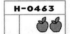

AHA/ACC Scientific Statement: Guide to Preventive Cardiology for Women   This Scientific Statement, courtesy of the American Heart Association and the American College of Cardiology, acknowledges coronary heart disease as the leading cause of death in women. Recommendations on gender-specific risk factor management are reviewed. A literature review, treatment exploration, and available tables provide guidelines for risk reduction.

http://circ.ahajournals.org/cgi/content/full/99/18/2480

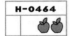

American Heart Association (AHA): Women, Heart Disease, and Stroke   Risk factors for heart disease are considered at this online fact sheet, linking users to information on both modifiable and nonmodifiable risk factors. Factors contributing to heart disease that may be specific to women are discussed, including menopause/estrogen loss and birth control pills.

http://216.185.112.5/presenter.jhtml?identifier=4786

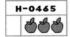

Postgraduate Medicine: Heart Disease in Women: Gender-Specific Statistics and Prevention Strategies for a Population at Risk   Emphasizing that coronary artery disease affects a diverse patient population, this article discusses the distinct diagnostic and therapeutic challenges of heart disease in women. Specific causes and risk factors, prevention strategies, and gender-specific disease characteristics are examined, as well as the effects of gender-biased research. Obesity, smoking, lipid levels, lifestyle, and additional risk factors are addressed, with a table at the page outlining major, moderate, and minor predictors of coronary artery disease.

http://www.postgradmed.com/issues/2000/05_00/rosenfeld.htm

SMOKING CESSATION

American Heart Association (AHA): Smoking Cessation Presenting the organization's scientific position on the subject, this document highlights the importance of smoking cessation in medical management as well as the Surgeon General's findings on the subject. The AHA advocacy position is stated.
http://216.185.112.5/presenter.jhtml?identifier=4731

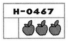

National Library of Medicine (NLM): Counseling to Prevent Tobacco Use A recommendation of the NIH is offered at this page, describing smoking cessation counseling, nicotine substitute supplements and anti-tobacco education. The efficacy of these risk reduction methods is discussed and supported by a review of the literature. Recommendations from several other major health organizations are included.
http://text.nlm.nih.gov/cps/www/cps.60.html#CH54

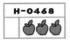

Virtual Office of the Surgeon General: Tobacco Cessation Guidelines Sets of material geared toward both consumer and clinician audiences are available at this address, including information on recently developed drugs and counseling techniques for treatment of tobacco dependence. Fact sheets, clinical practice guidelines, support group listings, and links to additional sites offering smoking cessation resources are provided. Many articles can be viewed with the use of Adobe Acrobat Reader, and some Spanish-language material is available.
http://www.surgeongeneral.gov/tobacco/

6.4 SIGNS AND SYMPTOMS

GENERAL RESOURCES

American Heart Association (AHA): Heart Attack and Stroke Warning Signs The warning signs of heart attack and stroke are outlined at this page of the AHA, with information on less common symptoms included. Links are provided to a stroke risk factor calculator and additional information about stroke and heart attack.
http://216.185.112.5/presenter.jhtml;
jsessionid=NCP3SGG1UYVBXWFZOAGSCZQ?identifier=3053

Continuum Health Partners: Symptoms and Types of Heart Disease This site lists symptoms of heart attack, including a brief discussion of the causes of this condition. The origins of angina, key differences between angina and a heart attack, and types of angina are defined.
http://www.bimc.edu/services/cardiology/symptoms.html

Merck Manual of Diagnosis and Therapy: Approach to the Cardiac Patient This chapter of the *Merck Manual of Diagnosis and Therapy* offers a guide to the cardiac history and physical examination. A variety of clues to diagnosis are discussed, including pain, cardiac dyspnea, weakness and fatigue, palpitations, and syncope. Abnormalities in vital signs and pulses, percussion, auscultation, and heart sounds are reviewed, and links to related chapters in the publication can be accessed.

http://www.merck.com/pubs/mmanual/section16/chapter197/197a.htm

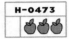 **University of Alabama: Cardiovascular Symptoms Clinical Resources** Provided by the Clinical Digital Libraries Project, this site offers links to clinical resources for cardiovascular symptoms by subtopic, with textbook entries, article links, and additional sources of information on bradycardia, chest pain, conduction disturbances, dyspnea, hypertension, murmurs, palpitations, shock, syncope, and tachycardia.

http://www.slis.ua.edu/cdlp/unthsc/clinical/cardiology/symptoms/index.htm

BRADYCARDIA

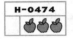 **eMedicine: Sinus Bradycardia** The eMedicine online journal offers this page describing the background, pathophysiology, and clinical presentation of bradycardia. Causes, medications causing symptoms, and sinus bradycardia as a symptom of various conditions are mentioned. Differential diagnostic links are provided, as well as overviews of the diagnostic workup.

http://www.emedicine.com/emerg/topic534.htm

 Virtual Hospital: Bradycardia Algorithm Externally peer reviewed, this site from University of Iowa Health Care provides a flowchart of steps to take in cases of bradycardia of a patient not in cardiac arrest. The algorithm is excerpted from AHA guidelines published in the *Journal of the American Medical Association* and includes intervention sequences and cautionary statements.

http://www.vh.org/Providers/ClinRef/FPHandbook/Chapter01/figures01/fig1-4.html

CAROTID BRUIT

 American Heart Association (AHA): Carotid Bruit Carotid bruit, a clear sign of increased stroke risk, is reviewed at this AHA site. A list of related Scientific Statements and fact sheets is provided at the site and can be accessed by using the site's search engine.

http://216.185.112.5/presenter.jhtml?identifier=4480

CHEST PAIN/ANGINA

 American Heart Association (AHA): Coronary Artery Spasm Coronary artery spasms and angina pectoris are discussed at this page of the AHA Web site. A discussion concerning possible complications and prevention,

Web site. A discussion concerning possible complications and prevention, along with a list of related publications of the AHA, is provided.
http://216.185.112.5/presenter.jhtml?identifier=4520

eMedicine: Chest Pain Chest pain originating from various parts of the chest is discussed at this online tutorial, including a list of potentially life-threatening and non-life-threatening etiologies. Links to differentials, descriptions of chest pain types, and several other sections on diagnosis and management are presented.
http://www.emedicine.com/aaem/topic103.htm

CLAUDICATION

Familydoctor.org: Claudication Provided by the American Academy of Family Physicians, this article offers consumers general information on claudication, its causes, and tests used in diagnosis. Three treatment steps are outlined at the page, which also contains a similar Spanish-language publication.
http://familydoctor.org/handouts/008.html

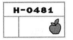

PhysicianWeb: Claudication A definition of claudication is found at this fact sheet, accompanied by an outline of causes, signs and symptoms, risk factors, and prevention. General measures for diagnosis and treatment are stated.
http://www.physicianweb.net/ptinfo/disease/claudication.html

CYANOSIS

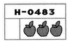

Merck Manual of Diagnosis and Therapy: Cyanosis Peripheral and central cyanosis are defined at this *Merck Manual* subchapter, which also briefly discusses the causes of cyanosis and diagnostic recommendations.
http://www.merck.com/pubs/mmanual/section6/chapter63/63h.htm

DYSPNEA

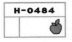

American Family Physician: Diagnostic Evaluation of Dyspnea Presented by the American Academy of Family Physicians, this online article explores the differential diagnosis of this common symptom, along with discussion of the pathophysiology of dyspnea. A table outlining the cardiac, pulmonary, mixed, and noncardiac/nonpulmonary etiologies are listed. Recommendations regarding the history, physical, and diagnostic examination are presented.
http://www.aafp.org/afp/980215ap/morgan.html

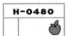

HealthAnswers: Shortness of Breath A definition of dyspnea is found at this consumer fact sheet, as well as information on the signs and symptoms of the condition, causes and risks, and prevention. Diagnosis of specific conditions associated with shortness of breath, treatment details, and monitoring are introduced. http://www.healthanswers.com/library/MedEnc/enc/3099.asp

Merck Manual of Diagnosis and Therapy: Dyspnea Common types of dyspnea are described at this site, including physiologic, pulmonary, and cardiac varieties. Circulatory dyspnea, dyspnea as a result of diabetic acidosis, dyspnea with cerebral lesions, and psychogenic causes are examined.
http://www.merck.com/pubs/mmanual/section6/chapter63/63c.htm

FATIGUE

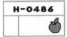

Cardiovascular Institute of the South: Unexplained Fatigue and Bradycardia Written by Richard P. Abben, M.D., this article describes the dangers of unexplained fatigue, especially for patients taking medications for heart disease. Information on the possibility of bradycardia and further diagnostics are offered.
http://www.cardio.com/articles/bradycrd.htm

GENDER-SPECIFIC SYMPTOMS

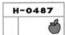

American Heart Association (AHA): Sex Differences in Heart Attack Reviewing a study published in the *New England Journal of Medicine,* this page introduces sex differences in heart attack causes, symptoms, and incidence. Conclusions with regard to the healthcare community's understanding of these factors are stated. http://216.185.112.5/presenter.jhtml?identifier=3069

MURMURS

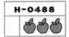

HealthCyclopedia: Heart Murmurs An extensive collection of online resources can be accessed from this site, including information from HealthAnswers, PersonalMD, and the American Heart Association on heart murmur definitions, sounds, variations, and news. Connections include an atlas of online murmurs, the "Auscultation Assistant," a brief discussion of the functional murmur, and heart murmurs in children and adolescents.
http://www.healthcyclopedia.com/heart_murmurs.html

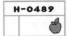

Merck Manual of Diagnosis and Therapy: Murmurs Analysis of heart murmurs is the focus of this chapter, which reviews a variety of systolic, diastolic, and continuous murmurs. Definition of the pericardial friction rub and a table grading murmurs according to intensity are available.
http://www.merck.com/pubs/mmanual/section16/chapter197/197c.htm#A016-197-0073

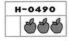

University of Alabama: Murmurs Part of the Clinical Digital Libraries Project, this site provides links to clinical resources concerning heart murmurs. Resources include chapters from Harrison's Online, the *Merck Manual,*

MDConsult Reference Books, and CliniWeb. Pediatric resources, clinical guidelines, and miscellaneous health reviews and heart murmur resources for healthcare professionals and educators are provided.

(some features fee-based) http://www.slis.ua.edu/cdlp/unthsc/clinical/cardiology/murmurs.html

PALPITATIONS

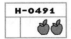

Doctor's Guide: Palpitations A listing of hyperlinks relating to the topic of palpitations is available at this Doctor's Guide site, including a wide variety of news articles and research information sites. Identification of causes, stories on diagnostic modalities, and new treatments for various palpitations and tachyarrhythmias are some of the topics addressed at this chronological listing.

http://www.docguide.com/news/content.nsf/$$SearchNews?SearchView&Query=Palpitatio
ns&SearchOrder=3&SearchMax=100&id=48dde4a73e09a969852568880078c249

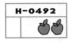

Temple University Hospital: Palpitations As part of Temple University's online patient education program, this site provides a definition of palpitations and explains reasons for their occurrence. Medical conditions related to palpitations are listed, and symptoms, diagnosis, and treatment are discussed.

http://www.temple.edu/heart/html/palpitations.html

SYNCOPE

American Heart Association (AHA): Syncope This AHA fact sheet provides background information on syncope, with particular reference to neurally mediated syncope and research on hormones that regulate blood pressure.

http://216.185.112.5/presenter.jhtml?identifier=4749

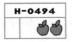

Diagnosis of Syncope The etiology of syncope and an outline of neurocardiogenic, cardiac, arrhythmic, and structural heart diseases that may cause this relatively common symptom are presented at this site, sponsored by Medtronic. The challenges of syncope diagnosis and a review of clinical evaluation are provided in this Technical Concept Paper on diagnostic cardiac monitoring.

http://www.medtronic.com/reveal/paper.html

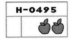

Merck Manual of Diagnosis and Therapy: Syncope (Fainting) Various cardiovascular and noncardiovascular causes of syncope are discussed at this online textbook page, including bradyarrhythmias and supraventricular or ventricular tachyarrhythmias. Symptoms and signs of a syncopal patient, a related link to orthostatic syncope, and diagnosis and physical findings of specific conditions are summarized.

http://www.merck.com/pubs/mmanual/section16/chapter200/200b.htm

6.5 DIAGNOSTICS

GENERAL RESOURCES

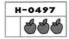

Cardiac HealthWeb: Diagnostic Procedures   Produced by the Blacksburg Electronic Village Health Center, this site contains links to information regarding cardiac catheterization, ambulatory electrocardiography, arteriography, blood pressure testing and measurement, and vital sign interpretation. A guideline of the American College of Cardiology and the American Heart Association can be accessed, and consumer information sheets are available.
http://www.bev.net/health/cardiac/treatment.html

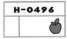

Cardiology.org   At Cardiology.org practitioners may access a lengthy list of common ECG abnormalities and find guidelines for treatment. In addition to the internal search engine, medical tools for assessment of body mass index (BMI), risk of cardiac events, Duke treadmill score, and diagnostic test evaluation are provided. ECG educational highlights, international symposium information, and additional updates in cardiology diagnostics are provided.
http://www.cardiology.org

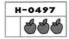

Chest Pain Perspectives   The mission of Chest Pain Perspectives is to provide a forum for healthcare professionals to enhance the efficiency and accuracy of diagnosing patients who complain of chest pain not typical of myocardial infarction. The site features an interactive series of case studies that illustrate the current challenges faced by clinicians. Information regarding cardiac markers and further review of cardiac diagnostics are offered, as well as a collection of related cardiology links.
http://www.chestpainperspectives.com

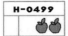

New York Online Access to Health (NOAH): Tests for Heart Disease
This portion of the NOAH Web site provides articles regarding cardiology diagnostics, including ambulatory electrocardiography, arteriography, blood pressure testing, carotid bruit, cardiac catheterization, computer imaging, heart damage detection, lumbar puncture, and tests for stroke. Sources include the American Heart Association and the Franklin Institute Science Museum.
http://www.noah-health.org/english/illness/heart_disease/heartdisease.html#TESTS

ANGIOGRAPHY, GENERAL

ACC/AHA Guidelines for Coronary Angiography   This management guideline, provided as a service of the American College of Cardiology and the American Heart Association, contains detailed information about the use of coronary angiography for specific conditions, including known or suspected coronary artery disease, valvular heart disease, congenital heart disease, congestive heart failure, and other conditions. The entire document may be downloaded for use off-line. Five appendices, including anatomic angiographic terminology, contrast agent selection, and elements of a coronary angiographic report, are included.

http://216.185.112.5/presenter.jhtml?identifier=1966

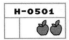

Diagnostic Angiography: Introduction and Procedure Description
Angiography, a principal diagnostic modality for evaluation of both arteries and veins, is reviewed at this site, with discussion of technological advances and implications for the procedure's use. A step-by-step description up to catheterization of the patient, commonly used sedating agents, and the option to read the site in "Plain Talk" for patients or "MedSpeak," for a more technical presentation, are available.

http://www.idsonline.com/gcm/anintrms.htm

Society for Cardiac Angiography and Interventions The focus of this
site is the Society Laboratory Survey Program, which addresses quality of clinical care delivery. Also available at this site is information regarding membership, society meetings, research awards, and publications. Links to related cardiology societies, journals, courses, and meetings are provided.

http://www.scai.org

APEXCARDIOGRAPHY

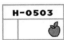

MDAdvice.com: Apexcardiography (ACG) The use of apexcardiography
as an aid in the evaluation of heart function is introduced at this online reference, drawn from the *Complete Guide to Medical Tests*. Readers will find a general introduction to the procedure and a listing of what abnormal results may indicate.

http://www.mdadvice.com/library/test/medtest28.html

ARTERIOGRAPHY

Medical College of Georgia: Arteriogram Providing basic information
to healthcare consumers, this site offers a definition of the arteriogram as well as a step-by-step review of the procedure.

http://www.mcghealthcare.org/radiology/Arteriogram__Angiogram_/arteriogram__angiogram_.htm

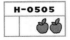

MEDLINEplus Medical Encyclopedia: Extremity Arteriography
General information on angiography of the extremities is provided at this MEDLINEplus resource, supplied by the National Library of Medicine. Alternative names for the test, its diagnostic capabilities, how the test is performed, and risks associated with the procedure are reviewed. The site also offers consumer information on normal and abnormal results and links to further information on conditions under which the test may be performed.

http://www.nlm.nih.gov/medlineplus/ency/article/003772.htm

ASSESSMENT OF FUNCTIONAL CAPACITY

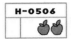

American Heart Association (AHA): Revisions to Classification of Functional Capacity and Objective Assessment of Patients with Diseases of the Heart   The AHA presents a classification system at this site for assessing patients with cardiac diseases. This classification system, originally published by the New York Heart Association, has been updated and approved by the AHA.
http://216.185.112.5/presenter.jhtml?identifier=1712

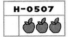

Medscape: A Shuttle Walk Test for Assessing Heart Failure   At this online article of the *American Heart Journal* a six-minute walk test and shuttle walk test (SWT) are evaluated and compared for their efficacy in assessment of functional capacity in chronic heart failure. The authors analyze the usefulness of these tests in clinically stable heart failure patients, exploring safety and greater usefulness of the SWT.
http://www.cs.columbia.edu/~noemie/to_classify/pnt-ahj1382.09.mora.html

AUSCULTATION

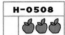

Heart Murmurs and Defects   Created by Synapse Publishing, Inc., this site contains a recorded collection of heart murmurs, heart defects, and other conditions. Downloadable audio files include normal heart sounds, functional murmurs, ventricular septal defect, atrial septal defect, aortic stenosis, pulmonary stenosis, mitral stenosis, mitral prolapse syndrome, and coarctation of the aorta.   http://www.medlib.com/spi/coolstuff2.htm

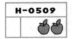

McGill University: Virtual Stethoscope   An educational resource of McGill University, this site contains a tutorial on the physical exam with an emphasis on auscultation. A summary of selected physiology and pathophysiology topics, a virtual stethoscope interface for auscultating normal and abnormal cardiac and respiratory sounds, and quiz reviews of presented material are provided.   http://sprojects.mmip.mcgill.ca/MVS/MVSTETH.HTM

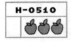

University of California Los Angeles (UCLA): Auscultation Assistant
The distinctive characteristics of heart and breath sounds may be heard at this site, designed by a fourth- year medical student. In addition, overviews of murmurs, normal heart sounds, and variations are provided, as well as audio files of several systolic murmurs, diastolic murmurs, and mixed murmurs. Examples of normal breathing, crackles, and wheezes are presented, along with detailed descriptions of each.
http://www.wilkes.med.ucla.edu/intro.html

BLOOD PRESSURE

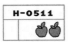

American Heart Association (AHA): Blood Pressure Levels An explanation of blood pressure measurement, geared toward consumers, is found at this AHA Web site and includes categories of blood pressure values and recommended follow-up. Related AHA publications are listed at the page, including those addressing causes of high blood pressure, statistics, and high blood pressure in children, and can be accessed by using the site's search engine.
http://216.185.112.5/presenter.jhtml?identifier=4450

Blood Pressure The history of blood pressure measurement and its recognition as an important diagnostic tool in the management and prevention of heart disease are discussed at this site, with an emphasis on current techniques and devices. Issues in blood pressure management, such as conditions preventing accurate readings, are reviewed, and specific types of measurements are introduced. Basic information on clinical values, self-measurement, and ambulatory 24-hour readings is offered, as well as discussion of issues in patient management. Hypertension management software may be ordered from the site.
http://www.iem.de/e/informationen/i_0.htm

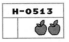

Canadian Medical Association (CMA): Accurate Blood Pressure Measurement The article at this address, excerpted from the *Canadian Medical Association Journal,* discusses the common pitfalls of inaccurate blood pressure assessments. Included in the review are problems associated with overdiagnosis or underdiagnosis of hypertension due to lack of attention to patient factors and standardized measurement protocols. Visitors may connect to a table outlining the various activities that often impact blood pressure readings, which also includes information regarding physicians' general adherence to the measurement recommendations of the American Heart Association. The article emphasizes the inability to provide effective therapy without consistency in technique and adequate operating equipment.
http://www.cma.ca/cmaj/vol-161/issue-3/0277.htm

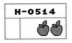

Measurement of Blood Pressure Accurate blood pressure measurement procedures are outlined at this information sheet, with guidelines for utilizing the three common devices for indirect reading. Specific instructions regarding the mercury meniscus and sphygmomanometer cuff are reviewed, as a service of the Malaysian Society of Hypertension. The measurement technique for auscultatory systolic and diastolic pressures is presented, as well as the particular indications of ambulatory pressure monitoring, including recognition of "white-coat syndrome" and other inconsistencies in readings.
http://www.msh.org.my/html/measurement_bp.htm

Body Composition Tests

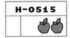 **American Heart Association (AHA): Body Composition Tests** The AHA provides information regarding body composition tests at this subsite, including waist circumference and body mass index (BMI). Background information on the tests' correlation with body fat and cardiovascular disease risk are discussed, and a table outlining BMI risk levels is provided.
http://216.185.112.5/presenter.jhtml?identifier=4489

C-Reactive Protein Screening

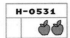 **American Heart Association (AHA): Inflammation, Heart Disease, and Stroke: The Role of C-Reactive Protein** Courtesy of the American Heart Association, this site offers information on the role of C-reactive protein in inflammation, heart disease, and stroke. A discussion of the role of C-reactive protein in predicting risk and a section on the causes of low-grade inflammation and measurement of C-reactive proteins are found.
http://216.185.112.5/presenter.jhtml?identifier=4648

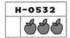 **Blood Levels of C-Reactive Protein May Predict Heart Attack and Stroke** Medical news from Mie University School of Medicine reviews the recent recognition of ultrasensitive tests for C-reactive protein and their value for predicting heart damage and heart attacks. The use of C-reactive protein as a sensitive marker of inflammation is discussed, with researchers of Brigham and Women's Hospital and Harvard Medical School commenting on the test's ability to detect the level of underlying atherosclerosis. Discussion of the test's benefit in studies specific to both men and women is reviewed, with a possible link between menopause and the inflammatory process noted.
http://www.medic.mie-u.ac.jp/newsbank/1998/980824crp.html

Calcium

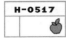 **Calcium, Serum** The use of serum calcium measurement and several causes of elevated serum concentrations are reviewed at this page, presented as a service of the Laboratory Corporation of America and Lexi-Comp. Possible meanings of decreased values and additional information pertaining to the differential diagnosis are presented.
http://www.labcorp.com/datasets/labcorp/html/chapter/mono/pr001700.htm

Cardiac Catheterization

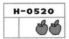 **Cardiac Catheterization Image Archives** Enlargeable thumbnail images at the site offer several views of cardiac catheterization, as well as close-up ex-

amples of the carotid and pulmonary angiogram, courtesy of Lowell General Hospital. http://www.lowellgeneral.org/html/Cath.html

Cardiologychannel: Cardiac Catheterization This discussion of cardiac catheterization includes generally accepted indications for the procedure, risks of cardiac catheterization, and additional links to details on the procedure itself and postprocedural care. Blood tests and other diagnostic tests scheduled in conjunction with cardiac catheterization are reviewed.
http://www.cardiologychannel.com/cardiaccath/

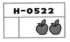

YourSurgery.com: Cardiac Catheterization Offering images and procedure explanations, this site provides a comprehensive overview of heart catheterization. Heart anatomy, pathology, and a description of surgical intervention are reviewed, accompanied by videos of angioplasty procedures. Complications and postcatheterization care are addressed.
http://www.yoursurgery.com/data/Procedures/cardiac_cath/p_cardiac_cath.cfm

CARDIAC GLYCOSIDES

Digoxin Serum testing for cardiac glycosides is the focus of this laboratory information sheet, provided by the Laboratory Corporation of America and Lexi-Comp. Limitations of testing are reviewed, with additional information on testing accuracy and the primary causes of digoxin toxicity included. The most likely causes of elevated levels are explored.
http://www.labcorp.com/datasets/labcorp/html/chapter/mono/ri013200.htm

CARDIAC IMAGING, GENERAL

North American Society for Cardiac Imaging The North American Society for Cardiac Imaging is a nonprofit, professional association dedicated to the advancement of cardiac and cardiovascular imaging. The site contains information regarding upcoming meetings and conferences, membership details, and previous meeting highlights. Also offered is a link to the online *International Journal of Cardiac Imaging*. The site maintains a history of the organization and a page of links to related sites.
http://www.nasci.org

CARDIOTOCOGRAPHY

Cochrane Library: Cardiotocography for Antepartum Fetal Assessment Maintained by the Cochrane Collaboration, this abstract describes a study on the use of cardiotocography for antepartum fetal assessment. It includes background, objectives, search strategy, selection criteria, data collection

and analysis, main results, and reviewer conclusions. Full text of the review is available in the Cochrane Library.
http://www.cochrane.de/cc/cochrane/revabstr/ab001068.htm

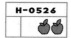

OBGYN.net: Cardiotocography (Fetal Monitoring)   Cardiotocography is described in this article, originally published in the *Textbook of Perinatal Medicine*. A history of the diagnostic procedure is followed by a discussion of normal and abnormal fetal heart rate patterns, recent criticisms of fetal heart rate pattern as a diagnostic tool, and the future of this diagnostic modality. Criticisms and areas for improvement in cardiotocography are presented in table format, and reference citations are available.
http://www.obgyn.net/FM/articles/cardiotocographya998-def.htm

COMPUTED TOMOGRAPHY (CT SCAN)

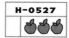

ACC/AHA Expert Consensus Document on Electron-Beam Computed Tomography for the Diagnosis and Prognosis of Coronary Artery Disease   This Expert Consensus Document provides a discussion regarding the use of electron-beam computed tomography in the detection of coronary artery calcification and in the screening of asymptomatic individuals assessed to be at risk for heart disease. Review of the literature, assessment of diagnostic accuracy, and the predictive value of this test compared with alternative methods of diagnosis are examined. Gaps in the current state of knowledge and the need for further research of the role of electron-beam computed tomography are addressed.
http://circ.ahajournals.org/cgi/content/full/102/1/126

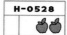

MedicineNet.com: Computerized Axial Tomography (CAT Scan/CT Scan)   Information on the computed tomography (CT) scan, links to related medical procedures and tests, related news and updates, and professional answers to patients' questions are available at the MedicineNet resource. A detailed description of the CT scan, intended for consumer readers, includes reasons for the procedure, any risks involved, and patient preparation. Details of the actual process are also available.
http://www.focusoncancer.com/script/main/art.asp?articlekey=315

CONTRAST ECHOCARDIOGRAPHY

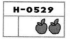

Contrast Echocardiography Workshops   Information on contrast echocardiography and the future of its use in the echocardiography laboratory is provided at this site, along with an outline of the ideal contrast agent, equipment innovations, and indications for its use. Preparation and machine settings, dosing and scanning review, and side effects of the contrast agent are mentioned.   http://www.acclakelouise.com/acc99/htm/work3.htm

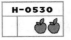

University of Virginia Health Systems: Novel Screening Test for Heart Disease Detection From the University of Virginia Health Systems, this site contains a news article regarding the safety and convenience of myocardial contrast echocardiography. The test's ability to measure the velocity of blood flow through the heart and its reliability in heart disease detection compared with other testing procedures are discussed.
http://www.med.virginia.edu/newstips/Archives99/mce.html

CORONARY CALCIFICATION SCORING

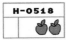

Cardiac Calcification Scoring This Web page lists identified risk factors for coronary artery disease that may lead to a heart attack, as cited by the AHA. A description of cardiac scanning required and a table at the site provide information on the clinical value of this testing. Images of a typical exam are displayed.
http://www.pruenergang.de/patinfos/cardiac_e.html

Coronary Calcium Scanning Coronary artery calcification scanning for identification of underlying heart disease, also known as heart scoring, is reviewed at this online article, courtesy of the Center for Diagnostic Imaging. Guidelines for its measurement are presented in table format, as well as respective implications for cardiovascular disease risk according to plaque burden and other factors. Capabilities and limitations of the test are examined, and discussion of its relation to other cardiac diagnostic procedures is provided. Additional information on calcium scoring technology and an algorithm for patient management are available.
http://www.heartct.com/forphysi.htm

ECHOCARDIOGRAPHY

ACC/AHA: Guidelines for the Clinical Application of Echocardiography This report, issued by the American College of Cardiology and the American Heart Association, was developed in collaboration with the American Society of Echocardiography. The entire report is available online and can be accessed by selecting specific topical chapters from the table of contents, including murmurs and valvular heart disease, ischemic heart disease, pericardial disease, cardiac masses and tumors, systemic hypertension, and arrhythmias and palpitations. Guidelines for echocardiography in the pediatric patient and in the critically ill are provided.
http://www.acc.org/clinical/guidelines/echo/

American Society of Echocardiography With over 5,500 members, the American Society of Echocardiography participates in research activities, the monitoring of federal agencies, and the development of standard documents and educational materials in the field. The site offers information about the organization, available research and grants, upcoming events, and a list of documents and materials that can be purchased. A monthly case study may be accessed, and a list of links to related sites is provided. The members-only section requires the use of a password.

(some features fee-based) http://asecho.org

 University of Medicine and Dentistry of New Jersey: Echocardiography Journal An electronic journal of cardiac ultrasound is available at this site, which includes alphabetically and chronologically organized medical articles and ultrasound images. Intended for use by physicians and other healthcare professionals, the site provides full-text disease descriptions, echocardiographic aspects, access to practice guidelines, and labeled images.

http://www2.umdnj.edu/~shindler/echo.html

ELECTRO-MAPPING

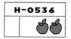 **University of Iowa Health Care: Electro-mapping of the Heart in Adults and Children** This article from *Currents,* a University of Iowa newsletter, discusses highlights of the recently developed noncontact catheter mapping and radiofrequency ablation. The new system, developed by Endocardial Solutions, Inc., is described at the page, with a link to a view of the noncontact mapping catheter. Information on insertion techniques, an example computer-generated image, and indications for its use are presented.

http://www.uihealthcare.com/news/currents/vol2issue2/electromap.html

ELECTROCARDIOGRAPHY

 AHA Medical/Scientific Statement: Recommendations for Safe Current Limits for Electrocardiographs Provided by the American Heart Association, this site is aimed at healthcare professionals who need to review the safety standards for electrocardiography. The site contains the association's recommendations and guidelines and includes an extensive reference list.

http://216.185.112.5/presenter.jhtml?identifier=1739

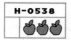 **American College of Cardiology (ACC): Guidelines for Electrocardiography** Courtesy of the American College of Cardiology and an American Heart Association Task Force, these guidelines for electrocardiography include a terminology review and indications for electrocardiography in different patient populations. Review of the general diagnostic considerations for each patient classification is provided.

http://www.acc.org/clinical/guidelines/electro

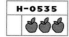 **EKG World Encyclopedia** A wealth of indexed material is found at this site, edited by Dr. Michael Rosengarten. Topics include myocardial infarction, conduction abnormalities, implanted devices, arrhythmias, invasive cardiac electrophysiology, ventricular hypertrophy, and the normal EKG artifact. Search engines, an EKG quiz, and case presentations are offered.

http://www.mmip.mcgill.ca/heart/egcyhome.html

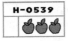

Internet Medical Education, Inc.: Electrocardiographic Rhythms This site provides descriptions of conditions diagnosed using electrocardiography. Abnormalities include accelerated ventricular rhythm, atrial multiform couplet, atrial couplet, junctional premature complex, parasystole, sinus arrhythmia, and ventricular fibrillation, with each synopsis containing diagnostic details and hyperlinks to related information.
http://www.med-edu.com/physician/arrhythmia/rhythms.html

ELECTROPHYSIOLOGY STUDIES

Electrophysiology Studies Indications for the use of electrophysiology study are reviewed at this site, as a service of Virginia Mason Medical Center. Patient preparatory procedures for electrical signal recording and electrode catheter pacing are discussed, including the various monitoring devices used and clinical management options.
http://www.vmmc.com/dbCardiology/sec373.htm

Florida Cardiovascular Institute: Electrophysiologic Studies An online information sheet offers review of the electrical system of the heart, conditions causing changes in heart rhythms, and information on patient preparation. Details of the electrophysiologic study, including important patient preparatory information, are provided.
http://www.fciheart.com/electrophysiologic_studies.htm

University of Michigan: Electrophysiology Study A description of the role of electrophysiology studies in determining the precise cause of arrhythmia is found at this site, including information about risks, preparation, obtaining results, and follow-up management procedures.
http://www.med.umich.edu/hcp/pa_info/diagnos.htm

EVENT RECORDING/TRANSTELEPHONIC ECG

University of Michigan: Transtelephonic ECG Transtelephonic ECG is explained at this University of Michigan informational brochure. Different types of monitors are described, and the test's usefulness in the pediatric population is discussed.
http://www.med.umich.edu/1libr/tests/teste22.htm

EXERCISE STRESS TESTING

ACC/AHA Guidelines for Exercise Testing Produced by the American College of Cardiology and the American Heart Association, this site provides clinical guidelines for exercise testing. The contents include an introduction to the testing procedure, exercise testing in diagnosis of obstructive coronary artery disease, risk assessment and prognosis, and exercise testing using ventilatory gas analysis. Pediatric testing and diagnosis in additional patient populations are reviewed. Explanatory tables and graphs are included, as well as an exhaustive list of references.

http://www.acc.org/clinical/guidelines/exercise/jac5074ref.htm

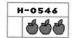

American Family Physician: Postexercise Systolic Blood Pressure Response: Clinical Application to the Assessment of Ischemic Heart Disease This article, provided as a courtesy of the American Academy of Family Physicians, outlines the three-minute systolic blood pressure ratio, a significant indicator of coronary artery disease. Analysis of abnormal values and their prognostic implications are reviewed at the site.

http://www.aafp.org/afp/981001ap/taylor.html

Mount Sinai School of Medicine: Exercise Stress Testing The Cardiovascular Institute of the Mount Sinai School of Medicine offers patient information about exercise stress testing and answers to commonly asked questions about the procedure. Questions relate to the purpose and nature of the test, risks involved, preparations required, duration and course of the test, and posttesting procedures. Details about nuclear stress testing, stress echocardiograms, and Dobutamine stress echocardiograms are provided.

http://www.mssm.edu/cvi/exstress.shtml

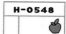

University of British Columbia: Exercise Stress Testing From the Healthy Heart Program at St. Paul's Hospital, this site offers information about the graded exercise stress test. A general explanation is provided, followed by information on test expectations and preparatory procedures.

http://healthyheart.org/Education/workshop/module2.htm

FETAL CARDIOLOGY IMAGING

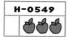

Fetal Echocardiography The detection of congenital heart disease in utero via echocardiography is discussed at this online article, with review of the indications for its use and specific techniques of fetal examination. The use of echocardiography for detection of heart disease in the presence of extracardiac anomalies or fetal distress, as well as in the case of identified chromosomal abnormalities, is summarized. Fetal cardiac arrhythmias and other indications warranting examination are reviewed. Links to two-dimensional echo examination images are provided, and other diagnostic methods, such as the M mode examination and Doppler techniques, are reviewed.

http://www.siuh.edu/pediatrics/articles/doc14.html

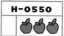

University College London: 3-D and 4-D Imaging of Fetal Heart From the Department of Medical Physics and Bioengineering, this site provides multi-dimensional ultrasound images of the fetal heart, as well as 3-D magnetic resonance imaging of the prenatal fetal heart. Images are labeled, and close-up shots may be viewed by clicking on the respective text.

http://www.medphys.ucl.ac.uk/mgi/jdeng/index.htm

HIS-BUNDLE ELECTROGRAPHY

MEDLINEplus Medical Encyclopedia: HIS-Bundle Electrography Part of the adam.com medical encyclopedia, this patient information sheet offers an introduction to testing purposes, risks and precautions, and other important details about HIS-bundle electrography. What to expect during testing and a listing of equipment used are included, as well as a test description and normal values. Factors that may affect test results are listed.
http://www.nlm.nih.gov/medlineplus/ency/article/003391.htm

HOLTER MONITORING/AMBULATORY ELECTROCARDIOGRAPHY

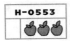

ACC/AHA Guidelines for Ambulatory Electrocardiography A complete guide to ambulatory electrocardiography is found at this site, which addresses both continuous and intermittent monitoring procedures. Chapters examine methods of electrode preparation, optimal duration of recording, methods of analysis, and emerging technologies. General considerations with regard to heart rate variability and assessment of symptoms that may be related to disturbances of heart rhythm are reviewed. The assessment of risk in patients without symptoms of arrhythmias, monitoring of myocardial ischemia, and evaluation in the pediatric population are discussed.
http://www.acc.org/clinical/guidelines/ae/ae4A.htm

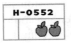

Torrance Memorial Medical Center: Holter Monitor Holter monitoring is described at this consumer fact sheet, including a detailed overview of the procedure, reasons for the procedure, patient safety suggestions during the monitoring period, and patient preparation.
http://www.torrancememorial.org/carholt.htm

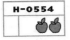

University of Alabama: Electrocardiography Clinical Resources The Health Sciences Digital Libraries Project of the University of Alabama offers this series of clinical resources pertaining to electrocardiography principles and practice. Subscription publications and free online material are both available, including clinical guidelines from the American Heart Association, clinical trial details, and online textbooks. General cardiovascular disorders clinical resources can be accessed. (some features fee-based)
http://www.slis.ua.edu/dls/cchs/main/
clinical/cardiology/procedures/electrocardiography.htm

LIPID-LEVEL PROFILE TESTING

Guidelines for Lipid Testing The Working Group on Hypercholesterolemia and Dyslipidemia provides guidelines at this site for lipid testing as it relates to the screening, diagnosis, and treatment of dyslipidemia. The principles provided by this group, sponsored by the Ontario Association of Medical Laboratories, advocate assessing various individual risk factors, rather than total cholesterol values alone, and may also be applied to atherosclerotic cardiovascular disease. Total cholesterol, high-density lipoprotein cholesterol, low-density lipoprotein cholesterol, and triglyceride measurements, with appropriate ratio calculation, are reviewed. Indications for screening, interpretation in light of additional risk factors, and a table outlining the number of risk factors and correlating coronary heart disease risk categories are shown. Patient monitoring guidelines are recommended.

http://www.oaml.com/clp017.html

Laboratory Corporation of America: Testing for Lipoprotein (a)

Information on testing to determine levels of lipoprotein(a) in patients with premature atherosclerosis or who have a family history of coronary heart disease, as well as in other specific circumstances, is provided at this laboratory Web site. Limitations of testing and additional information on lipoprotein(a) as a predictor of atherosclerotic vascular disease and as an independent risk factor for premature coronary heart disease are presented.

http://www.labcorp.com/datasets/labcorp/html/chapter/mono/sc025200.htm

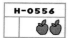

National Institutes of Health (NIH): Screening for High Blood Cholesterol and Other Lipid Abnormalities

Recommendations for blood lipid-level screenings across a variety of populations are specified at this in-depth publication, courtesy of the National Institutes of Health. Epidemiologic, pathologic, and genetic clinical studies that have pointed to causal relationships between blood lipids and heart disease are reviewed at the site, in addition to other lipid constituents and their relationships to coronary disease. Screening test accuracy, the positive results of early detection and intervention, and multi-center trials of cholesterol lowering agents are presented. Dietary management and specific reference to cholesterol lowering strategies in women, children, and young adults are summarized.

http://text.nlm.nih.gov/cps/www/cps.8.html

LUMBAR PUNCTURE

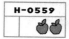

American Heart Association (AHA): Lumbar Puncture and Stroke

The process of lumbar puncture for the diagnosis of stroke is reviewed at this AHA fact sheet. Discussion includes reasons for the analysis of cerebrospinal fluid and the test's unique ability to quantify pressure within the central nervous system. Additional review of diagnostics that may be safely and effectively used during acute stroke is provided.

http://216.185.112.5/presenter.jhtml?identifier=4649

MAGNETIC RESONANCE ANGIOGRAPHY (MRA)

Magnetic Resonance Angiography: Update on Applications for Extracranial Arteries A Scientific Statement of the American Heart Association is available at this online edition of *Circulation*. Recent advances in magnetic resonance technologies and imaging of the extracranial arteries are reviewed at this page, along with a discussion of the future clinical applications of the technique. MRA of the carotid artery, MRA of the thoracic and abdominal aorta, renal MRA, peripheral MRA, and MRA of the pulmonary and coronary arteries are discussed, including current applications, summaries of recent research, and a table outlining concluding recommendations.
http://circ.ahajournals.org/cgi/content/full/100/22/2284

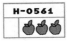

MR Imaging and MR Angiography The principles and protocols of MRA and magnetic resonance imaging (MRI) are presented at the site, which offers a series of downloadable slides and lecture material. Nearly a dozen MRA protocols provide imaging, timing, and guidelines for other parameters. Common indications, with positioning diagrams and sample typical dictation, are also provided. Specific clinical information on starting intravenous lines is offered, and technical review on the principles of 3-D gadolinium-enhanced MRA and the identification of pathological entities is provided.
http://www.mrprotocols.com

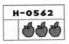

Volume Visualization in Magnetic Resonance Angiography The advantages of MRA over traditional X-ray projections are discussed at the site. Review of volume visualization techniques for 3-D organ viewing and its application to MRA data is offered. Several 3-D blood vessel visualizations are seen at the page and are accompanied by discussion of their applications in clinical practice, courtesy of professionals of the Institute of Mathematics and Computer Science in Medicine, Germany.
http://www.uke.uni-hamburg.de/institute/imdm/idv/publikationen/cga1992/

MAGNETIC RESONANCE IMAGING (MRI)

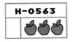

Cardiovascular Imaging Educational Site Clinical information pertaining to cardiovascular imaging of the heart with MRI is available at the site, with normal anatomical sections followed by diseases of the thoracic aorta, the heart, pulmonary arteries, and abdominal and peripheral vessels. Normal and pathological moving images are viewable at this educational MR teaching file, with discussion of new intravascular magnetic resonance contrast agents.
http://www.cardiac-mri.com

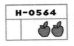

MedicineNet.com: Magnetic Resonance Imaging Scan An MRI fact sheet is found at this address, including a connection to the site's "MRI Scan Forum." A detailed overview of magnetic resonance imaging is found, with rea-

sons for the procedure, risks, patient preparation, and result interpretation details offered.
http://www.focusoncancer.com/script/main/art.asp?articlekey=421

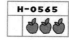

Society for Cardiovascular Magnetic Resonance The Society for Cardiovascular Magnetic Resonance (SCMR) brings visitors up-to-date news about the organization with its online newsletters, as well as updates of its annual scientific sessions and related meetings. Issue contents and article abstracts of SCMR's official publication, the *Journal of Cardiovascular Magnetic Resonance,* are available at the site, as well as information on society membership opportunities. The education link offers literature reviews, an online "Case of the Month," and a magnetic resonance atlas tutorial.
http://www.scmr.org

MYOCARDIAL BIOPSY

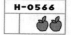

Cardiovascular Research Institute of Southern California: Heart Biopsy (Endomyocardial Biopsy) The nature and purpose of heart biopsy, patient preparation, details of the procedure, and patient recovery are summarized in this consumer fact sheet.
http://www.cvmg.com/education/test/biopsy.html

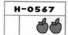

Hemodynamics This tutorial provides an introduction to hemodynamic waveforms at the basic level and gives examples and illustrations for the user. Venous, atrial, and arterial pressure tracings are available, as well as descriptions of common rhythms and their effects on cardiovascular hemodynamics, courtesy of the University of Tasmania Faculty of Health Science.
http://www.healthsci.utas.edu.au/physiol/tute1/hd.html

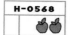

MEDLINEplus Medical Encyclopedia: Myocardial Biopsy Illustrations of the heart and basic information about the myocardial biopsy are supplied at this page of the National Library of Medicine. Why the test is performed, risks involved, and information on the meaning of abnormal results are outlined at this consumer-oriented reference. Additional links to conditions this test may reveal provide review of their symptoms, signs, diagnosis, and treatment.
http://www.nlm.nih.gov/medlineplus/ency/article/003873.htm

MYOCARDIAL INFARCTION SCAN

Ohio State University: Myocardial Infarction Scan Provided in PDF format, this consumer-oriented fact sheet introduces basic information about the myocardial infarction scan, including reasons the test is ordered and an overview of the procedure. Equipment used and warnings about radiation are addressed.
http://www.osu.edu/units/osuhosp/patedu/
homedocs.pdf/diagnost.pdf/nuclear.pdf/mi-scan.pdf

NUCLEAR IMAGING/MYOCARDIAL PERFUSION, GENERAL

Advances in Myocardial Perfusion Imaging   Provided by Siemens in the United Kingdom, this article addresses developments in myocardial perfusion imaging over the last decade. Information on newer pharmaceuticals used, advancements in positron emission tomography, and imaging protocols are discussed. Comparisons of myocardial perfusion agents, instrumentation and software advances in the field of cardiac nuclear medicine, the advent of pharmacological stress testing, and additional developments are reviewed.
http://www.siemens.co.uk/med/news/features/myocardial.htm

BrighamRAD: Atlas of Myocardial Perfusion SPECT   Presented by Brigham and Women's Hospital and Harvard Medical School, this online atlas offers general tutorials on normal myocardial perfusion single photon emission tomography (SPECT) imaging, cardiac pathophysiology, and basic imaging quality control. Chapters on radiopharmaceuticals used, stress protocols, imaging protocols, and quantification are included. Additionally, the site hosts several teaching cases that offer patient histories, text explanations, and annotated images. Normal heart variants, myocardial infarction, myocardial ischemia, and multivessel disease cases are available, in addition to a large selection of additional case studies and particularly challenging topics.
http://brighamrad.harvard.edu/education/online/Cardiac/main.html

NUCLEAR IMAGING: EXERCISE STRESS TEST

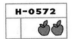

Deborah Heart and Lung Center: Nuclear Exercise Stress Testing
Intended for patients, this site offers a thorough explanation of nuclear exercise stress testing, including a description of isotopes used, special instructions, other types of exercise testing, and answers to FAQs.
http://www.deborah.org/consumer/nstress.html

Ohio State University: Stress Sestamibi Scan   Available in PDF format, this site offers a consumer information sheet on the stress sestamibi scan. Reasons the test may be ordered, precautions regarding radiation, and what to expect during the procedure are discussed.
http://www.osu.edu/units/osuhosp/patedu/
homedocs.pdf/diagnost.pdf/nuclear.pdf/stre-ses.pdf

Penn State: Thallium Stress Testing   From the Milton S. Hershey Medical Center, this site offers patient information about thallium stress testing, including a general description of the test, purpose, preparation, and posttest management instructions. Links to related articles are provided.
http://www.hersheyheart.com/pat_ed/pe123.htm

Prognostic Value of a Thallium Scan   The page at this Web address, authored by Scott Williams, M.D., presents clinical criteria for selecting patients

requiring further risk stratification and evaluates the usefulness of thallium scan imaging in unstable angina, post-myocardial infarction, and coronary artery disease. Assessment of a patient's likelihood for postoperative complications and the implications regarding further myocardial imaging studies are explored.
http://www.nmc.dote.hu/williams/NucMed/CV07.htm

NUCLEAR IMAGING: GATED BLOOD POOL SCAN (MUGA)

First Pass MUGA   Authored by Scott Williams, M.D., this article outlines radiopharmaceuticals used, technique, and findings for left to right shunt, right to left shunt, and stroke volume index.
http://www.indyrad.iupui.edu/public/lectures/HTML/NM-RM/NUCMED/CV16.HTM

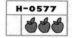

Frequently Asked Questions about Multi-Unit Gated Acquisition Scans   Answers to the most frequently asked questions regarding blood pool studies are provided at this Web address, with descriptions of the procedure and simple explanations of test preparations. Unique features of the site allow visitors to access an audible presentation of the procedure and to view an example scan and computer analysis data.
http://ns3.octet.com/~mikety/PtEd/Exams/MUGAQ.html

Mount Sinai School of Medicine: Gated Blood Pool Imaging   General information on gated blood pool imaging, also known as multi-unit gated acquisition (MUGA), is reviewed at this online fact sheet, with description of the test's ability to measure the ejection fraction of blood pumped. Reasons for ordering the test and differentiation between the resting and exercise MUGA are discussed. Preparations for exercise gated blood pool imaging and expectations regarding testing procedures are described, as a service of the Cardiovascular Institute.   http://www.mssm.edu/cvi/gated.shtml

Ohio State University: Resting MUGA   Available in PDF format, this document offers consumers an overview of resting MUGA testing and provides answers to commonly asked questions about radiation, test preparations, equipment, and procedures.
http://www.osu.edu/units/osuhosp/patedu/
homedocs.pdf/diagnost.pdf/nuclear.pdf/rest-mug.pdf

Ohio State University: Stress MUGA   Reasons why a stress MUGA test may be ordered and other information about test preparation are offered at this fact sheet, provided by the Ohio State University Department of Nuclear Medicine. Equipment used and what to expect during testing are discussed, as part of a Medical Center consumer information series.
http://www.osu.edu/units/osuhosp/patedu/
homedocs.pdf/diagnost.pdf/nuclear.pdf/stre-mug.pdf

NUCLEAR IMAGING: PHARMACOLOGIC STRESS TEST

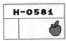

IV Persantine-Thallium Stress Test Offered by Torrance Memorial Medical Center, this site describes the IV Persantine-thallium stress test (IVP), including a definition and description of the test, its purpose, and necessary patient preparation.
http://www.torrancememorial.org/carivp.htm

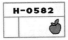

Ohio State University: Dipyridamole Stress Sestamibi Scan The dipyridamole stress sestamibi scan is discussed at this PDF document, courtesy of the Ohio State University Medical Center Department of Nuclear Medicine. Answers are provided to patient questions regarding purpose, radiation concerns, preparations, and equipment used.
http://www.osu.edu/units/osuhosp/patedu/
homedocs.pdf/diagnost.pdf/nuclear.pdf/dipy.pdf

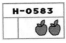

University of Michigan Health System: Adenosine Thallium Scan This fact sheet describes the adenosine thallium scan procedure, including information obtained, details of the process, patient monitoring activities, patient preparation, and preexisting conditions contraindicating the use of adenosine.
http://www.med.umich.edu/1libr/tests/testa02.htm

PERICARDIOCENTESIS

MEDLINEplus Medical Encyclopedia: Pericardiocentesis Presented by Adam.com, the site contains an overview of pericardiocentesis, also referred to as the pericardial tap. Details regarding test performance and sensory expectations; specific preparatory guidelines; depending upon age of patient; and a link to a listing of associated risks are provided. Abnormal causes of pericardial fluid accumulation are reviewed, as well as the anatomy and physiology of the heart and the pericardial sac.
http://www.nlm.nih.gov/medlineplus/ency/article/003872.htm

Technique of Pericardiocentesis Excerpted from the *Journal of Critical Illness,* this page reviews drainage of pericardial fluid for treatment of cardiac tamponade. Ideal tap location, needle insertion, and successful fluid removal are discussed and illustrated, and results of successful aspiration are stated.
http://icu-10.med.usyd.edu.au/ce/case1/pericardtext.html

PHARMACOLOGIC STRESS ECHOCARDIOGRAPHY

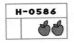

Florida Cardiovascular Institute: Dobutamine Stress Echocardiography Dobutamine stress echocardiography is summarized in this online information sheet, with an overview of the procedure, information on patient preparation, details of the process, and a discussion of results provided.
http://www.fciheart.com/DSE.htm

MCP Hahnemann University: Pharmacological Stress Echocardiography Dobutamine stress echocardiography and its usefulness in establishing a diagnosis of coronary artery disease or degree of myocardial ischemia in those unable to fully exercise is reviewed at this site of MCP Hahnemann University's Division of Continuing Medical Education. A description of the dobutamine infusion and additional procedural details are summarized. Additionally, the use of dobutamine stress echocardiography and its accuracy in myocardial viability detection are reviewed.
http://www.mcphu.edu/continuing/cme/medicine/v1n1/pharmacologic.htm

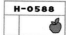

University of Michigan: Dobutamine Echocardiogram and Doppler Echocardiogram This University of Michigan site describes the dobutamine and Doppler electrocardiograms, including the risks involved, the procedure, and posttest management.
http://www.med.umich.edu/1libr/tests/testd08.htm

PHONOCARDIOGRAPHY

MDAdvice.com: Phonocardiography The various uses for phonocardiography are listed at this page, along with sensory factors, equipment used, and other descriptive test information. Intended for a consumer audience, this fact sheet includes information on what abnormal test results may indicate.
http://www.mdadvice.com/library/test/medtest287.html

POSITRON EMISSION TOMOGRAPHY (PET) SCAN

Crump Institute for Molecular Imaging: Clinical Positron Emission Tomography—Cardiology This tutorial from the University of California Los Angeles contains PET images that depict proper visualization of cardiac anatomy, with some anatomic labeling provided. The tutorial provides a framework for interpretation of cardiac pathology via PET scan, with simplification of images initially introduced. Modifications of the technique, views for various planes and the corresponding polar map, and enlargeable images of single and double vessel disease are shown. The lesson is completed by descriptions of tools for the assessment of myocardial metabolism and directions for identification of ischemia and idiopathic dilated cardiomyopathy.
http://www.crump.ucla.edu/lpp/clinpetcardio/evaluation.html

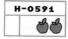

PET Research in Cardiology Provided by a Belgium PET laboratory, this site describes historical points of interest related to positron emission tomography in cardiac pathologies. Tracers used for cardiac imaging and problems specific to imaging in cardiovascular disease are introduced.
http://topo.topo.ucl.ac.be/cardiology.html

Tutorial: Clinical PET—Cardiology Homogeneous flow and metabolism patterns are displayed at this page, dedicated to clinical PET in cardiology. The

case presentation illustrates perfusion abnormalities under a state of increased myocardial stress.
http://nucmed.richis.org/case/CV/LPPh05.htm

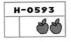

University of California Los Angeles (UCLA): The Power of Molecular Imaging   The UCLA Department of Molecular and Medical Pharmacology offers this 12-page PDF brochure on positron emission tomography, which describes the procedure's use in relation to coronary artery disease, cardiac transplantation, and bypass surgery. The site also provides links to other PET-related sites. http://www.nuc.ucla.edu/html_docs/frame_pet.html

POTASSIUM

MEDLINEplus Medical Encyclopedia: Potassium Test   Offered as a service of the National Library of Medicine, this encyclopedia entry reviews test preparations for children and reasons why serum potassium may be measured. Normal values are listed, as well as a link listing of disorders occurring with abnormally elevated or decreased levels. Additional conditions under which the test may be performed are included.
http://www.nlm.nih.gov/medlineplus/ency/article/003484.htm

RADIOGRAPHY

MDAdvice.com: Cardiac Radiography   Drawn from Yale University's *Complete Guide to Medical Tests,* this fact sheet reviews basic test components, test results, and possible meanings of an abnormal cardiac X-ray. Factors that may affect test accuracy are listed.
http://www.mdadvice.com/library/test/medtest122.html

SERUM CARDIAC MARKERS, GENERAL

American Heart Association (AHA): Blood Tests for Rapid Detection of Heart Attack   The AHA *Heart and Stroke Guide* provides this general presentation on the background of these tests, goals of rapid detection programs, steps for evaluating chest pain, and evaluation recommendations.
http://216.185.112.5/presenter.jhtml?identifier=4477

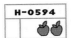

DrugBase: Blood and Genetic Tests Used to Determine Heart Disease Risk   Brief descriptions for six blood tests commonly used to assess a patient's level of heart disease risk are provided at the site. Included are triglyceride levels and additional measurement of substances known to be associated with blood clotting, cholesterol levels, and the genetic propensity towards heart disease. http://www.medinfo.co.za/data/med_info/tests.htm

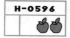

Medical University of South Carolina: Serum Cardiac Markers
Outlines at this page review the advantages and disadvantages of total creatine kinase, creatine kinase-MB isoenzyme, lactate dehydrogenase, troponin, and myoglobin cardiac markers. Related figures illustrate varying serum levels of each marker from onset of myocardial infarction.
http://www.musc.edu/~neilseea/scm.htm

Postgraduate Medicine: Role of Cardiac Markers in Evaluation of Suspected Myocardial Infarction Factors affecting choice and comparison of several cardiac markers are addressed, including a table rating characteristics of the ideal marker. Guidelines for selection of each marker, according to specificity, sensitivity, analytical factors, diagnostic and prognostic use, ease of measurement, and turnaround time for results, are offered.
http://www.postgradmed.com/issues/1997/11_97/mercer.htm

SIGNAL-AVERAGED ELECTROCARDIOGRAM

Clinical Cardiology: Signal-Averaged Electrocardiogram *Clinical Cardiology* offers this article abstract comparing the signal-averaged electrocardiogram (SAECG) to the standard 12-lead test. The greater sensitivity of SAECG markers for the detection of myocardial ischemia is explained.
http://clinical-cardiology.org/briefs/9906briefs/22-403.shtml

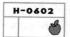

New York-Presbyterian: Signal-Averaged Electrocardiogram The university hospitals of Columbia and Cornell present this page of an online manual of diagnostic procedures. A brief review of the indications for the signal-averaged electrocardiogram, such as syncope or post - myocardial infarction risk assessment, is presented.
http://infonet.med.cornell.edu/lab/ancillary/
CGRAPH_Signal_Averaged_Electrocardiogram.htm

SINGLE PHOTON EMISSION COMPUTED TOMOGRAPHY (SPECT)

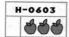

BrighamRAD: Atlas of Myocardial Perfusion SPECT From Brigham and Women's Hospital and Harvard Medical School comes this online atlas of myocardial perfusion single photon emission computed tomography (SPECT), containing more than 60 teaching cases, annotated images accompanied by text explanations, and a variety of navigational options. Normal SPECT imaging, cardiac pathophysiology, and imaging protocols are reviewed, as well as the histories, findings, and comments for fixed perfusion defects, myocardial ischemia, multivessel disease, and several other disease categories. The various radiopharmaceutical advantages and disadvantages are summarized, and special cases and techniques are discussed. The tutorial includes a glossary of abbreviations, a preview slide show of the various cases, and a quiz to test the user's diagnostic knowledge.
http://brighamrad.harvard.edu/education/online/Cardiac/Cardiac.html

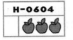

Emission Tomography This site provides a tutorial on emission tomography, along with a flowchart illustrating the stages of the diagnostic process. Also found are discussions on radioactivity and radionuclides used in medical imaging, measurement of the detected radiation, and tomographic imaging.
http://jura.stir.ac.uk/teaching/spect/web-tec.html

Stroke Tests

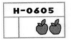

American Heart Association (AHA): Stroke Tests This section of the AHA *Heart and Stroke Guide* describes advances in medical diagnostics for stroke, including review of carotid phonoangiography, computerized axial tomographic scan, digital subtraction angiography, Doppler ultrasound, and evoked response tests. In addition, visitors will find a list of related Scientific Statements of the AHA and clinical practice guidelines for diagnostic imaging of transient ischemic attacks and stroke.
http://216.185.112.5/presenter.jhtml?identifier=4711

Tilt Table Test (TTT)

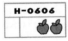

HeartSite.com: Tilt Table Test Questions regarding the tilt table test, used for the purpose of neurally mediated syncope diagnosis, are answered at this online brochure, provided as a service of the Heart Site. A review of the anatomy, physiology, and interaction of the sympathetic and parasympathetic nervous systems is summarized. Test performance details and photographs, with information on both positional change and sympathetic nervous system stimulation, are presented.
http://www.heartsite.com/html/tilt_test.html

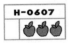

Postgraduate Medicine: Head-Upright Tilt Table Testing A discussion of the American College of Cardiology's consensus statement regarding how and when to evaluate patients with the tilt table technique is reviewed at this in-depth *Postgraduate Medicine* article. A summary of the current clinical understanding of vasovagal syncope, an overview of its evaluation, and complete review of the two basic tilt table testing methods are presented, including upright testing and isoproterenol infusion for increased sensitivity. Preparatory, positioning, and recording procedures are discussed, with definitions of five abnormal response patterns found.
http://www.postgradmed.com/issues/1998/01_98/grubb.htm

Transesophageal Echocardiogram (TEE)

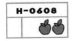

Florida Cardiovascular Institute: Transesophageal Echocardiography
A definition and detailed overview of transesophageal electrocardiogram are

available in this patient fact sheet, including details regarding patient preparation, a step-by-step procedural review, and information on test results.
http://www.fciheart.com/tee.htm

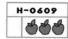

HeartSite.com: Transesophageal Echocardiogram   The differences between a standard echocardiogram and the transesophageal method are reviewed at this online brochure, courtesy of the Heart Site evaluation pages. Limitations of the ultrasound beams in transthoracic assessment are discussed, with patient preparatory procedures and the special indications of a transesophageal electrocardiogram reviewed. Moving images are available of a patient with a left atrial myxoma (heart tumor) before and after its removal.
http://www.heartsite.com/html/tee.html

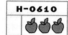

Place of Transesophageal Echocardiography in the Operating Room
The variety of uses for preoperative and intraoperative transesophageal electrocardiogram and other technological assessments of this diagnostic tool are reviewed at this in-depth article. Advancements in probe design and the test's unique ability to noninvasively assess cardiac structure and function are described, with future developments in image definition discussed. Category I, II, and III indications and guidelines recently published for perioperative procedures are noted, and further summaries on TEE's value during surgical procedures are presented. The test's application for monitoring myocardial ischemia and embolism and its general reliability in diagnosing most acute, perioperative hemodynamic problems are discussed.
http://www.md.ucl.ac.be/virtanes/pastedit/pe%20mar%2099.html

VENTRICULOGRAPHY

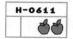

MEDLINEplus Medical Encyclopedia: Left Heart Ventricular Angiography   A definition of this diagnostic procedure, related illustrations of the heart, and information on how the test is performed are supplied at this National Library of Medicine resource. Offered by Adam.com, risks involved and information on normal and abnormal values are provided, as well as a link to the related left heart catheterization procedure.
http://www.nlm.nih.gov/medlineplus/ency/article/003875.htm

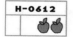

MEDLINEplus Medical Encyclopedia: Right Heart Ventriculography
Illustrations of the heart and catheter positioning are found at this patient reference site, as well as a definition of this angiography procedure and details on how the test is performed. Readers will find additional information on associated risks, links to related information, and the implications of abnormal results.   http://www.nlm.nih.gov/medlineplus/ency/article/003874.htm

6.6 PATHOLOGY AND CASE STUDIES

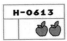

BrighamRAD: Acute Cerebral Infarction Computed tomography (CT), magnetic resonance imaging (MRI), and magnetic resonance angiography (MRA) of the head reveal findings consistent with acute cerebral infarct. Labeled descriptions and a detailed diagnostic discussion are provided, courtesy of Brigham and Women's Hospital and Harvard Medical School.
http://www.brighamrad.harvard.edu/Cases/bwh/hcache/93/full.html

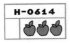

BrighamRAD: Atlas of Myocardial Perfusion SPECT This atlas, a part of the BrighamRAD project of Brigham and Women's Hospital and Harvard University, contains 70 clinical teaching cases. Information includes case history, imaging data, and myocardial perfusion single photon emission computed tomography (SPECT) images, with text explanations and tutorials on normal myocardial perfusion SPECT imaging, cardiac pathophysiology, basic imaging quality control, radiopharmaceuticals, stress protocols, imaging protocols, and quantification. The site provides links to other radiology and nuclear medicine-related sites. http://brighamrad.harvard.edu/education/online/Cardiac/Cardiac.html

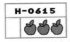

BrighamRAD: Carotid Artery Stenosis A case example of carotid artery stenosis is presented at this site of the Brigham and Women's Hospital and Harvard Medical School Teaching Case Database, with a collection of nine diagnostic images presented. A review of the findings is offered, and details are offered for each echocardiogram image. Other potential causes of elevated peak systolic and diastolic velocities are suggested.
http://www.brighamrad.harvard.edu/Cases/bwh/hcache/6/full.html

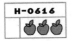

BrighamRAD: Cases This MedShare query result returns a list of cases involving disorders of the heart and great vessels, including aortic transection, coarctation of the aorta, right atrial myxoma, scimitar vein syndrome, thoracic outlet syndrome, and unilateral absence of pulmonary artery perfusion. Each presentation offers enlargeable imaging findings and a discussion of the diagnosis, courtesy of Brigham and Women's Hospital and Harvard University.
http://www.brighamrad.harvard.edu/cgi-bin/rc-report/query.py

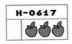

BrighamRAD: Partial Obstruction of the Superior Vena Cava A plain radiograph of the chest and contrast-enhanced computed tomography (CT) images reveal superior vena cava obstruction at this online case example, courtesy of the Brigham and Women's Hospital and Harvard Medical School Teaching Case Database. A description and discussion of the findings are offered, noting the frequency of malignant causes.
http://www.brighamrad.harvard.edu/Cases/bwh/hcache/58/full.html

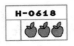

CARDIAX CARDIAX is a computer-aided instructional program of 20 planned cases in basic cardiology. The program uses text, digital images, audio, and QuickTime videos to teach the fundamentals of cardiac diagnosis. Included are plain film radiography, EKGs, heart sounds, ultrasound videos, and video vignettes. Intended users include medical students, residents, and practicing physicians. http://www.med.umich.edu/lrc/cardiax/cardiax.html

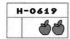

Chest Radiographs   This site, providing links to chest radiographs of patients with cardiac lesions, includes images of the normal chest, several views of mitral stenosis, cardiomyopathy, pericardial effusion, aortic stenosis, aortic regurgitation, mitral regurgitation, tetralogy of Fallot, atrial septal defect, ventricular septal defect, patent ductus, pulmonary valve stenosis, coarctation of the aorta, and atrial septal defect. A clinical discussion accompanies each image at the site, provided by South Bank University.
http://www.sbu.ac.uk/~dirt/museum/gs-first.html

Echo-Vascular.com   Showcasing the field of cardiovascular ultrasound, this site contains images, case studies, and links to echocardiography and vascular imaging case studies. An image index is available for those wishing to see images without accompanying text. Alternatively, visitors can choose to read more about particular images, in which cases individual case histories and discussions of image findings can be accessed. Related links are found at the end of each case presentation, as well as at the CME resource page.
http://www.wvc.net/~williams/daves/frame.htm

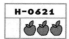

Electrocardiogram (ECG, EKG) Library   The ECG Library, a collection of realistic ECG recordings created by Stephen Gerred and Churchill Livingstone, provides healthcare professionals with the opportunity to improve their diagnostic skills. Categories of images include ischemic heart disease, hypertrophy patterns, atrioventricular block, bundle branch block, supraventricular rhythms, ventricular rhythms, pacemakers, and Wolff Parkinson White syndrome. An image of the normal adult 12-lead ECG is found, accompanied by a lengthy description. Hyperlinks to other library images are provided, and ECG-related sites on the World Wide Web can be accessed.
http://homepages.enterprise.net/djenkins/ecghome.html

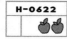

Emergency Medicine and Primary Care: EKG File Room   Irregularities and abnormalities in EKG readings are accessible from the site, which contains links to actual EKG tracings. Abnormal sinus rhythms, atrial fibrillations and flutters, myocardial infarction, and rhythms consistent with metabolic abnormalities can be viewed.
http://www.embbs.com/ekg/fileroom.html

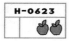

Heartpumper.com: Cardiac Pathology   Information on a selection of more than 20 congenital cardiac disorders is provided at this site. For each disorder, the site provides a definition and outlines clinical features and correction procedure options.
http://www.heartpumper.com/cardiac_pathology.html

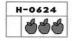

Internet Medical Education, Inc.: Physician Education Site for Cardiovascular Diseases   Intended for clinicians, this site offers an interactive tutorial on the electrocardiogram, complete with quizzes and an expert system for helping to diagnose dysrhythmias. Physician discussion forums and several subject reviews in cardiovascular diseases are offered, as well as two free search engines to the current medical literature. All tutorial materials and discussion groups are fully indexed.

http://www.med-edu.com/physician/index.html

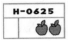

McGill Medical Informatics: Medical Teaching   Part of the *Online Journal of Cardiology,* this site contains links to the EKG World Encyclopedia, the "Virtual Stethoscope," echocardiograph and X-ray images, teaching videos, nuclear images, and multiple medical search engines.

http://www.mmip.mcgill.ca/heart/medt.html

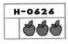

MDchoice.com: ECG Rounds   These ECG presentations offer professionals the opportunity to review more than a dozen example cases, including patients presenting with chest pain, anorexia, and palpitations. The ECG makes the diagnosis in each case, with links found to the 12-lead reading, higher resolution 12-lead ECG, and views of ECGs after appropriate treatment. The analysis links provide detailed explanations of ECG abnormalities.

http://www.mdchoice.com/ekg/ekg.asp

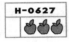

Med Files: Cardiovascular Links   Designed for healthcare professionals, this site contains cardiovascular case presentations and teaching files from various sources. Links are divided into cardiovascular topics, cardiovascular cases, and images. Pathophysiology files include angina, aortic insufficiency, aortic stenosis, atherosclerosis, carditis, congestive heart failure, endocarditis, hypertension, and vasculitis.

http://www.geocities.com/HotSprings/2255/heart.html

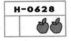

Medical Imaging: Cardiac Images   Pictures of the heart, captured from the Toshiba biplane cardiac catheterization system, are available for viewing at this site. Nearly a dozen clinical scenarios are depicted, including severe coronary artery disease, proximal coronary artery disease, coronary artery stent, and coronary atherectomy.

http://www.cvmg.com/education/images.html

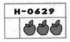

Radiology of Congenital Heart Disease in Neonates   Provided by South Bank University, this site's categories of images include transposition of the great arteries, hypoplasia and atresia, shunt situations, and anomalous pulmonary venous drainage. Numerous images are indexed under each category.

http://www.sbu.ac.uk/~dirt/museum/gs-fourth.html

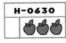

Society for Cardiovascular Pathology   Devoted to the advancement of the study of cardiovascular disorders, this society has over 200 active members with a wide range of interests in the field. The site provides information about the organization, including membership, meetings, announcements, and publications. Links to educational material, case studies, and additional cardiovascular pathology sites are found.

http://scvp.net/

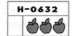 **University of Iowa College of Medicine: Case Studies of Aortic Aneurysms and Dissection** The case examples at this site of the University of Iowa Division of Physiological Imaging offer seven reviews of aortic aneurysm and dissection. Patient history, computed tomographic (CT) images, and reported measurements are provided. Volumetric imaging analysis and additional imaging methods allow further examination and optimal approaches for reduction of surgical risks. The site features additional file access to volumetric tools applied and online movies of CT data sets, oblique images, and shaded surface display (SSD).

http://everest.radiology.uiowa.edu/nlm/app/aorta/casestud.html

 University of Utah: Cardiovascular Pathology Index Part of the Pathology Laboratory for Medical Education, this site contains 130 images related to the heart and cardiovascular disease, including atherosclerotic cardiovascular disease, arterial dissection, infective endocarditis, myocarditis, congenital heart disease, cardiomyopathies, and arterial and venous diseases. Each image is accompanied by a clinical description. Views of the normal heart and a tutorial on myocardial infarction are provided.

http://www-medlib.med.utah.edu/WebPath/CVHTML/CVIDX.html#9

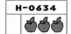 **Urbana Atlas of Pathology: Cardiovascular Volume** This extensive collection of online images, courtesy of the University of Illinois, offers a database in cardiovascular pathology. The assortment of over 40 topics and images ranges from aneurysms to tumor embolism, with each entry providing an enlargeable thumbnail image and slide description.

http://www.med.uiuc.edu/PathAtlasf/titlePage.html#vol2contents

6.7 PHARMACOLOGY

GENERAL RESOURCES

 British Medical Journal: ABC of Heart Failure Management: Digoxin and Other Inotropes, Beta Blockers, and Antiarrhythmic and Antithrombotic Treatment This technical article offers a detailed discussion of the use of digoxin and other inotropes, beta blockers, antithrombotic treatments, and antiarrhythmic treatments in the management of heart failure. Each therapeutic section is supported by graphs and tables illustrating results from clinical and demographic studies. Important clinical considerations of some therapies are summarized. The article also offers a review of the discussion in table format and a list of reference citations.

http://www.bmj.com/cgi/content/full/320/7233/495

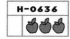 **British Medical Journal: ABC of Heart Failure Management: Diuretics, ACE Inhibitors, and Nitrates** This well-organized, article offers a summary of heart failure management goals, followed by individual assess-

ments of diuretics, ACE inhibitors, angiotensin receptor antagonists, oral nitrates and hydralazine, and other vasodilators. Tables, charts, and images accompany the discussions, and visitors can conduct PubMed searches for related articles referenced throughout the site.
http://www.bmj.com/cgi/content/full/320/7232/428

Cardiac HealthWeb: Heart Disease Medications
Part of the Cardiac HealthWeb, this site provides links to information from the American Heart Association detailing several types of cardiac medications. Included are anticoagulants, aspirin, cholesterol-lowering drugs, digitalis, heart attack treatments, potassium, and hormone replacement therapy. The RxList interaction check of the top 200 drugs is accessible from the site.
http://www.bev.net/health/cardiac/treatment.html

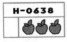

NetPharmacology
Contents of this online teaching center include six individual modules on cardiovascular pharmacology. Lecture notes introduce users to cardiovascular pharmacology and offer separate chapters on calcium channel blockers, antianginals, diuretics, antihypertensives, drugs used to treat congestive heart failure, and antiarrhythmics. A test question module, glossary, and a listing of figures, animations, and structures found in the tutorial are provided. The properties of prototypical cardiovascular drugs, categorized according to therapeutic application and mechanism of action, are reviewed at the cardiovascular drug list.
http://lysine.pharm.utah.edu/netpharm/

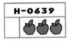

PDR.net
Departments for consumers, physicians, and other healthcare professionals are available from the home page of PDR.net. For consumers, PDR's "Getting Well Network" offers disease and drug information addressing a variety of medical concerns. Major advancements in pharmacology are available at the physician link, as well as free access to a number of publications, following a free registration process. Instant, online CME opportunities; several newsletters across a variety of medical specialties; and the MedEc Bookstore are additional features of the PDR.net pages, published by Medical Economics, Inc. Access to drug monographs from the _Physicians' Desk Reference and entry to the online version of *Stedman's Medical Dictionary* are available to registered visitors. (some features fee-based) http://www.pdr.net/

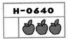

PharmLinks: Cardiovascular Drugs
Antithrombotics, antiarrhythmics, blood-lipid-lowering agents, antihypertensives, antianginals, calcium-entry blocking agents, and drugs for therapy of congestive heart failure are all examined at this online tutorial. Information on prototypes and other drugs is provided and includes actions, therapeutic effects, and nontherapeutic effects as well as toxicities for each. Links to example indications and uses are found, offering further details on prescribing.
http://www.md.huji.ac.il/mirrors/netpharm/dlmaster.htm

Aldosterone Antagonists (Spironolactone)

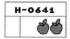

RxList: Spironolactone   From this page, viewers can access complete information on spironolactone, including a basic product description, clinical pharmacology, indications and dosage, side effects and drug interactions, warnings, contraindications, and a related patient FAQ and monograph. Several hyperlinked definitions are available, extracted and abridged from *Taber's Online*.
http://www.rxlist.com/cgi/generic/spiron.htm

Alpha Blockers

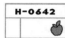

aHealthyMe: Alpha1-Adrenergic Blockers   Intended for consumers, this fact sheet reviews the purpose of alpha blockers in controlling high blood pressure, as well as other uses for these drugs. A summary of recommended dosage and administration, common side effects and those warranting attention from a physician, and key drug interactions are discussed.
http://www.ahealthyme.com/topic/topic100586413

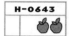

HealthEvolution.com: Alpha Blockers   An overview of adrenergic antagonists is presented at this site, with specific information on alpha blockers and indications for their use. Mode of action, possible side effects, drug interactions, and special conditions to observe are stated.
http://www.healthevolution.com/Articles/AlphaBlockers.html

Angiotensin Converting Enzyme (ACE) Inhibitors

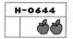

ACE Inhibitors   A list of chemical and brand names for nearly a dozen ACE inhibitors is followed by a brief discussion of treatment with these drugs. The site describes the action of ACE inhibitors and alternatives to ACE inhibitors, including angiotensin blockers, nitrates, and hydralazine. Links are available to detailed information on these drugs, courtesy of Cardiovascular Consultants Medical Group.
http://healthyhearts.com/acei.htm

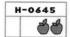

HealthInformatics.com: ACE Inhibitors   Providing health education on the Internet, this site offers data specifically on ACE inhibitors. Information, presented by Donald L. Warkentin, M.D., includes a general explanation of the medication, when it should be used, what dosage should be given, and risks associated with the drug.
http://www.healthinformatics.com/docs/english/CA/aceinhib.car.asp

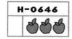

MEDLINEplus Health Information: Angiotensin Converting Enzyme Inhibitors (Systemic)   Brand names, drug categories, and a thorough description of ACE inhibitors are presented at this site, supplied by the National

Library of Medicine. Drug warnings, interactions, and proper medication usage are provided, as well as more common, less common, and rare side effects. http://www.nlm.nih.gov/medlineplus/ druginfo/angiotensinconvertingenzymeace202044.html

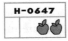

Partners for Healthy Aging: ACE Inhibitors Details of ACE inhibitors available from this fact sheet include brand and generic names, proper use, possible side effects and drug interactions, and other important points about these drugs. Special warnings are also listed. http://www.merck-medco.com/medco/myhealth/article_router.jsp?OID=9687

ANGIOTENSIN II INHIBITORS

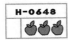

American Family Physician: Angiotensin II Receptor Antagonists This clinical pharmacology article, courtesy of the American Academy of Family Physicians, reviews angiotensin II receptor antagonists and their current role in antihypertensive therapy. Discussion of the renin-angiotensin-aldosterone system, specific angiotensin II receptor antagonists, their pharmacokinetic parameters, and dosing considerations for each are presented in text and table formats. Side effects and drug interactions are reviewed, and a discussion of investigations into the use of angiotensin II receptor antagonists in the treatment of heart failure is provided. http://www.aafp.org/afp/990600ap/3140.html

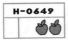

University of British Columbia: Angiotensin II Receptor Blockers Part of the evidence-based drug therapy Therapeutics Initiative, this issue of the *Therapeutics Letter* offers review of the indications, mechanism of action, and evidence for use of angiotensin II receptor blocker agents in hypertension management. A table of drugs outlines basic properties of each, and evidence for use in congestive heart failure, adverse events, and cost considerations are introduced. http://www.ti.ubc.ca/pages/letter28.htm

ANTIANGINAL AGENTS, GENERAL

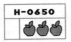

Agency for Healthcare Research and Quality (AHRQ): Evaluation of Beta-Blockers, Calcium Antagonists, Nitrates, and Alternative Therapies for Stable Angina A discussion of first-line choices for antianginal treatment is provided at this site, which offers a systematic review of the literature. Researched by investigators at the University of California San Francisco-Stanford Evidence-based Practice Center, the efficacy and safety data for beta blockers, calcium antagonists, and long-acting nitrates and information on alternative treatments are provided. A summary of findings and implications for future research are presented, with access to the full report available from the site. http://www.ahcpr.gov/clinic/anginasu.htm

NetPharmacology: Antianginal Agents   NetPharmacology of the University of Utah offers this collection of cardiovascular teaching materials, specific to antianginal agents. Links to information on nitrovasodilators, calcium channel blockers, and beta-adrenergic antagonists are found, along with review of mechanism of action, therapeutic effects, and nontherapeutic effects and toxicities of each. Indications, contraindications, drug interactions, and miscellaneous drug information are offered. Additional features of the site include molecular structure diagrams, pronunciation audio files, and hyperlinks to related information throughout the pages.
http://lysine.pharm.utah.edu/netpharm/netpharm_00/druglist/dl_ang.htm

Oklahoma College of Pharmacy: Chemistry of Antianginal Agents and Peripheral Vasodilators   Including information on organic nitrates/nitrites, calcium channel blockers, peripheral vasodilators, and beta blockers, this slide tutorial reviews the properties and mechanisms of actions of the various antianginal agents. Pharmacologic names, chemical composition, and key information about each drug are noted.
http://www.pharmacy.ouhsc.edu/basmadjian/Slides/Antianginal7824_files/frame.htm

ANTIARRHYTHMIC AGENTS, GENERAL

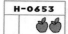

Antiarrhythmic Agents   Antiarrhythmic agents are summarized at this site, which provides a list of chemical and brand names and is followed by a discussion of therapeutic uses. The advantages of these drugs for the treatment of fast heart rhythms, alternatives to antiarrhythmic agents, side effects, and proper diagnosis and treatment decisions are discussed, courtesy of Cardiovascular Consultants Medical Group. Links are available to information on related drugs and other topics.   http://healthyhearts.com/antiarrh.htm

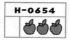

Arrhythmia.net   The Arrhythmia.net home page offers a large collection of links for antiarrhythmic agents, case histories and studies, publications, and international meeting information. Treatment pages on acute atrial fibrillation and ventricular arrhythmias are found, and clinical use of several antiarrhythmic agents is detailed. Manuscript abstracts of published randomized trials and adverse event analyses are viewable, as well as patient management histories and online treatment manuals. An A-to-Z guide to cardiology offers a list of 35 pharmacology and disorder topics, with accessible outlines of clinical significance, including implantable defibrillators, restenosis, specific drug details, and long QT syndrome. At the home page, connections to related links provide resources on management of abnormal heart rhythms, advances in biomedical research, ischemic stroke treatment, and molecular cardiology.
http://www.arrhythmia.net

Anticoagulants

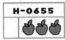

AHA Medical/Scientific Statement: Guide to Anticoagulant Therapy Part 1: Heparin Heparin is the focus of this scientific document, including a review of the thrombotic process and its complications. The clinical consequences of thrombosis, the need for anticoagulant therapy, and pharmacokinetics and pharmacodynamics of therapy are discussed. Preferred routes of administration and limitations of heparin usage are described, with several supporting tables and figures.
http://216.185.112.5/presenter.jhtml?identifier=1257

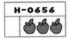

Anticoagulants Anticoagulant and thrombolytic agents are reviewed at this site, which explains the properties of these drugs, their mechanisms of action, and the differences between the clot-dissolving intravenous heparin and the subcutaneously administered low molecular weight heparins (LMWH). A discussion regarding oral coumadin and the necessity of monitoring via the International Normalized Ratio (INR) is found. A link to further facts about thrombolytic agents is also available, courtesy of Cardiovascular Consultants Medical Group. http://www.cardiacconsultants.com/anticoag.htm

Antihypertensives, General

HeartCenterOnline: Antihypertensives Intended for a consumer audience, this address offers a summary of antihypertensive medications, which includes a multimedia presentation on the mechanisms associated with high blood pressure. By scrolling through the pages, viewers will find basic information on diuretics, alpha blockers, beta blockers, and vasodilator medications. Links to more in-depth information about specific drugs are provided, as well as a discussion of how physicians make appropriate drug selections. Both general and specific listings of side effects are offered. A printer-friendly version of this site can be viewed.
http://www.heartcenteronline.com/myheartdr/common/articles.cfm?artid=382

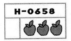

NetPharmacology: Antihypertensive Agents This comprehensive guide to antihypertensive drugs is provided as part of the University of Utah's Net-Pharmacology tutorial and offers information on specific antihypertensives and clinical strategies in patient management. A hypertension treatment algorithm outlines initial drug selection, lifestyle modifications, and indications for specific drugs. Considerations for choosing treatments across a variety of populations, along with pharmacologic details specific to diuretics, calcium channel blockers, sympatholytics, vasodilators, angiotensin converting enzyme (ACE) inhibitors, and angiotensin II antagonists, are presented.
http://lysine.pharm.utah.edu/netpharm/netpharm_00/notes/antihypertensives.html

The Pharmaceutical Journal: Drug Interactions That Matter, Antihypertensives Derived from CME material from *The Pharmaceutical Jour-*

nal, this page offers an article on the drug interactions of antihypertensives. Given the large number of prescription drugs offered and written, the article is dedicated to providing clinicians with awareness of both more and less common events that occur in clinical practice. Mechanisms of drug interactions for diuretics, beta-blockers, calcium channel blockers, drugs affecting the renin-angiotensin system, centrally acting antihypertensives, alpha blockers, and vasodilator antihypertensives are considered.

http://www.pharmj.com/Editorial/19990417/education/antihypertensives.html

ANTIPLATELET AGENTS/ASPIRIN

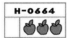

AHA Medical/Scientific Statement: Aspirin as a Therapeutic Agent in Cardiovascular Disease This paper, intended for healthcare professionals, contains a summary and recommendations for use of aspirin in the treatment of cardiovascular disease. Aspirin therapy for acute myocardial infarction, secondary prevention, and primary prevention are considered.

http://216.185.112.5/presenter.jhtml?identifier=1760

American Heart Association (AHA): Aspirin in Heart Attack and Stroke Prevention AHA recommendations concerning the use of aspirin in patients who have suffered a myocardial infarction, unstable angina, ischemic stroke, or transient ischemic attack are summarized at this consumer fact sheet. The site lists clinical indications of regular aspirin use and possible contraindications to prolonged therapy. Recommendations on the use of aspirin in primary prevention are presented, and cautions related to aspirin therapy and alcohol use are summarized. Related AHA topics are listed and can be accessed through the site's search engine.

http://216.185.112.5/presenter.jhtml?identifier=4456

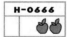

Antiplatelet Agents Antiplatelet agents discussed in this consumer fact sheet include aspirin, ticlopidine, clopidogrel, aggrenox, cilostazol, and abciximab, courtesy of the Cardiovascular Consultants Medical Group. Chemical and brand names are listed, and a brief discussion of platelets, the coagulation system, and platelet inhibition is available. Links are provided to discussions of related topics.

http://healthyhearts.com/antiplat.htm

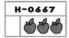

Aspirin Foundation of America A brief history of aspirin therapy is found at this site, which serves as a central source of information on aspirin and aspirin products. The site is divided into three sections, covering news, consumer information, and professional review. Each department offers information concerning the drug's mechanism of action, pain relief, and use in heart attack and stroke prevention, with both fundamental and clinical details provided. Press releases regarding the use of aspirin and related products are accessible.

http://www.aspirin.org

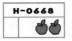

SpringNet: Glycoprotein Inhibitors and Acute Coronary Syndromes

This site offers a tutorial on glycoprotein inhibitors and their effects in easing acute coronary syndromes. An example case assessment and a checklist for monitoring patients during antiplatelet therapy are provided. Contraindications, similar to those for thrombolytic agents, and information on reducing complications are offered.

http://www.springnet.com/ce/p912b.htm

ANTITHROMBOTIC AGENTS, GENERAL

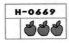

Oregon Health Sciences University (OHSU): Antithrombotic Therapy

The article at this site, authored by a physician at Oregon Health Sciences University, discusses the use of the antithrombotic, heparin; use of low molecular weight heparin (LMWH); and drug complications, such as heparin-induced thrombocytopenia (HIT). Warfarin therapy guided by prothrombin time is examined, and the advantages of the International Normalized Ration (INR), complications of the drug, and recommendations regarding phytonadione (vitamin K) dosing and INR reversal in these cases are outlined. Review of several antiplatelet agents and a summary of indications for antithrombotic therapy are provided, including special situations related to atrial fibrillation, acute myocardial infarction, rheumatic valve disease, and primary prevention.

http://www.ohsu.edu/som-hemonc/handouts/deloughery/antianti.shtml

BETA BLOCKERS

Beta Blockers

The therapeutic uses of beta blockers, possible side effects, and the function of these medications are summarized in this fact sheet, courtesy of the Cardiovascular Consultants Medical Group. A chart lists generic and brand names of many beta blockers, and links are available to information on lowering cholesterol levels.

http://healthyhearts.com/beta.htm

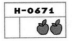

Medscape Cardiology: Beta-blockers in the Management of Cardiovascular Disease

A CME activity is available free-of-charge, following Medscape's free registration process. Chapters of the program, sponsored by Johns Hopkins, address physiology of the adrenergic system, beta-blockers in heart failure, beta-blockers in hypertension, and fixed-dose combination therapy.

http://www.medscape.com/medscape/
cardiology/TreatmentUpdate2000/tu01/public/toc-tu01.html

CALCIUM CHANNEL BLOCKERS

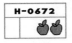

Calcium Channel Blockers

General information on calcium channel blockers is available at this consumer fact sheet, including a list of therapeutic

uses, physiologic actions of the medication, and possible side effects. The site offers a chart summarizing generic and brand names of calcium channel blockers, as a service of the Cardiovascular Consultants Medical Group.
http://healthyhearts.com/ccb.htm

Emory University: Calcium Channel Blockers Revisited An extensive study and slide presentation on the use of calcium channel blockers is found at this site, including discussion of antihypertensive agents and cardiovascular risk and selection of antihypertensive therapy for elderly patients. These topics and several subtopics can be accessed using the site's table of contents. The slide presentation is fully indexed, and a selection of CME information is offered.
http://www.cc.emory.edu/WHSC/MED/CME/CCB/toc.html

Centrally Acting Agents (Antihypertensives)

Prescriptions and Health: Centrally Acting Agents Centrally acting agents, used in the treatment of high blood pressure, are reviewed at this consumer fact sheet, courtesy of Merck-Medcot. Brand and generic names, proper use, possible side effects, drug interactions, additional clinical uses, and special patient warnings are listed. The site emphasizes that these drugs are seldom used in the elderly.
http://www.merckmedco.com/medco/myhealth/article_router.jsp?OID=9697

Chelation Therapy

American Heart Association (AHA): Chelation Therapy From the American Heart Association's *Heart and Stroke Guide,* this site offers questions and answers relating to chelation therapy, as well as a discussion regarding the lack of adequate, controlled scientific studies to support this therapy for coronary artery disease.
http://216.185.112.5/presenter.jhtml?identifier=4493

Coenzyme Q10

American Heart Association (AHA): Coenzyme Q10 Details on this antioxidant, fat-soluble substance and its function in the body are reviewed, as part of the AHA's consumer education series. The need for further evaluation of the safety and effectiveness of coenzyme Q10 as a therapeutic intervention is stressed, and a list of related publications on antioxidant vitamins and dietary/lifestyle interventions is provided, with documents accessible via the site's search engine.
http://216.185.112.5/presenter.jhtml?identifier=4564

WebMDHealth: Coenzyme Q10 Information from advocates of coenzyme Q10 is presented at this site, including its possible benefits and a basic description of its role in energy production. Good dietary sources of the substance, special precautions, and typical dosage are introduced.
http://my.webmd.com/content/article/3187.13545

CONGESTIVE HEART FAILURE DRUGS, GENERAL

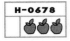

American Family Physician: The Importance of Beta Blockers in the Treatment of Heart Failure From the Practical Therapeutics series, this article of the American Academy of Family Physicians offers general information on heart failure and review of studies suggesting significant benefits of the addition of beta blockers in heart failure therapy. Comparisons of various treatments used in mortality trials in patients with heart failure are presented, as well as details on patient selection, agent selection and dosing, adjunct pharmacologic therapy, and contraindications to beta blocker treatment. A related editorial can be accessed.
http://www.aafp.org/afp/20001201/2453.html

Huffington Center on Aging: Commonly Used Drugs in the Management of Congestive Heart Failure A convenient online table outlines the dosages, principal site of action, target dose, and adverse effects associated with nine categories of congestive heart failure treatments. Direct vasodilators, nitrates, ACE inhibitors, digitalis glycosides, and thiazides are included.
http://www.hcoa.org/hcoacme/drug.htm

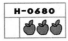

Postgraduate Medicine: Drug Therapy for Congestive Heart Failure
This portion of a *Postgraduate Medicine* symposium offers discussion of several appropriate choices for prognostic improvement in patients with congestive heart failure. Treatment goals, the effects of various medications, and suggestions for management and follow-up are reviewed. A summary of the Agency for Healthcare Policy Research and Quality (AHRQ)guidelines, discussion of diuretic resistance, and practices with combination therapy are presented.
http://www.postgradmed.com/issues/1997/01_97/sorr2.htm

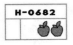

Virtualdrugstore.com: Congestive Heart Failure Fact sheets on two investigational therapies for the treatment of congestive heart failure are found at this site of the Virtualdrugstore. Product monographs outline drug usage, side effects and precautions, and current literature references.
http://www.virtualdrugstore.com/CHF/index.html

DIGOXIN/CARDIAC GLYCOSIDES

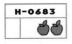

Familydoctor.org: Digoxin Published by the American Academy of Family Physicians, this consumer fact sheet outlines the uses of digoxin and states recommendations for dosing. Additional information includes medicines and foods

that can decrease drug absorption, possible side effects, and recommendations regarding when to contact a healthcare provider.
http://familydoctor.org/handouts/241.html

RxList: Digoxin Providing information on the generic digoxin, this RxList site offers comprehensive information on this cardiac glycoside. A general description is found and information on how the drug is supplied is included. Categories, brand name and foreign brand availability, cost considerations, and a complete review of clinical pharmacology are presented. A related patient FAQ and drug monograph can be accessed.
http://www.rxlist.com/cgi/generic/dig.htm

DIURETICS, GENERAL

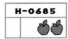

Diuretics Loop and thiazide diuretics are described at this fact sheet, including therapeutic uses, mechanisms of function, and possible side effects. Generic and brand names are listed in table format. Potassium sparing and combination diuretics are included, courtesy of the Cardiovascular Consultants Medical Group. http://healthyhearts.com/diuretic.htm

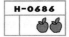

MEDLINEplus Medical Encyclopedia: Antihypertensives—Thiazide and Related Diuretics MEDLINE's Medical Encyclopedia includes this page addressing poisoning from a thiazide or related diuretic. Sources of toxicity, symptoms, and prognosis are examined.
http://www.nlm.nih.gov/medlineplus/ency/article/002577.htm

FOLIC ACID

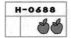

American Heart Association (AHA): Homocysteine, Folic Acid, and Cardiovascular Disease Offered as part of the AHA's online encyclopedia of publications, this page discusses recommendations of the organization regarding the role of folic acid and B vitamins in the reduction of heart disease and stroke. The relationship of homocysteine to cardiovascular disease is explained, with two reports cited that strengthen the evidence of the connection. Mechanisms by which folic acid and other B vitamins affect homocysteine levels are also introduced.
http://216.185.112.5/presenter.jhtml?identifier=4677

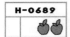

Linus Pauling Institute: CVD Prevention and Treatment by Diet and Supplements Focusing exclusively on the relationship between homocysteine, folic acid, and cardiovascular disease, this paper examines previous research on the connections. Possibilities with regard to correction of homocysteine levels and the need for clinical trial conclusions are stated.
http://www.orst.edu/dept/lpi/conference/malinow.html

HORMONE REPLACEMENT THERAPY/
ESTROGEN REPLACEMENT THERAPY

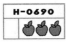

American Heart Association (AHA): Estrogen and Cardiovascular Diseases in Women   With the goal of keeping consumers aware of the issues related to hormone replacement therapy (HRT) and estrogen replacement therapy, this site offers a comprehensive introduction to the subject. Awaiting definitive clinical recommendations for the use of hormone replacement therapy or estrogen replacement therapy in the prevention of cardiovascular disease, this site examines the current state of knowledge on the subject. A link to key questions and answers regarding HRT summarizes new recommendations of the AHA, which can viewed in their entirety from a link at this site.
http://www.americanheart.org/Heart_and_Stroke_A_Z_Guide/estrogen.html

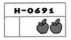

American Medical Association (AMA): Heart and Estrogen-Progestin Replacement Study (HERS)   A summary of the Heart and Estrogen-Progestin Replacement Study can be accessed from this page, discussing the lack of direct evidence connecting hormone replacement therapy and coronary heart disease risk reduction. Information on the Women's Health Initiative, which may serve to reconcile previously conflicting research, is provided.
http://www.ama-assn.org/cmeselec/part3/dt_estrofx3.htm#

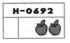

Doctor's Guide: Scientists Suggest Genetic Shutdown Links Estrogen with Heart Disease   The results of a recent Johns Hopkins study of heart disease and estrogen, published in *Cardiovascular Research,* are described in this article, posing questions about the benefits of hormone replacement therapy for individuals with existing coronary artery disease. Research focused on estrogen receptors in blood vessels and their inability to respond to estrogen's effects is discussed. An increase in the number of methylated genes as one ages is a possible explanation being explored and is discussed at this online article.
http://www.pslgroup.com/dg/1272c6.htm

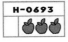

Facts about Hormone Replacement Therapy and Heart Disease: Postmenopausal Estrogen/Progestin Interventions (PEPI) Trial   Discussion of the accumulated evidence of coronary heart disease risk in postmenopausal women and facts regarding hormone replacement therapy are presented at the site, which provides results of the Postmenopausal Estrogen/Progestin Interventions Trial, sponsored by the National Heart, Lung, and Blood Institute (NHLBI) and other divisions of the National Institutes of Health (NIH). The goals of the study and a publication of its interpretation are found at the site. The document may be viewed online in plain text or PDF format. Multiple copies are available for purchase.
http://www.nhlbi.nih.gov/health/public/heart/other/hrt_pepi.htm

Inotropic Drugs, General

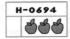

CVPharmacology: Inotropes   From the National University of Singapore, this site offers a definition of inotropic drugs. A discussion of cardiac glycosides pharmacologic action, information on beta adrenergic agonists, and an examination of phosphodiesterase inhibitors are presented.
http://www.med.nus.edu.sg/phar/medlect/inotropes.htm

Lipid Lowering Agents

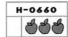

American Family Physician: Effective Use of Statins to Prevent Coronary Heart Disease   Authored by Michael A. Crouch, M.D., of Baylor College of Medicine, this American Academy of Family Physicians article discusses primary and secondary prevention trials of statins and their role in coronary event reduction. An overview of lipid management, pharmacologic treatment for primary prevention, pharmacologic intervention for secondary prevention, and a table of data derived from five major controlled trials of statins are presented. Drug selection, cost-effectiveness, and a related consumer information handout are available.
http://www.aafp.org/afp/20010115/309.html

American Heart Association (AHA): Cholesterol-Lowering Drugs   Intended for a consumer audience, this AHA publication offers general information on cholesterol-lowering drugs. Guidelines for those who qualify for therapy are outlined, and drugs most commonly prescribed are discussed. Additional drugs available for treatment of high cholesterol and the concepts behind combination therapy are introduced. Related pamphlets on dietary cholesterol, the cholesterol ratio, and cholesterol screening, as well as several other diagnosis and treatment guides, are available.
http://216.185.112.5/presenter.jhtml?identifier=163

Cholesterol-Lowering Medications   Cholesterol, heart disease risks, cholesterol-lowering drugs, and suggested lifestyle changes are reviewed at this site, in an effort to reduce cholesterol levels. Resins, fibrates, statins, and niacin are all described in detail, and a chart summarizes generic and brand names of these medications. Links are also available to discussions of related topics in heart disease management.
http://healthyhearts.com/cholmeds.htm

Magnesium Therapy

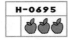

Clinical Cardiology: Magnesium Disorders and Cardiovascular Diseases   A professional article from East Carolina University, presenting research into magnesium disorders and cardiovascular diseases, is reviewed at this address. The article and review discuss the role of magnesium in the pathogene-

sis and treatment of heart disease. Epidemiology and specific diseases associated with magnesium deficiencies are discussed in detail, including ischemic heart disease, atherosclerosis, diabetes, dyslipidemia, hypertension, other coronary artery disease risk factors, coronary artery spasm, thrombosis, myocardial infarction, cardiomyopathy, congestive heart failure, and arrhythmias. Reference citations are provided.
http://www.execpc.com/~cc/disorder.html

MYOCARDIAL INFARCTION THERAPY, GENERAL

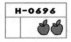

Heart Attack Survivors   Medications used to improve the outcome and survival of heart attack survivors are discussed at this Web site, sponsored by Cardiovascular Consultants Medical Group. In-depth information on antiplatelet agents, beta blockers, and angiotensin converting enzyme (ACE) inhibitors is found, as well as additional details on risk factor modification.
http://www.healthyhearts.com/misurvivor.htm

Postgraduate Medicine: Pharmacologic Therapy for Acute Myocardial Infarction   Authored by Elliot Rappaport, M.D., this part of an online symposium in myocardial infarction management addresses the pharmacologic aspects of treatment. Significant changes in management in recent years, the benefits of nitrates and recent studies of related mortality rates, and conclusions of the writer are presented. Similar information regarding aspirin in patients with unstable angina, the rationale behind beta blocker prescribing during early phases of acute myocardial infarction, and treatment recommendations are found. The article also offers review of clinical studies that have evaluated the role of ACE inhibition in both the acute and recovery phases of treatment.
http://www.postgradmed.com/issues/1997/11_97/rapaport.htm

NITRATES

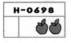

Nitrates   This fact sheet, provided by the Cardiovascular Consultants Medical Group, offers information on the mechanism of this class of drugs, dosage suggestions, and common side effects of nitrates. A list of generic and brand names is also available, in addition to links to information on related topics.
http://healthyhearts.com/nitrates.htm

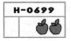

RxList: Nitroglycerin   The RxList provides clinical pharmacology information to professional readers, as well as details on indications and dosing, side effects, drug interactions, and overdosage of nitroglycerin. Related patient pages are available, answering frequently asked questions about the drug. The variety of brand names, foreign brand availability, and delivery systems used are reviewed.   http://www.rxlist.com/cgi/generic/ntg.htm

POTASSIUM

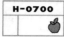

American Heart Association (AHA): Potassium   Basic information on the essential role of potassium in the body and details on causes of deficiency are cited at this consumer publication. Review of potassium supplementation and foods rich in the element are presented. Links to related brochures of the organization can be accessed, including those on dietary guidelines.
http://216.185.112.5/presenter.jhtml?identifier=4680

SYMPATHOLYTICS, GENERAL

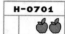

University of Manchester Hypertension Page: Sympatholytics   A general discussion on mechanisms of action of this drug class and seven main subclasses is presented at this site, which also addresses adverse effects and specific indications. Related figures are available throughout the text, illustrating drug effects.
http://www.teaching-
biomed.man.ac.uk/student_projects/2000/mnpm6ven/sympatholytics.htm

THROMBOLYTIC THERAPY

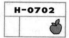

American Heart Association (AHA): Tissue Plasminogen Activator
The role of tissue plasminogen activator (tPA) in dissolving clots responsible for causing heart attacks is discussed at this page. This AHA site defines tPA, describes its benefits, and lists related publications and AHA guidelines.
http://216.185.112.5/presenter.jhtml?identifier=4751

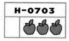

Circulation: Guidelines for Thrombolytic Therapy for Acute Stroke
These supplemental guidelines for the management of patients with acute ischemic stroke provide levels of evidence and grading of recommendations for treatment, in addition to results of recent clinical trials of various thrombolytic agents. Studies of the National Institute of Neurological Disorders and Stroke (NINDS) and other reputable sources are reviewed, as well as recommendations regarding management protocols in specific populations, in emergent care, and for complications of therapy. Risk ratios for long-term mortality and death are presented, and referenced MEDLINE abstracts are available from this AHA publication site.   http://circ.ahajournals.org/cgi/content/full/94/5/1167

Clot Dissolving Agents (Thrombolytic Agents)   Thrombolytic agents given intravenously to rapidly dissolve blood clots are profiled at this fact sheet. Therapeutic uses are summarized, and the use of thrombolytic agents versus emergency angioplasty is mentioned. The site, provided as a service of Cardiovascular Consultants Medical Group, also offers a list of generic and brand names of thrombolytic agents and a link to information on angioplasty.
http://healthyhearts.com/lytics.htm

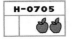

Internet Medical Education, Inc.: Thrombolytic ("Clot Buster") Therapy   The pharmacological method of eliminating blood clots is described at this site, with current medical theory discussed, criteria given, and contraindications to thrombolytic drugs reviewed. Debate over the use of thrombolytic agents in contrast to urgent surgical intervention is found.
http://www.med-edu.com/patient/cad/thrombolytics.html

VASODILATORS, GENERAL

Dr. Joseph F. Smith Medical Library: Vasodilators   The use of vasodilators in the treatment of hypertension is described at this page, in addition to recommended drug dosage and special precautions to consider while taking this medicine. Issues relating to allergies, pregnancy, drug interactions, and side effects are addressed.
http://www.chclibrary.org/micromed/00070010.html

Xrefer: Vasodilators   Differences between coronary vasodilators and peripheral vasodilators are discussed at this encyclopedia entry, as well as the main classes of vasodilator drugs. Common side effects are reviewed, courtesy of the Oxford University Press *Dictionary of Medicine*.
http://www.xrefer.com/entry/475948

6.8 PROCEDURES/THERAPIES

GENERAL RESOURCES

American College of Surgeons (ACS)   The American College of Surgeons is an association of professionals founded to improve the quality of patient care through education and the implementation of high standards. The site provides information about the organization, including its departments and divisions, board of regents, advisory councils, and board of governors. Education and surgical services, fellowships, publications, legislative affairs, and recent news are provided, as well as a link to public statements and guidelines published by the college.
http://www.facs.org

Cardiothoracic Surgery Network (CTSNet)   The goal of CTSNet is to provide a comprehensive source of information, news, and communication opportunities for professionals in the field of cardiothoracic surgery. The site contains a section on experts' techniques, in which the latest surgical procedures are described and illustrated with video clips. Resources for professionals include lists of surgeons, associates, organizations, journals, books, job opportunities, and upcoming events. A special section for residents, discussion forums, clinical

trials, a product forum, Web reviews, answers to frequently asked questions, and a chapter dedicated to the achievements of members are included.
http://www.ctsnet.org/doc/2172

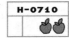

Coronary Artery Surgery Forum   Devoted to all those interested in coronary artery surgery, this site publishes surgical procedures, concepts, new ideas, proposed and completed research, and discussion of coronary artery surgery submissions collected from users. Topics submitted for discussion include shortness of breath, coronary stent failure, bypass surgery, and aneurysmal coronary artery disease. Submissions are posted on a message board and accessible to the public. The site also contains links to useful cardiology and general health sites.
http://coronary-artery-surg.com

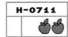

Developing Nations Cardiology and Cardio-Thoracic Surgery Forum
The international home page of the Developing Nations Cardiology and Cardio-Thoracic Surgery (DENCATS) Forum provides a discussion group dedicated to the special issues in cardiology and cardiothoracic surgery in developing nations of the world. The site features a discussion topic of the month, an online journal, a newsletter, and access to MEDLINE. A section for surgeons includes employment opportunities, meetings and conferences, a message board, and links to Internet resources.
http://www.dencats.org

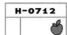

European Association for Cardio-Thoracic Surgery   The European Association for Cardio-Thoracic Surgery, a professional organization founded in 1986, offers information at its site regarding the society, membership, and upcoming events. The site contains archived and current editions of the group's newsletter and an online membership application form. A link is included to the *European Journal of Cardio-Thoracic Surgery.*
http://www.eacts.org

European Cardiac Surgical Registry   This registry is the cardiac surgery database of the European Association for Cardio-Thoracic Surgery and serves as a central repository for cardiac surgical data in Europe and other parts of the world. The site provides information about the registry and the database. Included are all the forms necessary for surgeons to submit data about themselves and their centers. Members may request software for entering patient data.
http://www.ecsur.ic.ac.uk

Heart Surgery Learning Center   The *Heart Surgery Forum,* an official publication of the International Society for Minimally Invasive Cardiac Surgery, provides explanations and information regarding cardiovascular diseases for patients and the general public. Topics discussed include minimally invasive cardiac surgery, heart disease in children, and heart disease in adults. Glossaries of medical terminology and lessons in cardiovascular anatomy are also available.
http://www.hsforum.com/learningctr

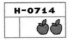

Heart-surgeon.com: Heart Surgery Information   Heart surgery information, including graphics and slide presentations, is provided at this site. Topics include coronary bypass surgery, aortic valve surgery, and mitral valve procedures. Discussions of individual topics include procedure images and graphs demonstrating the results. The site also links to current research topics, including in-vitro endotheliazation, coronary angiogenesis, and coronary bypass. A history of valve surgery is provided.
http://www.heart-surgeon.com/main.html

Medical and Surgical Intervention for Congenital and Acquired Disease   The table presented at this address lists cardiovascular therapeutic interventions, including associated pathologies and brief descriptions of the procedures. A link is available to a glossary of terms, which includes explanations of abbreviations and acronyms.
http://www.musc.edu/chp-clin/ect/interven.htm

Aortic Valve Surgery

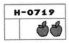

Heart-surgeon.com: Aortic Valve Replacement   Historical notes, indications, and a step-by-step, illustrated presentation of traditional aortic valve surgical techniques are presented at this site of Heart-surgeon.com. Diagrams and corresponding photographs accompany each process in the procedure, and additional sections on aortic valve replacement outcomes are provided. http://heart-surgeon.com/aortic-valve.html

Heartsurgeons.com: Aortic Valve Replacement   Provided by the Mid-Atlantic Surgical Associates, this site offers information about aortic valve replacement, intended for a variety of audiences. Ways in which damage to the aortic valve occurs are introduced, and advantages and disadvantages of both mechanical and tissue valves are examined. Figures at the site illustrate heart and aortic valve anatomy, aortic valve excision, and suturing.
http://www.heartsurgeons.com/pr4.html

Society of Thoracic Surgeons: Aortic Valve Replacement   Answers to frequently asked questions about aortic valve replacement are found at this fact sheet, which includes a series of illustrative images and hyperlinks to related terminology. Reasons for surgery, risks involved, and differences between mechanical and biological replacement valves are discussed.
http://www.sts.org/doc/3620

Arterial Catheterization

Arterial Catheterization   Common reasons for arterial catheterization are introduced at this site, sponsored by the Cardiovascular Clinical Associates group. Measurement of blood pressure with an arterial catheter line is described, and several risks of arterial catheterization are examined, including infections, blood clots, and bleeding.

http://www.heartdrs.com/procedure/ARTERIAL-CATHETERIZATION.htm

ARTERIAL GRAFTS

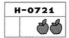

Cleveland Clinic: Arterial Coronary Artery Bypass Grafts Review of internal thoracic artery grafts, multiple vein bypass grafts, and operative comparisons is presented at this Cleveland Clinic Heart Center location. Searches for other bypass possibilities, including revival of the radial artery graft, are discussed.

http://www.clevelandclinic.org/heartcenter/pub/guide/disease/cad/lytle_arterialcabg.htm

ARTERIAL SWITCH

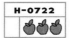

Canadian Cardiovascular Society: Congenitally Corrected Transposition of the Great Arteries This publication offers an in-depth look at the arterial switch, including background information on the transposition of the great arteries, grading descriptions of disease severity, diagnostic workup recommendations, and surgical and other interventional indications. By returning to the contents portion of the site, visitors will gain access to similar documents of the society on nearly 20 additional congenital heart defects and topics, such as tetralogy of Fallot, Ebstein's anomaly, and atrial septal defect, along with their management protocols and concomitant specialized techniques.

http://www.cachnet.org/consensus/ctga.htm

Cardiothoracic Surgery Network (CTSNet): Arterial Switch Operation Written by surgeons of the Riley Hospital for Children and Indiana University, this site of the Cardiothoracic Surgery Network offers the results of a study on the arterial switch operation and seeks to identify potential factors impacting current survival rates. The article includes discussion of objectives, methods, results, and conclusions.

http://www.ctsnet.org/abstract/1571

ATHERECTOMY

American Heart Association (AHA): Atherectomy A concise review of atherectomy is found at this fact sheet, including information on catheter insertion and other devices used in the procedure. Related AHA publications are listed and can be accessed via the site's search engine.

http://216.185.112.5/presenter.jhtml?identifier=4433

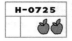

MCP Hahnemann University: Directional Coronary Atherectomy A patient guide to the directional coronary atherectomy procedure, which was de-

veloped for the management of coronary artery disease, is provided at this Web site, with general information on catheter insertion and plaque removal. Patient preparatory procedures and expectations are outlined, and a complete procedure guide is presented. Postcare information and follow-up instructions to hasten healing and prevent heart strain are provided, as a service of the Heart Hospital and MCP Hahnemann University.
http://husol.hahnemann.edu/dca.html

ATRIAL SWITCH

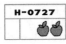

Mustard Page Although not commonly performed, the Mustard-Henning procedure, otherwise known as the atrial switch, is discussed at this site. Figures illustrating the procedure are shown, and a link to the "Mustard Diagram Page" depicts blood flow through the heart, transposition of the great arteries prior to the Mustard procedure, and post - atrial switch diagrams.
http://pw1.netcom.com/~stangboy/mstrd.html

BALLOON ANGIOPLASTY/PERCUTANEOUS TRANSLUMINAL CORONARY ANGIOPLASTY (PTCA)

AHA Medical/Scientific Statement: Carotid Stenting and Angioplasty Treatments for carotid artery stenosis are discussed in this professional statement, courtesy of various councils of the American Heart Association. Information on carotid surgical techniques and trials, medical compared with surgical interventions, and additional review of procedure risks and advantages are presented. http://216.185.112.5/presenter.jhtml?identifier=9185

American Heart Association (AHA): Angioplasty and Cardiac Revascularization Treatments and Statistics Part of the AHA *Heart and Stroke Guide,* this site offers statistics and guidelines for angioplasty and cardiac revascularization treatments, along with the AHA's scientific position on these procedures. http://216.185.112.5/presenter.jhtml?identifier=4439

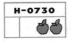

American Heart Association (AHA): Percutaneous Transluminal Coronary Angioplasty The scientific position of the AHA with regard to PTCA, as well as information on the guidelines established in a joint American College of Cardiology/American Heart Association report, are presented at this site. Related publications and Scientific Statements of the AHA can be accessed.
http://216.185.112.5/presenter.jhtml?identifier=4454

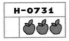

Angioplasty PTCA Home Page This award-winning site on percutaneous transluminal coronary angioplasty (PTCA) provides substantive information on interventional cardiology for medical professionals and patients alike. News on groundbreaking technologies and treatments and a forum for discussion of controversial issues are provided. For patients, the site contains a comprehensive

guide explaining the causes of coronary artery disease, in addition to common treatment and procedure summaries.
http://www.ptca.org

Internet Medical Education, Inc.: Angioplasty and Interventional Cardiology This site provides an explanation of percutaneous transcoronary angioplasty and includes a discussion of coronary artery bypass grafting surgery, an index link, a cardiology search engine, and cardiology-related news and forums. http://www.med-edu.com/patient/cad/intervention.html#angioplasty

Society of Cardiovascular and Interventional Radiology: Guidelines for Percutaneous Transluminal Angioplasty The Standards of Practice Committee of the Society of Cardiovascular and Interventional Radiology offers this guideline, intended to clarify the rationale and appropriate use of percutaneous transluminal angioplasty. Definitions of terms used to measure outcome are introduced, as well as factors determining clinical success. Determinants of patency, specific vascular lesions categories, and special information on brachiocephalic lesions are reviewed. Additional subgroups of patients are considered, including those needing renal, visceral, aortic, iliac, femoropopliteal, or infrapopliteal angioplasty. Intraoperative and outpatient procedures, as well as new devices for vascular intervention, are discussed.
http://www.scvir.org/clinical/T22.htm

Balloon Atrial Septostomy

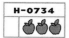

HeartCenterOnline: Balloon Atrial Septostomy Answers to frequently asked questions about balloon atrial septostomy are found at these consumer-oriented pages. History of the procedure, pre-procedural descriptions of blood flow and illustrations, an explanation of the procedure, and associated risks are described.
http://www.heartcenteronline.com/myheartdr/
Articles_about_the_heart/Balloon_Atrial_Septostomy.html

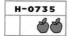

Staten Island University Hospital: Transesophageal Echocardiographic Guidance of Balloon Atrial Septostomy Written by George Kipel, M.D., Rica Arnon, M.D., and Samuel B. Ritter, M.D, this article describes transesophageal echocardiographic guidance of balloon atrial septostomy. Included are case reports, detailed discussions, and references. Hyperlinks to related electrocardiographic illustrations are provided.
http://siuh.edu/pediatrics/articles/doc6.html

Blalock-Taussig Shunt

Johns Hopkins University: Blalock-Taussig Shunt: That First Operation An online historical exhibit discusses the Blalock-Taussig diagnosis and anastomosis of cyanotic children, in addition to the success the procedure has

seen. Actual pages of the surgical record may be viewed online, as well as further explanation of this landmark operation. Archives of the *Journal of the American Medical Association* and other major news sources are shown that offer information on the procedure's origin via biographies of the internationally recognized surgeon and pediatric cardiologist.
http://www.med.jhu.edu/medarchives/nfirstor.htm

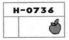

University of Chicago Children's Hospital: Blalock-Taussig Shunt   An explanation of this procedure, as well as details on the special risks involved in performance of the Blalock-Taussig shunt, is presented at this hospital Web page. Consumers, patients, and other interested readers will find a basic overview of the technique and links to information on congenital heart lesions.
http://www.ucch.org/sections/cardio/btshunt.html

CARDIAC CATHETERIZATION

American Heart Association (AHA): Cardiac Catheterization   A definition of cardiac catheterization is found at this site, part of the AHA's online publication collection, along with a listing of related AHA publications and Scientific Statements.
http://216.185.112.5/presenter.jhtml?identifier=752

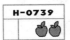

Internet Medical Education, Inc.: Cardiac Catheterization   This section of Internet Medical Education, Inc., includes discussions on cardiac catheterization generally, as well as specific details regarding left heart and coronary angiography, pressure measurements during cardiac catheterization, and coronary and cardiac angiography. The risks of left heart catheterization, reasons for performing right heart catheterization, and the advantages of simultaneous right and left heart measurements of blood flow rate and pressure are discussed. The cardiac biopsy and procedure risks are explained.
http://www.med-edu.com/patient/cad/cardiac-cath.html

CARDIAC PACEMAKER/IMPLANTABLE
ANTIARRHYTHMIC DEVICES, GENERAL

AHA Medical/Scientific Statement: Clinical Investigation of Antiarrhythmic Devices   Clinical investigation of antiarrhythmic devices is discussed at this site, as a service of the AHA and other professional organizations. Evaluatory review of cardiac pacemakers, implantable cardioverter-defibrillators, and electrode catheter systems is found, as well as discussion regarding diagnostic and therapeutic advances in the field, distinct processes involved in the regulatory assessment of safety and efficacy of procedures, and details regarding the phases of clinical investigation. A review of past guidelines and the evolution of antiarrhythmic therapy is presented.
http://216.185.112.5/presenter.jhtml?identifier=1255

American College of Cardiology (ACC): ACC/AHA Guidelines for Implantation of Cardiac Pacemakers and Antiarrhythmia Devices

Presented by the American College of Cardiology/American Heart Association Task Force on Practice Guidelines, this paper provides clinicians with a comprehensive reference to pacemaker and cardioverter-defibrillator therapies. Indications for permanent pacing are addressed, with a variety of specific conditions examined. The clinical efficacy of the therapies, alternatives to these treatments, comparisons of drugs and devices, and information specific to the pediatric population are included. The document is available for both online viewing and printing in Adobe Acrobat format.

http://www.acc.org/clinical/guidelines/april98/dirIndex.htm

American Family Physician: Implantable Cardioverter-Defibrillators

A clinical discussion of implantable cardioverter-defibrillators is found at this online article, courtesy of *American Family Physician*. Topics include components and implantation, detection and treatment of arrhythmias, the technology of the lead system, implantation approach and complications, efficacy of implantable cardioverter-defibrillators, indications, and general patient management. Environmental interference affecting proper function of the device is discussed, and ECG charts, device and radiology images, and tables enhance the review. http://www.aafp.org/afp/980115ap/groh.html

American Heart Association (AHA): Implantable Cardioverter-Defibrillator

The AHA offers this publication, providing consumers with general information on implantable cardioverter-defibrillators. Related AHA topics and sites are listed and can be accessed through the site's search engine. http://216.185.112.5/presenter.jhtml?identifier=11227

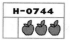

Arrhythmia Technologies Institute

The Arrhythmia Technologies Institute, an organization providing formal education for professionals in the rapidly advancing field of arrhythmias, cardiac device technology, and therapy, offers an online selection of CME information, device recalls, and safety alerts. The "Industry Views" subsite offers professionals information on current research findings of the institute. Patient fact sheets and articles on implantable devices are found, including *So You or a Loved One Are Getting a Pacemaker.*

http://www.arrhythmiatech.com

eMedicine: Pacemaker and Automatic Internal Cardiac Defibrillator

As a service of the eMedicine database, this site provides a profile of pacemakers and automatic internal cardiac defibrillators. The usual indications, issues encountered with these devices, and troubleshooting techniques are explained, as well as the code developed for various pacing modes. Major complications of pacemakers and internal cardiac defibrillators, along with images of heart rhythms and pacemaker codes, are provided.

http://www.emedicine.com/emerg/topic805.htm

McGill Medical Informatics: Pacemakers, Defibrillators, and Electrocardiograms

This site provides information about cardiac pacemakers, defi-

brillation and cardioversion, and electrocardiograms. A review of cardiac pacing and examples of different pacing modes are provided, as well as examples of external cardioversion and recordings from implantable defibrillators.
http://www.mmip.mcgill.ca/heart/ecgPindex.html

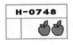

North American Society of Pacing and Electrophysiology   The NASPE is a professional society devoted to the study and management of cardiac arrhythmias. Tailored for both patients and professionals, the site offers patient information on heart anatomy and physiology, arrhythmia symptoms, various heart disorders, diagnostic tests, and therapeutic, antiarrhythmic options. The professional Web link, entitled "Medical Community," provides clinical trial review, case studies, and current news on defibrillators and other therapeutic devices. A feature case is found, and information on the annual scientific sessions is provided, in addition to a calendar of upcoming NASPE events.
http://www.naspe.org

Public Access Defibrillation League   The Public Access Defibrillation League is dedicated to saving lives through increasing the availability of automated external defibrillator (AED) units. The group advocates laws mandating public access to these devices. Their Web site provides articles and press releases, information about AEDs, AED legislation, and a donor registry.
http://www.padl.org

CARDIOMYOPLASTY

American Heart Association (AHA): Cardiomyoplasty   A description of this procedure, used to increase the heart's pumping ability, is presented at this AHA fact sheet. Related publications of the organization on cardiomyopathy and heart failure are listed.
http://216.185.112.5/presenter.jhtml?identifier=4474

CARDIOPULMONARY RESUSCITATION (CPR)

Advanced Cardiac Life Support Unofficial Guide: Focus on Interposed Abdominal Compression CPR (IAC-CPR)   A summary of new CPR modalities and recommendations with regard to interposed abdominal compression as an adjunct to traditional techniques are presented at this page. A description of the procedure, studies demonstrating its benefits, contraindications, and method are presented.
http://www.acls2000.org/new_cpr_technique.htm

American Heart Association (AHA): Cardiopulmonary Resuscitation   The AHA offers this page highlighting AHA and American Red Cross recommendations regarding CPR. Recent changes of method are introduced, and contact information for an alternative CPR learning method is found. Related AHA

publications, including *CPR and Emergency Care* and AHA Scientific Statements, are listed at the site.
http://216.185.112.5/presenter.jhtml?identifier=4479

CPR+Net This site features a tool that allows visitors to find the closest geographic location of a class providing CPR, automated external defibrillator (AED), or first aid training within the United States. Visitors need only click on their state of residence.
http://www.cprplusnet.com

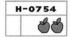

Less Stress Instructional Services: CPR Simulator This resource site offers adult, child, and infant CPR simulators that require visitors to choose the correct sequence of life-saving actions. Also included is an Automated Defibrillation Simulator.
http://www.lessstress.com/cprintro.htm

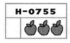

University of Washington: CPR Information and Training Resources
This informative site presents separate illustrated guides to performing standard CPR on adults, children, and infants. An alternative Quick CPR guide, which demonstrates the procedure in three simple steps, is also provided. After browsing through the additional sections on CPR facts, reading about the History of CPR, and viewing the CPR video, visitors may take an online quiz. The site provides first aid information for both conscious and unconscious choking victims, as well as a printable version of a CPR Pocket Guide, courtesy of the University of Washington School of Medicine.
http://www.learncpr.org

CARDIOVERSION

ACC/AHA Clinical Competence Statement on Invasive Electrophysiology A report of the American College of Cardiology, the American Heart Association, and the American College of Physicians-American Society of Internal Medicine Task Force on Clinical Competence is found at this link, which was developed in collaboration with the North American Society of Pacing and Electrophysiology. From the table of contents readers can access individual chapters, created to assist in the assessment of the education and skills necessary for competent performance of invasive electrophysiology studies, catheter ablation, and cardioversion. Recommendations for training, as well as necessary technical and cognitive skills, are outlined.
http://www.acc.org/clinical/competence/invasive/index.htm

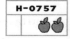

Cardioversion An online therapeutic procedure manual provides this outline of cardioversion techniques, used for the correction of abnormal heart rhythms. Indications for synchronized and unsynchronized cardioversion/defibrillation are listed, and management standards and checkpoints are provided. Special considerations regarding electrical current delivery at a predetermined point in the cardiac cycle are mentioned. A complete equipment listing, a step-by-step

procedure description, and postprocedure observations and documentation items are included.
http://216.94.9.122/clinical/ICU/procedures/cardiovn.html

Johns Hopkins Bayview Medical Center: Electrical Cardioversion
This health information page from Johns Hopkins Bayview Medical Center offers a description of cardioversion procedures, intended for consumer readers. Preparation needed, what to expect during the procedure, possible complications, and additional information regarding procedure success are presented at the page, which can be downloaded in Adobe Acrobat PDF format.
http://www.jhbmc.jhu.edu/healthy/healthconditions/cardio/cardiove.html

Virginia Mason Medical Center: Cardioversion   Cardioversion, a treatment for the correction of cardiac arrhythmias, is the subject of this information sheet, courtesy of Virginia Mason Medical Center. A brief description of the treatment and patient preparation necessary for this 30-minute procedure is provided.   http://www.vmmc.com/dbCardiology/sec375.htm

CAROTID ENDARTERECTOMY

American Family Physician: When to Operate in Carotid Artery Disease   Maintained by the American Academy of Family Physicians, this site reviews the benefits of carotid endarterectomy, its indications, surgical risks, and related study outcomes. Overall results and their dependence on surgical risk are emphasized, with appropriate patient selection, preoperative control of risk factors, and other medical strategies recommended.
http://www.aafp.org/afp/20000115/400.html

Canadian Medical Association Journal: Guidelines for the Use of Carotid Endarterectomy   Provided by the Canadian Neurosurgical Society, this document contains guidelines on patient selection for carotid endarterectomy. The table of contents includes an abstract, an introduction, methods, findings, recommendations, and reference citations.
http://www.cma.ca/cmaj/vol-157/issue-6/0653.htm

CATHETER ABLATION

American College of Cardiology (ACC): ACC/AHA Guidelines for Clinical Intracardiac Electrophysiological and Catheter Ablation Procedures   This report from the American College of Cardiology and the American Heart Association offers guidelines related to the role of catheter ablation in the diagnosis and management of cardiovascular disease. Its contribution to the field, specificity, indications and contraindications, cost-effectiveness, procedure details, and therapeutic benefits are reviewed. The role of electrophysiological study in the evaluation of sinus node function, in patients with acquired atrioventricular block, with chronic intraventricular conduction delay, with unexplained palpitations, in survivors of cardiac arrest, with

with unexplained palpitations, in survivors of cardiac arrest, with unexplained syncope, with prolonged Q-T intervals, with wide QRS complex tachycardias, and in other conditions is detailed.

http://www.acc.org/clinical/guidelines/ablation/dirIndex.htm

American Heart Association (AHA): Radiofrequency Ablation A definition of radiofrequency ablation, additional information about irregular heart rhythms, and a list of several related AHA publications are available at this site of the AHA's publication collection.

http://216.185.112.5/presenter.jhtml?identifier=4682

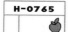

Catheter Ablation A breakdown and description of arrhythmia types are found at this site, which discusses their discovery via electrophysiology study and provides information on catheter ablation procedures. Risks that the procedures pose and important points to keep in mind when preparing patients for catheter ablation are reviewed, courtesy of Almaviva.

http://www.almaviva.it/abl.htm

Internet Medical Education, Inc.: Catheter-Mediated Radiofrequency Ablation This treatment of choice for many of the supraventricular tachycardias and several types of ventricular tachycardia is discussed at this site of the portion of Internet Medical Education's review of tachyarrhythmias. Cardiac rhythms that can be cured by radiofrequency catheter ablation and those whose symptoms may be reduced are discussed, with information on the procedure in the elderly and long-term complications included.

http://www.med-edu.com/patient/arrhythmia/arrhythmia-treatments.html#rfa

Postgraduate Medicine: Catheter Ablation for Atrial Flutter and Fibrillation *Postgraduate Medicine* presents a review of alternative treatment in patients with atrial flutter and fibrillation who are refractory to traditional pharmacological interventions. The success of radiofrequency catheter ablation and recent advances in its use are introduced, with sections on atrial tachycardia, descriptions of ablation techniques, and a review of its purposes. The limitations of radiofrequency ablation and the need for continuation of pharmacologic therapy are discussed.

http://www.postgradmed.com/issues/1998/01_98/kosinski.htm

Radiofrequency Ablation The Research Foundation of the Florida Cardiovascular Institute offers descriptions of catheter ablation, the heart's electrical system, and diagnosis of arrhythmias at this presentation. Abnormal rapid heart rhythms, including supraventricular tachycardia, Wolf-Parkinson-White syndrome, atrial fibrillation, and ventricular tachycardia, are described, and the use of catheter ablation in the treatment of rapid heart rhythms is discussed in detail. Patient preparation for the procedure, details of the actual process, a description of what patients can expect during the procedure, possible risks, potential benefits, and details regarding recovery are available.

http://www.fciheart.com/rf_ablation.htm

CENTRAL VENOUS CATHETERIZATION

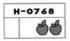

Society of Cardiovascular and Interventional Radiology: Quality Improvement Guidelines for Central Venous Access The Standards of Practice Committee of the Society of Cardiovascular and Interventional Radiology provides review of image-guided placement of central venous lines and ports, with an emphasis on patient selection, proper procedure performance, and patient monitoring. Indicators for assessment of efficacy are discussed, as well as indications for central venous access and definitions of complications.
http://www.scvir.org/clinical/T27.htm

COIL CLOSURE OF PATENT DUCTUS ARTERIOSUS

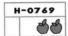

Oschner Clinic and Hospital: Coil Closure of Patent Ductus Arteriosus The new snare device technique of transcatheter patent ductus arteriosus (PDA) occlusion is described at this site of the Oschner Pediatric Heart Institute. Details regarding research results indicate several advantages of the coil procedure over traditional surgical methods.
http://www.ochsner.org/pedcard/coil.htm

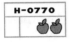

University of Michigan: PDA Coil Registry Created in 1994 to provide information to pediatric cardiac interventionalists on PDA coil occlusion, this site contains both clinical data and a large database of participating institutions. Useful information includes success rates, common and unusual complications, and patient- and procedure-related factors that may influence outcome. A section for questions and comments and a form for submitting patient information into the database are provided.
http://www.med.umich.edu/pdc/pdacoil/pda_main.htm

CONGENITAL HEART DISEASE TREATMENTS, GENERAL

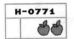

American Heart Association (AHA): Congenital Cardiovascular Disease Treatments From the AHA, this site offers a description of several treatments for congenital cardiovascular disease. Procedures discussed include the arterial switch, balloon atrial septostomy, balloon valvuloplasty, the Damus-Kaye-Stansel procedure, the Fontan procedure, pulmonary artery banding, the Ross procedure, the shunting procedure, and venous switch.
http://216.185.112.5/presenter.jhtml?identifier=4580

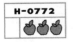

PediHeart: Operative Procedures Offering a list of congenital heart disease procedures, this site details important points in several of the more complicated operations available. Procedure preparations, stages, and completion are discussed in detail for each link, including operation variations according to individual heart defect. Repair of tetralogy of Fallot, the Fontan operation, the arterial switch, and several additional repairs are available for review.
http://www.pediheart.org/practitioners/operations/index.html

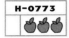

Perfusion Line: Palliative Procedures Nine palliative procedures to increase the capacity of the left atrium and ventricle until more permanent repairs can safely be made are introduced at this site. Definitions, advantages and disadvantages, and indications for the Blalock-Taussig shunt and other procedures that increase the flow of blood to the pulmonary system and aid with oxygenation of desaturated venous blood are summarized.
http://www.perfline.com/student/palliative.html

Coronary Artery Bypass Grafting (CABG)

ACC/AHA Guidelines for Coronary Artery Bypass Graft Surgery This joint venture of the American College of Cardiology and the American Heart Association contains more than 70 chapters, intended to assist clinicians in healthcare decision-making. Elaboration on a wide variety of approaches for diagnosis and management of coronary artery bypass surgery is provided, including therapeutic techniques and comparisons, maximization of postoperative benefits, CABG in special patient subsets, and the evolution of CABG technology. The entire guideline can be downloaded in PDF format.
http://www.acc.org/clinical/guidelines/bypass

American Heart Association (AHA): Bypass Surgery, Coronary Artery A patient information resource on coronary artery bypass surgery is presented at the site, as a service of the AHA. Basic anatomic review, procedural explanation, and postoperative expectations are detailed. Alternatives to coronary artery bypass surgery and related publications of the AHA are noted.
http://americanheart.org/Heart_and_Stroke_A_Z_Guide/bypass.html

Bypass Heart Surgery A wide variety of resources are offered at this site of the Global Justice Search from Madison in Wisconsin, a national information coalition, which provides an extensive collection of links relating to the latest advances in coronary bypass surgery. Patient information sheets, encyclopedic entries, clinical trial review, and news on related medications and technological advances are accessible. Information ranges from surgical overviews to technical information on developing techniques.
http://www.gjs.net/web-bphs.htm

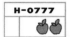

Coronary Artery Surgery Forum Dedicated to those with an interest in coronary artery surgery, this site outlines concepts, new approaches, surgical procedures, and research and offers topical discussion opportunities via the site's "Coronary Artery Surgery Message Board." Links to other useful sites include the Heart Surgery Forum.
http://coronary-artery-surg.com

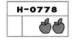

Society of Thoracic Surgeons: Coronary Artery Bypass Grafting This subsite of the Society of Thoracic Surgeons contains a patient information brochure on CABG, with sections on its indications, risks, new techniques, and

alternatives to the procedure. Discussions regarding the likelihood of long-term success and postsurgical expectations are provided.
http://www.sts.org/doc/3705

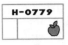

University of Michigan: Coronary Artery Bypass   The coronary artery bypass, a procedure used to treat atherosclerosis, is described at this site, courtesy of the University of Michigan. Explanations of procedure performance and postprocedural expectations are reviewed.
http://www.med.umich.edu/1libr/heart/surg01.htm

DAMUS-KAYE-STANSEL OPERATION

PediHeart: Damus-Kaye-Stansel Operation   A technical discussion of the Damus-Kaye-Stansel operation, a technique in which a congenital transposition of the great arteries is repaired by dividing the pulmonary artery in two and attaching it to both the ascending aorta and the right ventricle, is presented at this PediHeart subsite. Pre-cardiopulmonary bypass considerations, cannulation, and the dissection of the aorta, pulmonary artery, and head vessels are described at the site, with resection techniques completely reviewed.
http://www.pediheart.org/practitioners/operations/damus.html

ENDOSCOPIC VEIN HARVESTING

heartsurgery-usa.com: Endoscopic Vein Harvesting   This component of bypass surgery is discussed and illustrated, providing patients with general information on endoscopic procedures. Benefits and goals of surgery are explained, and two online videos are available for download using RealPlayer technology.
http://www.heartsurgery-usa.com/What_s_New/ENDO
VEIN/body_endoscopic_vein_harvesting.html

ENDOVASCULAR GRAFT

Food and Drug Administration (FDA): FDA Approves Two New Devices for Aneurysm Repair   FDA-based approval of endograft devices for repair of aortic aneurysms is the focus of this FDA Talk Paper. A summary of clinical studies, their success, and the need for additional research are addressed.   http://www.fda.gov/bbs/topics/ANSWERS/ANS00978.html

Society of Cardiovascular and Interventional Radiology: Stent-Graft Repair of Abdominal Aortic Aneurysms   This multipage site offers an overview of abdominal aortic aneurysms and information on image-guided stent-graft repair, intended for a consumer audience. Treatment of aortic aneurysm with medication, surgical repair, and minimally invasive techniques is presented, and comparisons and illustrations are found.
http://www.scvir.org/patient/aaa/home.htm

ENHANCED EXTERNAL COUNTERPULSATION (EECP)

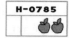

American College of Cardiology (ACC): Chronic Stable Angina: Does Enhanced External Counter Pulsation Work? Online CME material of the ACC includes this conference excerpt from a forum on chronic stable angina. Addressing the benefits of external counterpulsation, the discussion reviews this hot topic in cardiology and discusses results of a multicenter, randomized trial. Evaluation of the treatment's efficacy and the need for further research are addressed.
http://www.acc.org/education/online/hawaii/chronic.htm

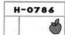

American Heart Association (AHA): External Counterpulsation (ECP) This site from the AHA describes external counterpulsation, with its purposes and technique outlined. Mention of when the procedure is employed and related AHA documents is found.
http://216.185.112.5/presenter.jhtml?identifier=4577

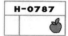

Enhanced External Counterpulsation Enhanced external counterpulsation, a noninvasive, atraumatic procedure that reduces the symptoms of angina pectoris by increasing coronary blood flow in ischemic areas of the heart, is reviewed at this illustrated site. Depictions of ECG signals, and connection to the Heart and Vascular Center home page are provided.
http://www.heartcenter.com/eecp.html

FONTAN PROCEDURE

Adult Congenital Heart Association: A Brief Overview of the Fontan Procedure The purpose of the Fontan procedure in patients with complex congenital heart defects is reviewed at the site, with an accessible labeled diagram of a univentricular heart. The rerouting of blood from the vena cava to restore segregation of oxygenated and deoxygenated blood is discussed, as well as the resulting improvements in exercise and descriptions of appropriate candidates for the procedure. Drawbacks that may be associated with the surgery are introduced, such as arrhythmias and protein-losing enteropathy.
http://www.achaheart.org/newsletter/fontan.shtml

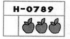

Fontan Procedure Several articles found at the site detail various aspects of the Fontan procedure for complex congenital heart defects. Brief reviews of the technique and its purpose, discussion of recent modifications to the procedure, and an in-depth publication reporting postsurgical outcome data are accessible, as a service of the Developing Nations Cardiology and Cardio-Thoracic Surgery (DENCATS) Forum.
http://www.dencats.org/fontan/fontan.htm

GENE THERAPY

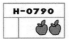

American Heart Association (AHA): Gene Therapy   A brief discussion of gene therapy in the treatment of heart disease is presented at this fact sheet. Examples of successful experimental therapy and areas of current research are mentioned, including gene insertion for the treatment of hypercholesterolemia, blood clot defenses, angiogenesis, and atherosclerosis.
http://216.185.112.5/presenter.jhtml?identifier=4566

University of Virginia: Gene Therapy Shows Promise in Protecting Hearts during Surgery   This news article offers a summary of research on the use of gene therapy in the protection of the heart muscle during surgery. The technique genetically increases the number of adenosine receptors on the heart. Discussion regarding replication of the therapy in humans and details concerning the principal investigator's research into the effects of adenosine receptor increases are provided.
http://www.newswise.com/articles/1998/5/HEARTGEN.UVM.html

INTERVENTIONAL RADIOLOGY

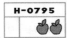

Cardiovascular and Interventional Radiological Society of Europe
The Cardiovascular and Interventional Radiological Society of Europe is an educational and scientific association of doctors, scientists, and others interested in interventional radiology and cardiovascular imaging techniques. The site contains links to two online journals, *Eurorad* and *Cardiovascular and Interventional Radiology,* in addition to upcoming conference information. Links to related sites, such as the Radiological Society of North America and the Society of Cardiovascular and Interventional Radiology, are provided. A portion of the site is restricted to members.
(some features fee-based) http://www.cirse.org

Society of Cardiovascular and Interventional Radiology   The Society of Cardiovascular and Interventional Radiology is a professional association of doctors whose specialty is interventional or minimally invasive procedures. The site contains information for healthcare professionals and consumers alike, with the latest medical advances in imaging and cardiovascular procedures presented. This site contains a section featuring the latest related news articles and information about forthcoming meetings and conferences. A members-only department features slide sets and online case studies, with valuable links to related Web resources included.
(some features fee-based) http://www.scvir.org

INTRACORONARY ARTERY RADIATION

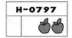

British Medical Journal: Radiation of the Arteries Can Reduce Narrowing The reduction of restenosis after angioplasty through the use of intracoronary artery radiation is discussed in this online news article. Mechanisms of restenosis are described in detail, and traditional treatment strategies are summarized. A review of recent research on the use of intracoronary artery radiation at Scripps Clinic is presented, describing patient inclusion criteria, radiation administration, posttreatment surveillance, and clinical results.
http://www.bmj.com/cgi/content/full/320/7232/402/a

LEFT VENTRICULAR ASSIST DEVICES (LVAD)

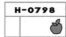

American Heart Association (AHA): Left Ventricular Assist Device Typically implanted prior to receiving a donor heart for transplantation, the left ventricular assist devices are discussed at this page. Additional, related publications of the AHA are listed at site, including those on congestive heart failure, heart transplants, and organ donation.
http://216.185.112.5/presenter.jhtml?identifier=4599

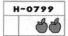

Society of Thoracic Surgeons: Ventricular Assist Devices Authored by William S. Pierce, M.D., of Penn State University, this FAQ page discusses types of ventricular assist devices, major differences among them, and the status of permanent ventricular assist pumps. Details on the HeartMate, the Thoratec assist pump, and the Novacor ventricular assist pump are found, and related information on the artificial heart and patient eligibility for these devices is introduced. http://www.sts.org/education/faqs/faqvassist.html

LEFT VENTRICULAR REDUCTION/BATISTA PROCEDURE

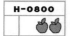

American Heart Association (AHA): Batista Heart Failure Procedure A potential alternative to heart transplantation is discussed at this online information sheet, courtesy of the AHA. An explanation of the procedure's ability to improve the heart's efficiency is found, in addition to a list of available related AHA publications.
http://216.185.112.5/presenter.jhtml?identifier=4466

MAZE PROCEDURE

Society of Thoracic Surgeons: The Maze Procedure The Society of Thoracic Surgeons patient information pages include this site on the Maze procedure, which addresses atrial fibrillation causes and resulting problems. The surgical procedure is described and a schematic of the "maze" and incisions made in the heart to accomplish its goals are illustrated. Indications, risks, and results are introduced.
http://www.sts.org/doc/4512

MINIMALLY INVASIVE DIRECT CORONARY ARTERY BYPASS (MIDCAB)

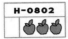

Brown University: Minimally Invasive Direct Coronary Artery Bypass

Part of the Brown University Minimally Invasive Heart Surgery series, this page details components of the MIDCAB procedure and offers a variety of operative images. Difficulties involved in the surgery are enumerated, and special considerations regarding technique and instrumentation are examined. A comparison between MIDCAB and traditional heart surgery methods is presented, including serious complications of the heart lung machine, disadvantages of conventional methods, and recent studies suggesting significant benefits of minimally invasive techniques. MIDCAB's disadvantages, its comparison with angioplasty alone, and further details on cost and patient selection are presented.

http://biomed.brown.edu/Courses/BI108/BI108_2000_Groups/Heart_Surgery/MIDCAB.html

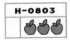

Clinical Update: Minimally Invasive Direct Coronary Artery Bypass

The emergence of MIDCAB as an equally effective and cost-containing surgical alternative to a variety of traditional cardiovascular procedures is discussed at this online article, excerpted from the *Medical Journal of Allina*. An understanding of the consequences of interrupted blood flow and experience gained from procedures performed on a beating heart have led to the development of this revolutionary treatment, which is outlined in terms of its goals, indications, and limitations of use. A summary of studies that have examined the limited access approach are referenced, and the authors' own MIDCAB study, with a focus on development of direct visualization for both coronary artery and valvular procedures, is outlined. MIDCAB's success and the advent of related, ever-evolving techniques are summarized.

http://www.allina.com/Allina_Journal/Spring1997/arom.html

MINIMALLY INVASIVE HEART SURGERY, GENERAL

American College of Cardiology (ACC): ACC/AHA Guidelines for Coronary Artery Bypass Graft Surgery

The impact of evolving technology on traditional coronary artery bypass techniques is the focus of this clinical guideline, created by the American College of Cardiology and the American Heart Association. Potential benefits of less invasive methods, including off-pump coronary artery bypass, minimally invasive direct coronary artery bypass, and port access procedures, are examined. Encouraging clinical results and cautionary statements are presented for these and other methods, including video-assisted operations, arterial and alternate conduits, and technological improvements in percutaneous technology.

http://www.acc.org/clinical/guidelines/bypass/bypass6.htm

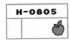

American Heart Association (AHA): Minimally Invasive Heart Surgery

Two approaches currently used in minimally invasive heart surgery

are reviewed at this fact sheet of the AHA. Recommendations of the organization regarding these promising new therapies are found, as well as an extensive listing of related AHA publications.
http://216.185.112.5/presenter.jhtml?identifier=1875

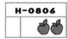

Circulation: Minimally Invasive Heart Surgery Drawn from the AHA's clinical journal, this report offers a description of techniques, examination of current knowledge of the field, and the future potential of new approaches. Links to MEDLINE abstracts and full texts of cited references are provided.
http://circ.ahajournals.org/cgi/content/full/94/10/2669

MITRAL VALVE SURGERY

Cardiothoracic Surgery Network (CTSNet): Minimally Invasive Mitral Valve Surgery A technical discussion of minimally invasive mitral valve surgery is available at this article. Topics include operative steps, equipment preferences, and important tips and pitfalls. Detailed illustrations accompany the discussion, and reference citations are provided.
http://www.ctsnet.org/doc/3308

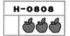

Heart-surgeon.com: Mitral Valve Surgery Historical information related to open heart surgery, descriptions of artificial valves, and a discussion of mitral valve replacement versus valve repair only are available from this online article. Charts summarize structural deterioration and valve-related complications, as well as survival rates associated with both mitral valve replacement and valve repair operations. Descriptions and accompanying diagrams of mitral valve repair techniques are provided, followed by a general summary of clinical outcomes. Mitral valve surgical slides are also available.
http://heart-surgeon.com/mitral-surgery.html

Heartsurgeons.com: Mitral Valve Replacement and Repair At this illustrated site of the Mid-Atlantic Surgical Associates, viewers will find discussions of procedures for treating diseased mitral valves. Anatomy and function of the mitral valve are reviewed, and distinct advantages and disadvantages of both mechanical and tissue valves are addressed. A description of surgical procedures is accompanied by illustrations of methods.
http://www.heartsurgeons.com/pr3.html

Society of Thoracic Surgeons: Mitral Valve Repair Information on mitral valve repair procedures is found at this illustrated Web site, intended for a consumer audience. Reasons for surgery, results of mitral valve repair, and what to expect following surgery are discussed. The site offers links to definitions of related medical terminology.
http://www.sts.org/doc/4107

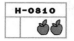

Society of Thoracic Surgeons: Mitral Valve Replacement An illustrated document is found at this page that provides well-rounded information to consumers on mechanical and biological valves for mitral valve disease. Causes of mitral valve problems, surgical options to consider, and associated risks are introduced.

http://www.sts.org/doc/4101

Norwood Operation

PediHeart: Norwood Operation The multistage Norwood operation and its usefulness in a variety of congenital heart defects are explained at this Pedi-Heart Web site. An operating room procedure review contains details on preoperative medication administration, dissection, cardiopulmonary bypass reinstitution, and restoration of the pulmonary blood flow.

http://www.pediheart.org/practitioners/operations/norwood.htm

Off-Pump Coronary Artery Bypass (OPCAB)

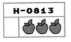

Brown University: Off Pump Coronary Artery Bypass Introduction to the off-pump technique is offered at this address, with a discussion of procedure history and development provided. Information on techniques and instrumentation used to operate on a beating heart and coverage of surgery comparisons are found. Additionally, readers will find moving images of the procedure and a video library link, offering several presentations of the off-pump technique and material on related operative procedures. Links to further safety and reliability studies are available.

http://biomed.brown.edu/Courses/BI108/BI108_2000_Groups/Heart_Surgery/OPCAB.htm

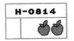

heartsurgery-usa.com: Off Pump An overview of this alternative to traditional bypass surgery is found at this Web site, which describes benefits of the procedure and reasons for its selection. The meaning of minimally invasive techniques, a description of this particular method, and distinctions between two techniques available in off-pump coronary artery bypass are introduced. Animations of various chest incisions can be viewed with the use of RealPlayer software.

http://www.heartsurgery-usa.com/Off_Pump_Beating_Heart_Surgery/off_pump_beating_heart_surgery.html

Percutaneous Balloon Commissurotomy

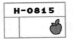

University of Chicago Cardiology Department: Non-Surgical Management for Mitral Stenosis A clinical discussion of the use of percutaneous balloon commissurotomy, a noninvasive alternative to surgical thoracotomy, is available from this address. Current numbers of patients undergoing surgical commissurotomy and progress in balloon commissurotomy are summarized.

Links are available to conference details, and a brief description of mitral steno-sis, with reference citations, is provided.
http://cardiology.uchicago.edu/pages/cathlab/mitralstenosis.html

Percutaneous Coronary Intervention, General

American College of Cardiology (ACC): ACC/AHA Guidelines for Percutaneous Coronary Intervention Printable in PDF format, this online revision of the 1993 guidelines includes recommendations concerning appropriate use of technology for diagnosis and intervention of those with cardiovascular disease. The document addresses percutaneous transluminal coronary angioplasty (PTCA), as well as additional techniques for reducing artery narrowing. Rotational atherectomy, directional atherectomy, extraction atherectomy, laser angioplasty, intracoronary stent implantation, and implantation of additional catheter devices are examined. Information on procedural complications, outcome, predictors of success, and several other chapters concerning specific technical considerations of procedures and follow-up are available.
http://www.acc.org/clinical/guidelines/percutaneous/percutaneous_l.htm

Perfusion

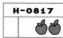

American Academy of Cardiovascular Perfusion The AACP strives to stimulate research and provide education in the field. Visitors who join AACP gain access to PERFSearch, which cites itself as the largest and most comprehensive database for perfusion-related journal articles, and PERFClass, which offers online perfusion courses. Information regarding the organization's speakers bureau, event schedules, and perfusion journals can be accessed from the site, in addition to a variety of professional publications. The site also features the newsletter of the AACP and a directory of related links.
http://members.aol.com/OfficeAACP/

American Board of Cardiovascular Perfusion The American Board of Cardiovascular Perfusion is a credentialing institution for clinical perfusionists. The site offers information on certification, recertification, and examination schedules. Visitors can download the "Clinical Activity Recertification Report" and the "Professional Activity Recertification Report." A listing of perfusion links is included. http://www.abcp.org

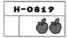

European Board of Cardiovascular Perfusion The European Board of Cardiovascular Perfusion aims to unite European perfusionists in an effort to establish, monitor, and maintain standards in perfusion education and training. The site offers concise information on accreditation and recertification and features a Perfusion Checklist and Examination Guide. Moreover, the site provides listings of members, committees, and related links.
http://www.ebcp.org

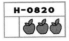

Perfusion Home Page This frequently visited Web site provides information on events, publications, employment, standards and guidelines, and clinical techniques related to perfusion. Additional features include scientific forums, a mailing list, access to perfusion software, and a conference server. The services section contains information on perfusion services and equipment sales, as well as an online bookstore. A comprehensive page on perfusion education maintains perfusion certification requirements and additional career-oriented details. http://www.perfusion.com

PERIPHERALLY INSERTED CENTRAL CATHETER (PICC)

Warren Grant Magnuson Clinical Center: Peripherally Inserted Central Catheter Placement Uses of the PICC, preparation before placement, procedures for insertion, and what to expect after catheter insertion are concisely reviewed at this online information handout. Special instructions for care of the line and other information intended for patients is presented. http://www.cc.nih.gov/ccc/patient_education/procdiag/PICC.pdf

PORT ACCESS CORONARY ARTERY BYPASS (PORTCAB/PACAB)

Brown University: The Port Access Technique The port access technique, allowing surgeons to eliminate the traditional sternotomy, is reviewed at this Brown University site, which contains information on instrumentation, the procedure itself, and the benefits of the procedure, as well as a complete series of related images and figures. A bulleted list of postoperative benefits is found, and a comparison page is available that outlines variables in surgery for minimally invasive direct coronary artery bypass (MIDCAB), port access (PACAB), off pump coronary artery bypass (OPCAB), and conventional methods. Popular instrumentation systems, a listing of procedures with port access, and discussions of safety data are available. http://biomed.brown.edu/Courses/BI108/BI108_2000_Groups/Heart_Surgery/PACAB.html

PREVENTIVE THERAPY

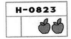

American Heart Association (AHA): Primary Prevention The AHA's primary prevention program for heart attack and stroke is outlined at this site. Recommendations are offered for education, smoking cessation, blood pressure control, cholesterol management, physical activity, weight management, and estrogens. http://216.185.112.5/presenter.jhtml?identifier=4704

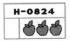

American Heart Association (AHA): Secondary Prevention Secondary prevention of heart attack and stroke involves identifying people at high risk and treating them. This site outlines the AHA's recommendations for secondary prevention, including smoking cessation, lipid management, physical activity, weight management, antiplatelet agents, angiotensin-converting enzyme (ACE)

inhibitors, beta blockers, and blood pressure control. Links to related AHA documents on primary prevention of coronary artery disease are found. http://216.185.112.5/presenter.jhtml?identifier=2746

PULMONARY ARTERY BANDING

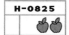

University of Chicago Children's Hospital: Pulmonary Artery Banding As part of the Pediatric Cardiac Surgical Procedures pages, this University of Chicago site offers discussion of various heart defects in which too much blood flow to the lungs occurs and surgical repair is necessary. Diagrams at the site illustrate pulmonary artery band placement in cases of multiple ventricular septal defects and in a single ventricle defect. Special risks of the procedure are introduced. http://www.ucch.org/sections/cardio/paband.html

PULMONARY ARTERY CATHETERIZATION

American Society of Anesthesiologists: Practice Guidelines for Pulmonary Artery Catheterization Published in *Anesthesiology,* this page offers an introduction to the pulmonary artery catheter and appropriate indications for its use. Important adverse effects are examined, and information on scientific evidence of its effectiveness is considered. Benefits, including effects on treatment decisions with its use, are emphasized, and outcomes of its use with cardiac surgery, peripheral vascular surgery, abdominal aortic reconstruction, and in the pediatric population are examined. Complications, expert opinion on effectiveness, public policy, and cost considerations are also covered in part of the discussion.
http://www.asahq.org/practice/pulm/pulm_artery.html

REPAIR OF DOUBLE OUTLET RIGHT VENTRICLE

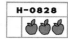

PediHeart: Repair of Double Outlet Right Ventricle Nine procedures used in the repair of double outlet right ventricle are explained in technical detail at this PediHeart subsite, with discussion of the arterial switch operation and complete review of the Rastelli technique for transposition of the great arteries with a ventricular septal defect and pulmonary stenosis. Aortic translocation via the Nikaidoh procedure and details on Kawashima's ventricular repair are offered. The goals of pulmonary translocation with this heart defect are outlined, and complex risk factors that warrant modification of these procedures are reviewed.
http://www.pediheart.org/practitioners/operations/DORV.html

Repair of Interrupted Aortic Arch

PediHeart: Repair of Interrupted Aortic Arch Palliative procedures for interrupted aortic arch repair, such as pulmonary artery banding and ventricular septal defect closure, are summarized at the site, with surgical details regarding aortic conduit placement. Medical and anesthetic considerations, dissection of the great vessels and head vessels, protection of the heart and brain, and the actual repair are outlined. An alternative procedure, in the case of left ventricular outflow tract obstruction, is described, and general principles regarding incorporation of growth potential in biventricular repair are reviewed.
http://www.pediheart.org/practitioners/operations/IAA.html

Repair of Tetralogy of Fallot

PediHeart: Repair of Tetralogy of Fallot Preparatory procedures for transventricular repair of tetralogy of Fallot with pulmonary stenosis are reviewed at this PediHeart Web site, with infundibulotomy and division of obstructing muscle bundles and ventricular septal defect closure detailed. The overall goals and procedure details intended for repair of tetralogy of Fallot with pulmonary atresia are included.
http://www.pediheart.org/practitioners/operations/TOF.htm

Repair of Truncus Arteriosus

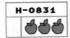

PediHeart: Repair of Truncus Arteriosus Preparation and repair of a simple truncus arteriosus are reviewed at the Web site. Excision of the pulmonary arteries from the truncal root, truncal root defect closure, and ventricular and atrial septal defect closure are discussed. Complete reconstruction of the right ventricular outflow tract is explained.
http://www.pediheart.org/practitioners/operations/truncus.html

Reperfusion Therapy

American Family Physician: ACC/AHA Guidelines on the Management of Acute Myocardial Infarction The American Academy of Family Physicians offers a summary of practice guidelines at this site, addressing reperfusion therapy as well as discharge and long-term management of acute myocardial infarction. Pharmacology is comprehensively covered, and new information on the use of glycoprotein IIb/IIIa inhibitors, the role of serum cardiac markers, angioplasty, and heparin following fibrinolytic agent administration are discussed. Full- text guidelines can be accessed at the ACC or AHA Web site. http://www.aafp.org/afp/20000315/practice.html

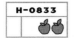

American Heart Association (AHA): Heart Attack Treatments
Treatments for heart attack are reviewed at this AHA site, including the advantages of thrombolysis therapies. Related AHA patient documents and professional guidelines for prevention and the management of patients with acute myocardial infarction are listed at the site.
http://216.185.112.5/presenter.jhtml?identifier=4601

ROSS PROCEDURE

CTSNet Experts' Techniques: The Ross Procedure A discussion of pulmonary autograft replacement of the aortic valve is found at this CTSNet Experts' article, authored by Robert C. Elkins, M.D. Patient selection and operative steps are described, and a series of enlargeable figures illustrate the procedure. Steps in root replacement, operative procedure for the inclusion cylinder, and annulus reduction and fixation modifications are examined.
http://www.ctsnet.org/doc/2380

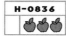

PediHeart: Ross Operation A technical review of the Ross procedure, also known as the pulmonary autograft, for pulmonary valve translocation is presented at this subsite of PediHeart. A step-by-step operative description is offered. http://www.pediheart.org/practitioners/operations/ross.html

STENT IMPLANTATION

American College of Cardiology (ACC): ACC Expert Consensus Document on Coronary Artery Stents Printable in PDF format, this electronic guideline offers clinicians the opportunity to review the technology, indications, patient selection, placement, and treatment details for coronary stents. Adjunctive therapy approaches and cost consideration chapters are included at this comprehensive document of the ACC, which contains figures, tables, and references. Data on safety, efficacy, and long-term outcome are part of this online analysis.
http://www.acc.org/clinical/consensus/coronary/jac5902gtc.htm

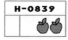

Coronary Stent Implantation Details regarding coronary stent implantation are presented at this fact sheet, including a definition, patient preparation, and complete process description. Two specific stent designs are explained, and additional information on patient expectations, safety, and benefits is provided, courtesy of the Florida Cardiovascular Institute. Information on the recovery period, including commonly prescribed medications and lifestyle changes.
http://www.fciheart.com/stent.htm

Superior Cavopulmonary Anastomosis (BDG Shunt)

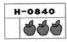

PediHeart: Superior Cavopulmonary Anastomosis Superior cavopulmonary anastomosis, often performed as an intermediary palliation in infants with a single functional ventricle, is described in clinical detail at this site. Information on the hemi-Fontan procedure and the bi-directional Glenn anastomosis, with directions for dissection and operation completion, is reviewed.
http://www.pediheart.org/practitioners/operations/BDG.html

Transmyocardial Laser Revascularization (TMR)

American Heart Association (AHA): Laser Angioplasty Laser angioplasty is described at this page of the AHA *Heart and Stroke Guide*. A list of related fact sheets, any of which can be accessed through the AHA search engine, is presented. http://216.185.112.5/presenter.jhtml?identifier=4446

Annals of Thoracic Surgery: Transmyocardial Laser Revascularization
This full-text article offers a thorough discussion of transmyocardial laser revascularization (TMR), a recent therapeutic option for patients suffering from severe diffuse coronary artery disease refractory to conventional therapies. Patient selection and methods are described in detail, and results are presented up to one year after the procedure. The investigators conclude that TMR offers symptomatic and quality of life improvement, as well as improvements in patients' ability to undergo stress.
http://www.ctsnet.org/journal/ats/67/432

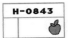

Harvard Medical School: Laser Myocardial Revascularization From the Harvard University Department of Interventional Radiology, this site offers information on experimental laser myocardial revascularization (LMR) procedures. Details on the development of percutaneous LMR and recent data on previous benefits seen are introduced, including a slide presentation of a randomized clinical trial and the likelihood of placebo effects.
http://angiogenesis.bidmc.harvard.edu/
Interventional/Laser%20Myocardial%20Revascularization.asp

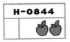

University of Missouri Health Care: Transmyocardial Laser Revascularization A general discussion of transmyocardial laser revascularization is available at this useful fact sheet, intended for patients and families. The presentation offers a thorough description of the procedure, and a review of indications for this procedure is provided. Details of the operation and additional sources of information are cited.
http://tribble.missouri.edu/tmr/public.htm

VALVE REPLACEMENT SURGERY, GENERAL

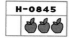

Cedars-Sinai Medical Center: Prosthetic Heart Valve Information Information on artificial heart valves, including characteristics of different heart devices, is found at this address. Links to manufacturers, anticoagulation protocols, echocardiographic and hemodynamic data, outcome data, and protocols for thrombolytic therapy in heart valve procedures are found. In addition, information regarding the prevention of bacterial endocarditis and new developments in the field of prosthetic heart valves is provided.
http://www.csmc.edu/cvs/md/valve/default.htm

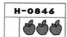

MEDLINEplus Tutorial: Heart Valve Replacement Created through a collaboration between the National Library of Medicine and the Patient Education Institute, this online tutorial guides viewers through a series of slides that explain the anatomy and symptoms of heart valve disease and the treatment options, procedures, and risks involved. This interactive tool contains graphics as well as audio features and provides convenient navigation tools and instructions for use. http://www.nlm.nih.gov/medlineplus/tutorials/heartvalvereplacement.html

YourSurgery.com: Surgery of the Heart Valves Surgery of the heart valves is described at this site, which includes anatomical illustration, discussion of pathology, and components of the history and physical examination. Diagnostic tests, example radiologic images, and indications for surgery are reviewed. Intended for a variety of audiences, the site describes the surgical procedure and offers a series of operative photographs and figures. Special considerations, complications, and postoperative recovery information are included at this comprehensive online resource.
http://www.yoursurgery.com/data/Procedures/heart_valve/p_heart_valve.cfm

VALVOTOMY

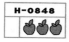

PediHeart: Pulmonary Valvotomy Information is presented on pulmonary valvotomy for pulmonary atresia with intact ventricular septum, as well as surgical relief in neonatal pulmonary stenosis. Procedures for each are fully reviewed, with a discussion of the positive results often achieved using balloon techniques in infants.
http://www.pediheart.org/practitioners/operations/valvotomy.html

VALVULOPLASTY

Annals of Thoracic Surgery: Long-Term Results of Surgical Valvuloplasty for Congenital Valvular Aortic Stenosis in Children This full-text article presents results of a retrospective study determining the long-term survival, incidence of valve restenosis or insufficiency, and incidence of reoperation or valve replacement in children undergoing surgical aortic valvu-

loplasty for congenital aortic valve stenosis. This study resulted in the conclusion that surgical valvuloplasty is safe and effective, benefiting the majority of patients for over 20 years.
http://www.ctsnet.org/journal/ats/68/1356

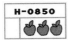

Children's Health Information Network: Pulmonic Stenosis and Balloon Valvuloplasty A cardiologist from Cedars-Sinai Medical Center in Los Angeles reviews the pathology and symptoms of valvular pulmonic stenosis, with historical treatment information and recent advancements regarding balloon pulmonary valvuloplasty via cardiac catheterization. Diagrams depicting the obstruction to normal blood flow in the pulmonary arterial system and balloon positioning and inflation are found, as well as a discussion of potential surgical complications.
http://www.tchin.org/resources/resorm/c_art_02.htm

Pennsylvania State University Geisinger Cardiovascular Center: Valvuloplasty Valvuloplasty, a procedure performed to open narrowed heart valves, is presented in this article, with information including what to expect before, during, and after the surgery; activity restrictions and follow-up care; and symptoms following the surgery that require medical attention. Links are available to related articles.
http://www.hersheyheart.com/pat_ed/pe119.htm

VENTRICLE-AND-A-HALF REPAIRS

PediHeart: Ventricle-and-a-Half Repairs Connection of the dysfunctional ventricle to the pulmonary artery and a superior cavopulmonary anastomosis for ventricle-and-a-half repairs are reviewed at this site, which includes stepwise investigatory considerations of the patient's former surgical interventions for optimization of procedure choices. The operation, from start to finish, is described in elaborate, clinical detail.
http://www.pediheart.org/practitioners/operations/ventHalf.html

6.9 TRANSPLANTATION

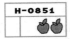

AHA Medical/Scientific Statement: Selection and Treatment of Candidates for Heart Transplantation A statement for healthcare professionals is available at this page, created by the Committee on Heart Failure and Cardiac Transplantation of the Council on Clinical Cardiology. The evaluation of patients with severe heart failure for heart transplantation is reviewed, with long-term management goals, the creation of specializd medical facilities, and the evolution of management discussed. Analysis of factors related to prognosis, data from clinical trials of medical therapies, and referral and evaluation are included. http://216.185.112.5/presenter.jhtml?identifier=1298

American Society for Artificial Organs Extensive information is available at this site of the American Society for Artificial Organs, which promotes the application and awareness of organ technologies to enhance the quality and duration of life. Information regarding the organization's annual conference and membership is found, as well as archived editions of the association's newsletter that deal with public policy issues surrounding the use of artificial organs. Links to related medical and bioengineering sites, along with advocacy organizations, can be found.

http://asaio.com

American Society of Transplantation The American Society of Transplantation consists of 1,300 transplant physicians and scientists active in research and management of patient care from the onset of end-stage disease to posttransplantation. The site contains information about the organization, meetings, publications, awards, certification, and public policy. A restricted section contains a member directory, education transcripts, a newsletter, slide lectures, and committee reports. Links to sites regarding general medicine, health news, and transplantation, along with links to newsgroups and LISTSERVs, are provided. (some features fee-based) http://www.a-s-t.org/index.htm

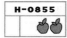

Association of Organ Procurement Organizations The Association of Organ Procurement Organizations (AOPO) is a private organization recognized as a national representative of organ procurement organizations. Their mission is to represent and serve these organizations through advocacy, support, and development of activities that will maximize the availability of organs and tissues and improve the quality, effectiveness, and integrity of the donation process. The site provides information about the AOPO, including membership information, organization activities, upcoming events, and news updates in the field of organ procurement. Links to donation and transplantation resources, such as the American Association of Tissue Banks and the Coalition on Donation, are provided, as well as connections to federal government agencies and individual AOPO member Web sites.

http://www.aopo.org

Cambridge and Oxford Heart Transplantation Foundation The Cambridge and Oxford Heart Transplantation Foundation is dedicated to the advancement of research in heart transplantation, the promotion of education in relation to heart disease, and the relief of illness. Their Web site contains information about the foundation and transplantation as well as details regarding the procedure's history. Research topics, including xenotransplantation, artificial hearts, tissue engineering, and cloning, are discussed, and a guide to transplantation includes answers to frequently asked questions.

http://www.heart-transplant.org

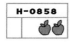

CenterSpan A collaborative project of the American Society of Transplantation and the American Society of Transplant Surgeons, CenterSpan provides transplant surgeons and physicians with essential information and resources.

The site contains information about the group, its objectives, membership, organization and structure, background, and board. A link is provided to Transplant News Network (TNN), a service of CenterSpan. Updated twice monthly, TNN gives the latest political, scientific, and industrial developments. Links to abstracts, publications, mailing lists, and outside Web sites are also provided, and registered members may access information about transplant registries. http://www.centerspan.org

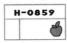

Children's Organ Transplant Association   The goal of the Children's Organ Transplant Association is to ensure that no individual in the United States is denied access to needed organs due to lack of financial resources. The site provides information about the group's campaigns, services, history, and procedures. An online newsletter and links to related sites are offered. http://www.cota.org

Eurotransplant   Eurotransplant acts as a clearinghouse and coordinates the international exchange of donor organs across a region with 116 million inhabitants. Information about potential recipients, indexed by blood group, tissue type, cause of illness, and clinical urgency, is provided, as well as extensive information about the foundation's working methods and board members. The site also contains news, links to other sites, and transplant information. http://www.transplant.org

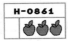

MEDLINEplus Health Information: Heart Transplantation   Informative heart transplantation links, selected by the National Library of Medicine, are provided at this MEDLINEplus health information Web site, offering everything from the latest legislation and news on organ transplantation to current research initiatives and rehabilitation advances. A link to the primary institute for heart disease at the National Institutes of Health is provided, and several connections to other government-related resources are found. Fact sheets on heart transplants, basic research regarding immune tolerance and transplantation, and a transplant glossary are accessible. A link to the United Network for Organ Sharing offers current news about the world's most technologically advanced transplant system, with current and past press releases and articles available. Medicare transplant regulations and other laws and policy regarding organ allocation, courtesy of the Health Resources and Services Administration, are found, and additional news-related and statistical sites are provided. http://www.nlm.nih.gov/medlineplus/hearttransplantation.html

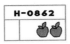

National Transplant Assistance Fund   The National Transplant Assistance Fund serves organ and tissue transplant patients, their families, and the healthcare professionals who treat them. Education, fundraising information, and financial support through medical assistance grants are provided. The site contains patient and family information that answers questions regarding expenses, insurance coverage, and help available through the National Transplant Assistance Fund. Information for medical professionals and potential contributors is provided. http://www.transplantfund.org

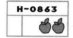

Transplant Living As a patient's connection to the transplant community, this site offers an introductory course for potential transplant patients, which includes answers to the most frequently asked questions. Patients may access information about waiting lists, donors, organ distribution, and finances. The site also contains an extensive database of transplant information, which may be searched by organ and state or institution. Statistics, organized according to race, age, and gender, provide information regarding the number of patients on the waiting list, how many received transplants, how many died, and how many were removed for other reasons. Links to related organizations are accessible.
http://www.patients.unos.org

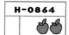

Transplant Recipients International Organization The Transplant Recipients International Organization (TRIO) works to improve the quality of life of transplant candidates, recipients, their families, and donor families. Information on the organization's mission, conferences, and chapters is provided, and services offered by the group, including a bimonthly newsletter, educational scholarships for transplant recipients, and a program for the promotion of organ donation, are found. A collection of educational and medical literature regarding donor awareness and transplantation is provided by the organization.
http://transweb.org/people/recips/resources/support/bkuptrio_main.html

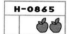

TransWeb.org Offering up-to-date information on transplantation and donation, this site educates visitors regarding the ethical and clinical issues surrounding organ and tissue donation and transplantation. The site contains questions and answers, the top 10 myths, and the latest headlines about donation and transplantation. Also located at this page are links to articles, books, newsletters, and transplant center Internet site listings.
http://www.transweb.org

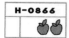

United Network for Organ Sharing The United Network for Organ Sharing (UNOS) was founded to advance organ availability and transplantation through education, technology, and policy development. This site explains the political and economic framework for organ donation and transplantation in the United States and offers information about transplant volume, organ procurement organizations, and waiting lists. Current headlines, links to articles related to organ procurement, statistical reports, and related Web site connections are provided.
http://www.unos.org/frame_Default.asp

6.10 CARDIAC REHABILITATION

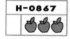

Agency for Healthcare Research and Quality (AHRQ): Clinical Guideline for Cardiac Rehabilitation By viewing the table of contents link, visitors can access sections of this document that address the effects of cardiac rehabilitation exercise training; cardiac rehabilitation education, counseling, and behavior modification; and organizational issues of cardiac rehabili-

tation programs. References, acronym definitions, tables and figures, and an online glossary provide a comprehensive clinical practice guideline, defining the scientific basis for cardiac rehabilitation recommendations.
http://text.nlm.nih.gov/ftrs/pick?ftrsK=0&collect=ahcpr&dbName=crpc&t=891494685

Agency for Healthcare Research and Quality (AHRQ): Guidelines for Post-Stroke Rehabilitation
This clinical guide to post-stroke rehabilitation, courtesy of the Agency for Healthcare Research and Quality, reviews assessment methods for stroke patients, rehabilitation during acute care, and screening for rehabilitation and appropriate setting choices. A glossary, a page of acronyms and abbreviations, and associated tables and figures accompany this clinical guide, which may be downloaded in its entirety.
http://text.nlm.nih.gov/ftrs/pick?dbName=psrc&
ftrsK=61924&cp=1&t=960777499&collect=ahcpr

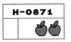

Agency for Healthcare Research and Quality (AHRQ): Recovering from Heart Problems through Cardiac Rehabilitation
This guide to cardiac rehabilitation offers an interactive table of contents, including sections on risk factors, cardiac rehabilitation team members, safety, benefits, alternate plans, and tips for success. Other sources of information and support are listed.
http://text.nlm.nih.gov/ftrs/pick?collect=ahcpr&dbName=crpp&cd=1&t=958682489

AHA Medical/Scientific Statement: Cardiac Rehabilitation Programs
This document, intended for healthcare professionals, offers information on cardiac rehabilitation programs, with discussions of program components, risk factor modification, psychosocial interventions, and current research. An extensive listing of references is included.
http://216.185.112.5/presenter.jhtml?identifier=1222

American Association of Cardiovascular and Pulmonary Rehabilitation
The mission of the American Association of Cardiovascular and Pulmonary Rehabilitation is to reduce morbidity, mortality, and disability from cardiovascular and pulmonary diseases through education, prevention, rehabilitation, and aggressive disease management. Used as a resource for healthcare professionals, this Web site offers links to association meetings, job and internship postings, and relevant publications. Connections to cardiovascular and pulmonary resources, professional organizations, and other related sites are provided.
http://www.aacvpr.org

American Heart Association (AHA): Cardiovascular Rehabilitation
The principles of cardiac rehabilitation and AHA recommendations for patients with congenital or acquired heart disease are presented at this site, along with a listing of related publications.
http://216.185.112.5/presenter.jhtml?identifier=4490

Johns Hopkins Heart Health at Bayview: Cardiac Rehabilitation
This site provides information about the cardiac rehabilitation and prevention program available at Johns Hopkins Bayview Medical Center. With a focus on diet

and heart disease, the benefits of cardiac rehabilitation are detailed. Educational information for both patients and healthcare professionals is provided, in addition to data regarding related clinical research.
http://www.jhbmc.jhu.edu/cardiology/rehab/rehab.html

6.11 CLINICAL PRACTICE GUIDELINES
AND DISEASE MANAGEMENT

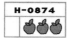

Agency for Healthcare Research and Quality (AHRQ): Clinical Practice Guidelines Clinical practice guidelines, quick reference guides for clinicians, and consumer guides in both English and Spanish are accessible from this site of the Agency for Healthcare Research and Quality (AHRQ), formerly the Agency for Health Care Policy and Research (AHCPR). By entering a topic of interest in one of the three publication categories, visitors are returned guidelines on management of acute pain, heart failure, and post-stroke rehabilitation. Unstable angina and cardiac rehabilitation topics are also available in clinical guideline or quick reference formats.
http://text.nlm.nih.gov/ftrs/pick?dbK=&ftrsK=34752&t=944420085&collect=ahcpr

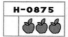

American College of Cardiology (ACC): Clinical Statements/Guidelines Free access to clinical documents is provided at this ACC Web site, which includes a variety of evidence-based statements and guidelines, issued by authorities in the field of cardiovascular medicine. A complete list of guidelines can be searched at the A-to-Z guide, and a quick pocket guideline reference is available. Newly released practice parameters for percutaneous coronary intervention and catheterization standards are accessible, as well as consensus documents and guidelines across a variety of cardiovascular topics.
http://www.acc.org/clinical/statements.htm

American Heart Association (AHA): Scientific Statements A chronological listing of active Medical and Scientific Statements from the American College of Cardiology and the American Heart Association is available at this site. Hundreds of titles pertaining to the management of various heart conditions, as well as guidelines for implementation of treatments and diagnostic procedures, are found. Included are advisory statements, executive committee summaries, and full-text guidelines for comprehensive clinical management reference. http://216.185.112.5/presenter.jhtml?identifier=9181

Columbia University: PULSE: The Heart Disease Management Center PULSE is a heart disease management center for medical professionals, offering a collection of news and features, a journal club with abstracts, editorial comments on particular aspects of heart disease, and focused bibliographies. Professional education resources include tutorials, case studies, slide shows, and clinical trials, as well as links to reviewed cardiology Web sites.
http://www.pulseonline.org

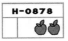

Medscape: Cardiology Practice Guidelines Acceptable practice for a variety of topics in cardiology is available at this address, which hosts medical management statements from National Institutes of Health divisions, the American College of Chest Physicians, and the National High Blood Pressure Education Program Committee. Practice guidelines in the areas of coronary artery disease, hypertension, lipid control, venous thromboembolism and pulmonary embolism, cardiovascular disease in women, physical fitness, and cardiovascular health are included among the available documents. (free registration)
http://www.medscape.com/Home/Topics/
cardiology/directories/dir-CARD.PracticeGuide.html

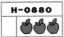

National Guideline Clearinghouse (NGC) Sponsored by the Agency for Healthcare Research and Quality (AHRQ) in partnership with the American Medical Association (AMA) and the American Association of Health Plans (AAHP), this site serves as an extensive public resource of evidence-based clinical practice guidelines. The database provides guidelines for both diseases/conditions and treatments/interventions. The site also includes a listing of FAQs and an electronic forum for professional exchange of information on clinical practice guidelines. More than 50 guidelines related to cardiovascular diseases are currently listed.
http://www.guideline.gov

University of Alabama: Cardiovascular Disorders Clinical Resources
Clinical resources in cardiovascular disease management are organized by topic at this page of the Clinical Digital Libraries Project, courtesy of the University of Alabama. Cardiovascular symptoms, pericardial disease, congestive heart failure, and more than 10 additional disorder and diagnostic procedure category links connect visitors to an extensive collection of online textbooks and documents in the particular field. Chapters of the online *Merck Manual,* eMedicine's online textbook, the *Family Practice Handbook,* and an assortment of additional reference links, pediatric resources, and clinical guidelines can be retrieved. Some documents and texts may require an online subscription.
(some features fee-based)
http://www.slis.ua.edu/cdlp/WebDLCore/clinical/cardiology/index.htm

University of California San Francisco (UCSF): Primary Care Clinical Practice Guidelines: Cardiovascular System Hyperlinks to guidelines and practice statements found at this site represent a variety of conditions in cardiovascular management and include documents from the National Guideline Clearinghouse, the World Health Organization, the American Heart Association, and several divisions of the National Institutes of Health. Guidelines are listed according to disorder or practice topic and include management summaries for hypertension, cardiac surgical procedures, coronary heart disease, pericardial disease, heart failure, stroke, arrhythmias, and valvular disease.
http://medicine.ucsf.edu/resources/guidelines/guide7.html

OTHER TOPICAL
RESOURCES

7.1 ADVOCACY AND PUBLIC POLICY

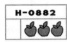

American College of Cardiology (ACC): Advocacy The advocacy page of the ACC offers access to *Advocacy Weekly,* a weekly newsletter intended to provide information on the latest legislative and regulatory developments of interest to college members. Archived issues can be viewed from the site, as well as coverage of the ACC's advocacy agenda. A State Action Center and resource links for becoming more familiar with health policy topics are available.
http://www.acc.org/advocacy/advocacy.htm

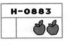

American Heart Association (AHA): Clean Indoor Air Laws An AHA advocacy position regarding the enactment of more stringent clean indoor air laws is discussed at this page. High public health standards, findings of the U.S. Surgeon General and the National Institute of Occupational Safety and Health regarding protection of nonsmokers, and recommendations for clean air statutes are introduced. Several related guides are listed, and can be accessed using the AHA search engine.
http://216.185.112.5/presenter.jhtml?identifier=4573

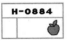

American Heart Association (AHA): Community Support for Exercise (Physical Activity) Steps that many communities can take to encourage physical activity are discussed at this page from the AHA. A list of related AHA publications and consumer guides is provided, including those addressing exercise in children, exercise for older people, and obesity and overweight conditions. A fact sheet on the National Coalition for Promoting Physical Activity is also available.
http://216.185.112.5/presenter.jhtml?identifier=4531

American Heart Association (AHA): Federal Regulation of Tobacco The status of regulations promulgated by the Food and Drug Administration asserting jurisdiction over tobacco products is discussed at this page from the AHA, and the AHA's advocacy position on the subject is introduced. A list of related publications is included.
http://216.185.112.5/presenter.jhtml?identifier=11223

7.2 Air Pollution

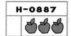

American Heart Association (AHA): Air Pollution, Heart Disease, and Stroke   The need for investigations into the possible effects of environmental air pollution on the incidence of cardiovascular diseases and stroke is the focus of this AHA article. Background information on the relationship of chronic exposure to air pollution and disease, several environmental pollutants to be aware of, and specific information on carbon monoxide, nitrogen dioxide, and particulate matter and sulfur dioxide are provided. Related documents include coverage of environmental tobacco smoke and clean indoor air laws.
http://216.185.112.5/presenter.jhtml?identifier=4419

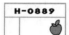

American Heart Association (AHA): Environmental Tobacco Smoke   The ongoing debate about environmental tobacco smoke and its effect on cardiovascular health is discussed at this online brochure. The scientific position of the AHA, including the goal of further educating the public about this issue; the AHA advocacy position; and background information on the effects of environmental tobacco smoke on the health of nonsmokers are presented, citing a 1986 report of the Surgeon General, studies by the National Academy of Science, and more recent published literature on the subject.
http://216.185.112.5/presenter.jhtml?identifier=4521

WebMDHealth: Air Pollution Linked to Heart Problems, Deaths
WebMD Medical News offers this information on a recent study conducted by researchers at Harvard Medical School. A previously suspected association between air pollution and increases in heart attacks and deaths due to other heart-related causes is examined, with connections between fine particles and ozone linked to effects on the heart. Recognition of air pollution as a public health concern and information on future investigations are introduced.
http://my.webmd.com/content/article/1728.55867

7.3 Anesthesiology

European Association of Cardiothoracic Anesthesiologists   The goal of the European Association of Cardiothoracic Anesthesiologists is to provide an international forum for scientific dialogue and to promote education in the field. The Web site contains information about the organization, its annual meetings, and membership, as well as details regarding abstract submission for conferences. Additionally, links to other anesthesiology-related sites, including the Society of Cardiovascular Anesthesiologists and the American Society of Anesthesiologists, are provided.
http://www.eacta.org

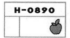

Society of Cardiovascular Anesthesiologists   Society event listings, current and archived newsletters of the association, and fellowship and grant programs and details are available for review at the Society of Cardiovascular

Anesthesiologists Web page. Details regarding the future of its online CME program and two presentations on echocardiographic assessment and cardiopulmonary bypass are presented. A variety of links to related anesthesiology organizations and journals are accessible, as well as connections to a variety of diagnostic and disease management sites.
http://www.scahq.org

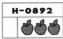

Virtual Anaesthesia Textbook: Anaesthesia for Cardiothoracic Surgery The Virtual Anaesthesia Textbook offers a comprehensive guide to anesthesia for cardiothoracic surgery, including preoperative assessment, monitoring, anesthetic choices, myocardial revascularization, valvular disorders, thoracic surgery, cardiopulmonary bypass, circulatory assist devices, and postoperative care. Additionally, the site provides links to related resources, such as the practice guidelines of the American Society of Anesthesiology and anesthetic drug information.
http://www.virtual-anaesthesia-textbook.com/vat/cardiac.html

7.4 Artificial Hearts

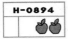

Cambridge and Oxford Heart Transplantation Foundation: Artificial Hearts The effectiveness of a new type of artificial heart, a plastic pump that fits directly into the left ventricle, is discussed at this site. Mechanical circulatory support, external centrifugal and roller pumps, external pulsatile ventricular assist devices, implantable left ventricular assist systems, and biventricular replacement prostheses are reviewed in terms of indications and their differences. http://www.heart-transplant.org/research/artificial.htm

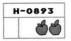

USA Today: Artificial Hearts Pumping Ahead This reprint of a *USA Today* article reviews recent advancements in artificial heart technology. The future of assist pumps and their potential as permanent implants, improvements of new pumps over older versions, and historical perspectives in the development of a mechanical heart are included.
http://www.usatoday.com/life/health/heart/lhhea150.htm

7.5 Autoimmunity

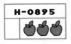

American Autoimmune Related Diseases Association, Inc. The American Autoimmune Related Diseases Association, Inc., was created to work toward the eradication of autoimmune disease and to alleviate suffering through education, research, and patient services. The site provides details about the organization, its mission, and activities. Patient information on autoimmune diseases, such as cardiomyopathy and Raynaud's phenomenon, is found, and press releases, informative articles from archived newsletters, answers to frequently asked questions, and gender-specific information are pro-

vided. Research reports and information regarding the group's position on related legislation are accessible, in addition to related resource links.
http://www.aarda.org

7.6 COMPUTERS IN CARDIOLOGY

Artificial Intelligence Systems in Routine Clinical Use This well-indexed site contains summaries of nearly 40 artificial intelligence systems that have been in routine use in medical settings. A lengthy history of the use of artificial intelligence in medicine is provided, along with links to research groups, journals, and other resources in the field.
http://www.coiera.com/ailist/list.html

Computer Applications in Clinical Care Computer-assisted reports of electrocardiograms (CARE) and the three main areas of ECG computer processing and analysis are discussed at the site, in addition to other uses of computers in cardiological care. The 24-hour ECG and descriptions of technological methods are reviewed, as well as the exercise ECG and the computerized signal processing of the signal-averaged ECG.
http://students.dcs.gla.ac.uk/courses/MSc_IT/cacc/bishopa/cardiology.html

Computer Simulation and Visualization in the Cardiovascular System These examples of computer visualization offer a look at a way in which computers may provide a better understanding of cardiovascular components and interaction. The video discussed offers animated sequences of simulated hemodynamics and fluctuations in blood pressure and flow through the cardiovascular system. The images shown at the site reference the video's vessel change simulations, with color-coded markings to illustrate flow rate, pressure, and tensed or relaxed states.
http://www.ncsa.uiuc.edu/SCMS/DigLib/text/biology/Cardiovascular-System-Clark.html

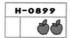

Computers in Cardiology Computers in Cardiology is a nonprofit corporation composed of scientists in the fields of medicine, physics, engineering, and computer science, providing a forum for presentations of computer applications in clinical cardiology and cardiovascular research. Users may access conference information and preliminary program details at the site in addition to an organized list of topics presented at Computers in Cardiology conferences. Topics are organized under several subheadings, including ECG, electrophysiology, modeling and simulation, cardiovascular mechanics, cardiovascular imaging, and medical informatics. Information for obtaining proceedings of Computers in Cardiology conferences is found, in addition to award details and an author's kit for manuscript preparation.
http://www.cinc.org

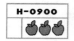

Heart Throb: Modeling Cardiac Fluid Dynamics An enlargeable aortic GIF image and discussion of the visualized results of computational model heart anatomy are offered at the Heart Throb Web site. A 3-D version of the heart, its valves, and nearby vessels are discussed, and images of computed flow patterns at different times during a single heartbeat are viewable at the site. Downloadable from the page are animated educational videos depicting muscle fibers of the heart wall and the mitral and aortic valves. Also available is the image of a simulated heartbeat with blood ejected into the aorta upon left ventricle contraction.

http://www.psc.edu/MetaCenter/MetaScience/Articles/Peskin/Peskin.html

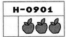

Heart: The Engine of Life Educational Software *The Heart: The Engine of Life* educational software is described at this site, with several reviews of this notable 3-D tutorial on human heart function. System requirements are discussed, and a free shareware version of the program is available for downloading from the site. Assistance with writing a program shortcut and answers to frequently asked technical questions are provided.

http://www.animatedsoftware.com/ascodesc/hartdesc.htm

7.7 CRITICAL CARE MEDICINE

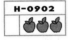

AHA Medical/Scientific Statement: Advisory Statements on the International Liaison Committee on Resuscitation Intended for consideration by national and international expert bodies, the AHA presents this Scientific Statement on resuscitation. Chapters on single-rescuer adult basic life support, a universal advanced life support algorithm, early defibrillation by emergency practitioners and other personnel, and special review of pediatric resuscitation are discussed. Coverage of special resuscitation situations, as seen in cases of electrolyte abnormalities, cardiac arrest due to toxic substances, and near-drowning experiences, is provided.

http://216.185.112.5/presenter.jhtml?identifier=1841

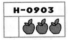

American Heart Association (AHA): Emergency Cardiovascular Care The Emergency Cardiovascular Care program of the AHA delivers training in acute care treatment to lay rescuers as well as emergency room physicians nationwide. Components of the program, cardiopulmonary resuscitation and automated external defibrillator treatment, and information on basic life support and advanced courses are discussed at the site. Online resources that support the scientific basis and recommendations of the AHA for emergency cardiovascular care are accessible, in addition to the emergency cardiovascular care newsletter, *Currents*.

http://www.cpr-ecc.org/

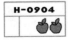

Clinical Information and Concepts in Chestpain Centers The clinical and professional information offered at this site includes review of the shifting paradigm to early heart attack care (EHAC), with several futuristic articles regarding chest pain awareness, emergency care, and the importance of prodromal symptom recognition. Modules for emergency cardiac care, examples of clinical tracks for hospitalized patients, and scientific articles on chest pain in emergency departments are found. A discussion of clinical pathways disease management is found, along with several accessible articles and abstracts on chest pain center care and strategies.

http://jumpstart.chestpaincenters.org/chestpaincenters/default.cfm

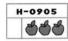

Pediatric Critical Care Medicine   The Pediatric Critical Care Medicine site provides a peer-reviewed, multidisciplinary educational guide for pediatric critical care, with original content and links to notable Internet resources. The site's news link offers information on an upcoming critical care colloquium, as well as journal article reviews and details on additional conferences and events. A clinical practice tutorial is available from the site, in addition to clinical publications, a comprehensive index of case reports, software review, and collaborative, clinical trial information for critically ill patients.

http://PedsCCM.wustl.edu

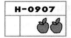

Society of Critical Care Medicine   Critical care news, activities of the Society of Critical Care Medicine (SCCM), and educational critical care events nationwide are discussed at the Web site. A connection to the consultative body of the SCCM, the American College of Critical Care Medicine (ACCM), provides complete access to all guidelines and clinical parameters for the critical care practitioner. Details regarding SCCM's Project IMPACT, for standardization of critical care data, and access to the newsletters of the Coalition for Critical Care Excellence, a critical care clinical investigation network, are provided. Access to the SCCM bookstore allows visitors to order any of the publications of the organization and its consultative branch.

http://www.sccm.org/

7.8 DRUG ABUSE

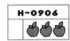

National Institute of Drug Abuse (NIDA): Commonly Abused Drugs
The table found at this address outlines common categories of commercial and street drugs of abuse, including cannabinoids, depressants, dissociative anesthetics, hallucinogens, opioids and morphine derivatives, stimulants, and miscellaneous drugs of abuse. Schedule category, modes of administration, and both intoxication potentials and health consequences are reviewed. Additionally, principles of drug addiction and a link outlining the criteria for substance dependence diagnosis are offered.

http://www.drugabuse.gov/DrugsofAbuse.html

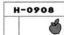

WebMDHealth: Pot Impacts Heart, Study Shows   Possible increased heart attack risk with marijuana use is the focus of this online story, a result of research initiated based on a report recommendation of the Institute of Medicine. Significant information derived from the research is stated.

http://my.webmd.com/content/article/1728.55387

7.9 EPIDEMIOLOGY AND BIOSTATISTICS

Emory Center for Outcomes Research The Emory Center for Outcomes Research (ECOR) serves as a coordinating center for clinical trials in diagnostic and therapeutic areas and provides specific expertise in the application of their research to quality-of-life and cost-effectiveness evaluations. Current clinical trials in electrophysiology, treatment of angina, and the Women's Ischemia Syndrome Evaluation are included. Further information at the site includes the ECOR newsletter and useful resource links regarding outcomes research.
http://www.emory.edu/WHSC/CARDIOLOGY/CVEC

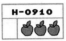

Global Cardiovascular InfoBase A group of scientists, including physicians and epidemiologists, created this site to prevent the epidemic of cardiovascular diseases in developing parts of the world. Headed by the World Health Organization, this project involved the construction and maintenance of a large database, accessible at this site. The InfoBase contains current statistics on demographics, mortality, morbidity, risk factors, and related healthcare variables. Data is linked to country maps and may be displayed in multiple formats.
http://cvdinfobase.ic.gc.ca

National Heart, Lung, and Blood Institute (NHLBI): Division of Epidemiology and Clinical Applications Epidemiological studies, basic and applied behavioral research, demonstration and education research, and projects for disease prevention and health promotion, including clinical trials, are conducted within this division of the NHLBI. Detailed summaries of the Clinical Applications and Prevention Program, the Epidemiology and Biometry Program, and the Office of Biostatistics Research are available, as well as contact information and an abbreviated staff directory.
http://www.nhlbi.nih.gov/about/deca/index.htm

7.10 EXTRACORPOREAL TECHNOLOGY/LIFE SUPPORT

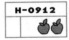

Advanced Cardiac Life Support Created as a resource for nurses seeking certification in advanced cardiac life support, this Web site offers tutorial material about medical procedures to be followed. Information includes the identification of cardiopulmonary arrest and initial patient assessment, ventricular fibrillation, and procedures following cessation of ventricular fibrillation. There is also information about ventricular tachycardia, automatic external defibrillators, sinus bradycardia, AV block, supraventricular tachyarrhythmias, sinus tachycardia, paroxysmal supraventricular tachycardia, and multifocal atrial tachycardia. Hyperlinks to information about drugs used in the outlined procedures are provided.
http://cyber-nurse.com/veetac/cham4.htm

American Society of Extra-Corporeal Technology (AmSECT) A professional society, AmSECT fosters improved patient care by providing continuing education and standards in the field of extracorporeal technology. Though one portion of the site is restricted to members, most of the site is open to the public and contains information about the organization, meetings, and events, as well as job opportunities, scholarships, and grants. There is a section dedicated to the Pediatric Perfusion Committee of AmSECT, as well as a section for consumers, which includes a lengthy glossary of terms and explains common perfusion services, cardiopulmonary bypass, and extracorporeal membrane oxygenation.

(some features fee-based) http://www.amsect.org

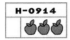

University of Michigan: Extracorporeal Life Support Organization

The Extracorporeal Life Support Organization maintains a large central database of extracorporeal life support cases, devices and complications, follow-up information, and active centers. This Web site provides information about their research laboratory, available educational materials, meetings, and staff. The site also contains informative family guides to extracorporeal life support and provides references and links to related organizations, medical centers, and Internet resources. http://www.med.umich.edu/ecmo

7.11 FETAL/NEONATAL CARDIOLOGY

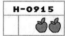

Childbirth.org: Monitoring Resources   This Web address offers links to

patient information about fetal monitoring. Resources include answers to frequently asked questions about fetal monitoring, abstracts on monitoring, related studies, and articles.

http://www.childbirth.org/articles/efm.html

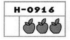

Kansas University Medical Center: Fetal and Neonatal Cardiology

Illustrations and diagnostic images of a variety of fetal and neonatal heart abnormalities are collected at this site, sponsored by the Children's Center at the University of Kansas Medical Center. Diagrams of patent ductus arteriosus, patent foramen ovale, persistence of the fetal circulation, traditional auscultation areas, and the cardiac cycle are found, as well as a large variety of echocardiogram videos and still frames. Both normal and pathologic imaging are provided. http://www.kumc.edu/kumcpeds/cardiology/fetaldfct.html

Perinatal Cardiology   This page contains information about fetal cardiology

and neonatal cardiology, providing an introduction to fetal cardiography and its value in the diagnosis of fetal heart defects. It answers questions frequently asked by expectant mothers during consultations and provides a hyperlink to information about the management of fetal arrhythmias. Neonatal cardiology information includes a discussion of neonatal ductus arteriosus and a link to an AHA document on the prevention of bacterial endocarditis.

http://www.unich.it/percar/main.htm

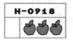

University of Pennsylvania: Fetal Echocardiography   The "Library of

Images" presented at this site offers typical views of a normal and an abnormal heart, with pathological images including Ebstein's anomaly and hypoplastic left heart syndrome. The "Library of Cases" covers aortic atresia, mitral stenosis, congenital cystic adenomatoid malformation, and tetralogy of Fallot. The site also features a gestational age calculator, a discussion forum, and a listing of related links.

http://www.med.upenn.edu/fetus/echo.htm

7.12 GENETICS AND GENOMICS

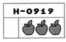

American Heart Association (AHA): Genome-Based Resource An excerpt from *Circulation* is found at this page of the AHA, which is offered as several PDF documents, available with Adobe Acrobat Reader. An analysis of cardiovascular gene expression, functional gene classification, and applications in the identification of developmental or disease states of the cardiovascular system are examined. The future of genome research and its use in the investigations of cardiovascular biology and disease are the focus of this resource.

http://216.185.112.5/presenter.jhtml?identifier=626

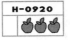

Applications of Gene Therapy in Cardiovascular Medicine The article at this site, authored by Ernest DeGidio, addresses concepts in gene therapy and transfer and their applications in the field of cardiovascular medicine. Review of the first successful gene transfer and newer techniques is provided, along with information on gene delivery to cardiac myocytes, heart transplant applications, angiogenesis for more efficient blood delivery, and the possibilities of gene therapy in preventing restenosis.

http://oak.cats.ohiou.edu/~ed170793/paper.htm

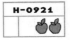

Cholesterol, Genetics, and Heart Disease Institute The Cholesterol, Genetics, and Heart Disease Institute is a nonprofit organization dedicated to research, education, training, and clinical heart disease treatment and prevention. The site provides information about the institution's activities and events, late-breaking trials from the AHA, case studies, abstracts, and publications and presentations. The site provides links to other clinics, research studies, and educational programs.

http://www.heartdisease.org

Medicine at Oxford: Molecular Genetics and Molecular Biology of Heart Muscle Disease The value of genetic approaches in the evaluation of the etiology of heart muscle phenotypes is summarized in this molecular genetics review. The methodology for studying heart muscle phenotypes and the work of related research groups are explored. Discussion includes the future of heart muscle phenotype research directions and current, collaborative studies on the genetic determinants of heart disease.

http://www.medicine.ox.ac.uk/cardiov/molgen.htm

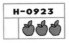

Online Mendelian Inheritance in Man (OMIM) By entering one or more search terms, visitors can access hundreds of database entries explaining the ge-

netic expression of thousands of disease states. Fifty entries are displayed on each page, with connections available to the clinical synopsis entry, biochemical disease features, modes of inheritance, and allelic variant discussion.
http://www3.ncbi.nlm.nih.gov/Omim/

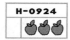

University of Kansas: Genetics Education Center This site provides a search engine for the Genetics Education Center, which permits the user to access human and clinical genetics information, research, and educational resources. There are also links to nearly 20 additional search engines, accompanied by valuable tips on searching.
http://www.kumc.edu/gec/search.html

7.13 GERIATRIC CARDIOLOGY

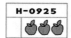

American Family Physician: Hypertension Treatment and the Prevention of Coronary Artery Disease in the Elderly Hypertension and its relation to coronary artery disease and congestive heart failure in the elderly is the focus of this article, provided by the American Academy of Family Physicians. Authored by a physician at Yale University School of Medicine, the article discusses major risk factors in the aging population, specific antihypertensive therapies that may prevent or reduce the risk of complex heart disease, and pharmacological trials related to lowering blood pressure.
http://www.aafp.org/afp/990301ap/1248.html

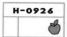

Society of Geriatric Cardiology The Society of Geriatric Cardiology was founded to address the problems associated with cardiovascular diseases in the increasing number of aging people in the United States and around the world. The site provides information about the society, including membership information and applications, personnel directories, society news, and a calendar of events. Authors of medical articles may access information about submitting articles, papers, and abstracts.
http://www.sgcard.org

7.14 HEART STUDIES

Below are links to selected research study details and headlines in the field of cardiology. Readers are encouraged to consult the "Clinical Studies and Trials" section of the Quick Reference chapter for access to more complete listings of both government- and industry-sponsored research.

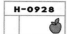

Antioxidant Helps the Heart A report on a three-year study is found at this site, sponsored by The Age Company, Ltd. The effects of coenzyme Q10 on the heart muscle tissue of heart bypass surgery patients are described at this summary of a clinical trial, presented at the World Congress of the International Co-enzyme Q10 Association in Frankfurt, Germany.
http://www.theage.com.au/news/2000/12/20/FFX8PGUFWGC.html

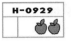

Bogalusa Heart Study   Information from Tulane University on the Bogalusa Heart study offers details concerning cardiovascular disease risk factor research. Details on substudies, a bibliography of hundreds of published papers on the research, and significant accomplishments of the research are cited.
http://www.som.tulane.edu/cardiohealth/bog.htm

British Heart Foundation: Family Heart Study   Information on this genetic research being conducted in the Family Heart Study is presented at the page, with basic components of the project and key reasons for genetic research offered. The importance of getting involved in this long-term study is emphasized, and contact information for the University of Leeds team is offered.
http://www.leeds.ac.uk/reporter/461/factsheet.htm

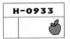

Bypass Angioplasty Revascularization Investigation (BARI)   News on a published study is found at this site, which provides information on a recent report published in *Circulation*. A new analysis of the BARI study and benefits of bypass over angioplasty for diabetic patients are discussed, courtesy of the Heart Information Network.
http://www.heartinfo.com/news97/bari101397.htm

Cardiovascular Disease in Familial Forms of Hypertriglyceridemia: A 20-Year Prospective Study   Further information on this study, designed to estimate cardiovascular disease mortality risk among relatives of those with familial combined hyperlipidemia and familial hypertriglyceridemia, is found at this *Circulation* article, part of the American Heart Association Web site. The full text of the article, a PDF reprint, and links to other collections under which this article is cited can be accessed.
http://circ.ahajournals.org/cgi/content/abstract/101/24/2777

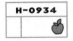

Coronary Primary Prevention Trial   Details on this landmark study and brief statements about several related research projects demonstrating a correlation between cholesterol levels and cardiovascular mortality are found at this address of the American Heart Association. Several related guides of the organization are available.
http://www.americanheart.org/Heart_and_Stroke_A_Z_Guide/corpp.html

Criteria Underestimate Heart Disease Risk in People under 50   Sponsored by drkoop.com and the American Council on Science and Health, this page addresses questions raised about the National Cholesterol Education Program's assumptions concerning cholesterol elevations in younger populations. Components of the analysis are reviewed, and recommendations with regard to prevention guidelines are stated.
http://www.drkoop.com/news/focus/april/young_hearts.html

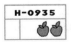

Dietary Approaches to Stop Hypertension (DASH)   Findings from the DASH study are available for viewing online in PDF format. Alternatively, users can order printed copies online, by telephone, fax, or e-mail. Included in the publication is a description of the DASH diet, a step-by-step eating plan, sample menus, tips to reduce sodium intake, and recommendations for food label comparison. http://www.nhlbi.nih.gov/health/public/heart/hbp/dash/index.htm

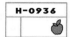

Duke Study Finds Key Heart Drug Underutilized   The underutilization of an effective cardiology drug is the focus of this discussion offered by Duke University Medical Center. The safety and effectiveness of angiotensin converting enzyme (ACE) inhibitors and the lag time demonstrated between positive clinical trials of the drug and widespread acceptance and prescribing are discussed. The need for education in the field and possibilities for future usage studies are mentioned.
http://www.dukenews.duke.edu/Med/mcguraha.htm

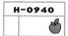

Foundation-Funded Study Links Improved Heart Failure Outcome to Pharmacist Involvement   This study, funded in part by the American Society of Health-System Pharmacists Foundation, reviews the role that pharmacists play in a multidisciplinary healthcare team. Outcomes of heart failure patients who benefited from pharmacist intervention are emphasized.
http://www.ashpfoundation.org/news/nlspr00/heartstudy.htm

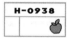

Heart Damage and Muscular Dystrophy   Information on a potential preventative treatment for the heart damage associated with muscular dystrophy is provided at this page, reporting on recent research at the University of Iowa. A new understanding of the disease process and its implications for pharamacotherapeutic interventions are introduced.
http://www.uiowa.edu/~ournews/2001/january/0112heart-damage.html

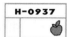

INSPIRE Study: VA Assesses Benefit of Cardiac Catheterization Following Heart Attack   Presented by the Medical College of Georgia, this site offers a look at whether or not cardiac catheterization following heart attack reduces death and disability. The INSPIRE study and its comparison of cardiac catheterization a medication-only regimen is presented, along with a discussion of the goals of the INSPIRE research and the purpose of resting and stress versions of myocardial perfusion imaging in study participants.
http://www.mcg.edu/news/2000NewsRel/cardiac_cath.html

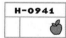

Iron and Heart Disease   The *Heart and Stroke Guide* of the American Heart Association introduces information on the possible link between iron stores and heart disease. Information on the original theory, posed by Jerome L. Sullivan, M.D., Ph.D.; past failures to replicate the findings; and more recent research that presents largely inconclusive information about the association are discussed. http://www.americanheart.org/Heart_and_Stroke_A_Z_Guide/iron.html

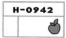

Jackson Heart Study   Sponsored by the National Institutes of Health, this page describes research intended to discover risk factors for cardiovascular disease in African Americans. Additional goals of the research, accomplished through collaborative efforts of major teaching institutions, are discussed at this page of the University of North Carolina at Chapel Hill.
http://www-bios.sph.unc.edu/units/cscc/JHSW/jhswdesc.html

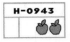

Lyon Diet Heart Study Information on this Mediterranean-type diet and its relation to the incidence of coronary events is presented at this American Heart Association site, which briefly describes the results of recent research and its implications. A description of the analysis performed of the Mediterranean-style diet and details on dietary guidelines developed by the National Cholesterol Education Program and the AHA are provided. Lyon diet details, results of the study, limitations of the information, and conclusions reached about this dietary pattern are discussed.
http://www.americanheart.org/Heart_and_Stroke_A_Z_Guide/lyondietheart.html

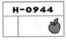

Magnesium in Coronaries (MAGIC) Designed to evaluate the clinical effectiveness of early administration of magnesium sulfate following myocardial infarction, the MAGIC study is introduced at this page. Potential risks and benefits, patient recruitment information, inclusion and exclusion criteria, and study objectives are summarized, courtesy of the National Heart, Lung, and Blood Institute.
http://www.nhlbi.nih.gov/studies/magicweb.htm

Multi-Ethnic Study of Atherosclerosis (MESA) Study design, primary aims of the MESA study, and details on the dietary assessment component of this research are discussed at this site of Northwestern University. Potential of the study to identify risk factors and prevent the progression of subclinical to clinical heart disease is addressed, as well as other research goals.
http://www.galter.nwu.edu/nutrition/prevent/multi.htm

Muscatine Heart Study General objectives of the Muscatine Heart Study are reviewed at this site of the University of Iowa, which commemorates 30 years of cardiovascular research. Information on the research projects of the study, funded by the National Institutes of Health, is provided, and related links and stories are available.
http://www.public-health.uiowa.edu/perspective/Muscatine study/

Normative Aging Study—1963-1998 Published by MultiMedia Health Care, this electronicversion of a *Clinical Geriatrics* article offers study cohorts and measurement, information on statistical methods, and conclusions with respect to risk factors and percentile distributions for cardiovascular illness in the aged. Recognized predictors of cardiovascular events are discussed, and comparisons to related research are found.
http://www.mmhc.com/cg/articles/CG9909/lee.html

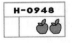

Ornish Treatment Studies authored by Dean Ornish, M.D., published in both the *Lancet* and the *American Journal of Cardiology,* are discussed at this page, including the American Heart Association's response to Ornish's research and many components of the Ornish treatment plan. Comparison of the Ornish plan with the Step I and II diets of the AHA and the National Cholesterol Education Program is found, and questions raised by the Ornish research are posed.
http://www.americanheart.org/Heart_and_Stroke_A_Z_Guide/ornish.html

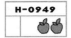

Physicians' Health Study: Baldness Is Cardiovascular Risk Factor A review of research originally published in the *Archives of Internal Medicine* is found at this site, addressing the differences between vertex and frontal baldness and their associated risks of coronary heart disease. The possible connection between baldness and increased androgen receptors and higher testosterone levels is discussed, as well as the usefulness of baldness as a clinical marker to identify men at increased risk, courtesy of the *Pharmaceutical Journal*.
http://www.pharmj.com/Editorial/20000212/clinical/baldness.html

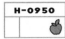

Prevention of Recurrent Venous Thromboembolism (PREVENT) Trial Sponsored by the National Heart, Lung, and Blood Institute, the multicenter Prevent trial is discussed at this site. Basic information on venous thromboembolism, treatment of deep vein thrombosis and pulmonary embolism, inclusion and exclusion criteria, treatment, and trial status are introduced.
http://www.nhlbi.nih.gov/studies/prevent1.htm

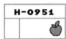

Prospective Study of Egg Consumption and Risk of Cardiovascular Disease in Men and Women Recent research examining a possible association between egg consumption and risk of coronary heart disease is reviewed at this site, which includes study objectives, outcome measures, and research conclusions. Provided by the *Journal of the American Medical Association,* the full text of the article is available to regular subscribers or on a pay-per-view basis.
(some features fee-based) http://jama.ama-assn.org/issues/v281n15/abs/joc81683.html

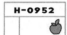

Research in Congenital Heart Defects Sponsored by the National Heart, Lung, and Blood Institute, this site of the University of Iowa provides details concerning recruitment of families for participation in this research, intended to prevent heart defects in future generations. Requirements of the research and contact information are included.
http://www.uihealthcare.com/depts/med/pediatrics/congenitalheart/

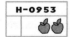

Researchers Study Cardiac Energetics with Fluorescence and Spectroscopy Provided by OriginLab, this site discusses research recently conducted at Loyola University Chicago, utilizing fluorescence spectroscopy to monitor mitochondrial nicotineamide adenine dinucleotide (NADH). Information on the various control signals, hypothesized to serve as mechanisms for energy regulation in the heart, is presented, along with conclusions regarding energy deprivation and its relationship to certain cardiac conditions.
http://www.originlab.com/www/resources/case_studies/Loyola1.asp

Strong Heart Family Study The Southwest Foundation for Biomedical Research offers this page, which discusses population-based epidemiologic study of cardiovascular disease risk factors in American Indians. New components of the project and details on the heritability of cardiovascular risk factors are introduced. http://www.sfbr.org/sfbr/public/research/strongheart.html

Study Finds Heart Benefits from Apples and Juice Research conducted at the University of California Davis is cited at this Healthwho news

story. Study methods are described, and potential cardiovascular benefits of the compounds found in apples and apple juice are discussed.
http://www.healthwho.com/newsUpdate/NU_Feb01_088.cfm

Study Links Heart Attacks to Heavy Meals A report of the American Heart Association's 73rd Scientific Session is reviewed at this Newswise page, which cites having a heavy meal as a risk factor for triggering a heart attack. Possible explanations for how a heavy meal may be related to a heart attack and differences between this and risk factors for coronary artery disease development are discussed.
http://www.newswise.com/articles/2000/11/HEART2.VAR.html

Study May Help Explain More Cardiovascular Disease in African Americans Released at the AHA's 70th Scientific Session, the information offered at this address of the University of Georgia includes results on research of saphenous vein tissue from bypass patients. Implications about the cardiovascular disease process in African American patients and the use of antioxidants in the treatment of cardiovascular disease are presented.
http://www.gtri.gatech.edu/grtm/cardio.htm

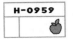

Study Shows Breastfeeding Reduces Risk Factors for Cardiovascular Disease Examining the association between infant feeding method and cardiovascular disease in later life, this site reports of Naturalchildbirth.org reports on research originally published in the *Archives of Disease in Childhood*. Differences between bottle-fed and breastfed subjects are stated, as well as implications regarding future cardiovascular conditions.
http://www.naturalchildbirth.org/natural/resources/breastfeeding/breastfeeding22.htm

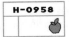

Study Shows Higher Cardiac Death Rates in Major U.S. Cities, Rural South Research conducted by the Centers for Disease Control and Prevention in Atlanta provides information on a study of heart disease prevalence according to region, race, and ethnic origin. Debunking the misconception that heart disease is not a major concern for women, the study reviews annual mortality rates and great disparities in prevalence according to U.S. region. Probable reasons for differences in both the rural South and several urban cities are cited, including social and lifestyle conditions.
http://www.wsws.org/articles/2000/feb2000/hdis-f22.shtml

Viagra Increases Nerve Activity Associated with Cardiovascular Function Examining the effect of Viagra on the cardiovascular system, this news release reports on recent research from the University of Iowa Cardiovascular Research Center. Results of the research reinforce previous recommendations of the AHA and the American College of Cardiology on the use of Viagra in those with cardiovascular disease.
http://www.uiowa.edu/~ournews/2001/january/0103viagra.html

7.15   HISTORY OF CARDIOLOGY

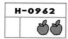

Franklin Institute Online: Milestones in Cardiology   "Famous Firsts" in the field of cardiology are listed at this site, from the first description of blood circulation to the first artificial heart implantation. A connection to the "Heart History" page offers a review of events that have led to recent increases in heart disease and important investigations and developments in the field.
http://sln.fi.edu/biosci/history/firsts.html

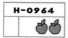

University of Iowa Health Care Medical Museum: A History of Cardiology   A virtual tour of this University exhibit addresses the history, diagnosis, therapy, and prevention of heart disease through a series of exhibitions and programs at this address. Discoveries in anatomy and function of the heart, a look at the first stethoscopes, advancements in EKG technology, and the origin of pacemakers are a sampling of what viewers will find. Pharmaceutical developments and technological advancements in surgical procedures are also discussed. All portions of the site are accompanied by historical images of equipment and instruments.
http://www.uihealthcare.com/depts/
medmuseum/beatgoesonhistory/beatgoesonhistory.html

7.16   MEDICAL INFORMATICS

Healthcare Information and Management Systems Society   This nonprofit organization represents professionals involved in the development of healthcare-related clinical systems, information systems, management engineering, and telecommunications. Society members develop technologies in telemedicine, computer-based patient records, community health information networks, and portable/wireless healthcare computing. This site offers details of the organization, membership information, and contact information for individual chapters. News, an online bookstore, a mailing list, links to related sites, and details of the annual meeting, including resources for participating exhibitors, are available. The site also provides details of advocacy activities and professional education programs. One section of the site is reserved for members.
(some features fee-based) http://www.himss.org

National Library of Medicine (NLM): Research Programs   Visitors to this site will find links to National Library of Medicine centers for research; computational molecular biology resources, including molecular biology databases; and other online molecular tools and informatics resources. Additional materials available through this site are relevant to digital computing and communications, digital library research, interactive multimedia technology, and medical informatics training. The Visible Human Project is discussed, along with details of extramural funding opportunities.
http://www.nlm.nih.gov/resprog.html

7.17 NUCLEAR CARDIOLOGY

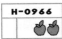

American Board of Nuclear Medicine The American Board of Nuclear Medicine is dedicated to the advancement of health through the establishment and maintenance of standards of training, education, and qualification of physicians. Their site contains information about the specialty, history and structure of the society, as well as about the significance of certification. Details on licensure, training programs, examinations, fees, and policies and procedures are reviewed.
http://www.abnm.org

American College of Nuclear Medicine The American College of Nuclear Medicine was created to advance the science of nuclear medicine, improve the benefits to patients, and encourage continuing education in the field. The site contains links to recent newsletters, information about annual meetings, and applications for membership.
http://www.acnucmed.org

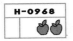

American College of Nuclear Physicians The American College of Nuclear Physicians is composed of physicians, scientists, and corporate members dedicated to enhancing the practical applications of nuclear medicine through study, educational events, and improvement of clinical practice. The site contains information on publications, quality assurance programs, professional and public information programs, press releases, government relations, meetings and events, and CME opportunities. Links to government organizations, corporate committee members, and additional nuclear medicine associations are found. http://www.acnponline.org/

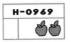

American Society of Nuclear Cardiology The American Society of Nuclear Cardiology seeks to facilitate communication between members worldwide to advance clinical and research excellence in the field of nuclear cardiology. The site contains information about society organization and activities, its products, and membership. The latest news, policy statements, and updated details regarding accreditation and certification are offered at the site, in addition to a bulletin board, online educational materials, and a list of links to related sites. http://www.asnc.org

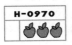

Society of Nuclear Medicine The Society of Nuclear Medicine is an international association dedicated to promoting the science, technology, and practical application of nuclear medicine. Their site provides information about the organization, including annual meeting information, directories, publications, and current events. Details regarding research, fellowships, continuing education, certification, and practice updates are provided, as well as a general overview of nuclear medicine and tests.
http://www.snm.org

7.18 NUTRITION

About.com: The Mediterranean Diet   An article written for a consumer audience is posted at this page of the About Web guide, describing the fundamentals of the Mediterranean diet and offering reviews from various organizations on its benefits. A bulleted list provides the basic components of the diet. Links at the site lead to further definition and articles on related information, such as omega-3 fatty acids and the Mediterranean diet pyramid.
http://nutrition.about.com/library/weekly/aa100499.htm

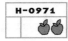

American Academy of Family Physicians (AAFP): Role of Nutrition in Chronic Disease Care   The American Academy of Family Physicians, the American Dietetic Association, and the National Council on the Aging present this online manual, courtesy of the Nutrition Screening Initiative (NSI), which provides healthcare professionals with the latest in nutrition science for the management of patients with several chronic diseases, including hypertension, congestive heart failure, and coronary artery disease. The research, compiled and authored by health and nutrition experts from across the health continuum, may be downloaded from the site in PDF format.
http://www.aafp.org/nsi/manual/index.html

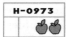

American Heart Association (AHA): Enjoy Eating   Produced by the AHA, this site contains a user-friendly manual for a healthy lifestyle, providing dietary guidelines and goals and information regarding fat, cholesterol, and sodium intake. Tips on grocery shopping and food labels, a cookbook for heart-healthy recipes, and recommendations on cooking methods, seasonings, and substitutions are provided. The brochure contains guidelines for staying fit and assistance in following AHA-recommended diet plans.
http://www.deliciousdecisions.org/ee/wbd_easy_main.html

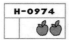

American Heart Association (AHA): Fiber   This AHA fact sheet on dietary fiber offers a discussion of the health benefits of both soluble and insoluble dietary fiber, including recommended daily total fiber intake and important food sources of both types of fiber. A list of related AHA dietary topics is available.   http://216.185.112.5/presenter.jhtml?identifier=4574

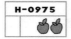

American Heart Association (AHA): Phytochemicals and Cardiovascular Disease   An introduction to chemicals found in plants and other micronutrients is the focus of this introduction to phytochemicals. The AHA's recommendations with regard to further research in this area and related publications of the organization are available. The discussion includes information on the possible benefits of plant sterols, flavanoids, and plant sulfur compounds, as well as information demonstrating positive, yet inconclusive, benefits.
http://216.185.112.5/presenter.jhtml?identifier=4722

Cardiovascular Institute of the South: Vitamins and the Treatment of Heart Disease   The place of vitamins in heart disease treatment is reviewed at this article, created by the director of the Prevention Center for Cardiovascular Disease. Several nutrients currently under investigation for their ability to lower unhealthy cholesterol levels and to provide antioxidant protection are discussed.

http://www.cardio.com/articles/vitamins.htm

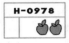

Heart Information Network: HeartInfo Nutrition Guide   The nutrition guide at this site provides links to articles on many different topics, including healthy dining, general nutrition tips, nutrition and heart disease, and nutrition and high blood pressure. The table provided at the site offers viewers the opportunity to read article content descriptions before accessing information.

http://208.133.254.45/search/display.asp?Id=459&caller=455

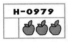

Heart Information Network: Soy and Cardiovascular Disease   Soy products and their benefits in the prevention of heart disease are discussed in this consumer article. Possible explanations for the effectiveness of soy in cardiovascular risk reduction are presented, in addition to recommended daily soy servings for different risk groups and AHA guidelines for including soy in the American diet.

http://www.heartinfo.org/nutrition/soy012800.htm

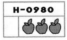

International Food Information Council Foundation   The International Food Information Council Foundation was created to communicate science-based information on food safety and nutrition to health and nutrition professionals, government officials, and journalists. Food safety and nutrition news releases, questions and answers, and links to the group's online journal are found. Information for educators, online ordering of publications, and links to additional resources are provided.

http://ificinfo.health.org

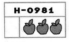

National Heart, Lung, and Blood Institute (NHLBI): Eating to Lower Your High Blood Cholesterol   This comprehensive consumer guide to diet modifications for lowering cholesterol offers general facts about high blood cholesterol and heart disease as well as rules for diet, physical activity, and weight loss. Tables offer summaries of nutritional content in different foods, including fat content, cholesterol content, serving sizes, and details of calories burned during different physical activities. Other suggested publications are listed, with contact details for catalogs and orders provided.

http://www.nhlbi.nih.gov/health/public/heart/chol/sbs-chol/

New York Online Access to Health (NOAH): Diet and Heart Disease This portion of the New York Online Access to Health (NOAH) Web site provides links to articles about diet and heart disease from several sources, including the American Heart Association, the Franklin Institute Science Museum, and the National Heart, Lung, and Blood Institute. Accessible articles offer information regarding dietary cholesterol, antioxidant vitamin intake, and the relation of certain diets and dietary habits to heart disease risk.

http://www.noah-health.org/english/illness/heart_disease/heartdisease.html#DIET

The Diet Channel: Over 100 Diet and Heart Disease Articles   More than 115 links to Internet resources devoted to diet, nutrition, and heart disease are listed in this online directory, courtesy of the AHA, prominent educational institutions, and other professional organizations. Categories include general diet and heart disease information, fats, cholesterol, triglycerides, trans fats, dietary supplements, salt/sodium, diet, blood pressure, stroke, modifying unhealthy recipes, and recommended diets, such as Dean Ornish's program and the DASH diet. Heart disease links devoted to weight loss, dining out, soy and tofu, antioxidants, and phytochemicals are provided.
http://www.thedietchannel.com/dietandheart.htm

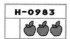

Tufts University: Nutrition Navigator   Provided by Tufts University Center on Nutrition Communication, School of Nutrition Science and Policy, the Nutrition Navigator was designed to help users find accurate, useful nutrition information from credible sources. Sites are categorized, summarized, and rated on a 25-point scale, with detailed information about the rating system provided. Categories include sites for children, women, parents, journalists, health professionals, and educators. The National Food Safety Database, the American Dietetic Association, and the FDA Center for Food Safety and Applied Nutrition are among the professional resource sites offered.
http://www.navigator.tufts.edu

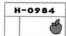

WellnessWeb: Heart Disease and Diet   This site describes the relationship between heart disease and diet. Topics discussed include a balanced diet, water-soluble dietary fibers, fructo-oligosaccharides, antioxidants, minerals, and herbals.
http://www.wellweb.com/nutri/heartanddiet.htm

7.19 PATIENT EDUCATION AND SUPPORT

Agency for Healthcare Research and Quality (AHRQ): Consumer's Guide to Heart Failure   Guidelines for living with heart disease are offered at this site, which includes chapters on heart failure, diagnosis and evaluation, managing heart failure, chest pain, heart surgery, monitoring progress, and the future of heart disease management. Additional resources are provided.
http://text.nlm.nih.gov/ftrs/pick?ftrsK=0&collect=ahcpr&dbName=lvdp&t=891494233

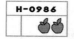

Cardiac Arrhythmias Research and Education Foundation   CARE dedicates their Web site to the memory of children and young adults who lost their lives to sudden cardiac death. The site provides information about foundation events and contains links to relevant articles including *Gender Differences in Long QT—What Are They?, The Long QT Syndrome and Pregnancy,* and *New Horizons in LQT Research.*
(some features fee-based) http://www.longqt.org

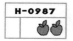

Center for Current Research   This service offers patients summaries of recent medical research on specified disease topics. Databases at the National

Library of Medicine are searched for recent research studies published in leading medical journals. Users can choose from a wide range of disease topics found at the site, such as angina or hypertension, or request information on an unlisted topic. The service also offers a thorough overview of the disease, designed for patients and consumers. A fee is required for these resources, and the site includes ordering details and a description of all features of the service.
(some features fee-based) http://www.lifestages.com/health/index.html

Children's Heart Society The Children's Heart Society is a nonprofit organization that supports families of children with heart disease. This site contains information about the group, its goals, fundraising efforts, and membership. Information about upcoming events, monthly meetings, and one-on-one support is provided. A newsletter, answers to FAQs, references, and links to other sites are included.
http://www.childrensheart.org

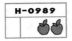

Congenital Heart Disease Support Organizations This resource for patients and their families offers links and contact information to numerous support organizations. Links are specific to individual disorders and include connections to Barth syndrome, cardiomyopathy, CHARGE syndrome, Holt-Oram syndrome, hypoplastic left heart syndrome, long QT syndrome, and Marfan syndrome support pages and contacts.
http://208.234.163.107/sheri/support-other.html

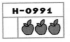

CuriousHeart.com At this Web address visitors will find information about heart disease, the prevention and treatment of heart disorders, and other general health issues. The main page provides access to additional material on the heart, a bookstore, a discussion group and a collection of links to heart-related Internet sources.
http://www.curiousheart.com

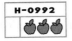

Heart Care Index Presented by Advocate Health Care, the Heart Care Index provides a comprehensive directory of links to cardiac information for patients. Topics covered at the site include how the heart works, reducing risk factors, common heart problems, non-invasive diagnostics, medical treatment, invasive procedure review, surgery, and recovery.
http://www.advocatehealth.com/healthinfo/articles/heartcare//index.html#medtreat

Heart Connection The Heart Connection is a support group for adults with congenital heart disease. The group seeks to provide opportunities for heart patients to share experiences, relate challenges, and give support and encouragement to other adults with congenital heart disease. The site provides a summary of the disease and a history of the Heart Connection organization. Information about meetings and upcoming events is provided, as well as links to related Internet resources.
http://users.lanminds.com/joyce

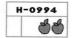

Heart Disease Online This site includes patient information about normal heart structure and function and diagnostic tests used by physicians. Congenital heart defects, valvular defects, coronary artery disease, heart failure, and minimally invasive surgery are discussed in detail. In addition, heart-related news, references on heart disease, and an online heart community are found.
http://www.dencats.org/heart/index.htm

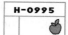

Heart Link An independent source of support, this site offers practical help, advice, and comfort. It provides information on risk factor reduction, blood pressure, cholesterol, pharmacology, stress, aspirin, and smoking, along with a section on pediatric cardiology. The site also offers information about several procedures and conditions as well as a patient forum and a list of links to related Web sites.
http://www.heartlink.org.uk/

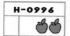

Heart Patient Support This site provides a nonclinical perspective on experiencing heart disease. Included is information about heart attacks, angiograms, angioplasty, and bypass surgery. The site contains outside links to medical resources, health services, bypass procedures, cardiovascular rehabilitation, bypass recovery, and balloon angioplasty.
http://www.netcore.ca/~billk/heart.html

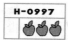

Heartmates Heartmates is an online resource for the friends and family of heart patients and for cardiac healthcare professionals. The site includes "Interactive Connections," a forum for online communication with other people affected by heart disease and healthcare professionals, as well as Heartmate resources and current news about heart disease. Downloadable support publications are accessible from the site, in addition to information on ordering an award-winning video series.
http://www.heartmates.com

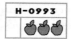

HeartPoint HeartPoint provides reliable health information for consumers and the general public, including commentary from professionals about heart-related topics. Information about heart-healthy diets, health tips, and related news items are found, in addition to the "HeartPoint Gallery," which consists of several multimedia presentations on a number of cardiology topics, including smoking, heart disease, ventricular arrhythmias, and atrial fibrillation.
http://www.heartpoint.com

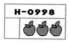

Mended Hearts, Inc. Affiliated with the AHA, this organization is committed to helping heart disease patients and their families and caregivers. The group offers support and encouragement during lifestyle changes, recovery, and depression. The site contains membership information, national activities and awards, and information about the Endowment Fund. Information heart patients should know, articles on healthy living, information about specific hospitals, and links to pediatric support sites are included.
http://www.mendedhearts.org

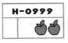

Patient Education in Cardiology A library of printable information is presented at the PULSE patient education Web site, with articles on diagnostics, therapeutic procedures, and commonly diagnosed cardiovascular conditions. Review of blood pressure categories in adults and a glossary of heart-related terms are provided.

http://www.pulseonline.org/patient_ed

Phillip's Heartpage Links at this site are divided into seven categories such as congenital heart disease, hypoplastic left heart syndrome, transplantation, surgeries for congenital heart disease, LISTSERVs, heart stories, and heart medication information. Each category contains links to cardiology almanacs, preeminent hospitals and teaching institutions, heart disease Web ring sites, and additional Web resources.

http://www.execpc.com/~markc/links.html

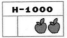

Pulmonary Hypertension Association The purpose of the Pulmonary Hypertension Association is to provide emotional and educational support to patients and families with an interest in pulmonary hypertension. This site contains information about the society, including details about membership, advocacy, and scientific advisors. The resource section provides a physician registry, a bibliography, and links to related Web sites. For support, the site includes a message board, an e-mail directory, a LISTSERV, and a list of regional support groups. http://www.phassociation.org/

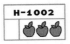

Yale University School of Medicine Heart Book The *Yale University School of Medicine Heart Book,* a project of Yale University Medical Library, is a valuable guide for patients and consumers. Section titles include "The Heart and How It Works," "How to Lower Your Risk of Heart Disease," and "Steps in Making a Diagnosis." A chapter on major cardiovascular disorders, sections on heart disease in specific populations, and reviews of treatment methods are offered. A glossary of terms, a directory of resources, a selected bibliography, and an index are all accessible. The text requires Adobe Acrobat Reader software for viewing.

http://www.med.yale.edu/library/heartbk/welcome.html

7.20 PEDIATRIC CARDIOLOGY

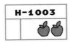

American Pediatric Surgical Association The American Pediatric Surgical Association was founded in 1970 and focuses on patient care, research, and teaching. Its site provides information about the association, including membership information and bylaws, along with information about committees, officers, and future meetings. The visitor will find information about training programs in pediatric surgery and an international pediatric surgery LISTSERV. Patient information regarding pediatric surgery and links to sites of interest to professionals are also available.

http://www.eapsa.org/

Association for European Paediatric Cardiology The Association for European Paediatric Cardiology recognizes the rapid increase over the past decades in possibilities for treating children who suffer from heart disease. This site provides detailed information on the role of the pediatric cardiologist, including duties such as patient care, noninvasive and invasive diagnosis, treatment of the disorders of cardiac and vascular function, electroregulation, and catheter intervention. The site also contains information regarding the society's structure, its membership, training and institute requirements, meetings, and grants. http://www.aepc.org/home.htm

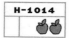

Children's Health Information Network: PDHeart This site of the Children's Health Information Network is an online support and discussion forum for parents and family members of those afflicted with congenital heart disease. An opportunity for personal introduction and access to the community chats are found at the site. The resource room provides reviews of relevant publications and an event listing, and the Internet connections offer specific educational material for both families and healthcare professionals. http://www.tchin.org/pdheart.htm

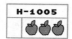

Children's Health Information Network: Pediatric Cardiology Departments This site provides links to the home pages of national and international pediatric cardiology departments in the United States, Australia, Canada, and Germany. Specialty centers, such as the Mount Sinai Pediatric Arrhythmia Center, are accessible, as well as congenital heart surgery clinics nationwide. http://www.tchin.org/ilinks/cardio/c_cardio.htm

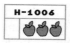

Children's Health Information Network: Support Groups Part of the Children's Health Information Network, this site provides links to the home pages of support groups for families of pediatric heart disease patients in the United States, Australia, Belgium, Canada, Germany, Netherlands, Newfoundland, New Zealand, Scotland, Singapore, Switzerland, and the United Kingdom. Complete contact information and e-mail addresses of organizations are provided. http://www.tchin.org/resources/support/c_support.htm

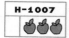

Children's HeartLink Children's HeartLink provides treatment and prevention programs for needy children around the world suffering from or at risk for developing heart disease. This site offers information about their programs, which include treatment, prevention, education, training of medical staff, technical assistance, and acquisition of medical equipment and supplies. Links to upcoming events and the latest success story are included. http://www.childrensheartlink.org

Heart to Heart International Heart to Heart International is dedicated to helping children in developing countries who suffer from congenital heart defects by bringing those children to the United States for treatment. The site provides information about the history of the organization, its programs, patients, and successes. Information for medical professionals, translators, and the gen-

eral public about volunteering time, technical skills, and housing for children staying in the United States is outlined.
http://www.uab.edu/hearttoheart/mission.htm

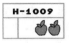

International Children's Heart Foundation The International Children's Heart Foundation is dedicated to helping children with congenital heart defects in developing countries around the world. To achieve its goal, the organization seeks to educate healthcare professionals in those countries and bring them to the United States for advanced study. The site provides information about activities, trips, successes, and financial needs.
http://www.babyhearts.com

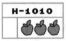

Internet Resources for Pediatric Cardiologists An extensive assortment of clinical resources in pediatric cardiology is available at this page, including pediatric reference material, procedure reviews in the field, teaching materials in clinical management, and links to relevant journals and meetings related to childhood heart disease. Pediatric cardiology divisions on the World Wide Web, training programs in pediatric cardiology, and individual hospital departments of pediatrics are all accessible from the site. A connection to PediHeart, which provides Internet mailing lists for practicing physicians, is provided, as are specialty resources in areas related to pediatric cardiology, such as heart transplantation. http://www.geocities.com/HotSprings/Spa/2192

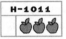

Johns Hopkins Bayview Medical Center: Cardiovascular Health Promotion for Children This site from Johns Hopkins Bayview Medical Center promotes heart-healthy lifestyles for children, including a healthy diet, physical activity, and abstinence from smoking. By clicking on "Health Tips" the user gains access to articles on convenience foods, children and obesity, helping kids make healthy choices, healthy ideas for summer, resistance training for adolescents, and smoke-free kids. Also included at the site is a slide presentation about children and high-fat diets.
http://www.jhbmc.jhu.edu/cardiology/partnership/kids/kids.html

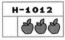

Kids Cardiology: Pediatric Web Sites A listing of links to pediatric cardiology sites on the Internet offers connections for both patients and professionals, courtesy of Seacoast Children's Cardiology. Sites for consumers include the home page of the AHA, and medical resources for healthcare professionals offer connections to algorithms in pediatric cardiology, scientific statements, and multimedia teaching files. Patient education and support site listings are provided. http://www.kidscardiology.com/links.htm

North American Society for Pediatric Exercise Medicine The North American Society for Pediatric Exercise Medicine is devoted to promoting exercise science, physical activity, and fitness in the health and medical care of children and adolescents. Membership is limited to professionals and academic institutions interested in exercise science as it relates to children and adolescents. This site provides information about future meetings and conferences, research grants, and presentations at the American College of Sports Medicine. A list of books and abstracts, important contacts, and links to related sites are included. http://www.NASPEM.org

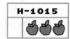

Pediatric Cardiology Almanac   This educational resource on pediatric cardiology, a service of the Tulane Hospital for Children, offers links to information on pediatric heart transplantation, heart murmurs, diagnostic imaging, and specific congenital heart defects. Each multimedia educational module contains images, discussion, and MEDLINE references for common pediatric cardiac conditions. Textbooks, atlases, and digital anatomical cineangiograms are found, as well as the online "Cyberquiz.
http://www.neosoft.com/~rlpierce/pc.htm

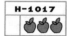

Pediatric Surgery Update   *Pediatric Surgery Update* is an electronic newsletter for primary physicians, pediatricians, surgeons, students, and healthcare professionals interested in current topics related to pediatric surgery. The site provides links to current and past issues of the newsletter and an alphabetical index to specific disorder-related articles. The pediatric surgery handbook for residents and medical students highlights new techniques in pediatric surgery, along with case studies, information about upcoming meetings, and a surgery journal club.
http://home.coqui.net/titolugo

PediHeart   Divided into three sections, this site contains information for children with heart disease, for parents of children with heart disease, and for medical practitioners. The "Kidzone" provides information about the heart and links to related Web sites, as well as a form for children to submit questions about their disorder. For parents, information about common congenital heart defects and cardiac tests and studies is provided. Links to informational sites, to children's hospitals around the world, and to medical journals are also available. The area for practitioners provides comprehensive treatment information for congenital heart defects, with an emphasis on anatomy, segmental analysis, and surgical techniques.
http://www.pediheart.org

PEDINFO: Congenital Heart Diseases   PEDINFO, an index of online pediatric information sources, provides this page of links to congenital heart disease resources, including CliniWeb, the Children's Health Information Network, and PDHeart. Links to interactive, disorder-specific courses; an online cardiology almanac; and congenital heart disease teaching diagrams are provided. http://www.pedinfo.org/DiseasesCongenital.html#Heart

7.21 RADIOLOGY/IMAGING

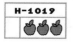

American College of Radiology   The American College of Radiology (ACR) provides strict standards in the field. Its site contains information about the organization, its governance, meetings, and publications. Of particular

value is the opportunity provided to access the ACR "Appropriateness Criteria for Imaging and Treatment Decisions," which requires free registration. Additionally, visitors will find information about CME opportunities, government and public relations, and ongoing research. Links to state chapters and related sites are also provided.

http://www.acr.org

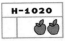

American Roentgen Ray Society The American Roentgen Ray Society (ARRS) provides information about the group's annual meeting, membership, scholarships and awards, radiology meetings, and announcements. Opportunities to diagnose the case of the week are available, as is the current online issue of the *American Journal of Roentgenology,* featuring full-text articles and radiology case reports. The ARRS pressroom offers press releases regarding awards, current trends in diagnosis, and information on the benefits of radiographic technology.

http://www.arrs.org

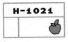

Association of Vascular and Interventional Radiographers The Association of Vascular and Interventional Radiographers was created to establish and maintain high professional standards of medical and ethical performance for cardiovascular and interventional radiographers. Its Web site contains information about the priorities of the society, meetings, board members, chapters, and job listings, along with interventional institutes and test review materials. http://www.avir.org

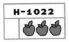

Radiological Society of North America The Radiological Society of North America (RSNA) created this Web site for physicians and other healthcare professionals, educators, and patients. The site contains extensive information about the organization, including membership, meetings, and related societies, in addition to a section for patients entitled "Radiology Resource," which provides current and concise information about radiologic science and procedures. Research reviews, professional publications, educational resources, practice resources, and hospital listings are provided.

http://www.rsna.org

Society for Pediatric Radiology The Society for Pediatric Radiology is committed to advancing the care of pediatric patients through improving the quality of diagnostic medical imaging in the treatment of neonates, infants, children, and adolescents. Its site provides information about the society, meetings, communications, and committees, along with educational materials for radiology residents. The site also provides links to related societies, journals, and hospitals.

http://www.pedrad.org

Society of Thoracic Radiology The Society of Thoracic Radiology was created as an inclusive organization of radiologists dedicated to cardiopulmonary radiology. Its site contains news and information about the organization and its meetings, as well as information on radiology fellowships offered around the country. Educational resources, such as the complete syllabus and downloadable abstracts from the organization's annual meeting, are found, in addition to resources available exclusively to members of the society. A listing of related sites provides connections to additional professional organizations.

(some features fee-based) http://www.thoracicrad.org/str2000/default.asp

7.22 Sexual Activity and Heart Disease

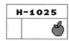

American Heart Association (AHA): Sexual Activity and Heart Disease or Stroke The AHA's recommendations regarding sexual activity following serious heart disease are reviewed at this information sheet, geared toward a consumer audience. General guidelines for couples to follow, information for stroke survivors, and related publication listings are available.

http://216.185.112.5/presenter.jhtml?identifier=4714

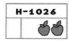

Clinical Cardiology: The Cardiovascular Response to Sexual Activity: Do We Know Enough? Authored by Rodney H. Falk, M.D., of Boston University School of Medicine, the *Clinical Cardiology* article addresses investigations into the cardiac response to sexual intercourse for purposes of advising patients following myocardial infarction or cardiac surgery. The current state of knowledge and several areas where more information is needed are discussed. A table available from the site outlines published research on the subject.

http://www.clinical-cardiology.org/briefs/200104briefs/cc24-271.review.html

7.23 Transfusion Medicine

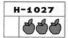

American Association of Blood Banks This international association of hospital and community blood centers and transfusion and transplantation services offers information at its Web site on blood banking, donor screening, blood components, autologous blood, transfusions, and transfusion-transmitted diseases. Patient guides to donating and receiving blood are provided, in addition to professional reviews and guidelines on transfusion practices, molecular methods for tissue typing, progress in understanding non-HLA antigens on blood cells, quality management product information, and blood banking. Additional sections offer information on education and training, publications, legislative issues, and products and services. A useful list of related Internet sites is included. http://www.aabb.org

Transfusion Practices The American Society of Anesthesiologists presents this online publication, providing answers to questions relating to transfusion practices. The entire manuscript may be viewed online and covers donor screening and testing, blood component therapy, and preparation and administration of blood products. Chapters on transmission risks and adverse effects, special considerations in massive transfusions, and specific indications and monitoring procedures for cardiac surgery are found. Clinically useful red blood cell substi-

tutes, such as hemoglobin-based oxygen carriers and volume expanders, are discussed, and a glossary of abbreviations is provided.
http://www.asahq.org/ProfInfo/Transfusion/TOC.html

7.24 VASCULAR MEDICINE

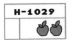

American Venous Forum   The American Venous Forum was designed to be an academic forum for physicians interested in research, education, and clinical investigation of venous diseases. Information about the organization is provided, as well as a list of upcoming events and a newsletter. In addition, visitors to the site will find information about CME programs, a case of the month, and links to other vascular sites.
http://www.venous-info.com

Endovascular Forum   The Endovascular Forum was created to be a physician resource for interactive information on circulatory disease. The physician section requires a free registration and provides access to monthly "Ask the Expert" opinions and editorials; virtual endovascular cases; a thrombolysis resource center containing reference materials on thrombolysis-related topics; and listings of meeting updates, forum news, and links of interest.
(free registration) http://www.endovascular.org

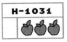

European Society for Vascular Surgery   The Web site of the European Society for Vascular Surgery offers online information regarding the society's annual meeting, current news review in the specialty, and a connection to the *European Journal of Vascular and Endovascular Surgery*. A world calendar of events, vascular surgery Web sites, and a "Who's Who" directory of prominent figures in vascular surgery are accessible. Vascular registry information, clinical trial reviews, and details regarding the availability of travel grants to the annual meeting are offered.
http://www.esvs.org

International Society of Endovascular Specialists   The International Society of Endovascular Specialists is a professional society created to meet the demands of 21st-century vascular medicine. Much of the site is accessible to members only. However, readers can tour the site and learn about endovascular surgery, the society, and how to apply for membership. For members, the site contains a bulletin for worldwide information exchange, announcements about upcoming meetings, member services, training sites, professional opportunity postings, and organization information.
(some features fee-based) http://www.socevsurg.org

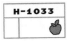

North American Vascular Biology Organization   The North American Vascular Biology Association (NAVBO) facilitates communication between members of different subspecialties within the field of vascular biology. Its site includes information about membership, recent announcements and additions to the site, newsletters, and a calendar of events. Additionally, information about the governance of the organization and links to related Web sites are found. http://www.navbo.org

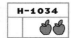

Society for Clinical Vascular Surgery   The mission of the Society for Clinical Vascular Surgery is to provide a forum for discussion of current scientific and technical information related to the field. Its Web site provides a history of the society, its objectives, information on the next annual symposium on vascular surgery, and current news about the organization.
http://www.vascsurg.org/doc/270.html

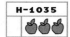

Society for Vascular Medicine and Biology   The Society for Vascular Medicine and Biology is an organization of vascular professionals. Its site contains information about the society, its mission, and activities, along with links to a newsletter and professional journal. Physicians may purchase CME materials at this site. A members-only section features case management consulting, and a section for patients offers answers to frequently asked questions about vascular disease. Links to other societies, organizations, and academic and clinical programs are provided.
(some features fee-based) http://www.svmb.org

Society for Vascular Surgery   The Society for Vascular Surgery provides an international forum for the presentation, discussion, and dissemination of the latest information about cardiovascular disease. The site offers membership information and guidelines, announcements, awards, and information about annual meetings.
http://www.vascsurg.org/doc/852.html

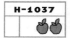

Society of Vascular Technology   This Web site provides information to Society of Vascular Technology (SVT) members, professionals in vascular technology and related fields, and the public. The association is dedicated to the advancement of noninvasive vascular technology in the diagnosis of vascular diseases. For patients and other interested parties, the "Legislative/Regulatory Watch" section addresses issues that have an impact on supervision, reimbursement, and quality of care. The latest developments in the vascular technology field are featured in SVT's journal and annual conference sections. A listing of association publications and connections to other vascular sites are available.
http://www.svtnet.org

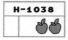

Vascular Disease Foundation   The Vascular Disease Foundation is dedicated to educating the public about prevention, diagnosis, and management of peripheral arterial disease. The site provides information about the foundation, including press releases and upcoming events. Patient resources about peripheral arterial disease include information about its progression and its relation to heart disease, diabetes, and stroke, as well as answeres to FAQs and recommendations on living with the disorder. Information about risk factors, symptoms, diagnosis, and treatment options is found, in addition to a glossary of terms and links to related sites.
http://www.vdf.org

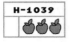

Vascular Surgical Societies   Created by the Society for Vascular Surgery and the North American Chapter of the International Society for Cardiovascular Surgery, this site is intended to facilitate the exchange of information between members of the medical profession. The site contains information about the organizations and affiliated societies, in addition to research and clinical case forums. A physician database is restricted to members and professional colleagues. Visitors will find links to other vascular societies and surgical groups, departments and divisions of vascular surgery, journals, technology, related government sites, and patient support services.

(some features fee-based) http://www.vascsurg.org

7.25 WOMEN'S CARDIAC HEALTH

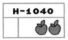

American Heart Association (AHA) Journals: Clinician's Guide to Fighting Cardiovascular Diseases in Women   Issues surrounding cardiovascular disease and women are addressed at a series of fact sheets available from this site. Sex differences in prevalence, causes, and symptoms of heart disease; clinician responsibilities; primary and secondary prevention guidelines; and a document addressing the need for patient compliance are included in the guide. Readers will also find a publication presenting several questions to be answered in future research.

http://216.185.112.5/presenter.jhtml?identifier=2780

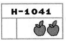

HeartStrong Woman   Gender-specific issues related to cardiovascular health, including the causes and symptoms of heart attacks, are reviewed at this public awareness Web site, sponsored by the American College of Obstetricians and Gynecologists. By completing a free registration, users can answer questions about heredity and lifestyle to assess individual risk factors. Results of a national survey regarding gender perceptions and healthcare and a link to the American Heart Association are found.

(free registration) http://www.heartstrongwoman.com

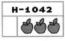

National Heart, Lung, and Blood Institute (NHLBI): Controlling High Blood Pressure: A Woman's Guide   This woman's guide to controlling high blood pressure contains commonsense tips that may be beneficial for both sexes. A basic understanding of what blood pressure measures, categories of high blood pressure, and self-management guidelines for lowering the numbers are presented. Information about smoking and weight management, tips for persons with diabetes mellitus, and physical activity suggestions are offered. Information on decreasing sodium intake, a sensible snack regimen, facts on fat consumption, and details regarding key nutrients are provided. High blood pressure drug listings and contact information for three consumer-oriented organizations are found, completing this comprehensive consumer reference.

http://www.nhlbi.nih.gov/health/public/heart/hbp/hbp_wmn.htm

ORGANIZATIONS AND INSTITUTIONS

8.1 ASSOCIATIONS AND SOCIETIES

Below are profiles of more than 80 associations and societies in the field of cardiology. Those organizations that have a specific focus appear a second time in this volume under particular diseases and disorders or under an appropriate topical heading.

Academy of Molecular Imaging   The Academy of Molecular Imaging is a nonprofit educational foundation created to advance the science of positron emission tomography (PET), optical imaging, magnetic resonance imaging (MRI), single photon emission tomography (SPECT), computed tomography (CT), and ultrasound, as well as their development in the clinical setting. Information about the organization, its meetings, and other activities is presented at the site. Additional information on the academy's three subdivisions is available, as well as details about the organization's annual meeting and educational programs. http://149.142.143.206/index.html

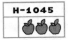

Adult Congenital Heart Association   The Adult Congenital Heart Association is a national organization for adults and adolescents with congenital heart disease. The site provides information about association events, a newsletter, a message board, and references. There is a list of clinics for adults with congenital heart disease in addition to links to chat rooms and support groups. The site also provides links to general information about congenital heart disease, American and international organizations, insurance information, and transplant sites.
http://www.achaheart.org

Alliance of Cardiovascular Professionals   The Alliance of Cardiovascular Professionals provides its members with standards in excellence, leadership in representation, and authoritative information about the profession. Membership includes practitioners, managers, and administrators with backgrounds in echocardiography, invasive procedures, management, noninvasive procedures, pulmonary, and cardiovascular healthcare. Organization information, including details on upcoming meetings and publications, is provided. A message board and links to related sites are found.
http://www.acp-online.org/

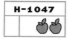

American Academy of Cardiovascular Perfusion   The American Academy of Cardiovascular Perfusion (AACP) strives to stimulate research and provide education in cardiovascular perfusion. Visitors who join AACP gain access to PERFSearch, which cites itself as the largest and most comprehensive database for perfusion-related journal articles, and PERFClass, which offers online perfusion courses. Information regarding the speakers bureau, event schedules, and perfusion journals is provided, as is access to various documents, including the annual Thomas G. Wharton Memorial Lecture series, the academy by-laws, standards of practice, and guidelines for authors. Links are provided to the comprehensive perfusion education page, AACP's newsletter, and a directory of related sites.
http://users.aol.com/OfficeAACP/home.html

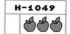

American Association for Thoracic Surgery   Topics in thoracic surgery are discussed at this organizations Web site, including surgical repair for hypoplastic left heart syndrome and additional in-depth commentary on important cardiovascular literature. The *CTSNet Newswire* provides articles of interest to professionals in the field, selected by Reuters Medical News and offering a wide range of clinical, scientific, and regulatory topics. Research grants and fellowships, annual meeting details, and a search engine for locating member surgeons are provided.
http://www.aats.org

American Association of Blood Banks   This international association of hospital and community blood centers and transfusion and transplantation services offers information at its Web site on blood banking, donor screening, blood components, autologous blood, transfusions, and transfusion-transmitted diseases. Patient guides to donating and receiving blood are provided, in addition to professional reviews and guidelines on transfusion practices, molecular methods for tissue typing, progress in understanding non-HLA antigens on blood cells, quality management product information, and blood banking. The current Parentage Testing Annual Report Summary is also available from the site. Additional sections offer information on education and training, publications, legislative issues, and products and services.
http://www.aabb.org

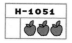

American Association of Cardiovascular and Pulmonary Rehabilitation   The mission of this association is to reduce morbidity, mortality, and disability from cardiovascular and pulmonary diseases through education, prevention, rehabilitation, and aggressive disease management. Used as a resource for healthcare professionals, this Web site offers links to association meetings, job and internship postings, and related publications. Links to cardiovascular and pulmonary resources, professional organizations, and related sites are provided.
http://www.aacvpr.org

American Autoimmune Related Diseases Association, Inc.   The American Autoimmune Related Diseases Association, Inc., was created to eradicate autoimmune disease and alleviate suffering through education, research, and patient services. The site provides information about the organization, its mission, and activities. Patient information on autoimmune diseases, such as cardiomyopathy and Raynaud's phenomenon, is found, and press releases, informative articles from archived newsletters, answers to frequently asked questions, and gender-specific information are provided. Research reports and information regarding the group's position on related legislation are accessible, in addition to related resource links.

http://www.aarda.org

American Board of Cardiovascular Perfusion Intended to provide information regarding certification and recertification to professionals practicing clinical perfusion, this site offers a description of certification requirements and eligibility criteria. Recent revisions of the recertification program, an examination schedule, and downloadable recertification forms can be accessed. Additional external links are offered to nonpracticing professionals and other interested visitors, providing information about the field and related career opportunities. http://www.abcp.org/

American Board of Nuclear Medicine The American Board of Nuclear Medicine is dedicated to the advancement of health through the establishment and maintenance of standards of training, education, and qualification of physicians. The site contains information about the specialty, the history and structure of the society, and the significance of certification. Information on certification, licensure, training programs, examinations, fees, policies and procedures, and board membership is also included.

http://www.abnm.org

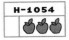

American College of Cardiology (ACC) A major professional society with more than 24,000 members from around the world, the ACC sets rigorous standards to improve the quality of care delivered by its members. The society actively participates in healthcare policy debate, and visitors may access information about its position on specific issues. A database of ACC publications, programs, and products is provided, along with links to clinical information, conferences, information on advocacy, industry relations, and patient education. Summaries from the ACC scientific session and downloadable medical guidelines are found. The site contains numerous links to heart and health resources, medical information, and cardiovascular specialists, all accessible after a simple, free registration process.

(free registration) http://www.acc.org

American College of Chest Physicians A professional organization related to all areas of chest medicine, the American College of Chest Physicians (ACCP) includes membership and organization information at its Web site. There are also links to publications, CME, products, clinical information, public affairs, and news related to the organization.

http://www.chestnet.org/

American College of Emergency Physicians Dedicated to maintaining high standards of care for patients in emergency situations, the American College of Emergency Physicians (ACEP) offers information about educational conferences, publications, legislation, advocacy, and research at its Web site. Recent headlines, a bookstore, a calendar of events, and relevant links are available.
http://www.acep.org

American Heart Association (AHA) The AHA is devoted to providing the public with valuable information on the prevention and treatment of heart disease and stroke. Resources available from this address include a list of warning signs, an interactive risk assessment tool, fact sheets on diseases, drug therapy, prevention, and biostatistical topics. Information on AHA education programs and on ordering AHA publications, nutrition and exercise suggestions, and details on local AHA chapters and activities are provided. Detailed information on cholesterol is available for both consumers and physicians, and additional professional resources are included. AHA journals, Scientific Statements, guidelines, conference and meeting details, professional fact sheets, and AHA research programs and funding review are discussed. Details of the AHA Pharmaceutical Roundtable, cardiovascular disease and stroke statistics, information on professional education opportunities, and professional health news are found at this comprehensive resource.
http://www.americanheart.org/presenter.jhtml?identifier=1200000

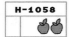

American Institute of Ultrasound in Medicine The American Institute of Ultrasound in Medicine is a multidisciplinary organization dedicated to advancing the art and science of ultrasound in medicine and research. The Web site contains links to official statements and reports, CME opportunities, committee details, publications and audiovisual materials, and related societies.
http://www.aium.org

American Medical Association (AMA) The American Medical Association has been setting the standards of medical practice since 1847. Its Web site offers extensive information about the organization's history and mission, policy and advocacy activities, ethics, public health, and accreditation programs. Information for physicians at the site includes an online data collection center, membership information, and member special interest groups. Additionally, the site offers general health, children's health, and interactive health information for patients, along with details on specific conditions, a hospital locator, and a doctor finder.
http://www.ama-assn.org

American Pediatric Surgical Association The American Pediatric Surgical Association, founded in 1970, focuses on patient care, research, and teaching. Aside from information regarding membership and future meetings, there is information about training programs in pediatric surgery and an international pediatric surgery LISTERV. Patient information about pediatric surgery and links to related sites are provided. http://www.eapsa.org/

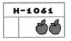

American Roentgen Ray Society The American Roentgen Ray Society (ARRS) provides information about the group's annual meeting, membership, scholarships and awards, radiology meetings, and announcements. Opportunities to diagnose a case of the week are available, as is the current online issue of the *American Journal of Roentgenology,* featuring full-text articles and radiology case reports. The ARRS pressroom offers press releases regarding awards, current trends in diagnosis, and information on the benefits of radiographic technology. http://www.arrs.org

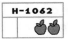

American Society for Artificial Organs Extensive information is available at this site from the American Society for Artificial Organs, which promotes the application and awareness of organ technologies to enhance the quality and duration of life. Included is information about the organization, its annual conference, membership, and by-laws, as well as archived editions of the group's newsletter, which deals with public policy issues surrounding the use of artificial organs. Links to cardiac and general medical sites on such topics as bioengineering and political advocacy are found.
http://www.asaio.com/

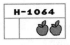

American Society of Echocardiography The American Society of Echocardiography is a professional society dedicated to maintaining excellence in the field of echocardiography. The site provides an overview of the practice and a calendar of the society's upcoming events. A different case study is presented each month, and access to diagnoses from recent cases is offered. Information about research and grants, industry developments, and online ordering for patient pamphlets and practice guidelines is included.
http://www.asecho.org

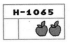

American Society of Extra-Corporeal Technology (AmSECT) As a professional society, AmSECT fosters improved patient care by providing continuing education and standards in the field of extracorporeal technology. Although one portion of the site is restricted to members, most of this site is open to the general public and contains organization information and details regarding meetings, events, job opportunities, scholarships, and grants. There is a section dedicated to the Pediatric Perfusion Committee of AmSECT, as well as a site for consumers explaining common perfusion services, cardiopulmonary bypass, and extra-corporeal membrane oxygenation. Connections to perfusion sites are provided. (some features fee-based) http://www.amsect.org

American Society of Gene Therapy Upcoming meetings and recent press releases are featured at the Web site of the American Society of Gene Therapy, along with membership information, policy and position statements, and links to sites of interest.
http://www.asgt.org

H-1066

American Society of Hypertension The American Society of Hypertension reports itself to be the largest organization in the United States devoted exclusively to hypertension and related diseases. Its site provides information

about the organization, organizational news, and details regarding upcoming conferences. Links to full-text articles from *Current Concepts in Hypertension* and the *American Journal of Hypertension* are found.
http://www.ash-us.org

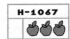

American Society of Nuclear Cardiology The American Society of Nuclear Cardiology seeks to facilitate communication between members worldwide to advance clinical and research excellence in the field of nuclear cardiology. The site contains information about society organization and activities, its products, and membership. The latest news, policy statements, and updated details regarding accreditation and certification are offered at the site, in addition to a bulletin board, online educational materials, and a list of links to related sites.
http://www.asnc.org

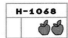

American Society of Transplantation The American Society of Transplantation consists of 1,300 transplant physicians and scientists active in research and management of patient care from the onset of end-stage disease to post-transplantation. The site contains information about the organization, meetings, publications, awards, certification, and public policy. A restricted section contains a member directory, education transcripts, a newsletter, slide lectures, and committee reports. Links to sites regarding general medicine, health news, and transplantation, along with links to newsgroups and LISTSERVs, are provided. (some features fee-based) http://www.a-s-t.org/index.htm

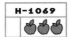

American Stroke Association The American Stroke Association, newly named to reflect a stronger commitment to stroke research and education, is a division of the American Heart Association. This comprehensive resource provides information about stroke risk factors, conditions and treatments, surgery and related procedures, and recovery. Extensive stroke-related statistics, gender-specific information, and links to more specific stroke and cardiovascular-related topics, including cardiovascular epidemiology, fitness, hypertension, nutrition, transplantation, and pediatric cardiology, are provided.
http://www.strokeassociation.org/presenter.jhtml?identifier=1200037

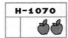

American Thoracic Society The American Thoracic Society (ATS) is a professional organization devoted to respiratory and critical care medicine. Its site provides information about the society, including its structure, staff, mission, leadership, board of directors, and by-laws, as well as information about assemblies, committees, local chapters, membership, and upcoming conferences. In addition, the site contains information about the group's public policy activities, publications, and research and also provides links to related sites and organizations, educational materials, documents, and laboratory products.
http://www.thoracic.org

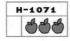

Association of Black Cardiologists The Association of Black Cardiologists is a volunteer organization created to improve access to quality healthcare for African Americans. Its Web site offers membership information, a calendar

of upcoming events and conferences, publications, details regarding organization programs, association news, and links to cardiovascular sites.
http://www.abcardio.org

Association of Organ Procurement Organizations The Association of Organ Procurement Organizations (AOPO) is a private organization recognized as a national representative of organ procurement organizations. Its mission is to represent and serve these organizations through advocacy, support, and development of activities that will maximize the availability of organs and tissues and improve the quality, effectiveness, and integrity of the donation process. The site provides information about the AOPO, including membership information, organization activities, upcoming events, and news updates in the field of organ procurement. Links to donation and transplantation resources, such as the American Association of Tissue Banks and the Coalition on Donation, are provided, as well as connections to federal government agencies and individual AOPO member Web sites. http://www.aopo.org

Brain Aneurysm Foundation The purpose of the Brain Aneurysm Foundation is to provide patients and their families with information on brain aneurysms and their treatment through support networks and educational materials. Information on the organization's public awareness campaigns, specific publication details, and access to a Web version of the organization's quarterly newsletter are provided.
http://neurosurgery.mgh.harvard.edu/baf/

British Cardiac Society The British Cardiac Society provides clinical documents related to many aspects of cardiology at this Web site. Information about electrophysiological techniques, guidelines for specialist training in cardiology, recommendations on prevention of coronary heart disease in clinical practice, and other useful articles are provided. Links to affiliated groups, information sources, and American and European cardiac societies are listed, as are conference and research fellowship details.
http://www.bcs.com/

Canadian Association for Williams Syndrome This site is dedicated to providing information about Williams syndrome. It includes a general overview of the disorder and information about diagnosis, physical characteristics, school age characteristics, adolescent and adult characteristics, psychological characteristics, current medical research, and patient management. The site also provides information about association events and links to other articles and Web sites about the disorder.
http://www.bmts.com/~williams

Canadian Cardiovascular Society Resources maintained by the Canadian Cardiovascular Society include position statements, government information, publications, conference summaries, clinical cases, and featured research, along with links to training centers, heart centers, and related Internet sites.
http://www.ccs.ca

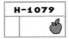

Canadian Hypertension Society   The objectives of the Canadian Hypertension Society include encouragement and coordination of research, dissemination of information and cooperation with other organizations with an interest in hypertension. The site contains information about the organization, membership, awards, literature, and meetings, as well as links to related organization Web sites.   http://www.chs.md/

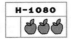

Canadian Marfan Association   The Canadian Marfan Association was created to improve the quality of life for patients with Marfan's syndrome. Information about the disorder includes a definition and discussion of causes, diagnosis, related medical problems, and treatment. Information about the association, membership information, upcoming events, featured articles, and links to related sites are also available.
http://www.marfan.ca

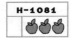

Cardiomyopathy Association   The purpose of this site is to explain the background, diagnosis, and treatment of cardiomyopathy using common medical terms. The site provides discussions of each of the four recognized conditions of cardiomyopathy, accompanied by illustrations.
http://www.cardiomyopathy.org

Cardiovascular and Interventional Radiological Society of Europe
The Cardiovascular and Interventional Radiological Society of Europe is an educational and scientific association of doctors, scientists, and others interested in interventional radiology and cardiovascular imaging techniques, with a portion of its Web site restricted to members. The site contains links to two online journals, *Eurorad* and *Cardiovascular and Interventional Radiology,* as well as conference information. Links to such sites as the Radiological Society of North America, Medic-Online, and the Society of Cardiovascular and Interventional Radiology are provided.
(some features fee-based)   http://www.cirse.org

Children's Heart Society   The Children's Heart Society is a nonprofit organization that supports families of children with heart disease. This site contains information about the association, its goals, fundraising efforts, and membership. Details regarding upcoming events, monthly meetings, and one-on-one support are provided, as are an online newsletter, FAQs, references, and links to related sites.   http://www.childrensheart.org/

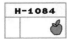

Children's Organ Transplant Association   The goal of the Children's Organ Transplant Association is to ensure that no individual in the United States is denied access to needed organs due to lack of financial resources. The site provides information about the group's campaigns, services, history, and procedures. An online newsletter and links to related sites are offered.
http://www.cota.org

Computers in Cardiology   This international organization of scientists and other professionals in the field sponsors annual scientific meetings focusing on

computer applications in the field of clinical cardiology. Topics presented at conferences are listed, as well as information on obtaining past proceedings. A link to the Working Group of the Computers in Cardiology of the European Society of Cardiology is found, offering information on new developments and an annual report of that group.
http://www.cinc.org/

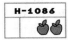

Congenital Heart Surgeons' Society   The data center for the Congenital Heart Surgeons' Society offers news, correspondence, staff listings, and membership information, along with information on current studies and a list of publications. http://www.chssdc.org

European Association of Cardiothoracic Anesthesiologists   The goal of the European Association of Cardiothoracic Anesthesiologists is to provide an international forum for scientific dialogue and to promote education in the field. The Web site contains information about the organization, its annual meetings, and membership, as well as details regarding abstract submission for conferences. Additionally, links to other anesthesiology-related sites, including the Society of Cardiovascular Anesthesiologists and the American Society of Anesthesiologists, are provided.
http://www.eacta.org

European Atherosclerosis Society   Devoted to advancing knowledge about the causes, natural history, treatment, and prevention of atherosclerosis, the European Atherosclerosis Society Web site provides information regarding membership and society meetings, as well as access to its online journal. Links to other societies, including the International Atherosclerosis Society and the American Heart Association, are provided.
http://www.elsevier.com/inca/homepage/sab/eas/menu.htm

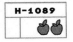

European Board of Cardiovascular Perfusion   The EBCP aims to unite European professionals practicing clinical perfusion in an effort to establish, monitor, and maintain high standards in perfusion education and training. The site offers concise information on accreditation and recertification, a perfusion checklist, and an examination guide. Listings of members, committees, and related links are also available.
http://www.ebcp.org

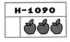

European Society of Cardiology   The European Society of Cardiology is dedicated to improving the quality of life and reducing the effects of cardiovascular disease. Its Web site contains information about the society, including history and goals, membership information, working groups, national societies, industry relationships, fellowships, congresses, and educational activities. Links to several related online journals, clinical guidelines, registries, study groups, task forces, clinical trials, and public information are available. A search engine and links to organizations, national societies, public administrations, patient information, cardiological specialties, and libraries are provided.
http://www.escardio.org/main.htm

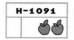

Healthcare Information and Management Systems Society   This nonprofit organization represents professionals involved in the development of healthcare-related clinical systems, information systems, management engineering, and telecommunications. Members develop technologies in telemedicine, computer-based patient records, community health information networks, and portable/wireless healthcare computing. The site offers details of the organization, as well as membership information. Current news, an online bookstore, a mailing list, and details of the annual meeting, including resources for participating exhibitors, are available. The site also provides details of advocacy activities and professional education programs. One section of the site is reserved for members. (some features fee-based) http://www.himss.org

Heart Failure Society of America   The Heart Failure Society of America seeks to provide a forum for heart failure professionals interested in heart function, heart failure, and congestive heart failure research. Its mission is to promote research, educate physicians, encourage preventive care, and enhance the quality and duration of life for those with heart failure. The site contains information about membership, the executive council, corporate support for the organization, and developments within the field. Conference details are provided. http://www.hfsa.org

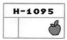

Hypertrophic Cardiomyopathy Association   The Hypertrophic Cardiomyopathy Association is a recently formed organization in the United States. The Web site provides membership information and details about the disorder, including a general overview and facts regarding occurrence rates, effects, causes, signs, symptoms, diagnosis, cures, treatments, complications, and research. The site contains illustrative graphics in many sections. http://www.kanter.com/hcm

Inter-American Society of Hypertension   The Inter-American Society of Hypertension is a nonprofit professional organization dedicated to understanding, preventing, and controlling hypertension and vascular diseases. The site contains information about the association, including its origin, objectives, challenges, committees, meetings, and newsletter. Links are listed to related organizations and centers. http://www.caduceus.com.pe/iash/iashe.htm

International Children's Heart Foundation   The International Children's Heart Foundation is a charitable organization devoted to helping children with heart disease receive the care they need, regardless of their ability to pay. The site offers information about the various programs, goals, and needs of the foundation as well as a description of its Memphis-based facilities. In addition, details about volunteer and donation opportunities, referrals for needy children, and becoming a host family to patients are provided. http://www.ichf.org

International Society for Adult Congenital Cardiac Disease   The purpose of the International Society for Adult Congenital Cardiac Disease is to

promote, pursue, and maintain excellence in the care of adults with congenital heart disease. Membership is open to health professionals involved in the care of these patients. The site contains general goals and objectives, opportunities for professional education, scientific programs, and patient issues.
http://www.cachnet.org/isaccd.html

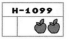

International Society for Applied Cardiovascular Biology
The International Society for Applied Cardiovascular Biology is dedicated to improving research in the field, enhancing communication between scientists, and providing a forum of meetings for the presentation of original work. Its site offers information about the organization, history, and objectives, along with membership information, upcoming conferences, and a biannual newsletter. Links to related sites are listed.
http://riker.neoucom.edu/isacb/index.shtml

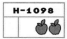

International Society for Endovascular Specialists
The International Society of Endovascular Specialists is a professional society created to meet the demands of 21st-century vascular medicine. Much of the site is accessible to members only. However, visitors may tour the site and learn about endovascular surgery, the society, and how to apply for membership. For members, the site contains a bulletin board for worldwide information exchange, announcements about upcoming meetings, member services, training sites, professional opportunity postings, and organization information.
(some features fee-based) http://www.socevsurg.org

International Society for Heart and Lung Transplantation
Membership in the International Society for Heart and Lung Transplantation includes cardiologists, cardiothoracic surgeons, immunologists, perfusionists, transplant coordinators, and other professionals. Its site includes information about the organization, an annual transplant registry, a heart failure registry, membership applications, and transplant notification follow-up forms. Details regarding additional programs and services, including a newsletter, journal, registry, scientific councils, grants and awards, and annual education and scientific meetings, are found.
http://www.ishlt.org

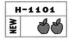

International Society for Heart Research
At this organization Web site viewers will find North American, Australasian, Chinese, and European division sites, as well as lecture material and a Webcast from past symposia. A full-text version of *Basic Research in Cardiology* is available from a site link, in addition to *Heart News and Views,* a research topics message board, and a calendar of events. http://www.ishrworld.org/

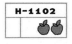

International Society for Minimally Invasive Cardiac Surgery
Links to upcoming meetings, abstract submissions, board members, and by-laws of this organization are available at this site. A link to the official journal of the association, *Heart Surgery Forum,* provides the complete text of clinical articles in

the field, accompanied by a navigational tool that allows visitors to go directly to commentary, figures and tables, and reprint information.
http://www.ismics.org/

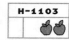

International Society on Thrombosis and Haemostasis The International Society on Thrombosis and Haemostasis(ISTH) is a nonprofit organization with over 2,000 members from more than 50 countries. The site provides information about the organization and membership, fellowship programs, upcoming meetings and conferences, and committees. Links to relevant registries and databases, working groups and liaison reports, and related sites are found. Scientific subcommittee reports are accessible.
http://www.med.unc.edu/isth/welcome

National Society for Mitral Valve Prolapse and Dysautonomia This page, created by the Mitral Valve Prolapse Center of Alabama, contains resources for information on mitral valve prolapse, including explanations of symptoms, treatment options available, and links to literature on the topic. The society publishes a newsletter, which is accessible directly from the site. Connections to support groups and related Web sites are also offered.
http://www.mvprolapse.com

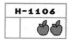

National Stroke Association Resources provided by the National Stroke Association include the Stroke Information Library, which offers review of types of stroke, symptom recognition, and additional online background volumes. The site's professional pages contain clinical publication access, including abstracts and tables of contents of the *Journal of Stroke and Cardiovascular Disease,* as well as information on evaluation and diagnostic testing of stroke. The Clinical Trials Acceleration Program, the Stroke Center Network, and additional activities of the organization are discussed, and stroke prevention guidelines, screenings, and the STROKE PREVENT tool for surveying seniors in managed-care populations are reviewed.
http://www.stroke.org

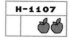

North American Society for Cardiac Imaging The North American Society for Cardiac Imaging is a professional association dedicated to the advancement of cardiac and cardiovascular imaging. The site contains information about upcoming meetings and conferences, membership, committees, sponsors, and review of previous meetings. A link to the online *International Journal of Cardiac Imaging* is provided, along with a history of the organization and links to related sites.
http://www.nasci.org

North American Society for Pediatric Exercise Medicine This organization is devoted to promoting exercise science, physical activity, and fitness in the health and medical care of children and adolescents. Membership is limited to professionals and academic institutions interested in exercise science as it relates to children and adolescents. This site provides information about future meetings and conferences, research grants, and presentations at the Ameri-

can College of Sports Medicine. A list of books and abstracts, important contacts, and links to related sites are included.
http://www.NASPEM.org

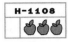

North American Society of Pacing and Electrophysiology   This professional society is devoted to the study and management of cardiac arrhythmias. Tailored for both patients and professional audiences, the site offers patient information on heart anatomy and physiology, arrhythmia symptoms, various heart disorders, diagnostic tests, and therapeutic, antiarrhythmic options. The professional Web link, entitled "Medical Community," provides clinical trial review, case studies, and current news on defibrillators and other therapeutic devices. A feature case is found, and information on the annual scientific sessions is provided, in addition to a calendar of upcoming society events.
http://www.naspe.org

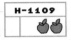

North American Vascular Biology Organization   The North American Vascular Biology Organization (NAVBO) facilitates communication between members of different subspecialties within the field of vascular biology. Its site includes information about membership, recent announcements and additions to the site, newsletters, and calendar of events. There is information about the governance of the organization, and links are provided to related Web sites.
http://www.navbo.org

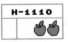

Primary Care Cardiovascular Society   The Primary Care Cardiovascular Society promotes quality cardiology care in the primary care setting. Membership services and benefits are described at the site, along with cardiovascular links and a membership application form.
http://www.pccs.org.uk/pccs.htm

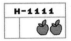

Pulmonary Hypertension Association   The purpose of the Pulmonary Hypertension Association is to provide emotional and educational support to patients and families with an interest in pulmonary hypertension. This searchable site contains information about the society, including information about membership, advocacy, and scientific advisors. The resource section provides a physician registry, bibliography, and links to related Web sites. For patient support, the site includes a message board, e-mail directory, LISTSERV, and regional support groups. http://www.phassociation.org/

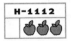

Radiological Society of North America   The Radiological Society of North America (RSNA) Web site as a resource to physicians and other healthcare professionals, educators, and patients. The site contains extensive information about the organization, including membership, committees, councils, meetings, and related societies. A section for patients provides current and concise information about radiologic science and procedures along with an extensive glossary. Research reviews, professional publications, educational resources, practice resources, and hospital listings are included.
http://www.rsna.org

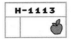

Society for Cardiac Angiography and Interventions The Society for Cardiac Angiography and Interventions promotes excellence through physician education and representation. It seeks the advancement of quality standards to improve patient care. The focus of this site is the group's Laboratory Survey Program, which addresses quality of clinical care delivery. Visitors will also find information regarding membership, society meetings, research awards, and professional publications. Links to related cardiology societies, journals, courses, and meetings are provided.
http://www.scai.org

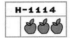

Society for Cardiovascular Pathology Devoted to the advancement of the study of cardiovascular disorders, this society has more than 200 active members with a wide range of interests. The site includes information about membership, meetings, announcements, and publications, along with links to educational material, case studies and other cardiovascular pathology sites.
http://scvp.net/

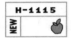

Society for Heart Valve Disease In addition to general information about the councils and committees of this organization, viewers will find a listing of working groups of the organization, details on scientific programming of the association's first biennial meeting, an events listing, and the index and table of contents for issues of the *Journal of Heart Valve Disease*. A downloadable membership form is provided.
http://www.shvd.org/

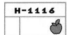

Society for Mitral Valve Prolapse Syndrome The goal of the Society for Mitral Valve Prolapse Syndrome is to reach out to sufferers and offer information and support. The society does not offer information online. Instead, the user fills out an online request form and free information is mailed within 10 days. The site also offers the 1998 Mitral Valve Prolapse Syndrome Seminar videotape, an organization newsletter, and additional publications.
http://www.mitralvalveprolapse.com

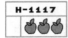

Society for Pediatric Radiology The Society for Pediatric Radiology is committed to improving the quality of diagnostic medical imaging in the treatment of neonates, infants, children, and adolescents. Its site provides information about the society, meetings, communications, and committees, along with educational materials for radiology residents. The site also provides links to related societies, journals, and hospitals.
http://www.pedrad.org

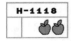

Society for Vascular Medicine and Biology The Society for Vascular Medicine and Biology is an organization of vascular professionals. Its site contains information about the society, its mission, and activities. There are links to a newsletter and professional journal, and physicians may purchase CME materials. There is a members-only section featuring case management consulting and a section for patients that seeks to answer questions about vascular disease.

Links to other societies, organizations, and academic and clinical programs are accessible. (some features fee-based) http://www.svmb.org

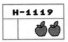

Society for Vascular Surgery The Society for Vascular Surgery provides an international forum for discussion, evaluation, and dissemination of the latest information about cardiovascular disease. The site provides membership information and guidelines, announcements, awards, and information about annual meetings. http://www.vascsurg.org/doc/852.html

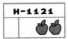

Society of Cardiovascular and Interventional Radiology The Web site of the Society of Cardiovascular and Interventional Radiology contains details for both healthcare professionals and consumers, with information available regarding the latest medical advances in treatment. Topics discussed include angiography, angioplasty and stent placement, as well as information specific to pediatric patients. A members-only section features slide sets and case studies. Access to the latest news articles, information about meetings and conferences, and links to other Web resources are also available.
http://www.scvir.org

Society of Cardiovascular Anesthesiologists The Society of Cardiovascular Anesthesiologists offers information regarding membership, upcoming events, fellowships, and grants, along with access to monthly, archived newsletter editions that include literature reviews, educational information, and event details. A collection of links to anesthesia societies, journals, search engines, cardiothoracic surgery sites, cardiology sites, echocardiology sites, perfusion sites, and practice guidelines is maintained.
http://www.scahq.org

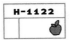

Society of Chest Pain Centers and Providers The Society of Chest Pain Centers and Providers encourages hospitals to develop a comprehensive triage approach to patients who complain of chest pain. The site contains information about the society's mission, objectives, and leadership. Resources at the site include early heart attack care information and chest pain centers.
http://www.scpcp.org/default2.cfm

Society of Critical Care Medicine Critical care news, activities of the Society of Critical Care Medicine (SCCM), and educational critical care events nationwide are discussed at the SCCM Web site. A connection to the consultative body of the SCCM, the American College of Critical Care Medicine (ACCM), provides complete access to all guidelines and clinical parameters for the critical care practitioner. Details regarding SCCM's Project IMPACT, for standardization of critical care data, and access to the newsletters of the Coalition for Critical Care Excellence, a critical care clinical investigation network, are provided. Access to the SCCM bookstore allows visitors to order any of the publications of the organization and its consultative branch.
http://www.sccm.org/home/sccm_home_set.html

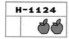

Society of Geriatric Cardiology   Formed to address cardiovascular problems in the elderly, the Society of Geriatric Cardiology maintains a Web site that provides information about the society, including membership information and applications, personnel directories, society news, and a calendar of events. Authors of medical articles may access information about submitting articles, papers, and abstracts. http://www.sgcard.org

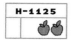

Society of Invasive Cardiovascular Professionals   The Society of Invasive Cardiovascular Professionals leads the effort to define a core curriculum for cardiovascular professionals, offering educational opportunities, participating in establishing standards for the field, and providing a communication forum for specialists. The library section of this site provides extremely useful information, and users will find links to patient care standards, orientation and employment standards, and society position statements regarding issues such as patient advocacy, drug testing of healthcare professionals, and ethics in cardiology research. http://www.sicp.com

Society of Nuclear Medicine   The Web site of the Society of Nuclear Medicine provides information about the organization, including annual meeting information, directories, publications, events, and organization details. The site also provides information about current research, fellowships, careers, government relations, continuing education, certification, and practice updates. For patients, the site offers a general overview of nuclear medicine and tests. http://www.snm.org

Society of Thoracic Radiology   The Society of Thoracic Radiology's membership consists of radiologists dedicated to cardiopulmonary radiology. Its site contains news and information about the organization and its meetings, as well as radiology fellowships, educational resources, and links to related Web sites. http://www.thoracicrad.org/str2000/default.asp

Society of Thoracic Surgeons   The Society of Thoracic Surgeons (STS) has more than 4,100 members. Its site includes details about the organization and the practice of cardiothoracic surgery, with extensive information offered on such topics as heart surgery, coronary artery bypass grafting, and aortic valve replacement. Recent news items related to cardiothoracic surgery, operative notes, a glossary, and links to related sites are found. http://www.ctsnet.org/doc/2189

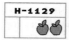

Society of Vascular Technology   This Web site provides information to Society of Vascular Technology (SVT) members, professionals in vascular technology and related fields, and the public. For patients and other interested parties, the "Legislative/Regulatory Watch" section addresses issues that have an impact on supervision, reimbursement, and quality of care. The latest developments in the vascular technology field are featured in SVT's journal, and annual conference sections are found. A listing of association publications and links to related vascular Web sites are found. http://www.svtnet.org

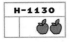

Thoracic Surgery Directors Association   The Thoracic Surgery Directors Association, established as an affiliate board of the American Board of Surgery, provides a comprehensive thoracic surgery curriculum at its site. Visitors are provided with free access to 15 online works-in-progress, covering the embryology and anatomy of normal systems, as well as major congenital anomalies. Unit objectives, curriculum outlines, and discussions of each chapter are provided. Information specifically geared toward residents, author guidelines, and educational program news are found.

(some features fee-based) http://www.tsda.org

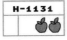

Transplant Recipients International Organization   The Transplant Recipients International Organization (TRIO) maintains a Web site that contains information about the organization's mission, conferences, chapters, officers, and services. Services include a bimonthly newsletter, educational scholarships for transplant recipients, the promotion of organ donation, and the collection and dissemination of educational and medical literature regarding donor awareness and transplantation.

http://www.trioweb.org/

University of Michigan: Extracorporeal Life Support Organization
The Extracorporeal Life Support Organization maintains a large central database of extracorporeal life support cases, devices and complications, follow-up information, and active centers. Information about the research laboratory, education materials, meetings, and staff, as well as informative family guides to extracorporeal life support are found. References and links to related organizations, other medical centers, and Internet resources are provided.

http://www.med.umich.edu/ecmo

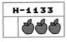

Williams Syndrome Association   This Web site contains the latest information on Williams syndrome, with facts about the disorder, information about diagnosis, answers to frequently asked questions, and updated medical guidelines. Information about the association includes a calendar of events, a mission statement, and a newsletter. Upcoming conference details and regional events, camps and workshops, and links to additional information about Williams syndrome are provided, including the Williams Syndrome Foundation, the Lili Claire Foundation, and the National Association for Music Therapy.

http://www.williams-syndrome.org

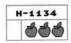

World Heart Federation   The World Heart Federation seeks to promote the study, prevention, and relief of cardiovascular disease. It consists of national societies of cardiology and heart foundations from over 80 countries. Information about organization members and the group's activities, such as World Heart Day, is found, as well as links to publications, guidelines, Webcasts, continental and national cardiology congresses, and upcoming meeting details. An extensive list of other Web sites, including Global Cardiology and the International Non-Governmental Coalition Against Tobacco, is provided.

http://www.worldheart.org

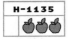

World Hypertension League The World Hypertension League maintains a Web site that includes information about the organization, its history, and membership of the league. For consumers, information is provided about understanding and measuring blood pressure, and there are links to articles written for the general public. Scientific articles and related sites on the Internet are found. http://www.mco.edu/whl/index.html

8.2 Cardiology Departments at Medical Schools and Hospitals

Baylor College of Medicine: Division of Pediatric Cardiology This Web site offers congenital heart surgery resources, a glossary of terms, and a clinical database of patients' records. Research programs include leukocyte biology, transplantation and transplant immunology, molecular genetics of cardiac disease, nuclear MRI, clinical hemodynamic research, and myocardial biology. Clinical facilities are located in Texas Children's Hospital in Houston, Texas. http://www.bcm.tmc.edu/pedi/cardio/index.html

Baylor College of Medicine: Section of Cardiology The Baylor cardiology Web site provides clinical services and patient information. Topics include acute coronary care, echocardiography, electrophysiology, genetic screening, heart failure and transplantation, invasive cardiology, nuclear cardiology, and preventive cardiology. Education programs, CME, and fellowship appointments are described, as are research projects. Current research focuses on the development of transvenous catheters for endocardial mapping and cardioversion; image processing; evaluation of stents, lasers, and other interventional devices; molecular mechanisms of reperfusion injury; magnetic resonance spectroscopy; cardiovascular pharmacology; markers of ischemic injury; cellular electrophysiology and biophysics; molecular genetics of hereditary cardiomyopathies; vascular biology; and gene therapy.
http://www.bcm.tmc.edu/cardio

Boston Medical Center: Coronary Health Unit The Coronary Health Unit, a specialized clinical research center at Boston Medical Center and Boston University School of Medicine, presents research regarding the effects of black tea and dietary iron on atherosclerosis. Additional studies examine the effect of dietary salt on blood pressure and the effect of cyclo-oxygenase-2 inhibitors (COX-2) on blood vessel function. The site also provides information about three recent vitamin C discoveries to treat coronary heart disease.
http://www.bmc.org/coronary/

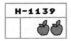

Boston University School of Medicine: Cardiovascular Medicine This Web site presents information about research programs, teaching conferences, and faculty profiles. Current topics of research include hypertension, prediction of stroke, echocardiography, and therapies for heart failure. An overview of fellowships and citations of recent department publications are available.
http://www.bumc.bu.edu/Departments/PageMain.asp?Page=3324&DepartmentID=76

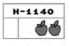

Carilion Health System: Cardiac Services Heart care resources offered through Carilion Health System, include the congestive heart failure clinic, cardiac rehabilitation, education and support groups, details of surgical procedures, pediatric cardiology, and diagnostic techniques. This medical center has become one of the first hospitals to use robotic surgery to treat heart patients. Clinical research focuses on new drugs, procedures, and devices to treat cardiac problems. http://www.carilion.com/cardiac/index.html

Cedars-Sinai Medical Center: Division of Cardiology The Cedars-Sinai Medical Center Division of Cardiology offers information on clinical research, advances in cardiovascular medicine, and vascular biology and gene therapy. Subdivisions of the Division of Cardiology, fellowship positions, clinical information, and research program review are available from the site, as well as CME opportunities and information for patients. Current research projects include those in preventive cardiology, nuclear cardiology, restenosis, atherosclerosis, image analysis, stenting, gene therapy, heart transplantation research, and electrophysiology. http://www.csmc.edu/cardiology

Cleveland Clinic: Heart Center Information on the Heart Center at Cleveland Clinic includes details of recent innovations, links to medical services and specialty pages, descriptions of current research and clinical trials, and educational programs for healthcare professionals. Research highlights include thoracic and cardiovascular surgery, echocardiography, and electrophysiology and cardiac paging. Visitors will find links to position papers, recent projects and technologies, real-time 3-D echocardiogram of an atrial septal defect, and topical review in the subspecialties. Recent, indexed articles and summaries of the current advances in thoracic and cardiovascular surgery are presented, including research related to transmyocardial revascularization, angiogenesis, topical hemostasis, allografts, and clinical investigations in valve surgery, revascularization, and postoperative complications. The "Heart Guide" offered at this site provides resources such as an "Ask the Doctor" forum, information on heart anatomy and diseases, medications, and tests and procedures.
http://www.clevelandclinic.org/heartcenter

Duke University Heart Center The Duke University Heart Center page provides information on the cardiac research, specific case numbers, and activities of this top-rated cardiac program. Major clinical research programs include the development of interventional cardiovascular devices; clinical trials of thrombolytic regimens; development of new noninvasive methodologies for the diagnosis, assessment, and management of cardiovascular disease; and the use of investigational pharmacologic agents, pacemakers, and automatic implantable defibrillators and electrophysiologic techniques in antiarrhythmic therapy.
http://heartcenter.mc.duke.edu/heartcenter.nsf?Open

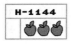

Duke University: Division of Cardiology The Duke University Division of Cardiology is currently developing interventional cardiovascular devices for managing chronic coronary artery disease and acute myocardial infarction.

Other research areas cover cardiac biochemistry, behavioral cardiology, cellular electrophysiology and pharmacology, clinical electrophysiology, clinical epidemiology, molecular biology of adenosine receptors, molecular biology of smooth muscle cell proliferation, nitric oxide related research, and vascular gene therapy. Clinical interests focus on echocardiography, peripheral vascular disease, adult congenital/valve disease, preventative cardiology and rehabilitation, chest pain, and coronary care.
http://dukecardiology.duke.edu/home.asp?divisionID=39

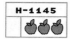

Emory University: Division of Cardiology The Emory University Division of Cardiology Web site contains information about clinical services, including heart failure; the heart and vascular center; nuclear cardiology; and epidemiology research. Laboratories serve research interests in the areas of angiotensin II signaling, atherosclerosis, hypertension, and vascular oxidative stress. Other components of this Web site are the Emory Center for Outcomes Research, the Emory Heart and Vascular Center, the Emory Center for Heart Failure Therapy, and links to fellowship program information.
http://www.heartmdphd.com/emorycardiology/

Georgetown University Hospital: Cardiology Division General information on this Department of Medicine Cardiology Division, located at the Pasquerilla Healthcare Center, is provided at the site. Clinical program links include descriptions of Georgetown's cardiac arrhythmia services, cardiac catheterization and interventional cardiology, lipid disorders, and nuclear cardiology divisions. Clinical research areas include heart failure, arrhythmias, lipid evaluation and therapy, cardiovascular effects of stress, estrogen and the cardiovascular system, and several other areas of study. The Interventional Cardiology Services site features a long list of clinical studies with brief descriptions of each. Some research initiatives examined include balloon angioplasty and atherectomy in plaque removal, tirofiban in restenosis, antithrombotic agents, intravascular ultrasound, and stent effectiveness.
http://www.georgetownuniversityhospital.org/depts/deptlisting.cfm?deptid=15

Harvard Medical School-Beth Israel Deaconess Medical Center: Angiogenesis Research Center and Interventional Cardiology Beth Israel Deaconess Medical Center, a major teaching affiliate of Harvard Medical School, has been recognized for excellence in patient care, biomedical research, teaching, and community service. This site offers treatment strategies for ischemic heart disease and peripheral vascular disease; details of research, education, and training programs; and information on health and wellness programs. http://angiogenesis.bidmc.harvard.edu/

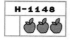

Harvard Medical School-Brigham and Women's Hospital: Cardiac Care Brigham and Women's Hospital, an affiliate of Harvard Medical School, offers visitor and healthcare information, links to information on primary care and specialty services and links to individual research programs. Several clinical departments and divisions related to cardiology may be accessed from the site,

including the Cardiac Center, the Department of Medicine Division of Cardiovascular Medicine, and the Division of Cardiac Surgery. The Cardiac Center offers a brief overview of research firsts in mitral valve surgery, direct current cardioversion for fibrillation, and the first heart transplant in New England. Visitors may access listings of ongoing clinical trials and basic scientific research, including clinical pharmacology, heart failure, oxidative stress, epidemiological studies, and PEACE (Prevention of Events with Angiotensin Converting Enzyme Inhibition), sponsored by the National Institutes of Health and the National Heart, Lung, and Blood Institute.
http://www.brighamandwomens.org/patient/dept_group.asp?dept_group=2

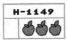

Harvard Medical School-Massachusetts General Hospital: Department of Cardiology

Massachusetts General Hospital, the oldest and largest teaching hospital of Harvard Medical School, offers patient and visitor information about the Department of Cardiology. The Division of Cardiac Surgery, the Cardiac Unit, and the Cardiovascular Research Center are accessible, and each departmental page offers information on its staff, services, and research. The Cardiovascular Research Center offers links to information on faculty research programs, research seminars, and an overview of the center, which discusses translational research, fundamental investigations in genetics and embryology, and molecular physiology and pathophysiology. Lists of current clinical trials in therapeutic areas, including cardiac surgery and cardiology, and investigations of therapeutics for heart valvular disease, cardiomyopathy, congestive heart failure, coronary artery disease, heart transplantation, and hypertension are found. http://cardiac.mgh.harvard.edu/default.htm

Henry Ford Health System: Heart Disease

Resources provided by this Web site include links to information on patient care, research, and education. Research in heart and vascular diseases focuses on congestive heart failure, coronary artery disease, and treatments for high blood pressure. Clinical information is provided for more than 40 topics related to heart disease.
http://www.henryfordhealth.org/body.cfm?id=38316

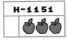

Indiana University School of Medicine: Clarian Cardiovascular Center

This Web site offers information about the Cardiovascular Center and the *Heart Healthy Handbook,* which provides details of cardiovascular care, research, and teaching. Visitors may access the Riley Hospital for Children with abstracts of clinical research trials involving the treatment of congenital tracheal stenosis with anterior pericardial tracheoplasty, the use of ultrafiltration techniques to reduce pulmonary hypertension after congenital heart disease operations, treatment of pulmonary hypertension, management of complete atrioventricular septal defects with surgical procedures, and surgical treatment of hypoplastic left heart syndrome. The latest advances in cardiovascular care include ECMO (extracorporeal membrane oxygenation), nitric oxide, and nonsurgical correction of some heart defects that previously required surgery. Clarian Health Partners is an organization that comprises the Krannert Institute of

Cardiology at Indiana University Medical School, the Indiana University Hospital, and the Riley Hospital for Children. http://cvcenter.clarian.com/

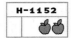

Indiana University School of Medicine: Section of Cardiothoracic Surgery This site provides details about the cardiovascular and thoracic surgery residency program at Indiana University, as well as general information about surgeries performed by members of this department. A link to the pediatric cardiovascular surgery Web page, maintained by Riley Hospital for Children, is offered. http://scalpel.med.iupui.edu/cardio.info.html

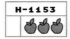

Inova Health System: Inova Heart Center Inova Fairfax Hospital, a teaching hospital in the Washington, D.C., area, is affiliated with the medical schools of Georgetown University, George Washington University, and the Medical College of Virginia. The Inova Heart Center Web site offers information on heart disease, including fact sheets on invasive and noninvasive diagnostic tests, defibrillators and pacemakers, and additional treatment options offered at the center. A physician link provides access to hospital CME, journals of the Inova Heart Institute, and the Inova Institute of Research and Education. Online access to the *Inova Institute Review* provides a listing of current clinical research trials, abstracts, and therapies, while additional links take visitors to an A-to-Z listing of general and NCI-sponsored protocols. Each study synopsis briefly describes the study design and lists the enrollment, sponsor, and principal investigator. Special mention is made of the Inova Institute's study on the effect of pistachio nuts on serum lipid levels in patients with hypercholesterolemia. http://63.111.58.138/heart/heartcenter.html

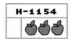

Johns Hopkins Medicine: Division of Cardiac Surgery As part of the Department of Medicine, the Division of Cardiac Surgery maintains this Web site which details faculty members' areas of specialty, including coronary artery bypass surgery, valve surgery, heart transplants, and pediatric surgery. Visitors may access the Cardiac Surgery Research Laboratory, which provides a listing of current projects, including mesenchymal stem cell grafting, heterotopic heart transplantation, spinal cord perfusion via the inferior vena cava, and molecular and physiological changes in conjunction with genetic engineering. http://www.csurg.som.jhmi.edu/

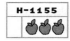

Johns Hopkins Medicine: Division of Cardiology Johns Hopkins Medicine is composed of faculty physicians and scientists from the Johns Hopkins University School of Medicine, as well as professionals from the Johns Hopkins Hospital and Health System. Visitors may search for researchers at Johns Hopkins; access individual research departments, including the Cardiac Surgery Research Laboratory; and find information on grants, funding, and a scientific calendar of events. Research departments and divisions include the projects of the Cardiac Surgery Research Laboratory related to left ventricular volume reduction, hypothermic circulatory arrest, spinal cord injury, minimally invasive cardiac surgery, transplantation immunology, mechanical assistance, and noninvasive flow technology. Funding information and a listing of representative, published articles are provided. http://www.cardiology.hopkinsmedicine.org/

Lahey Clinic: Cardiovascular Services   The Cardiovascular Services site of the Lahey Clinic offers links to the Sections of Cardiology, Vascular Medicine and Hypertension, and Cardiovascular and Thoracic Surgery. Information is presented on diagnostic modalities and the specialized therapies offered. Connections to arrhythmia, electrophysiology, and pacemaker services, as well as links to the Cardiac Rehabilitation Clinic, the Heart Failure Clinic, and the Lipid Clinic of Lahey, are found. Current and past research activities may be accessed, with information on clinical trials in percutaneous transluminal myocardial revascularization discussed. The Lipid Clinic, a teaching and research center, participates in significant studies that define the role of drug management in heart disease prevention.
http://www.lahey.org/Depts/Cardio/index_cardio.stm

Mayo Clinic: Division of Cardiovascular Diseases   The Division of Cardiovascular Diseases at the Mayo Clinic provides the opportunity to obtain further information about its laboratories, subspecialty programs, and preventive health services from the site by clicking on the respective links. Information on the activities of the cardiovascular subspecialty laboratories and clinics includes listings and links to more than 20 distinct divisions. The research link of the cardiovascular diseases division offers a listing of the principal areas of investigation, including atherosclerosis pathophysiology and prevention, heart failure, neurohormonal and vasoactive hormones and peptides, and restenosis physiology and prevention. Clinical research trials involving patients may be accessed at the subsite and list ongoing trials and a connection to the Mayo Physician Alliance for Clinical Trials (M-PACT), which is designed to manage and interpret clinical trials of significance. Each clinical trial synopsis offers concise information on its goals, as well as contact information of investigators.
http://www.mayo.edu/cv/wwwpg_cv/cv_hmpg.htm

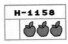

Mid America Heart Institute   The Web site of the Mid America Heart Institute discusses investigational equipment, drugs, and procedures and offers information on its clinical research programs. The institute's residency program in thoracic surgery and fellowships in cardiology, nuclear cardiology, and balloon angioplasty are discussed. Research includes treatment procedures, such as balloon angioplasty; laboratories for pacemaker implants and electrophysiologic development; and leadership in several new technologies, such as the use of radiofrequency ablation and automatic implantable cardiac defibrillators.
http://www.mahi.org

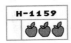

Mount Sinai School of Medicine: Cardiovascular Institute   Cardiac care resources at this site include extensive descriptions of causes, diagnosis, and treatments for common conditions. Detailed information is provided to patients for cardiac prevention, general symptoms, and numerous groups of medications. Directories of Mount Sinai cardiologists and cardiac and thoracic surgeons are available, along with connections to the school's clinical services, programs, which include the Cardiac Catheterization Laboratory, the Cardiac Rehabilitation Program, the Echocardiography Laboratory, the Electrophysiology and Arrhythmia Service, the Heart Failure and Transplant Program, Nuclear Cardiology and Stress Testing, and Hypertension Diagnosis and Management. Researchers will find information on cardiology fellowships, molecular and cellular cardiology training, and basic and clinical research.

http://www.mssm.edu/cvi

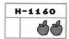

New England Medical Center: Heart Center   The New England Heart Center provides a listing of clinical activities, education, research, and staff profile links. A synopsis for each diagnostic and therapeutic unit is listed, including the Preventive Cardiology Center, the Heart Failure and Cardiac Transplant Center, Cardiothoracic Surgery, and the New England Cardiac Arrhythmia Center. A summary of research interests at the Molecular Cardiology Research Center is available. The major research focus involves molecular vascular biology, specifically signal transduction in vascular cells. Projects investigate the molecular mechanism of platelet function inhibition by endothelial-derived nitric oxide and the role of estrogen in cardiovascular disease.

http://www.nemc.org/medicine/card/

New York Weill Cornell Center: Department of Cardiothoracic Surgery   The New York Weill Cornell Center Department of Cardiothoracic Surgery is described at the Web site, with access to faculty biographies and current news regarding new approaches such as gene therapy to treat heart disease. Visitors have access to comprehensive information regarding various clinical, academic, and research endeavors of the center.

http://www.nycornell.org/cardiothoracic.surgery

New York-Presbyterian: Columbia Weill Cornell Heart Institute   Information on the Heart Institute is found at this Web site. Other resources include prevention measures, such as cholesterol monitoring, eating a nutritious diet, and arranging an exercise schedule. Diagnostic services focus on MRI, PET, echocardiography, and single photon emission computed tomography. Treatment procedures are detailed for coronary heart disease, heart failure, heart rhythms, vascular disease intervention, and valve disease. Advances in pediatric cardiology include heart transplant, left ventricular assist devices, interventional cardiac catheterization, and arrhythmia management.

http://www.nypheart.com/

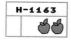

Northwestern University: Division of Cardiology   The Northwestern University Division of Cardiology Web site offers information on areas of faculty research interest, including acute coronary care, cardiac catheterization, cardiac electrophysiology, nuclear cardiology, magnetic resonance imaging, and heart failure. Weekly conference schedules, lecture series details, and cardiology grand rounds are also found, in addition to fellowship details.

http://www.medicine.northwestern.edu/
divisions/cardiology/divisions_cardiology_home.htm

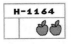

Ohio State University: Division of Cardiology This Web site offers information about the Heart and Lung Institute and the Heart Center of Ohio State University. Clinical services address the treatment of heart failure, congenital heart disease, pacemaker and implantable defibrillator follow-up, and interventional procedure follow-up and cardiac rehabilitation. Research interests focus on vascular cell abnormalities, angioplasty, angiotensin II receptors, and myocardial ischemia.
http://www.intmed.med.ohio-state.edu/Cardio/cardiology_homepage.htm

Oregon Health Sciences University (OHSU): Department of Medicine, Division of Cardiology This site includes a list of Oregon's cardiology subspecialties, such as heart failure, arrhythmia, ischemic heart disease, imaging/diagnosis, and congenital disease in adults. Fellowship programs in clinical cardiology and clinical electrophysiology are described online, and an application may be downloaded. Congenital heart disease and familial dilated cardiomyopathy are identified as primary research areas.
http://www.ohsu.edu/som-Cardiology

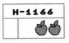

Oschner Foundation Hospital: Heart and Vascular Institute The Oschner Heart and Vascular Institute offers general information about the Oschner Medical Institution, physician details, specialties, and publications, as well as an overview of the diagnostic and treatment services provided. Cardiology specialties include clinical cardiology, electrophysiology and pacing, heart failure and cardiac transplantation, interventional cardiology, noninvasive imaging, and cardiac prevention and rehabilitation. Advanced therapy programs exist for patients with congestive heart failure, and the institute's achievements in transplantation, pulsed Doppler, and Doppler color flow imaging are noted.
http://www.ochsner.org/cardiology/index.html

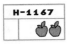

Regional Medical Center Bayonet Point: Heart Institute News articles, details of available services, and information on education and research programs are available at the Heart Institute Web page. Visitors may access a listing of invasive and noninvasive services and surgical procedures performed at the hospital, including left ventricular assist device implant. Clinical studies are summarized, including an investigation of a drug to dilate the arteries supplying the kidneys during cardiac catheterization and an additional study of heart attack patients utilizing thrombolytics and long-term clot prevention drugs upon admittance.
http://www.heartoftampa.com

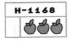

Rush-Presbyterian-St. Luke's Medical Center: Heart Institute The Rush Heart Institute, formed to provide excellence in both pediatric and adult cardiovascular care, offers advancements in cardiovascular services in the areas of pulmonary heart disease, the heart scan, positron emission tomography (PET), and transmyocardial laser revascularization (TMR). Links to the several networks, including pediatric cardiovascular services and those named above, may be found at the site. Research includes work in vascular biology and

mechanisms of reversible heart cell dysfunction, funded by the National Institutes of Health, the American Heart Association, and other major granting agencies. Visitors may access interventional cardiac catheterization studies; preventive cardiology studies; and the Electrophysiology, Arrhythmia, and Pacemaker Program.
http://www.rpslmc.edu/patients/heart/index.html

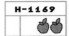

Scripps Clinic: Division of Cardiovascular Diseases Resources available at the site include details of clinical and surgical services, summaries of specialty Centers of Excellence and special programs, a physician directory, employment listings, and information on wellness programs, special events, and support groups. The Heart, Lung, and Vascular Center offers patient education, diagnosis, and treatment for hypertension, stroke, vascular disease, lung cancer, emphysema, other pulmonary diseases, coronary artery disease, rheumatic heart disease, and other cardiovascular conditions.
http://www.scrippsclinic.com/specialties/onedivision.cfm?ID=5650&div_type=div

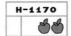

Sentara Norfolk General Hospital: Cardiac Services A description of Sentara's cardiac services presents the hospital's leadership in diagnostic testing, inpatient and outpatient cardiac care, and cardiac rehabilitation programs. Frequently performed procedures include the coronary artery bypass, valve replacement, and minimally invasive heart surgery, as well as diagnostic procedures. Details regarding its cardiopulmonary rehabilitation unit and links to a heart health information section, a glossary of cardiac terms, and an online research tool are provided.
http://www.sentara.com/peninsula/norfolk_cardiacdiagnostic.htm

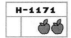

St. Louis University: Department of Cardiology The Division of Cardiology is recognized as a national and international leader in the diagnosis and treatment of cardiovascular disease. In addition to clinical cardiology services, the hospital offers a cardiac catheterization service, electrophysiology and pacing service, transplantation program, cardiovascular stress testing and nuclear cardiology service, electrocardiographic monitoring, and cardiac rehabilitation. By accessing the research study link, visitors will find information on current studies in cardiology, including the Cardiovascular Effects of Medication on Post-Menopausal Women, the Effects of Antibiotics on People with Heart Disease, and a study of women with high blood pressure to discover the effects of exercise on hypertension. Information is also found on the African-American Antiplatelet Stroke Prevention Study and research into the evaluation of aspirin in the prevention of stroke.
http://www.slucare.edu/clinical/card/index.shtml

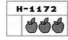

St. Luke's Episcopal Hospital: Texas Heart Institute The Texas Heart Institute provides information on the institute's educational programs, research agendas, and departments. The site also includes press releases, employment opportunities, and issues of the quarterly *Texas Heart Institute Journal*. Clinical studies with open enrollment are listed, including one investigating medical

treatment versus surgical intervention in congestive heart failure. The "Find educational information" link provides access to information on many cardiovascular topics such as arrhythmia, cholesterol, congenital heart disease, heart transplant, mitral valve prolapse, pericarditis, stroke, and valve disease.
http://www.texasheartinstitute.org

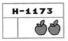

St. Luke's Hospital and Health Network: Heart Center Descriptions of the Heart Center at St. Luke's provide information on its Coronary Care Unit, the Cardiology/Respiratory Therapy/Clinical Vascular Laboratory, the Cardiac Catheterization Laboratory, the Cardiac Recovery Unit, the Cardiac Surgical Intensive Care Unit, and the cardio-respiratory home services. Aggressive protocols and management for lowering myocardial infarction mortality rates, successful completion of heart surgery procedures each year, and details regarding stentless aortic valves, arterial grafts, and endoscopic saphenous vein harvesting are provided. Visitors will find several links for the hospital's clinical research training program, the Research Institute's Secondary Data Archive, and to external research sites.
http://www.slhn-lehighvalley.org/programsandservices/cardio

St. Vincent Hospital and Health Center: Indiana Heart Institute A history of treatment at the Indiana Heart Institute is accessible from the site, from the first balloon angioplasty in Indiana in 1980 to the first in the state to perform percutaneous transmyocardial laser revascularization (PTMR). Diagnostic outpatient services, routine procedures and therapies, and information regarding the institute's commitment to applied research are discussed at the site. The institute is known for its excellence in the areas of device research, pharmacological investigations, and retrospective studies. Areas of research involve specialized percutaneous transluminal coronary angioplasty (PTCA) catheters, laser-assisted balloon angioplasty, stent placement, coronary atherectomy, electrophysiology, nuclear cardiology, pathology of restenosis post angioplasty, and pacemaker and automatic implantable cardioverter defibrillator placement. http://www.mdheart.org

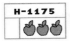

Stanford University: Department of Medicine, Division of Cardiovascular Medicine The Stanford University cardiovascular medicine Web pages include weekly, monthly, and occasional conference schedules; details about fellowship appointments; links to nearly 20 cardiovascular-related journals; and links to ACC/AHA Scientific Statements for more than 30 cardiovascular conditions. More than a dozen clinical services are listed, and the following include links to separate, descriptive pages: cardiothoracic surgery, noninvasive cardiovascular imaging, interventional cardiology, and lymphedema. The division cites 15 areas of research interest, including arrhythmia and electrophysiology, cardiac pathology, cardiac rehabilitation and disease, cardiovascular core analysis, cardiovascular interventions, exercise physiology, experimental angioplasty, and general cardiology.
http://cardiology.stanford.edu/

Don't type in long URLs – add the site number to the eMedguides URL: www.eMedguides.com/**G-1234**.

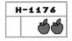

Summa Health System: Cardiac Care The Cardiac Care division of Summa Health System and its individual cardiac care units are discussed at this Web site, with details on cardiac diagnostics, the cardiac catheterization laboratory, and the William H. Falor Center for Vascular Studies. The site highlights information about coronary artery disease, noninvasive medical diagnostics, new clot-dissolving drugs, lifesaving therapies, and resources in surgical techniques and surgical cardiovascular intensive care. Research laboratories evaluate innovations in pharmacologic therapy, procedures, and surgical techniques. The William H. Falor Center for Vascular Studies has made discoveries that allow physicians to examine carotid arteries with highly accurate Doppler ultrasound techniques. New techniques in surgical care and wound healing are currently being studied at this laboratory.
http://www.summahealth.org/services/centers/heart/

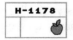

Thomas Jefferson University Hospital: Division of Cardiology The Division of Cardiology at Thomas Jefferson University Hospital offers a range of services in preventive and medical therapies, and the division is known for its innovative services in interventional cardiology. The use of catheter ablation techniques is a major focus of the department's electrophysiology program. The site describes the JeffSTAT transfer program for the critically ill and the FDA-approved endo-graft for prevention of aneurysm rupture. A connection to the Cardiac Treatment Program is accessible. Information on current clinical trials and research studies is available. Cardiovascular research at the hospital focuses on interventional cardiology, including several current national trials utilizing intracoronary stents for the treatment of coronary artery disease.
http://www.jeffersonhospital.org/cardiology2/e3front.dll?durki=3893

Tufts University School of Medicine: Division of Cardiothoracic Surgery The active clinical center and a discussion of Tufts-affiliated hospitals are reviewed at the site, with general information on the clinical investigation and basic research by faculty members provided. A listing of department faculty is accessible. Affiliated hospitals include Baystate Medical Center and the Lahey Clinic Medical Center. http://medicine.tufts.edu/dept/heart.cfm

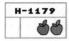

University Medical Center: Heart and Lung Care The University Medical Center in Tucson, Arizona, provides information on consultative services and its diagnostic and treatment facilities at the division Web page. A listing of areas of expertise, including implantable pacemakers and defibrillators, end-stage heart disease, digital subtraction, and cardiac transplantation, is provided. Nationally recognized cardiologists of the department are affiliated with Sarver Heart Center, where research teams study cardiopulmonary resuscitation techniques, ways in which new valve tissue may be developed, and treatments for congestive heart failure. The microbiology of cardiac enlargement, cardiothoracic transplantation, and new prevention strategies and treatments for stroke are studied, in addition to abnormal heart rhythms, studies in special populations, and heart disease prevention.
http://www.azumc.com/specialtycare/types/heartlung.htm

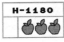

University of Alabama at Birmingham: Heart Center
The University of Alabama Heart Center specializes in the treatment of conditions such as diseases of the thoracic aorta, congenital heart disease, end-stage heart disease, and valvular heart disease exist. At the division page, visitors will find news about the Heart Center related to current research. Information on magnetic resonance imaging services, the Acute Chest Pain Center, and the Comprehensive Stoke Center may also be accessed from the left sidebar menu. A Cardiothoracic Surgery Clinic, cardiac rehabilitation program, critical care services, and a pediatric division are found. By accessing any one of the particular heart specialty departments, visitors will gain information on current state-of-the-art technology and treatments in that department. The Cardiovascular Research Trials page lists current trials, courtesy of the *UAB Insight* publication. Discussions of study on depression and heart disease, prevention of restenosis following angioplasty with intracoronary radiation, the effect of dietary lipids on chylomicron function, and an NIH-sponsored trial for patients with chest pain of unknown etiology are found. A complete government-sponsored clinical trials listing is accessible.
http://www.health.uab.edu/show.asp?durki=10066

University of California Los Angeles (UCLA): Division of Cardiology
This Web site allows access to the various sections of the cardiology division. Training programs consist of fellowship programs in cardiology and postdoctoral training combined with clinical fellowship training. Atherosclerosis research, cardiovascular research, and vascular biology provide the focus for the research units. Clinical programs, including adult congenital heart disease, cardiomyopathy, electrophysiology, and cholesterol and lipid management, are discussed, and a series of faculty profiles is provided.
http://www.med.ucla.edu/cardiology/cardiology/home.htm

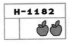

University of California San Diego (UCSD): Cardiovascular Sciences
An overview of the multidisciplinary postdoctoral program in cardiovascular physiology and pharmacology at UCSD is available at this Web site. A faculty roster gives background information on current research interests and offers readers links to more detailed profiles. There are links to other UCSD programs concerned with cardiovascular sciences, including bioengineering, biomedical sciences, and molecular mechanisms of cardiac hypertrophy and heart failure.
http://cardprint.ucsd.edu/cvtrain/tgp1.htm

University of California San Francisco (UCSF): Division of Cardiology
The University of California San Francisco offers a discussion of the range of programs and services offered in cardiology at UCSF Stanford Health Care. Recognized as a pioneer in heart, lung, and heart-lung transplants, the institution is a leader in the development of devices and procedures in cardiovascular practice and surgery. Coronary artery bypass grafting (CABG), repair of aneurysm, and treatment of heart tumors are among the services performed. Research projects feature arterial arrhythmia, electrophysiology, interventional cardiology, and vascular reactivity. Clinical areas are highlighted, including

heart failure evaluation and treatment, nuclear cardiology, enhanced external counterpulsation, intravascular ultrasound, and the Cardiovascular Health Assessment and Modification Program (CHAMP).
http://cardiology.ucsf.edu/

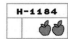

University of Chicago: Section of Cardiology   The goals of this top-rated cardiology program are outlined at this Web site. Examples of cutting-edge medical technologies include the development of three-dimensional, noninvasive imaging techniques, nonsurgical implantation of smart defibrillators, and discoveries concerning the basis of genetic heart diseases. Outpatient services, including the Center for Advanced Medicine, interventional cardiology, cardiac electrophysiology, and the heart failure management program, are reviewed at the site. The department conducts research into the basis of molecular biology, physiology, pharmacology, and biochemistry of the cardiovascular system in order to develop new heart disease therapeutics in the fields of hyperlipidemias, atherosclerosis, cardiac arrhythmias, and heart failure.
http://www.uchospitals.edu/areas/medicine.html

University of Cincinnati: Division of Cardiology   The Division of Cardiology provides background information on translational and clinical research and pharmaceutical and industry-sponsored research. A comprehensive look at the fellowship program identifies the program's aims and the expectations of research training, as well as providing an outline of the application process. Specific clinical programs focus on adult congenital heart disease, cardiac care, catheterization/intervention, echocardiography, electrocardiography, electrophysiology, exercise and nuclear cardiology, and heart failure/transplantation. http://www.med.uc.edu/cardiology

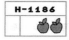

University of Colorado: Division of Cardiology   A description of the Division of Cardiology at the University of Colorado Department of Medicine is augmented by a list of faculty members, many of whom have individual pages that detail their clinical and research interests. The Heart Transplant Program provides care from the initial stages of treatment to posttransplant management. http://www.uchsc.edu/sm/deptmed/card.htm

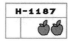

University of Florida: Division of Cardiovascular Medicine   Division sections within this cardiovascular medicine department include arrhythmia and electrophysiology, echocardiology and noninvasive treatment, heart failure and transplantation, interventional care, and vascular biology. A section devoted to descriptions of ongoing clinical trials can be found, in addition to CME information. Included are specialized research programs, a drug information center, and descriptions of fellowship programs.
http://www.medicine.ufl.edu/cardio/index.shtml

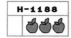

University of Iowa: Division of Cardiovascular Diseases   An outline at this site gives readers a quick, clear look at the department's specialty areas, patient care, and research. Fellowships are offered in cardiovascular diseases training, interventional cardiology, electrophysiology, and heart failure and cardiac transplantation. Areas of clinical and basic science research include arrhythmia therapy, heart failure therapy, cardiac imaging, cellular electrophysiology, and gene transfer and therapy.

http://www.int-med.uiowa.edu/Divisions/Cardiology

University of Maryland: Division of Cardiac Surgery
A fact sheet about this department's areas of expertise lists specialized treatments such as coronary artery bypass grafting (CABG), aortic and mitral valve repair and replacement, thoracic aortic aneurysm repair, and heart transplantation. Links to further information regarding the Ross procedure and trans-myocardial revascularization (TMR) are provided at this site.

http://www.umm.edu/surg-cardiac

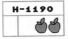

University of Maryland: Division of Cardiology
This division's Web site lists patient conditions and evaluations conducted, as well as special programs addressing preventive care. Information on the Maryland Heart Center, which focuses on evaluation and treatment of cardiac disease, and the Chest Pain Evaluation Center is provided. The research interests include mapping coronary blood flow and quantitative arteriography, medical arrhythmia suppression, drug therapies for congestive heart failure, management of hypercholesterolemia, and transesophageal echocardiography.

http://www.umm.edu/cardiology

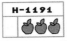

University of Michigan: Cardiovascular Center
This Web site offers lists of clinical services, a physician listing and referral service, and information for healthcare professionals, access to pediatric cardiology and the Michigan Congenital Heart Center, the preventive cardiology program, adult cardiology services, the congestive heart failure program, the Dyspnea Clinic, and the 10-bed Coronary Care Unit. The "Clinical Services" section offers information on open clinical trials, including current trials in cardiology.

http://www.med.umich.edu/hcp/

University of Minnesota: Cardiovascular Division
The Cardiovascular Division offers information about the different specialized clinical services available. The Rasmussen Heart Failure Clinic site provides information about the terminology of heart failure and treatment, patient care, and patient testimonials. The Cardiac Arrhythmia Center works with heart rhythm disturbances and devices such as pacemakers and implantable defibrillators. Other areas of interest include the Minnesota Vascular Diseases Center and the Heart Disease Prevention Clinic.

http://www.dept.med.umn.edu/medicine/Divisions_of_Medicine/DivCard/divcard.html

University of North Carolina at Chapel Hill: Division of Cardiology
Research, clinical services, and training programs are outlined at this site. The Experimental Cardiology Group offers research focuses in areas such as experimental cardiology training and ventricular fibrillation. Descriptions are provided of the Cardiac Physiology and In Situ Confocal Microscopy Laboratory, the Molecular Cardiology Laboratory, and the Langendorff Biomedical Labora-

tory and include information on current research and recent publications. Among the clinical service specialties are cardiac catheterization, echocardiography, nuclear cardiology, coronary care, and cardiac heart failure. Residency and fellowship programs are described.

http://www.med.unc.edu/wrkunits/2depts/medicine/cardiolo

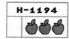

University of Pennsylvania: Cardiothoracic Surgery General areas of interest include cardiac surgery, pediatric surgery, trauma/critical care, thoracic surgery, and vascular surgery departments. Clinical care addresses adult congenital heart disease, arrhythmia surgery, coronary artery disease, and valvular heart disease. Specific research topics may be found by accessing researchers' individual profiles.

http://health.upenn.edu/surgery/clin/cardio.html

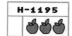

University of Pittsburgh Medical Center (UPMC) Presbyterian: Cardiovascular Institute The Cardiovascular Institute of the UPMC Health System has specialty departments in such areas as preventive cardiology, the Women's Heart Center, a cardiothoracic surgical specialty, and the Artificial Heart Program, along with routine diagnostic and outpatient services. Information on the cardiology fellowship program, basic science research, clinical trials, news releases, and faculty may be found. The institute offers gene therapy for the treatment of blood vessel blockages. Basic science research includes study of the physiology, biochemistry, and molecular biology of cardiovascular disease. The Cardiovascular Research Center (CVRC) contains facilities for cell culture, imaging, and statistical analysis, and its researchers are pursuing investigations into modern strategies for gene transfer. Information on clinical trials in arrhythmias, cardiothoracic surgery, congestive heart failure, coronary artery disease, imaging, exercise physiology, pacemakers, and pulmonary hypertension may be obtained by following the respective link. An overview of the cardiology fellowship program is provided at the site, with its goals and structure, teaching methods, and educational content reviewed.

http://www.upmc.edu/Cardiology

University of Rochester: Cardiology Unit At the Web site of the University of Rochester Cardiology Unit visitors have access to information on eight cardiac areas, including cardiac rehabilitation, clinical cardiology, nuclear cardiology, electrophysiology, echocardiology, and cardiac catheterization. Each of these areas presents a description of the subspecialty and services offered. Links are also available to information on educational opportunities and fellowships and to the Center for Cardiovascular Research.

http://www.urmc.rochester.edu/strong/cardio

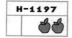

University of Southern California: Department of Cardiothoracic Surgery The Department of Cardiothoracic Surgery has expertise in the Ross procedure, donor-related lung transplantation, minimally invasive cardiac surgery, heart and lung transplantation, pediatric cardiac and thoracic surgery, and perfusion services. Specific programs within this department include adult car-

diac surgery, adult thoracic surgery, and video-assisted thoracic surgery. Further information at this site includes departmental educational programs, such as the cardiothoracic medical student rotation, a cardiothoracic student handout, and descriptions of the cardiothoracic and research fellowship programs.
http://www.surgery.usc.edu/divisions/ct/index.html

University of Southern California: Division of Cardiology   Visitors will find fellowships, residency programs and CME discussed at length, in addition to the clinical programs of interventional cardiology, electrophysiology, congestive heart failure and transplants, preventive cardiology, the Pacemaker Center, and adult congenital heart disease. Clinical and basic science research interests are identified as pharmacological therapies for acute coronary syndromes and interventional cardiology using anti-platelet therapy (GPIIb/IIIa inhibitors), anti-inflammatory growth factors, radiation therapy, basic research into the mechanism of restenosis, atherosclerosis research, and pharmacological treatments for high blood pressure and congestive heart failure.
http://www.usc.edu/schools/medicine/academic_departments/medicine/cardiology/

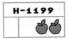

University of Texas Southwestern: Division of Cardiology   This page features information about cardiology at the University of Texas, Southwestern, such as managing heart disease and its risks and complications. Topics of research include stem cell populations and myogenic regeneration, mechanisms that coordinate cell cycle control with myogenic differentiation, and genetic immunization. Among the clinical interests are heart disease in pregnancy, cardiac catheterization, and rapid cardiac magnetic resonance imaging.
http://www.swmed.edu/home_pages/cardiology

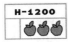

University of Utah: Division of Cardiology   An organized table of contents presents Internet connections for the University of Utah Division of Cardiology. The Family Lipid Clinic, as well as adult congenital heart disease, arrhythmia/electrophysiology, heart failure/cardiac transplantation, and general cardiology departments, is described within the clinical programs section. Research focuses on arrhythmias and sudden death, atherogenesis and coronary artery disease, heart failure and transplant immunology, and molecular genetics and epidemiology of cardiac disease. Medical student and fellowship programs are described in detail. Visitors will also find faculty and fellow rosters, facilities information, and an explanation of the Madsen Preventive Cardiology Program.
http://www.med.utah.edu/cardio

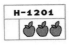

University of Virginia: Heart Center   A combination of clinical expertise and the latest technology is offered at the University of Virginia Heart Center. Clinical services provide information on the extensive array of procedures performed at the facility in the fields of general thoracic, cardiac, and vascular surgery. Research in eight designated areas may be accessed from the site, including investigations in cardiology, pediatric cardiology, surgery, and imaging. Links are provided to various Heart Center affiliates, the Tissue Adhesive Center, and the Cardiovascular Research Center. A multi-investigator program in the study

of gene transfer and gene therapy in the cardiovascular system is in progress at the Cardiovascular Research Center.
http://hsc.virginia.edu/docs/heart/

University of Washington: Division of Cardiology Within the fellowship program area are links to a faculty roster that identifies areas of research interest. Found in "Patient Care Services" are links to individual clinics, including cardiology outpatient, the adult congenital heart disease service, interventional cardiology, advanced heart failure/transplantation, arrhythmia services, and echocardiography. http://depts.washington.edu/cardweb

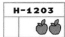

University of Washington: Regional Heart Center Cardiac services at the Regional Heart Center encompass cardiology, cardiac surgery, cardiac anesthesia, vascular surgery, and vascular basic science. The Web site lists studies regarding cardiac catheterization, the Azithromycin and Coronary Events Study (ACES), late-onset diabetes, and cholesterol medication trials.
http://www.washington.edu/medical/uwmc/uwmc_clinics/cardiac/index.html

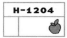

University of Wisconsin, Madison: Section of Cardiolovascular Medicine The Web site for the Section of Cardiolovascular Medicine begins with an overview and leads to contact information for specific clinics. The Arrhythmia Clinic and the Cardiac Arrhythmia Center, the Adult Congenital Heart Disease Clinic, the Cardiac Catheterization and Interventional Cardiology Center, Preventive Cardiology, the Lipid Clinic, and the Cardiac Rehabilitation Clinic are reviewed. The site also offers a list of faculty credentials and individual areas of interest as well as a roster of fellows.
http://www.medicine.wisc.edu/sections/cardiology

Vanderbilt Medical Center: Division of Cardiovascular Medicine The Vanderbilt Division of Cardiovascular Medicine provides information on the department, as well as listings of its research programs and current clinical research studies. The Research for Heart Disease Management and Research for Heart Disease Rehabilitation links connect visitors to study titles, details, and investigator names. Fellowship orientation and research opportunities, an online application, and faculty and staff listings are provided.
http://medicine.mc.vanderbilt.edu/divisions/cardiology

Wake Forest University Medical Center: Department of Cardiothoracic Surgery The clinical activities of the Department of Cardiothoracic Surgery are described along with information about the department's residency programs, a bibliography of publications, and overviews of current research interests. The research interests include myocardial ischemia, reperfusion injury, endothelial cell biology, strategies of myocardial protection, and clinical research projects, such as congenital heart disease surgical procedures, homograft aortic valve replacement, xenograft aortic valve replacement, and cerebral function following cardiopulmonary bypass. Information at this site also features descriptions of the department's Ventricular Assist Device (VAD) Program and illustrations of the devices. http://www.wfubmc.edu/surg-sci/ct/ct.html

Wake Forest University Medical Center: Heart Center Cardiology at the Heart Center's site is divided between adult and pediatric care, with details of adult care linked to pages on catheterization and interventional cardiology, electrophysiology/pacemakers, heart failure, and preventive and rehabilitative cardiology. The pediatric services presented are specific to arrhythmia, lipids, the Marfan's Clinic, and hypertension. Adult cardiothoracic surgery is focused on arrhythmia, coronary artery bypass, valvular heart surgery, and cardiothoracic transplantation. Other concerns include cardiothoracic anesthesia, hypertension and vascular disease, imaging services, vascular surgery, cardiac wellness, extracorporeal membrane oxygenation, and the Centralized Telemetry Surveillance Center (CTSC).
http://www.wfubmc.edu/HeartCenter

Washington University in St. Louis: Cardiovascular Division Research focuses primarily on the areas of myocyte growth and metabolism, cell-cell communication and electrical coupling, and biology of the vessel wall. Information is offered for clinical trials, such as electrophysiology studies, interventional trials, hypertension research, antithrombotic trials, cardiac imaging studies, and heart failure/cardiac transplantation research. The fellowship program description provides information on research interests, clinical training, and the training program in cardiovascular diseases.
http://internalmed.wustl.edu/divisions/cardiology/index.html

Yale University: Section of Cardiovascular Medicine Areas of research include new technology in coronary stents, atherectomy, laser angioplasty, cardiovascular thrombosis, transplant cardiology, risk factor modification in cardiovascular disease, diastolic function, immune mechanisms of vascular injury, and transplantation immunology. Fellowship and educational programs are described at this site, as are diagnostic clinical facilities and outpatient facilities.
http://info.med.yale.edu/intmed/cardio

8.3 FOUNDATIONS AND GRANT SUPPORT

Hundreds of major foundations offer financial support for research in medicine. Below are Web sites that provide access to foundation grants, grant organizations, areas of focus, eligibility, and other relevant data. In addition, several major sources of government research funding are provided, as well as Web sites for grants that are cataloged by specialized organizations and clearinghouses. Major associations and societies that appear in the "Associations and Societies" section frequently include information on research grants, and many offer annual awards for research and study.

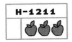

Foundation Center The Foundation Center provides links to thousands of grant-making organizations, including foundations, corporations, and public charities, along with a search engine to enable the user to locate sources of funding in specific fields. In addition, the site provides listings of the largest private foundations, corporate grant makers, and community foundations. Infor-

mation on funding trends, a newsletter, and grant-seeker orientation material are provided, and more than 900 grant-making organizations are accessible through this site.
http://fdncenter.org/

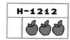

National Institutes of Health (NIH): Funding Opportunities   Funding opportunities for research, scholarship, and training are extensive within the federal government. At this site of the NIH, there is a "Grants Page" with information about NIH grants and fellowship programs, a "Research Contracts" page containing information on requests for proposals (RFPs), the "Research Training Opportunities" page offering opportunities in biomedical areas, and the *NIH Guide for Grants and Contracts*. The latter is the official document for announcing the availability of NIH funds for biomedical and behavioral research and research training policies. Links are provided to major divisions of NIH that have additional information on specialized grant programs.
http://www.nih.gov/grants/index.cfm

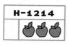

Polaris Grants Central   For the grant seeker, this site provides resources that are available from numerous organizations pertaining to grant identification and application. Books and other publications on grant sources, descriptions of grant information providers, clearinghouses for grant information, federal contacts, grant training materials, and resources on disk or CD-ROM are offered. Within the site, the "Tips and Hints" section offers suggestions on writing grant proposals, the "Grants News" section provides updates from different government agencies and other organizations, and the "Scholarships and Loans" section offers general information on obtaining individual educational grants. Information on grant workshops is also available.
http://www.polarisgrantscentral.net/

Society of Research Administrators GrantsWeb   The Society of Research Administrators has created this comprehensive grant information site, with extensive links to government resources, general resources, private funding, and policy/regulation sites. The section devoted to U.S., Canadian, and other international resources provides links to government agency funding sources, the commerce business daily, the Catalog of Federal Domestic Assistance, scientific agencies, research councils, and resources in individual fields, such as health and education. Grant/application procedures, regulations, and guidelines are provided throughout the site, and extensive legal information is provided through links to patent, intellectual property, and copyright offices. Associations providing funding and grant information are also listed, with direct links.
http://www.srainternational.org/cws/sra/resource.htm

8.4 SELECTED RESEARCH CENTERS

Research centers and institutes at major universities and hospitals appear in the "Selected Hospitals" and "Selected Medical School Departments" topics elsewhere in this section. Below are additional selected research facilities of interest.

CLINICAL RESEARCH CENTERS AND SERVICES

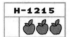

CenterWatch: Profiles of Centers Conducting Clinical Research in Cardiology/Vascular Diseases This site contains profiles of more than 150 research centers conducting clinical investigations in cardiology and vascular diseases. Profiles include descriptions of facilities and information on the credentials of clinical investigators and research staff.
http://www.centerwatch.com/procat1.htm

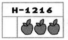

CenterWatch: Profiles of Industry Providers CenterWatch has cataloged an extensive listing of preclinical and clinical research, laboratory, monitoring, project management, trial design, patient recruitment, and post-marketing services and regulatory services providers in the United States, organized topically and geographically. For each industry provider, CenterWatch has prepared an in-depth profile listing services, facilities, and contact information.
http://www.centerwatch.com/provider/provlist.htm

SELECTED RESEARCH CENTER WEB SITES

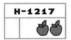

Baylor College of Medicine: Atherosclerosis and Lipoprotein Research Part of Baylor College of Medicine, the Section of Atherosclerosis and Lipoprotein Research provides access to information on interdisciplinary programs in atherogenesis, vascular biology, and lipid disorders. The site offers information about the institute, including research, education, and patient care, as well as links to recent publications and sources of funding.
http://www.bcm.tmc.edu/medicine/athero/index.html

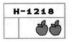

Cardiovascular Institute of the South The Cardiovascular Institute of the South provides a library of reports on cardiology topics, including prevention, diagnosis, and nonsurgical and surgical interventions for a multitude of cardiovascular disorders. This site offers information about the institute, contributing doctors' biographies, and a list of related sites.
http://www.cardio.com

Cardiovascular Research Institute of Southern California Now part of Access Clinical Trials, the Cardiovascular Research Institute of Southern California was established to discover better treatments through research programs involving clinical trials. The site provides links to information about studies in acute myocardial infarction, arrhythmia, cardiac catheterization, congestive heart failure, coronary artery disease, hyperlipidemia, hypertension, noninvasive testing, and peripheral vascular disease. Sections on cardiac imaging and education are included.

http://www.cvmg.com/cvri/index.html

Cleveland Clinic: Heart Center   This leading medical facility provides a combination of patient care, scientific research, and innovative treatment development in cardiovascular care. Critical elements of the Cleveland Clinic Heart Center in basic and clinical research include hundreds of current trials, ranging from basic cellular function study to artificial heart development. Current research efforts in thoracic and cardiovascular surgery include the transmyocardial revascularization (TMR) trials, injection of vascular endothelial growth factor trials, and homograft replacement for diseased aortic valves, as well as clinical studies in valve surgery and revascularization. Various echocardiographic cases are reviewed, and information on electrophysiological research laboratories of the institute and their principal investigators is provided. Heart Center news, educational material for physicians and patients, and innovations in minimally invasive procedures, coronary artery disease, valve disease, heart failure, and great vessel disease are presented.

http://www.ccf.org/heartcenter

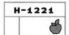

Columbia-Presbyterian Medical Center: Molecular Cardiology Program   A description of the Molecular Cardiology Program at the Columbia-Presbyterian Medical Center is found at this site, along with a detailed description of core facilities.

http://cpmcnet.columbia.edu/dept/cardiology/molecular

Duke Clinical Research Institute (DCRI)   This preeminent research organization, combining an academic environment with world-class clinical research, is affiliated with Duke University Medical Center. The institute provides a cardiovascular database, has sponsored over 4,000 investigators worldwide, and boasts the largest thrombolytic trial in history. Innovations in online trial coordination, evidence-based medicine, education of clinical researchers, and other institute services are described at the DCRI Web site. Statistics regarding trials conducted, information on landmark trials, such as the GUSTO and EPIC trials, and discussion of current, cutting-edge cardiovascular research areas are reviewed. Information on the research activities of the Center for Education and Research in Therapeutics (CERT) trials, the organization's national consortium of cardiologists in community and academic settings, and online investigation publications is available.

http://www.dcri.duke.edu

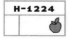

Hahnemann University: Institute for Cardiovascular Research   The Institute for Cardiovascular Research integrates cardiovascular physiology with cellular and molecular biology. The Web site provides an overview of the institute along with links to research projects and other institutes and centers at Hahnemann University.   http://www.auhs.edu/institutes/instcardio.html

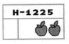

Heart Institute of Spokane The Heart Institute of Spokane offers information about the scope of research and cardiac care performed at the institute, along with details about its mechanical heart and thoracic organ transplant programs. Schedules of professional education seminars and activities are also provided. http://www.this.org

Howard Gilman Institute for Valvular Heart Diseases This research center specializes in the evaluation and treatment of valvular heart disease and participates in cellular and molecular research to increase the understanding of these heart conditions. Details on various diseases treated, descriptions of technological strategies for management, and a variety of case studies are available at the institute's home page. Goals of the institutes research are outlined, and conference information is provided.
http://www.gilmanheartvalve.org/

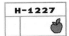

International Society for Heart Research The International Society for Heart Research fosters worldwide heart research in cardiovascular medicine and surgery. Its site provides information about the organization; its home in Winnipeg, Canada; meetings and conferences; and registration. Information about the World Congress of the International Society for Heart Research, which is scheduled to meet in 2001, is, additionally, provided.
http://www.heartconference.com/

James H. Quillen College of Medicine: Cardiovascular Research Institute The Cardiovascular Research Institute at the James H. Quillen College of Medicine promotes further study into cardiovascular diseases and their treatment. This Web site provides a discussion of the institute's mission, history, and recent developments, along with personnel profiles, project summaries, and details about grant funding, seminars, donations, and the medical student research program. A link to information on publications, abstracts, presentations, and grant submissions from grantees is included.
http://qcom.etsu-tn.edu/cvri/index.html

John M. Dalton Cardiovascular Research Center Part of the University of Missouri, the John M. Dalton Cardiovascular Research Center offers investigator profiles, seminar schedules, and cardiovascular news at its Web site, along with a message from the director.
http://web.missouri.edu/~dalton

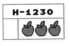

Johns Hopkins Bayview Medical Center: Division of Cardiology The Johns Hopkins Bayview Medical Center Division of Cardiology offers cardiac rehabilitation and prevention information at its Web site, including brochures for patients, clinical research studies, faculty presentations, position statements, conference and seminar details, and links to patient care topics. Other resources at the site include cardiovascular health promotion in children, clinical research information, and a newsletter.
http://www.jhbmc.jhu.edu/cardiology/cardiology.html

Massachusetts General Hospital: Cardiovascular Research Center

The Cardiovascular Research Center at Massachusetts General Hospital provides an overview of the center at this Web address. The site includes information about fundamental investigation, molecular physiology and pathophysiology, and translational research. Other resources offered include faculty research programs, a list of seminars, and a staff directory.
http://cvrc.mgh.harvard.edu

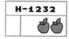

Miami Heart Research Institute

Established to promote, conduct, and disseminate results of cardiovascular research, the Miami Heart Research Institute presents a Web site with tutorials on the cardiovascular system, cells, heart, blood vessels, microcirculation, and genetics. Article archives, an events calendar, and information on sponsorship are provided.
http://www.miamiheartresearch.org

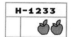

Midwest Heart Research Foundation

The Midwest Heart Research Foundation is principally concerned with knowledge related to the etiology, prevention, and management of cardiovascular disease. The site provides information about medical advances, affiliations, projects and interests, and protocol highlights.
http://www.midwestheart.com/visitor/services/mhrfound_pop.html

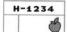

Northwestern University Medical School: Feinberg Cardiovascular Research Institute

The Feinberg Cardiovascular Research Institute is located at Northwestern University Medical School. Its Web site provides information about the group's mission, history, and founder, as well as its administrative office and members.
http://www.nums.nwu.edu/feinbergcardio/front.html

Oregon Health Sciences University (OHSU): Heart Research Center

The Heart Research Center at OHSU in Portland furthers research related to heart disease in adults and in children. The Web site includes information about the center's staff, events, and programs, along with archived editions of newsletters and links to related sites.
http://www.ohsu.edu/chrc

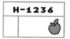

Thoracic Surgery Foundation for Research and Education

Organizational information is found at the Web site of the Thoracic Surgery Foundation for Research and Education, along with a newsletter, list of scholarships, research awards, and grant application forms.
http://www.tsfre.org

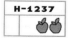

University of Arizona Foundation

The University of Arizona Foundation maintains the Andy Stoppelman Fund for Research in Right Ventricular Dysplasia. The foundation created a worldwide databank of patient information and statistics to coordinate the research efforts of investigators internationally. Its Web site contains information about the fund and the activities of the foundation. http://www.al.arizona.edu/foundation/home.html

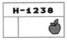

University of Calgary: Cardiovascular Research Group The University of Calgary Cardiovascular Research Group in Calgary, Alberta, Canada, is developing a program of research using patient-based studies and analysis of molecular processes. Its site provides a list of research activities and investigators, faculty e-mail listings, and information about its seminar series. Links to research opportunities and collaborating institutes, as well as connections to related sites, are found.
http://www.cvr.ucalgary.ca

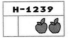

University of California Irvine: Heart Disease Prevention Program The Heart Disease Prevention Program at the University of California Irvine offers clinical research programs, publishes research on cardiovascular epidemiology and prevention, and operates community and individualized programs for prevention and reversal of heart disease. Its site features a relevant monograph and a slide show program on coronary calcium. Information about the program's faculty and staff, current clinical studies, and related heart disease links are offered. http://www.heart.uci.edu

University of California San Francisco (UCSF): Cardiovascular Research Institute The Cardiovascular Research Institute is organized under the University of California San Francisco. The Web site provides a description of the three components of the institute, which are research laboratories, training programs, and core facilities. In addition, there are links to publications and newsletters, as well as information about the faculty and administration.
http://cvri.ucsf.edu/default.html

University of California San Francisco (UCSF): Gladstone Institute of Cardiovascular Disease Areas of investigation are outlined at this research center page, including clinical molecular genetics, vascular and myocardial biology, molecular biology, and lipoprotein biochemistry metabolism. The individual focus of various laboratories is listed, as well as core facilities and outreach programs. A listing of research milestones and several related links are offered.
http://gweb1.ucsf.edu/gicd/

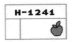

University of Colorado: Human Cardiovascular Research Laboratory The Human Cardiovascular Research Laboratory focuses its research on the effects of aging and regular physical activity on autonomic nervous system control of the circulation and overall cardiovascular health in humans. Its site provides a list of personnel, a list of current research projects, and information about current funding.
http://www.colorado.edu/kines/Lab/Cardiovascular.html

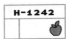

University of Iowa: Cardiovascular Research Center The Cardiovascular Research Center at the University of Iowa coordinates the cardiovascular programs of the college. The site provides a list of subunits of the center, including the Program Project Grant on Fatty Acids, Lipoproteins, and Lipid Oxidation; the Program Project Grant on Cerebral Blood Vessels; and the Program Project Grant on Integrative Neurobiology of Cardiovascular Disease

Project Grant on Integrative Neurobiology of Cardiovascular Disease Regulation. http://www.uiowa.edu/~vpr/research/organize/cardires.htm

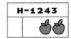

University of Rochester Medical Center: Center for Cardiovascular Research   The Center for Cardiovascular Research at the Aab Institute of Biomedical Sciences focuses on four areas of research: vascular and developmental biology, ischemic injury, molecular pharmacology, and signal transduction. The site lists several examples of current projects, along with information about faculty and links to news, events, and job opportunities.
http://www.urmc.rochester.edu/Aab/Cardio.htm

University of Toronto: Cardiac Gene Unit   Located on the University of Toronto campus, the Cardiac Gene Unit is focused on gene discovery and analysis. Its Web site provides maps of the 23 chromosomes and chromosome X, along with links to other gene discovery projects. In addition, the visitor will find an index of publications, and links to related Web resources.
http://www.tcgu.med.utoronto.ca

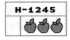

University of Virginia: Cardiovascular Research Center   The Cardiovascular Research Center at the University of Virginia offers an overview of the center, training information, employment opportunities, and faculty listings at its Web site, along with a calendar of upcoming events and summaries of recent seminars. Additionally, information about research activities and external funding opportunites is provided.
http://www.med.virginia.edu/medicine/inter-dis/cvrc

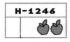

Victoria Heart Institute Foundation   A charitable organization, the Victoria Heart Institute Foundation supports cardiac research in Victoria, Canada. Its Web site offers information about the board of directors, staff, and ongoing clinical trials, along with links to related sites.
http://www.vhif.org

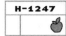

Washington University School of Medicine: Center for Cardiovascular Research   The Center for Cardiovascular Research at Washington University School of Medicine is engaged in research focused on the biologic processes of cardiovascular disease. Its Web site provides information on the center's research projects such as myocyte growth and metabolism, cell-cell communication and electrical coupling, and biology of the vessel wall. The site also provides information about fellowship programs, clinical trials, cardiology conferences, and faculty as well as links to related sites.
http://internalmed.wustl.edu/divisions/cardiology/ccr/index.html

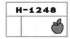

Yale University: Sumpio Laboratory   The Sumpio Laboratory at the Yale University School of Medicine is currently conducting studies on the role of hemodynamic forces in the biology of the vascular wall. Its Web site contains information about these studies, links to selected publications, and access to the Yale University Section of Vascular Surgery.
http://info.med.yale.edu/surgery/vascular/sumpio_lab

Diseases/Disorders

9.1 Adams-Stokes Disease

American Heart Association (AHA): Adams-Stokes Disease A description of this heart rhythm disorder is provided, courtesy of the American Heart Association. References to related publications within the AHA site are listed. http://216.185.112.5/presenter.jhtml?identifier=4418

9.2 Arrhythmias/ Dysrhythmias

General Resources

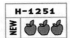

American Heart Association (AHA): What Are Arrhythmias? Offering a starting point for research on arrhythmias for both consumer and professional readers, this site includes comprehensive overviews of a variety of arrhythmias. Details on diagnosis, treatment, and long-term management are included at a series of online articles. Additional professional resources include AHA monographs, lifestyle information sheets, pharmaceutical roundtable proceedings, and related articles from *Circulation* and other noteworthy sources. A consumer education department includes discussion of important risk factors, medications, and self-care measures.
http://216.185.112.5/presenter.jhtml?identifier=560

Arrhythmias Adapted from the Heart and Stroke Foundation of Canada, this site offers patient information about cardiac arrhythmias. It includes a general overview of the condition and discussions of bradycardia and tachycardia. Information about treatment and hyperlinks to details about atrial fibrillation, medications, pacemakers, and implantable defibrillators are found, courtesy of Centenary Cardiology Associates.
http://www.centenarycardiology.com/Conditions/Arrhythmias.htm

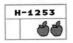

Cardiac Arrhythmia Advisory System By choosing a case from the Cardiac Arrhythmia Advisory System, visitors are provided access to long-distance learning regarding cardiac arrhythmias. The demonstration page provides access to analysis of various ECG cases, including an original ECG tracing, a GIF image, and the opportunity to examine the clinical electrophysiology data used to create the example.
http://www.med-edu.com/htdocs/einthoven.html

Internet Medical Education, Inc.: Arrhythmias Intended for patients, this site educates the user about many topics related to arrhythmia. Included are discussions of Holter monitoring and event recording. Sections on bradycardias and tachycardias, as well as information about sudden cardiac death, cardiac electrophysiology studies, and treatments for electrophysiological abnormalities, are included.
http://www.med-edu.com/patient/arrhythmia/arrhythmia.html

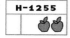

Manuals on Cardiac Arrhythmias This section of Einthoven's *Manuals on Cardiac Arrhythmias* offers chapters on the management of tachyarrhythmias in the emergency room, in addition to the correct use of propafenone. The epidemiology, diagnostic procedures, and specific tachycardias are discussed, and information is provided on the electrophysiological effects, as well as the pharmacological and pharmacokinetic considerations of cardiac arrhythmia management. http://www.aston.it/einthoven/eint0016.htm

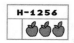

Merck Manual of Geriatrics: Arrhythmias and Conduction Disorders From the online *Merck Manual of Geriatrics,* this site discusses the incidence, significance, and treatment of cardiac arrhythmias in geriatric patients. Topics discussed include tachyarrhythmias and ectopic beats, specific arrhythmias, supraventricular ectopic beats, atrial tachycardias, ventricular ectopic beats, and general treatment considerations. The incidence of specific arrhythmias is discussed, and a table outlining the relationship of arrhythmias to age and mortality is provided, with appropriate interventions listed. Histological changes in the conduction system are reviewed, as are cardiac pacemakers and age-related changes in echocardiograms.
http://www.merck.com/pubs/mm_geriatrics/sec11/ch91.htm

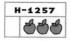

University of Alabama: Tachycardias Clinical Resources This site provides links to a wide variety of resources related to tachycardia. Topics include atrial flutter, ventricular fibrillation, multifocal atrial tachycardia, and atrial ectopic beats, with clinical resources including eMedicine, *Family Practice Handbook,* the online *Merck Manual,* and CliniWeb. Information specific to pediatric disorders and links to clinical guidelines and Scientific Statements of the American Heart Association may be accessed, as well as those of the National Guideline Clearinghouse.
http://www.slis.ua.edu/cdlp/WebDLCore/clinical/cardiology/arrhythmias/tachycardias.html

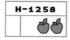

University of Florida: Arrhythmia Identification This site provides guidelines for identifying various cardiac arrhythmias. Information is divided into four diagnostic components: rate, rhythm, P wave, and QRS complex. For each component, links to possible diagnoses are provided.
http://www.med.ufl.edu/medinfo/baseline/arrhythm.html

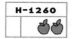

Virtual Hospital: Cardiac Arrhythmias Produced by the University of Iowa, this site of the *Family Practice Handbook* contains physician information about cardiac arrhythmias. Included is a discussion of atrial fibrillation with a hyperlink to advanced cardiac life support protocols for acute management of

atrial fibrillation with a rapid ventricular response. Information about paroxysmal supraventricular tachycardia, ventricular tachycardia, and sick sinus syndrome is offered.
http://www.vh.org/Providers/ClinRef/FPHandbook/Chapter02/04-2.html

ACCELERATED IDIOVENTRICULAR RHYTHM

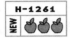

eMedicine: Accelerated Idioventricular Rhythm   The eMedicine online textbook offers a complete review of the pathophysiology, clinical presentation, physical findings, and diagnostic methods available for accelerated idioventricular rhythm at this 11-section site. Consultations, treatment, and dietary measures are considered, as well as several profiles of pharmacologic interventions.
http://www.eMedicine.com/med/topic12.htm

ATRIAL FIBRILLATION

Atrial Fibrillation   Authored by Scott Sakaguchi, M.D., of the University of Minnesota, this site provides CME education for physicians, accredited by the Accreditation Council for Continuing Medical Education. By accessing the table of contents, readers of this CME module will find information on navigating the pages, which include core content, case studies, clinical endpoints, and treatment planning in atrial fibrillation. An annotated bibliography and CME credit details are also available.
http://www.cmeprograms.umn.edu/bestpractice/afib/atrialfibrillationhome.html

eMedicine: Atrial Fibrillation   From eMedicine, this site provides an overview of atrial fibrillation. An introduction includes background details, pathophysiology, frequency, and information about mortality, sex, and age. Clinical review concerning the patient history, physical findings, and causes is provided, and workup review includes laboratory studies, imaging studies, and other diagnostic tests. Treatment modalities, medication, and follow-up procedures are recommended, and ECG images are provided.
http://www.eMedicine.com/emerg/topic46.htm

ATRIAL FLUTTER

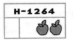

Merck Manual of Diagnosis and Therapy: Atrial Flutter   From the *Merck Manual of Diagnosis and Therapy,* this site provides a description of atrial flutter. It includes symptoms, signs, diagnosis, and treatment. Discussion regarding specific pharmacotherapeutic agents and radiofrequency ablation is found, and links to additional arrhythmia sites within the online publication are provided.   http://www.merck.com/pubs/mmanual/section16/chapter205/205c.htm

BRADYCARDIAS

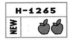

American Heart Association (AHA): Heart Block   A discussion of sinoatrial and atrioventricular nodes is found at this page, which offers a description of signal impairment of heart block. First-degree, second-degree, and third-degree heart block are discussed, and related publications and AHA Scientific Statements are available.
http://216.185.112.5/presenter.jhtml?identifier=42

Bradycardias   Provided as a service of the Texas Arrhythmia Institute, this Web page offers information on slow heart rates, including normal and abnormal variants. Particular attention to sick sinus syndrome and heart block (AV block) is found, including a definition of each, ECG tracings, and information on tolerability of slow heart rates.
http://www.txai.org/patient/bradycardias.html

eMedicine: Heart Block, First Degree   Authored by F.M. Brown, M.D., this eMedicine site reviews the pathophysiology of first-degree heart block. The clinical presentation and causes are outlined, and links to similar information on second and third-degree heart block are available. Laboratory studies, emergency department care, inpatient care, and possible complications are considered.   http://www.eMedicine.com/emerg/topic233.htm

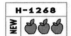

eMedicine: Sinus Bradycardia   Containing information on presentation, diagnosis, and treatment, this eMedicine site offers a thorough overview of slow sinus rhythm. Pathophysiology, dependent on underlying cause, is discussed, and an anticholinergic agent profile is included.
http://www.eMedicine.com/emerg/topic534.htm

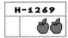

Merck Manual of Diagnosis and Therapy: Sick Sinus Syndrome   A variety of abnormalities of sinus node function are reviewed at this site of the online *Merck Manual of Diagnosis and Therapy,* including persistent sinus bradycardia, sinoatrial block manifested as sinoatrial Wenckebach, complete sinoatrial block, and sinus arrest. An important variant of sick sinus syndrome, bradycardia-tachycardia syndrome, is reviewed, and information on symptoms and diagnosis, as well as permanent pacing treatment, is provided.
http://www.merck.com/pubs/mmanual/section16/chapter205/205o.htm

Sinus Bradycardia   An ECG illustration of sinus bradycardia is provided, along with a table showing rate, P wave, QRS, conduction, and rhythm. Also included are a short description of the disorder, a list of possible treatments, and information on junctional rhythm.
http://www.rnceus.com/ekg/ekgsb.html

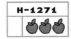

University of Alabama: Bradycardia Clinical Resources   Textbooks of cardiovascular medicine, such as eMedicine and the *Merck Manual of Diagnosis and Therapy,* as well as rhythm disorder listings from the *EKG World Ency-*

clopedia, are accessible online from this listing of clinical reference material, courtesy of the Clinical Digital Libraries Project. Clinical guidelines from the National Guideline Clearinghouse, health reviews for primary care providers, and recent journal article listings on abnormal bradycardia rhythms may be accessed from this comprehensive resource. Access to some material requires a subscription, although many free references are provided.

(some features fee-based)

http://www.slis.ua.edu/cdlp/uab/clinical/cardiology/arrhythmias/bradycardia.html

ECTOPIC BEATS

American Heart Association (AHA): Premature Beats The professional section of the AHA Web site includes this discussion of atrial rhythm disturbances. Specific information on the occurrence of premature beats is presented, as well as associated ECG findings and possible precipitating factors. A summary of ECG criteria is included.

http://216.185.112.5/presenter.jhtml?identifier=40

Merck Manual of Diagnosis and Therapy: Atrial Ectopic Beats The causes of premature beats are discussed at this summary from the *Merck Manual of Diagnosis and Therapy.* A link at the site leads to a representative ECG tracing of the disorder. Identification of precipitating factors and treatment are discussed, and related links in the "Arrhythmias" chapter are accessible.

http://www.merck.com/pubs/mmanual/section16/chapter205/205b.htm

University of Wisconsin Medical School: Escape and Premature Beats This site provides ECG examples of atrial escape, junctional escape, ventricular escape, premature atrial contraction, premature junctional contraction, and premature ventricular contraction. Images and explanations are provided. http://www.fammed.wisc.edu/pcc/ecg/rhythm.group2.html

JUNCTIONAL RHYTHM

eMedicine: Junctional Rhythm Descriptions of types of junctional rhythms are found at this page, including junctional bradycardia and accelerated junctional tachycardia. Causes, differential links, diagnostic tests and findings, and management information are reviewed, for a complete introduction to the topic. Example ECG tracings are included.

http://www.eMedicine.com/med/topic1212.htm

MULTIFOCAL ATRIAL TACHYCARDIA

eMedicine: Multifocal Atrial Tachycardia The cardiovascular chapter of the online eMedicine textbook includes this 10-part review of multifocal atrial tachycardia, authored by Robin R. Hemphill, M.D., of Vanderbilt University. The physical presentation and causes are outlined, and information on the diagnostic workup is provided. Links to differentials to be considered are included in the review, as well as a thorough treatment overview.

http://www.eMedicine.com/EMERG/topic320.htm

Merck Manual of Diagnosis and Therapy: Chaotic and Multifocal Atrial Tachycardia   From the online *Merck Manual of Diagnosis and Therapy,* this site provides a short description of chaotic and multifocal atrial tachycardia. Features of their occurrence and management options are reviewed, with links to related topics accessible from the site.

http://www.merck.no/pubs/mmanual/section16/chapter205/205f.htm

NARROW-QRS TACHYCARDIAS WITH REGULAR RHYTHM

Manuals on Cardiac Arrhythmias: Narrow-QRS Tachycardias with Regular Rhythm   From *Management of Tachyarrhythmias in the Emergency Room,* this site provides guidelines on treating narrow-QRS tachycardias with regular rhythm. The site includes flowcharts, tables, and diagrams. Discussion includes atrial tachycardia, atrial flutter classification, paroxysmal reentrant tachycardia, and drug therapy.

http://www.aston.it/einthoven/eint0138.htm

SUPRAVENTRICULAR TACHYCARDIAS

American Heart Journal: Supraventricular Tachycardia   A list of references and abstracts, this site contains more than 60 citations related to supraventricular tachycardia, courtesy of the *American Heart Journal.* Institutional contact information is provided for each study.

http://www.pediheart.org/searches/topic/svt.htm

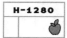

AV Nodal Reentry Tachycardia (AVNRT)   A fact sheet at this site provides general information regarding the most common type of paroxysmal supraventricular tachycardia, with general pathophysiology of the condition discussed.

http://www.arrhythmia.org/general/whatis/avnrt.html

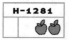

HeartWeb: Radiofrequency Ablation for Inappropriate Sinus Tachycardia Following Successful Ablation of Atrioventricular Nodal Reentrant Tachycardia   This full-text article from the University of Florida College of Medicine discusses successful radiofrequency ablation, potential complications of the procedure, and the possibility of inappropriate sinus tachycardia after radiofrequency ablation of other supraventricular tachycardias. Images, tables, and reference citations accompany the discussion.

http://www.heartweb.org/heartweb/0197/ep0001.htm

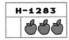

Postgraduate Medicine: Reentrant Tachycardias The first in a series of articles on clinical electrophysiology, this *Postgraduate Medicine* paper discusses the management of one of the most common sudden-onset supraventricular tachycardias, AV nodal reentrant tachycardia. The classic form of the condition is described, as well as its difficult diagnosis. Management, pharmacologic therapy, and the use of radiofrequency catheter ablation procedures are introduced. Additional forms of dysrhythmias involving the AV node or an accessory pathway and the use of ablation techniques for effective management of most supraventricular tachycardias are examined.

http://www.postgradmed.com/issues/1998/01_98/karas.htm

Sorting Out Supraventricular Tachycardias Distinctions are made at this SpringNet educational site between various tachycardias and supraventricular tachycardias (SVT), resulting from reentry, altered automaticity, or triggered activity. Information is provided on sinus tachycardia, the most familiar SVT; paroxysmal supraventricular tachycardia (PSVT); and methods of differentiating the various types of PSVT. An online test with instant processing is available.

http://www.springnet.com/ce/ccc98ce.htm

TACHYCARDIAS, GENERAL

Manuals on Cardiac Arrhythmias: Management of Tachyarrhythmias in the Emergency Room At this site index, users will find links to an introduction on epidemiology and diagnostic procedures; tutorials on narrow QRS tachycardias with regular and irregular rhythm; and a discussion of wide QRS tachycardias. Diagnostic and therapeutic algorithms are included for each, and pharmaceutical interventions are thoroughly detailed.

http://www.aston.it/einthoven/eint0136.htm

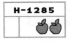

Tachycardia Therapy Information about normal conduction, including methods of control of tachycardia rhythms, is reviewed. Animated graphics at the site illustrate basic anatomy, conduction, and flow of blood through the heart. A connection to support group listings is provided.

http://www.studio-delos.com/tachy/tachy2.htm

TORSADE DE POINTES

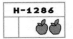

Clinical Cardiology: Practical Approach to Torsade de Pointes *Clinical Cardiology* presents this peer-reviewed discussion on clinical management of torsade de pointes. The most common cause of polymorphic ventricular tachycardia is discussed, along with general information regarding other settings in which it may occur. Electrocardiographic features are concisely reviewed, as are treatment modalities.

http://clinical-cardiology.org/briefs/9703briefs/cc20-285.shtml

eMedicine: Torsade de Pointes Authored by physicians at Mount Sinai Medical Center, this eMedicine site provides a complete introduction and detailed clinical information for torsade de pointes. Review includes pathophysiology, frequency, and mortality rates. Clinical material includes patient history, physical findings, causes of Q-T interval prolongation, workup, treatment, medications, and follow-up management. EKG images and MEDLINE reference links are provided.
http://www.eMedicine.com/EMERG/topic596.htm

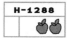

Internet Continuing Education Services: Torsade de Pointes This site provides an EKG tracing to illustrate torsade de pointes, an unusual ventricular tachycardia. The site also offers information about the mechanism of torsade de pointes, causes, and commonly associated agents.
http://wices.com/icescardiac23.htm

Internet Medical Education, Inc.: Torsade de Pointes Torsade de pointes is described at this site, along with treatment recommendations.
http://www.med-edu.com/patient/arrhythmia/arrhythmia-tachy-ventr.html#mVT

VENTRICULAR TACHYCARDIAS, GENERAL

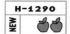

American Heart Association (AHA): Ventricular Rhythm Disturbances General information on ventricular arrhythmias is presented at this fact sheet, part of the AHA's online encyclopedia. The wide range of clinical pictures is presented, and scenarios known to be associated with sudden cardiac death are discussed. Additional pages can be accessed, providing general information, distinctions among types, treatment, and ECG criteria for ectopic ventricular complexes and ventricular tachycardias.
http://216.185.112.5/presenter.jhtml?identifier=1679

eMedicine: Ventricular Tachycardia This review of ventricular tachycardias, courtesy of eMedicine, offers background and clinical information, including main symptoms, risk factors, and physical findings associated with the disorder. Classifications according to electrocardiographic appearance; several diagnostic differential links for contrast and comparison; and listings of laboratory, imaging, and other diagnostic tests in establishing precise causative factors are discussed. Procedural information on diagnostic electrophysiological study, complete medical and surgical care reviews, and medication profiles for antiarrhythmics are provided. A variable prognosis is presented, as well as miscellaneous information on medical and legal pitfalls in management. Several enlargeable ECG tracings are available.
http://www.eMedicine.com/med/topic2367.htm

Internet Medical Education, Inc.: Monomorphic Ventricular Tachycardias The monomorphic ventricular tachycardias are defined at this site, part of Internet Medical Education, Inc., and treatment recommendations are given. http://www.med-edu.com/patient/arrhythmia/arrhythmia-tachy-ventr.html#mVT

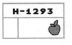

Internet Medical Education, Inc.: Polymorphic Ventricular Tachycardias This site defines the polymorphic ventricular tachycardias, and lists their common components. Treatment recommendations are included.
http://www.med-edu.com/patient/arrhythmia/arrhythmia-tachy-ventr.html#mVT

Ventricular Tachycardia Clinical Cases Clinical cases in ventricular tachycardia are available at this site, with each link offering case history details, diagnostic and procedural review, outcome, and follow-up comments. Enlargeable images are available.
http://www.cardima.com/vt_cases.html

WIDE-COMPLEX TACHYCARDIA

Management of Tachyarrhythmias in the Emergency Room: Wide-QRS Tachycardias This site provides guidelines on treating wide-QRS tachycardias and lists four common causes of the disorder. Figures, tables, and a schematic representation of two paroxysmal supraventricular reentry tachycardias with wide QRS are included. Regular and irregular rhythms are discussed, and algorithmic approaches to the patient with wide-QRS tachycardia are outlined in flowchart form.
http://www.aston.it/einthoven/eint0140.htm

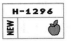

University of Medicine and Dentistry of New Jersey: Wide Complex Tachycardia (WCT) A three-part definition of wide-complex tachycardia is found at this clinical outline, which also introduces arrhythmia differentiation and management measures.
http://www2.umdnj.edu/medrpweb/pearls/cardio/WCT.htm

Yale University Cardiovascular Medicine: The Assessment of Wide Complex Tachycardia An algorithm for diagnosis, based on a clinical study found in *Circulation,* is available at the pages of this Yale University resource. Diagnostic considerations, electrocardiographic assessment, and a clinical case ECG tracing and discussion are provided.
http://revco.med.yale.edu/edux/wct/

9.3 ARTERIOSCLEROSIS

GENERAL RESOURCES

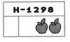

Arteriosclerosis Produced by Health Education Associates, this site contains patient information about arteriosclerosis. A general overview of the disease is included, as well as information about causative factors, including hypertension, diabetes mellitus, smoking, and obesity. Keys to recognizing arteriosclerosis, as well as information about its treatment, are highlighted.
http://well-net.com/cardiov/arterios.html

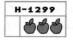

Atherosclerosis and Coronary Artery Disease Created by the Cardiac Prevention Research Centre, this page provides a discussion of atherosclerosis. Consumers may access information about atherosclerotic plaque, coronary arteries, angina, and heart attacks. Separate discussions for each of several risk factors, including high blood cholesterol, high blood pressure, smoking, lack of exercise, diabetes, obesity, and stress and hostility, are included, as well as nutrition information, risk factor statistics, and community resources for risk factor reduction. http://www.chebucto.ns.ca/Health/CPRC/home_pg.html

WellnessWeb: Arteriosclerosis A general overview of arteriosclerosis is available from this address, including definitions of distinct forms of the disease, risk factors, symptoms, and prevention. Current research studies and treatment strategies are also discussed, and reference citations are available. http://www.wellnessweb.com/masterindex/cardio/arterio.htm

ATHEROSCLEROSIS

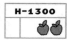

American Heart Association (AHA): A Definition of Advanced Types of Atherosclerotic Lesions From the American Heart Association, this medical statement gives a definition of advanced types of atherosclerotic lesions and a histological classification of atherosclerosis. The article provides an abstract and sections on atherosclerotic lesion types advanced by histology; type IV, type V, and type VI lesions; atherosclerotic aneurysms; histological classification of atherosclerotic lesions; history of classifications in pathology; and characterization of atherosclerotic lesions by clinical imaging. http://216.185.112.5/presenter.jhtml?identifier=1417

American Heart Association (AHA): Coronary Artery Calcification From the American Heart Association, this site offers information on the epidemiology, imaging methods, and clinical implications of coronary artery calcification. Topics discussed include the pathophysiology of coronary artery disease, in vivo imaging methods, epidemiological considerations, and practical applications of coronary calcium detection. http://216.185.112.5/presenter.jhtml?identifier=1684

eMedicine: Atherosclerosis Authored by James L. Orford of Harvard Medical School, this eMedicine review includes the background, pathophysiology, and demographic details for atherosclerosis. Highly variable symptoms are discussed, and information on luminal narrowing, angina pectoris, peripheral vascular disease, and related conditions is presented. Physical findings and review of epidemiological studies in North America and Europe are part of this article, along with coverage of established risk factors and treatment for hypertension and hyperlipidemia. Primary and secondary prevention measures are also reviewed. http://www.eMedicine.com/med/topic182.htm

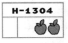

European Atherosclerosis Society Devoted to advancing knowledge concerning the causes, natural history, treatment, and prevention of atherosclerosis, the European Atherosclerosis Society provides information about the society's executive committee, membership, and meetings. A link to the group's online journal and related societal links are found, including the International Atherosclerosis Society and the American Heart Association.
http://www.elsevier.com/inca/homepage/sab/eas/menu.htm

Merck Manual of Diagnosis and Therapy: Atherosclerosis The pathology and pathogenesis, risk factors, symptoms and signs, diagnosis, prevention, and treatment of atherosclerosis are discussed in this comprehensive textbook chapter. Two hypotheses explaining pathogenesis and reversible risk factors are described in detail.
http://www.merck.com/pubs/mmanual/section16/chapter201/201b.htm

University of Alabama: Atherosclerosis Clinical Resources Visitors to this address will find links to general information, pathology images, clinical guidelines, scientific statements, and other miscellaneous resources related to atherosclerosis. Links to directories devoted to related topics are also available.
http://www.slis.ua.edu/cdlp/WebDLCore/
clinical/cardiology/cardiovascular/atherosclerosis.html

Nonatheromatous Arteriosclerosis

Merck Manual of Diagnosis and Therapy: Nonatheromatous Arteriosclerosis The nonatheromatous arteriosclerosis of aging is reviewed at this site of the online *Merck Manual of Diagnosis and Therapy,* with discussion found regarding the overall elasticity reduction in the vessel wall and Monckeberg's arteriosclerosis.
http://www.merck.no/pubs/mmanual/section16/chapter201/201c.htm

9.4 Cardiac Arrest

General Resources

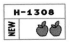

American Heart Association (AHA): Sudden Cardiac Death The AHA scientific position concerning cardiac arrest is summarized at this site, which includes causes of cardiac death and treatments for survivors. Citations to in-depth research on the subject are presented, as well as a listing of related AHA publications for both consumer and professional readers.
http://216.185.112.5/presenter.jhtml?identifier=14

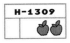

Current Concepts in the Management of Cardiac Arrest Review of an article against rigid management procedures in cardiac arrest is provided at this

site, with discussion of core interventions, such as blind defibrillation, endotracheal intubation, and additional measures. A summary of the proven benefit of direct current countershock in ventricular fibrillation and cardiopulmonary resuscitation followed by advanced life support is provided. The principles of basic cardiac life support and additional advanced measures requiring electrical defibrillation and intravenous drugs and fluids are outlined. All interventions are reviewed, emphasizing the rationale for high-dose adrenaline, management of specific dysrhythmias, and therapy specific to either ventricular defibrillation, asystole, or electro-mechanical dissociation.
http://www.australianprescriber.com/magazines/vol20no2/cardiac.htm

ASYSTOLE

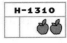

Asystole/Ventricular Standstill An EKG tracing demonstrating asystole, or ventricular standstill, is provided at this site. In addition, an explanation for the EKG and a discussion of possible interventions are included.
http://www.rnceus.com/ekg/ekgasystole.html

PULSELESS ELECTRICAL ACTIVITY

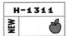

Family Practice Notebook.com: Pulseless Electrical Activity An online resource for physicians, the Family Practice Notebook offers an outline of both the causes and management of pulseless electrical activity at this site. Related links to emergency cardiovascular guidelines, conditions associated with pulseless electrical activity, and procedures in management are available.
http://www.fpnotebook.com/CV9.htm

VENTRICULAR FIBRILLATION/
PULSELESS VENTRICULAR TACHYCARDIA

Pediatric Ventricular Fibrillation and Pulseless Ventricular Tachycardia Common causes of cardiopulmonary arrest, as manifested by ventricular fibrillation or pulseless ventricular tachycardia, are reviewed at this site, with assessment and treatment protocols outlined. Basic, intermediate, and paramedic procedures are enumerated.
http://www.vgernet.net/bkand/state/pfib.html

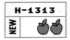

Ventricular Fibrillation/Pulseless Ventricular Tachycardia Provided by InterAccess, this Web site discusses the assessment and treatment priorities of ventricular fibrillation/pulseless ventricular tachycardia. Basic, intermediate, and emergency treatment protocols are reviewed.
http://www.vgernet.net/bkand/state/vfib.html

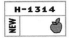

Virtual Hospital: Algorithm for Ventricular Fibrillation and Pulseless Ventricular Tachycardia   Externally peer-reviewed by Mosby, this online algorithm outlines emergency interventions for ventricular fibrillation and pulseless electrical activity. Information is derived from the Emergency Cardiac Care Committee and Subcommittees of the American Heart Association.
http://www.vh.org/Providers/ClinRef/FPHandbook/Chapter01/figures01/fig1-1.html

9.5 CARDIAC INFECTIOUS DISEASES

GENERAL RESOURCES

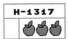

Weill Medical College of Cornell University: Vascular Infections   This site was produced by Dr. Richard B. Roberts of the Weill Medical College of Cornell University and contains nearly a dozen case studies of patients with vascular infections. Each case study offers images, answers diagnostic questions, and provides a summary of treatment recommended. A discussion of infective endocarditis is offered.
http://edcenter.med.cornell.edu/Pathophysiology_Cases/Vascular_Infections/VI_TOCs.html

CHAGAS' DISEASE

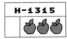

Trypanosoma cruzi   Maintained by the Ohio State University College of Biological Sciences, this site provides information about *Trypanosoma cruzi*, also known as Chagas' disease. The discussion includes origin, transmission, and progress of the disease. Hyperlinks to a map of geographic distribution, diagram of the life cycle of the parasite, and images of *Trypanosoma cruzi* are offered. http://www.biosci.ohio-state.edu/~parasite/chagas.html

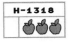

World Health Organization (WHO): Chagas' Disease Elimination
The World Health Organization's strategy for elimination of Chagas' disease is discussed at this site. The strategy includes controlling vector-transmitted infections and blood-transmitted infections. Information about the disease itself, disease situations, and disease control activity is provided, and links to related information sources, including the Centers for Disease Control and Prevention, are found. http://www.who.int/ctd/html/chag.html

CHLAMYDIA PNEUMONIAE AND CARDIOVASCULAR DISEASE

Emerging Infectious Diseases: *Chlamydia pneumoniae* and Cardiovascular Disease   A publication of the Centers for Disease Control and Prevention, this *Emerging Infectious Disease* issue examines the possible role of chronic infection in the development of cardiovascular disease, with particular attention to the pathogen *C. pneumoniae*. Evidence for the association is pre-

sented, including studies of the pathogen in atherosclerotic tissue and its suspected role in atherogenesis.
http://www.cdc.gov/ncidod/EID/vol4no4/campbell.htm

INFECTIVE ENDOCARDITIS

American College of Cardiology (ACC): Guidelines for the Management of Patients with Valvular Heart Disease This site contains a document section pertaining to the evaluation and management of infective endocarditis. Discussions include symptoms of endocarditis, common causative organisms, criteria for diagnosis, and recommendations for antimicrobial regimens. http://www.acc.org/clinical/guidelines/valvular/jac5929fla112.htm

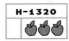

American Heart Association (AHA): Bacterial Endocarditis A description of bacterial endocarditis is presented at this site, along with a review of common causes and risk groups. The site contains links to AHA-related topics, including information about heart defects and rheumatic fever. Links to AHA medical and scientific statements relating to bacterial endocarditis are also found at the site, including a prevention guideline, antibiotic treatment, and diagnostic and management protocols.
http://216.185.112.5/presenter.jhtml?identifier=4436

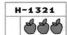

American Heart Association (AHA): Prevention of Bacterial Endocarditis From the American Heart Association, this Scientific Statement provides recommendations on the prevention of bacterial endocarditis, including discussions of cardiac conditions associated with endocarditis. Information about bacteremia-producing procedures, such as dental and oral, respiratory, gastrointestinal, and genitourinary tract procedures, is reviewed, as well as a number of predisposing circumstances.
http://216.185.112.5/presenter.jhtml?identifier=1729

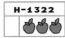

eMedicine: Endocarditis Authored by a physician from New York University Bellevue Medical Center, this eMedicine site contains frequently updated information about the disorder. Background information, including statistics on pathophysiology, frequency, mortality, sex, and age, and a clinical discussion of the illness, including symptoms, causes, and variations, are provided. Diagnostic differential links, guidelines for diagnosis, and information on drug treatment and follow-up management are included.
http://www.eMedicine.com/emerg/topic164.htm

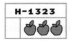

University of New South Wales: Infective Endocarditis An image of a preserved, opened human heart, revealing an infected mitral valve, is presented at this site. Detailed descriptions of specific areas of the image are available by clicking on an area of interest. A history of this specific illness and a description of the specimen are also provided.
http://www.med.unsw.edu.au/pathology/pathmus/F1004089.htm

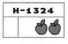

Unraveling the 'Mystery' of Endocarditis This general information article presents a valuable review regarding endocarditis in patients with congenital heart defects. Answers to questions about the relationship between congenital heart abnormalities and endocarditis are provided, as well as information on symptoms, diagnosis, treatment, and prevention. The effects of the illness on different body systems are reviewed.

http://www.cachnet.org/thebeat/thebeat_fall95.3.html

Vanderbilt Medical Center: Pediatric Infective Endocarditis A description of acute and subacute endocarditis, with a focus on the disease in children and infants, is available at this Web address. Causative organisms, risk factors, signs and symptoms, and diagnostic procedures are discussed in detail.

http://www.mc.vanderbilt.edu/peds/pidl/cardio/sbe.htm

Weill Medical College of Cornell University: Infective Endocarditis This summary lists common microorganisms associated with infective endocarditis, complications of endocarditis, and indications for surgery.

http://edcenter.med.cornell.edu/
Pathophysiology_Cases/Vascular_Infections/VI_Summary.html

Myocarditis, General

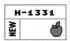

American Heart Association (AHA): Myocardium and Myocarditis Intended for a consumer audience, this page discusses the function of the myocardium and inflammation. Various causes are listed, and treatment is briefly introduced. Related pages of the AHA site are available.

http://216.185.112.5/presenter.jhtml?identifier=4729

eMedicine: Myocarditis The review of myocarditis at this site was authored by physicians of the University of Chicago. The article provides an introduction to the disorder as well as information about patient history, symptoms, physical presentation, and causes. A list of differential links and information about workup, treatment, medication, and follow-up care are provided.

http://www.eMedicine.com/emerg/topic326.htm

Myocarditis, Viral

eMedicine: Myocarditis, Viral Taken from the pediatric chapter of the eMedicine database, this page describes the more common viral pathophysiology of myocarditis and reviews variable clinical presentations and etiologic agents. Several differential links within the eMedicine database can be accessed from the page. Information at the site also includes pharmacologic profiles of various therapeutic agents.

http://www.eMedicine.com/ped/topic1534.htm

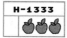

University of Nebraska Medical Center: Viral Myocarditis This site describes the role of non-poliovirus enteroviruses in human disease and focuses primarily on group B coxsackieviruses and their role in inflammatory heart disease. A discussion of current research, answers to frequently asked questions, articles about inflammatory heart disease, and personal accounts of survivors of this disease are provided. Other resources include links to related sites, additional information on viral heart disease, and a description of the group B coxsackieviruses and adenoviruses.
http://www.unmc.edu/Pathology/Myocarditis

PERICARDITIS, ACUTE

American Family Physician: Electrocardiographic Manifestations and Differential Diagnosis of Acute Pericarditis Typical symptoms and several etiologies of acute pericardial disease are discussed at this article, created by the American Academy of Family Physicians. An illustrative case study, ECG tracing, and discussion of ECG manifestations are offered. A table at the site outlines disease stages and related ECG findings. Other details on differential diagnosis and follow-up care are provided.
http://www.aafp.org/afp/980215ap/marinell.html

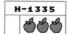

eMedicine: Pericarditis, Acute This eMedicine review offers comprehensive information on acute pericarditis resulting from a variety of viral or bacterial pathogens. Idiopathic causes; cases resulting from rheumatoid arthritis, systemic lupus erythematosus, and other connective tissue disease; and a variety of other causes are reviewed. Pericardial physiology, pathophysiology, symptoms, and physical signs, such as the pericardial friction rub, are presented.
http://eMedicine.com/MED/topic1781.htm

PERICARDITIS, VIRAL

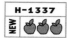

eMedicine: Pericarditis, Viral The pathogenesis of clinical manifestations in both adults and children is reviewed at this eMedicine site, along with an outline of symptoms, physical presentation, and several etiologic agents. Information on differentials to be considered can be accessed from hyperlinks at the page. Diagnostic tests and procedures are reviewed, in addition to complete medical management protocols.
http://www.eMedicine.com/ped/topic2524.htm

POSTPERICARDIOTOMY SYNDROME

eMedicine: Postpericardiotomy Syndrome Part of the eMedicine online textbook, this disease synopsis includes a discussion of etiologic infective agents following open pericardial surgery. History, physical presentation, and possible

causes are reviewed, and a list of diagnostic differential pages within the eMedicine domain can be accessed directly from the site. Outlines of the diagnostic workup and medical, surgical, and consultative care are presented, as well as profiles of mainstays of pharmacologic therapy.
http://www.eMedicine.com/ped/topic1875.htm

RHEUMATIC FEVER

HealthlinkUSA: Rheumatic Fever A variety of links to other Web sites related to causes, incidence, risk factors, diagnosis, prevention, signs and tests, statistics, and prognosis for rheumatic fever are available from this online collection. http://www.healthlinkusa.com/Rheumatic_Fever.htm

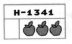

Rheumatic Fever Published by the South Dakota Department of Health, this site gives detailed, technical answers to questions about rheumatic fever. It explains rheumatic fever, describes the susceptible population, and outlines symptoms, exposure, diagnosis, treatment, precautions, and prevention. The site provides links to the health department's home page.
http://www.state.sd.us/doh/Pubs/rheumat.htm

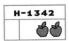

Virtual Hospital: Rheumatic Fever and Rheumatic Carditis Prepared by the University of Iowa, this excerpt from the *Family Practice Handbook* contains information about rheumatic fever and rheumatic carditis. Included is a discussion of etiology and present significance. Details concerning clinical signs and symptoms, cardiac manifestations, and treatment and prophylaxis are offered, as well as information about pharmacology.
http://www.vh.org/Providers/ClinRef/FPHandbook/Chapter02/05-2.html

9.6 CARDIAC TUMORS

GENERAL RESOURCES

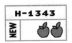

Cardiothoracic Surgery Notes: Cardiac Tumors This presentation of Cardiothoracic Surgery Notes, an online, interactive review, offers a complete listing of benign and cardiac tumors, with the morphology, location, clinical presentation, diagnostic tests, and surgical management techniques outlined. Image links are provided.
http://www.ctsnet.org/residents/ctsn/archives/31txt.html

Merck Manual of Diagnosis and Therapy: Cardiac Tumors A general description of primary cardiac tumors is found at this address, and information on their similarities in presentations to other heart disease is offered. More detailed discussions of both benign and malignant disease can be accessed from this page and include information on myxoma, rhabdomyoma, fibroma, teratoma, cardiac sarcoma, and cardiac metastases.

http://www.merck.com/pubs/mmanual/section16/chapter210/210a.htm

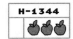

University of Alabama: Cardiovascular Neoplasms Clinical Resources

An extensive assortment of clinical resources related to cardiovascular neoplasms is provided by the University of Alabama at this site. References include chapters from Harrison's Online, the online *Merck Manual,* CHORUS (Collaborative Hypertext of Radiology), WebPath, MD Consult Reference Books, and CliniWeb, which offers preformatted MEDLINE searches and additional diagnostic and management tools. Links to clinical guidelines from MD Consult Practice Guidelines and the National Guideline Clearinghouse are provided, as well as links to WebMedLit and HealthWeb-Oncology. A large amount of free reference material is provided; however, some textbooks require an online subscription. (some features fee-based)

http://www.slis.ua.edu/cdlp/unthsc/clinical/oncology/cardiovascular/index.htm

CARDIAC ANGIOSARCOMA

Canadian Journal of Cardiology: Primary Cardiac Angiosarcoma

This abstract of a clinical article, available in both English and French, reviews the difficult diagnosis of cardiac angiosarcoma due to unusual presentations. Visitors can order the full text of this article from the site.

(some features fee-based) http://www.pulsus.com/CARDIOL/13_03/afza_ed.htm

CARDIAC FIBROMA

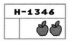

Pediatric Imaging Teaching Files: Cardiac Fibroma
A pediatric case of cardiac fibroma is presented at this site, including four representative diagnostic images and a detailed clinical discussion. A patient history, clinical findings, and discussion of cardiac fibromas are available, including details of pathologic biopsy. Reference citations are provided.

http://www.uhrad.com/pedsarc/peds023.htm

CARDIAC SARCOMA, GENERAL

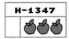

eMedicine: Cardiac Sarcoma
Authored by physicians of the University Hospitals of Cleveland, this eMedicine site provides an overview of cardiac sarcoma. The introduction includes demographic information and pathophysiology, and clinical summaries review patient history, physical findings, and causes. Workup procedures, treatment, and follow-up care guidelines are provided, in addition to several diagnostic differential links. Bibliographic references are listed, with access to correlating MEDLINE article abstracts.

http://www.eMedicine.com/med/topic282.htm

CARNEY COMPLEX

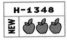

eMedicine: Carney Complex Background information on this rare, inherited syndrome is found at this page, providing professional coverage of pathophysiology and cardiac involvement. Clinical presentation is available, as well as links to differentials. Laboratory studies, additional diagnostic testing procedures, and protocol for treatment are reviewed. A case example at the site offers either a full-size echocardiographic image or eMedicine's "Zoom View" option. http://www.eMedicine.com/med/topic2941.htm

CYSTS

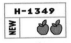

Clinical Cardiology: Pericardial Cyst An enlargeable chest X-ray displayed at this page demonstrates a presumptive diagnosis of pericardial cyst. Discussion of symptoms and additional magnetic resonance imaging are found, confirming original diagnostic findings.
http://www.clinical-cardiology.org/briefs/9803briefs/cc21-223.html

LIPOMA

Southern Medical Association: Primary Lipomatous Tumors of the Cardiac Valves A case report of a tricuspid valve mass is found at this site of the Southern Medical Association. The importance of including valvular tumors in the differential diagnosis is emphasized, along with discussion of additional reported cases in the literature. Images of the mass are accessible.
http://www.sma.org/smj/96oct20.htm

MYXOMA

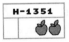

Brigham and Women's Hospital: Right Atrial Myxoma From Brigham and Women's Hospital and Harvard Medical School, this site provides a case study of right atrial myxoma. The study includes background information and history, imaging findings, differential diagnosis, diagnosis, discussion, and references. http://brighamrad.harvard.edu/Cases/bwh/hcache/46/full.html

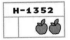

HealthCentral: Left Atrial Myxoma Part of the Health Central General Health Encyclopedia, this site offers an overview of left atrial myxoma. The table of contents includes alternative names, causes, incidence, and risk factors, prevention, symptoms, signs and tests, treatment, expectations, and potential complications.
http://planet-health.com/mhc/top/000196.cfm

University of Connnecticut: Myxoma A general gross description, histological description, and clinical correlations regarding left atrial myxoma

are conveyed at this concise outline on myxoma, maintained by the University of Connecticut Health Center.
http://radiology.uchc.edu/TMGEN/32188400.htm

RHABDOMYOMA

Cardiac Rhabdomyoma This site provides clinical information about rhabdomyoma. An overview includes synonyms, a definition, prevalence, etiology, pathogenesis, associated anomalies, resulting cardiac anomalies, differential diagnosis, prognosis, recurrence risk, and management. Two case examples with tables, diagrams, images, photographs, and discussions are presented, and extensive reference citations are provided.
http://www.thefetus.net/sections/articles/
Cardiovascular/Cardiac_rhabdomyoma_Dolkart_2127.html

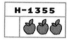

University of Illinois at Chicago: Cardiac Rhabdomyoma A synopsis of this disorder includes synonyms, definition, prevalence, etiology, pathogenesis, associated anomalies, differential diagnosis, prognosis, recurrence risk, and management protocol. A case study example, accompanied by images and tables, is provided, in addition to an extensive reference listing.
http://www.obgyn.uic.edu/mfm/tcase/case.htm

RHABDOMYOSARCOMA

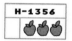

American Cancer Society (ACS): Rhabdomyosarcoma Resource Center The Rhabdomyosarcoma Resource Center provides information about prevention and risk factors, detection and symptoms, treatment, and survivorship. A review of cancer drugs, a glossary, and answers to frequently asked questions are also presented.
http://www3.cancer.org/cancerinfo/load_cont.asp?ct=53

Soft Tissue Sarcoma Committee The Children's Oncology Group Soft Tissue Sarcoma Committee designs and conducts clinical trials in the treatment of rhabdomyosarcoma. The site includes group details, information about clinical trials, answers to frequently asked questions, and links to additional sources of information. Anatomical locations of rhabdomyosarcoma, age occurrence of the disorder, types, staging, treatment, adult rhabdomyosarcoma, and images of the disorder are presented.
http://rhabdo.org/rhabdo/irsg.htm

St. Jude Children's Research Hospital: Rhabdomyosarcoma Patient information about rhabdomyosarcoma, including a general definition, details about incidence, influencing factors, treatment strategies, survival rates, and current research, is offered at this Internet location.
http://www.stjude.org/Medical/rhabdomyosar.htm

Don't type in long URLs – add the site number to the eMedguides URL: www.eMedguides.com/**G-1234**.

9.7 CARDIOVASCULAR SHOCK

GENERAL RESOURCES

Merck Manual of Diagnosis and Therapy: Shock Hypovolemic shock, vasodilatory shock, cardiogenic shock, and septic shock are described in this online clinical review. Symptoms and signs, possible complications, diagnosis, and prognosis and treatment of each condition are discussed in detail. A table outlining the mechanisms that cause cardiogenic shock; access to specific information on bacteremia and septic shock, as well as on coexisting pulmonary complications; and a connection to information on stabilization therapies are provided. Additional treatment links found throughout the text include cardiopulmonary resuscitation measures and oxygen administration.
http://www.merck.com/pubs/mmanual/section16/chapter204/204a.htm

ACUTE ADRENAL INSUFFICIENCY

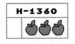

eMedicine: Adrenal Insufficiency and Adrenal Crisis Adrenal crisis and severe acute adrenocortical insufficiency are described in this CME article. Pathophysiology, frequency, morbidity and mortality, and demographics are offered in an introductory section. Clinical details, differential links, and typical diagnostic tests are listed, followed by details of treatment, medications, and follow-up care. Special medical concerns associated with the condition and reference citations are provided.
http://www.eMedicine.com/emerg/topic16.htm

MEDLINEplus Medical Encyclopedia: Acute Adrenal Crisis Maintained by the National Library of Medicine, this encyclopedia entry contains basic information on acute adrenal crisis, including causes, risks, symptoms, and diagnostic tests. Links to further details on related testing, treatment, and complications are offered at this site.
http://www.nlm.nih.gov/medlineplus/ency/article/000357.htm

ANAPHYLACTIC SHOCK

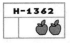

HealthlinkUSA: Anaphylactic Shock A listing of links is available at this address, providing visitors with access to various resources on anaphylactic shock. Most resources pertain to this reaction in children and are intended for consumers and parents.
http://www.healthlinkusa.com/15.html

CARDIOGENIC SHOCK

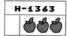

eMedicine: Cardiogenic Shock The clinical presentation, differential links, and diagnostic workup are all included at this eMedicine page, which provides a comprehensive guide to assessment and management of this physiologic state. Myocardial pathology, cellular pathology, reversible myocardial dysfunction, and cardiovascular mechanics of cardiogenic shock are discussed. Systemic effects are reviewed, and information on shock state, irrespective of etiology, is considered. A lengthy list of causes is found, and other problems to be considered during the initial clinical evaluation are introduced.
http://www.eMedicine.com/EMERG/topic530.htm

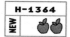

MEDLINEplus Medical Encyclopedia: Cardiogenic Shock A concise encylopedic review of cardiogenic shock is offered at this resource of the National Library of Medicine. Causes, risks, prevention, and diagnostic tests are listed, with hyperlinks thoughout the text connecting to related information. A treatment overview is provided.
http://www.nlm.nih.gov/medlineplus/ency/article/000185.htm

DRUG-INDUCED SHOCK

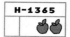

Update on Management of the Patient with Poisoning or Drug Overdose Specific management protocols for drug-induced hypotension are outlined at this CME module. Recognition of the severely poisoned patient, an emphasis on differences in treatment where drugs are concerned, and general management procedures for cardiovascular stability, ventilation, and other treatment considerations are provided. Poststudy questions and answers for CME credit are provided.
http://www.chestnet.org/education/pccu/vol12/lesson09.html

HYPOVOLEMIC SHOCK

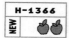

MEDLINEplus Medical Encyclopedia: Hypovolemic Shock Updated by Alan Greene, MD, this page offers information on hypovolemia as a cause of shock and presents details on causes, risks, and symptoms. Additional links to related information from this National Library of Medicine database are available, including examinations of diagnostic tests and interventions.
http://www.nlm.nih.gov/medlineplus/ency/article/000167.htm

SpringNet: Hypovolemic Shock This continuing education resource is a component of SpringNet's *Continuing Education Handbook*. Information is presented through discussion of three clinical hypovolemic case studies, created for this teaching module. Topics include actual versus relative hypovolemia, head-to-toe assessment, and appropriate intervention. Visitors can earn continuing education credit by completing a review test.
http://www.springnet.com/ce/p509a.htm

Obstructive Shock, General

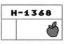

Cardiopulmonary Obstructive Shock Links to pulmonary embolism, pericardial tamponade, and additional disturbances of the cardiopulmonary circuit resulting in shock are listed at this medical glossary page. Specific conditions may be accessed for further details.
http://www.medhelp.org/glossary/new/GLS_0941.HTM

Pulmonary Embolism

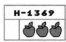

eMedicine: Pulmonary Embolism This CME article offers a discussion of pulmonary embolism, including background, pathophysiology, frequency, mortality and morbidity, clinical examinations and patient history, causes, differential links, laboratory studies and imaging, treatment and medications, possible complications, and medical and legal pitfalls.
http://www.eMedicine.com/emerg/topic490.htm

Pulmonary Embolism Diagnosed during a Cardiac Catheterization
This example case reports on an emergency situation in which shortness of breath and chest discomfort follow a syncopal episode. Enlargeable ECG images, resuscitative measures instituted, and a pulmonary angiogram, which reveals massive bilateral pulmonary emboli, are presented and outline the patient history and eventual cardiopulmonary collapse.
http://www.mmip.mcgill.ca/heart/xr981015R1.html

Septic Shock

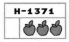

eMedicine: Septic Shock Septic shock is described in this technical CME article. An introduction to the condition includes pathophysiology, frequency, morbidity and mortality, and general demographic information. Clinical presentation and causes are discussed, followed by links to information on differential diagnoses. Diagnostic procedures, treatment, follow-up care, and prognosis are also presented. A table at the site provides information on common therapeutic medications, and CME review questions conclude the article.
http://www.eMedicine.com/EMERG/topic533.htm

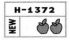

MEDLINEplus Medical Encyclopedia: Septic Shock Intended for consumer viewers, this site describes various components of septic shock. Links to related information within this National Library of Medicine reference are provided, including those on causes, risks, symptoms, and diagnosis.
http://www.nlm.nih.gov/medlineplus/ency/article/000668.htm

TENSION PNEUMOTHORAX

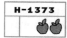

Colorado State University: Tension Pneumothorax   Background information on tension pneumothorax and the resultant blood pooling and ensuing cardiovascular collapse and shock are reviewed at this site. An online diagram illustrates the condition, and radiographic signs of tension pneumothorax are enumerated. Treatment to alleviate intrapleural pressure is summarized.
http://www.cvmbs.colostate.edu/clinsci/wing/trauma/tension.htm

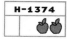

University of Maryland: Acute Closed Tension Pneumothorax   This site offers a case example of tension pneumothorax, emphasizing the necessity of its quick identification and discussing the cardiac output reduction that may rapidly ensue. A diagram illustrating the causes of shock is provided, and the hallmark signs and symptoms of the condition are listed. A treatment link provides access to information on intubation and mechanical ventilation procedures, additional oxygen administration techniques, pericardial drainage, needle thoracostomy, and intravenous fluid bolus administration.
http://nursing.umaryland.edu/students/~jkohl/scenario/tension2.htm

VASODILATORY SHOCK

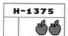

American Association for Thoracic Surgery: Management of Vasodilatory Shock after High-Risk Cardiac Surgery   This brief article summary offers an overview of the use of arginine vasopressin (AVP) in the treatment of vasodilatory shock and the clinical predictors of this condition in high-risk cardiac surgical patients. Background to the study, methods, results, and conclusions are presented.
http://www.aats.org/doc/1858

9.8 CEREBROVASCULAR DISEASE

GENERAL RESOURCES

Aneurysm and AVM Support   This comprehensive resource for patients features a large collection of personal stories. Visitors can read about the experiences of others with brain aneurysms, aortic aneurysm and dissection, and arteriovenous malformation. The site also allows visitors to submit questions to a neurosurgeon, vascular surgeon, or interventional radiologist. Moreover, a listing of regional brain-related support groups is provided, in addition to an online forum to exchange related information.
http://www.westga.edu/~wmaples/aneurysm.html

Massachusetts General Hospital: Brain Aneurysms/AVM Center   This site for patients and professionals offers various educational materials on aneurysms, arteriovenous and cavernous malformations, carotid disease, stroke, and transient ischemic attacks. Additional sections are devoted to neurovascular news, AVM support groups, booklets and publications, interventional neuroradiology, and cerebrovascular links. The site also offers brief descriptions of treatment guidelines.

http://neurosurgery.mgh.harvard.edu/vaschome.htm

ARTERIOVENOUS MALFORMATIONS (AVM)

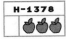

Brain Surgery Information Center: Arteriovenous Malformations Specific information for patients about arteriovenous malformations is found at this site, which includes illustrations to support a general description of the disorder. The page also contains a section on treatment options, addressing embolization and surgery.

http://www.brain-surgery.com/bsicavm.html

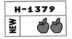

Columbia University: Arteriovenous Malformations The Cerebrovascular Center of the Neurological Institute provides this overview of the causes of arteriovenous malformations, dangers involved, and methods by which the diagnosis is made. Additional information includes review of treatments available and their various advantages and disadvantages. Specific information on embolization therapy and investigational studies is presented.

http://cpmcnet.columbia.edu/dept/cerebro/AVM.html

CENTRAL NERVOUS SYSTEM VASCULITIS

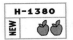

Cleveland Clinic: What You Need to Know about Central Nervous System Vasculitis Information on this rare vasculitic condition is presented at this site, as a service of the Department of Rheumatic and Immunologic Diseases of the Cleveland Clinic. Symptoms of central nervous system vasculitis, details on cerebral arteriography and other information on diagnosis, and treatment for biopsy-proven disease are introduced.

http://www.clevelandclinic.org/arthritis/treat/facts/cns.htm

HEMORRHAGIC SYNDROMES, GENERAL

Brain Aneurysm Foundation The Brain Aneurysm Foundation was developed by members of the Brain Aneurysm/AVM Center at Massachusetts General Hospital. The foundation offers resources to patients and families affected by brain aneurysms through support networks, a medical advisory board, newsletters, and educational programs. General information on brain aneurysms is provided, along with a description of the organization. A list of educational resources and an online newsletter are also available.

http://neurosurgery.mgh.harvard.edu/baf/baf-hp.htm

Brain Surgery Information Center: Aneurysm Surgery This general information site for patients provides a basic overview of aneurysms, with statistical information included. The site answers questions related to the prevention of a second hemorrhage, hydrocephalus, and vasospasm. Outcome prediction using the Hunt-Hess score is explained.
http://www.brain-surgery.com/aneurysm.html

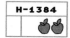

Intracranial Aneurysms An explanation of the development of aneurysms in vessel walls is provided at this site, accompanied by enlargeable computed tomography, angiography, and schematic representations. An artist's rendering of a clip applied across the neck of an aneurysm, arteriograms showing aneurysms of the posterior communicating artery, and illustrations of aneurysm types are shown. Discussion regarding vasospasm, embolization, and early intervention is provided as a service of the Buffalo Neurosurgery Group.
http://www.buffaloneuro.com/aneurysm/aneur.html

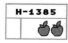

Mayo Clinic: Treatment of Unruptured Brain Aneurysms From the Mayo Clinic Rochester News, this site describes an international study, originally published in the *New England Journal of Medicine,* which suggests new treatment guidelines for small, unruptured brain aneurysms. The site describes the basis of the study, the overall lack of consensus regarding unruptured intracranial aneurysms, and the significant changes that may occur in the way these lesions are treated.
http://www.mayo.edu/comm/mcr/news/news_467.html

HEMORRHAGIC SYNDROMES, EPIDURAL HEMATOMA

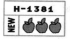

eMedicine: Epidural Hematoma Background information on the traumatic accumulation of blood in the epidural space is presented at this eMedicine article, as well as a summary of pathophysiology and introductions to diagnosis and treatment. Imaging modalities used, emergency care, and enlargeable computed tomography images are found.
http://www.emedicine.com/EMERG/topic167.htm

HEMORRHAGIC SYNDROMES, INTRACEREBRAL HEMORRHAGE

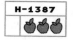

Brain Surgery Information Center: Intracerebral Hemorrhage A typical occurrence of intracerebral hemorrhage is described at this site, with discussions of other kinds of intracerebral hemorrhages, changing therapies, the current understanding of the disorder, improved imaging capabilities, and improved surgical techniques found.
http://www.brain-surgery.com/bsicintr.html

Current Approaches to Acute Stroke Management: Intracerebral Hemorrhage This article includes an overview and discussion of intracerebral hemorrhage, with coverage of epidemiology and risk factors, diagnostic

evaluation, prognosis, medical management, surgical management, and future approaches. Diagrams, references, and illustrative tables are found.
http://www.neuro-net.net/diseases/journals/acutestroke/intra.html

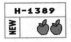

MEDLINEplus Medical Encyclopedia: Lobar Intracerebral Hemorrhage Presented by the National Library of Medicine and adam.com, this encyclopedia entry contains fundamental information on the causes, risks, diagnosis, and treatment of lobar intracerebral hemorrhage. A large selection of related links is available on tests for determining amount and cause of bleeding, confirmation of diagnosis, and treatment alternatives.
http://www.nlm.nih.gov/MEDLINEplus/ency/article/000718.htm

HEMORRHAGIC SYNDROMES, SUBARACHNOID HEMORRHAGE

Louisiana State University: Cerebral Vasospasms A review of cerebral vasospasm, a significant component of subarachnoid hemorrhage, is introduced at this page, along with a clinical definition and details on its pathophysiology and management. Primary treatment goals, aimed at preventing the severity of vasospasm, are introduced, and current and future treatments are discussed.
http://www.medschool.lsumc.edu/Nsurgery/spasm.html

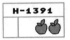

Massachusetts General Hospital: Clinical Review of Subarachnoid Hemorrhage A clinical review of subarachnoid hemorrhage is presented at this site of Massachusetts General Hospital. Causes are examined, with emphasis on the need for rapid diagnosis, and a summarized protocol for patients with the disorder is presented. Microscopic clipping of the lesion and other forms of treatment are discussed, in addition to the risks of developing vasospasm and the necessity for early recognition.
http://neurosurgery.mgh.harvard.edu/v-w-93-1.htm

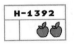

Massachusetts General Hospital: Subarachnoid Hemorrhage of Unknown Etiology Management of patients with angiogram-negative subarachnoid hemorrhage is the subject of this presentation, which includes causes of angiographically occult disease, recent advances in diagnosis, theory behind angiography failure, and discussion of additional diagnostic tools.
http://neurosurgery.mgh.harvard.edu/v-w-94-1.htm

HEMORRHAGIC SYNDROMES, SUBDURAL HEMATOMA

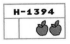

University of Missouri Health Care: Subdural Hematoma Found in the neuromedicine section of this Family health information guide, this page provides background information on subdural hematoma. An informative general overview is given, followed by a discussion of causes, signs and symptoms, diagnostic tests, treatment, and recovery after surgery.
http://muhealth.org/~neuromedicine/subdural.shtml

ISCHEMIC SYNDROMES

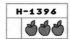

American Heart Association (AHA): Guidelines for the Management of Patients with Acute Ischemic Stroke Intended for a professional audience, this document offers information about current management protocols for acute ischemic stroke. Recommendations for immediate care are emphasized, as well as the future of therapy and its connection to very early disease recognition. http://216.185.112.5/presenter.jhtml?identifier=1227

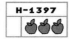

American Medical Association (AMA): Prevention of a First Stroke This online article from the *Journal of the American Medical Association* explores several interventions that may reduce treatable cardiovascular and cerebrovascular risk factors. These guidelines, a multidisciplinary consensus statement from the National Stroke Association, offer evidence for direct stroke reduction with hypertension treatment, use of warfarin under specific conditions, and performing carotid endarterectomy in certain patients. Additional observational studies are reported, providing information on the role of lifestyle risk factor modification in stroke prevention.
http://jama.ama-assn.org/issues/v281n12/ffull/jst80021.html

American Stroke Association The American Stroke Association, newly named to reflect a stronger commitment to stroke research and education, is a division of the American Heart Association. This comprehensive source provides information about stroke risk factors, conditions and treatments, surgery and related procedures, and recovery. Extensive stroke-related statistics, gender-specific information, and links to more specific stroke and cardiovascular-related topics, including cardiovascular epidemiology, fitness, hypertension, nutrition, transplantation, and pediatric cardiology, are provided.
http://www.strokeassociation.org/presenter.jhtml?identifier=1200037

Brain Attack Coalition This site provides tools for healthcare professionals working to develop systems that enable the rapid diagnosis and treatment of acute stroke. Management guidelines are available from numerous reputable sources, including the AHA and the NINDS. The Stroke Coding Guide of the American Academy of Neurology is found, in addition to Stroke Prevention Guidelines of the National Stroke Association. Coordinated care tracks, hospital admission orders, and diagnostic scales are found, including that of the NIH, the Modified Rankin Scale, and the Hunt-Hess Classification of Subarachnoid Hemorrhage. Patient education materials may be accessed, courtesy of the Stroke Belt Consortium, NINDS, and the AHA.
http://www.stroke-site.org

Cerebral Ischemia Written and maintained by the Neurodegeneration Research Group, this site offers a technical description of cerebral ischemia. A quantitative fluorescence image of a hippocampal slice culture subjected to artificial ischemia is included.
http://www.med.uio.no/imb/anatomi/gruppe_3/fluo.htm

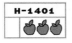

National Stroke Association   The goal of the National Stroke Association is to reduce the incidence and impact of stroke. Information about membership, donations, and materials is accessible at this site, as well as background information, prevention program details, and stroke information pages for patients. Professional information and links include the Stroke Center Network, clinical trials acceleration program, stroke prevention programs, professional meeting and event details, fellowships, and library services.

http://www.stroke.org

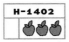

University of Alabama: Transient Ischemic Attack Clinical Resources
Textbook chapters and clinical consultative material, including the online *Merck Manual* and eMedicine's topical reviews, are available from this extensive collection of material on transient ischemic attack. The *Family Practice Handbook's* section on cerebrovascular disease, as well as pediatric resources, clinical guidelines, and Scientific Statements of the AMA, is provided. Although some material requires an online subscription, most of this clinical collection is free, courtesy of the Clinical Digital Libraries Project of the University of Alabama.

(some features fee-based)

http://www.slis.ua.edu/cdlp/uab/clinical/neurology/cerebrovascular/tia.htm

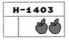

Virtual Hospital: Stroke and Brain Attack   This site, provided by the University of Iowa, offers general information about stroke and brain attack. Statistical facts about stroke and brain attack in the United States, links to additional Web resources, clinical treatment guidelines, and reference connections are provided, including those of the AHA and the online *Merck Manual of Diagnosis and Therapy*.

http://www.vh.org/Providers/ClinGuide/Stroke/

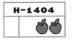

Wake Forest University: Stroke Index   Created and maintained by the Wake Forest University School of Medicine Department of Neurosurgery, this site provides links to information about many stroke-related topics. Links to information on carotid endarterectomy, support organizations, information guides, treatment guidelines, clinical trials, and teaching presentations are offered.   http://www.bgsm.edu/bgsm/surg-sci/ns/stroke.html

Washington University School of Medicine: Internet Stroke Center
The Internet Stroke Center is a Web resource for healthcare professionals, scientists, and consumers. General stroke information for patients and families, including links to stroke resources, major stroke organizations, stroke centers, and support and discussion groups, is provided, as well as connections to information about medication. Students and healthcare professionals will find news, professional management links, a calendar of scientific meetings and conferences, and training and employment opportunities. Current research, including clinical trials, therapies, and scales and tools, is offered, and connections to consensus statements, pharmacologic profiles, diagnostic procedures, syndromes, images, teaching links, and brain anatomy are available.

http://www.neuro.wustl.edu/stroke

Moya-Moya Disease

Columbia-Presbyterian Neurological Institute: Moya-Moya Accessible through the Pediatric Neurosurgery home page, this page was written specifically for parents and relatives of children with Moya-Moya. The site contains a description of the disease and its complications, in addition to diagnostic tests, operations performed, and prognosis.
http://cpmcnet.columbia.edu/dept/nsg/PNS/moyamoya.html

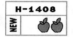

Massachusetts General Hospital: Moya-Moya Forum This non-moderated Web forum was designed to facilitate discussion and comment on Moya-Moya. New articles and informative links may be posted at the site, provided as a service of the Department of Neurology at Massachusetts General Hospital. http://neuro-www.mgh.harvard.edu/forum/MoyaMoyaMenu.html

Vascular Malformations, General

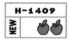

Intracranial Vascular Malformations Presented by James G. Smirniotopoulos, M.D., this article discusses the classic pathologic subtypes of intracranial vascular malformations, including the most common, arteriovenous malformations, as well as cavernous hemangioma, venous malformation, telangiectasia, and vein of Galen malformations. Characteristics of each lesion type, diagnosis, and diagnostic images are included.
http://radlinux1.usuf1.usuhs.mil/rad/home/vascmalf/malf0.html

Michigan State University: Vascular Malformations Characteristics, clinical signs, and consequences of vascular malformations are outlined at this site, which includes summaries of arteriovenous malformations and Sturge-Weber syndrome. An enlargeable image at the site depicts the microscopic appearance of arteriovenous malformations.
http://kobiljak.msu.edu/CAI/Pathology/Cerebrovascular_F/cerebrovascular_6.html

Wallenberg's Syndrome

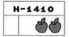

Johns Hopkins University: Lateral Medullary Syndrome Produced by Johns Hopkins University, this site offers clinical information about lateral medullary syndrome. Characteristic clinical manifestations are listed, and additional vascular syndromes to keep in mind for the differential diagnosis are discussed. http://www.bme.jhu.edu/labs/chb/disorders/wallenbe.html

9.9   CONDUCTION DISORDERS

ATRIOVENTRICULAR BLOCK

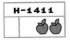

Atrioventricular Node Blocks   This site offers electrocardiographic depictions of first-, second-, and third-degree heart blocks. Explanations of each sample tracing are provided.
http://personalwebs.myriad.net/dan/EKG/blocks.htm

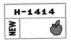

Bradycardia and Atrioventricular Block   Authored by Kent R. Olson, M.D., of the University of California San Francisco, this page provides a definition of bradycardia and atrioventricular block and offers important toxic and nontoxic causes. Clinical disorder features are discussed, and information on relevant investigations is included. In addition to observation, intravenous access, supplemental oxygen, and cardiac monitoring, specific measures to be taken with evidence of end-organ hypoperfusion are introduced.
http://www.intox.org/pagesource/treatment/english/bradycardia.htm

eMedicine: Atrioventricular Block   Background information on atrioventricular block is presented at this site of the eMedicine database, which contains peer-reviewed clinical articles on a variety of cardiology disorders. Pathophysiology is reviewed, and demographic details are included. The clinical presentation of first-, second-, and third-degree atrioventricular block is found, as well as physical findings and causes for each. Laboratory and imaging studies as well as other diagnostic modalities, are reviewed, and a profile of anticholinergic agents is included. Enlargeable ECG tracings are also available.
http://www.eMedicine.com/med/topic189.htm

MEDLINEplus Medical Encyclopedia: Atrioventricular Block, EKG Tracing   Provided as a service of the National Library of Medicine, an image at this page depicts the electrocardiogram tracing of a person with atrioventricular block. P and QRS wave descriptions and the absence of the heart contraction are introduced.
http://www.nlm.nih.gov/medlineplus/ency/imagepage/1429.htm

BUNDLE BRANCH BLOCK

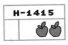

American Heart Association (AHA): Bundle Branch Block   This patient education fact sheet describes the normal travel of electrical impulses within the heart, as well as electrical travel where a bundle branch block inhibits normal function. Links are available to information on related topics and to the Medical and Scientific Statements of the AHA.
http://216.185.112.5/presenter.jhtml?identifier=4486

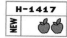

Bundle Branch Block   Provided by Cardionetics, this site describes the abnormalities of bundle branch block. Conduction diagrams of left and right bundle branch block, as well as examples of electrocardiogram readings for both blocks, are provided.

http://www.cardionetics.com/docs/healthcr/ecg/arrhy/0204_bd.htm

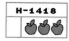

Yale University Cardiovascular Medicine: Bundle Branch Block Diagnostic Basics   Diagnostic basics of bundle branch block are contained at this reference site of Yale's Section of Cardiovascular Medicine. Description of a bundle branch blocked beat is found, as well as associated electrical activity and variations of the QRS axis.

http://revco.med.yale.edu/edux/wct/wct4a.html

HEMIBLOCK (FASCICULAR BLOCK)

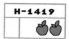

McGill Medical Informatics: Bundle Branch and Fascicular Blocks This site provides case studies of bundle branch and fascicular blocks. For each case study, an explanation and electrocardiogram are provided. Case examples illustrate intraventricular conduction defect, right bundle branch block, left bundle branch block, left anterior fascicular block, left posterior fascicular block, bifascicular block, alternating bundle branch block, and trifascicular block, with example tracings and treatment information.

http://www.mmip.mcgill.ca/heart/ecgCindex.html

University of Wisconsin Medical School: Fascicular Blocks   This site offers electrocardiographic images of fascicular blocks, which are part of the left bundle. Examples of fascicular blocks include anterior fascicular block, posterior fascicular block, and bifascicular block. Explanations accompany the illustrations.   http://www.fammed.wisc.edu/pcc/ecg/fasicular_block.html

HIS BUNDLE ARRHYTHMIAS

Merck Manual of Diagnosis and Therapy: His Bundle Arrhythmias   A description of regular rapid beats originating in the His bundle is provided as a courtesy of the *Merck Manual of Diagnosis and Therapy* online reference. An explanation of its occurrence and information on distinguishing true His bundle disturbances from other conduction abnormalities are found.

http://www.merck.com/pubs/mmanual/section16/chapter205/205j.htm

WOLFF-PARKINSON-WHITE SYNDROME

American Heart Association (AHA): Wolff-Parkinson-White Syndrome   The extra conduction pathway in Wolff-Parkinson-White syndrome,

treatment information for symptomatic patients, and links to related AHA publications are offered at this site of the American Heart Association.
http://216.185.112.5/presenter.jhtml?identifier=4785

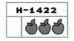

eMedicine: Wolff-Parkinson-White Syndrome   This eMedicine site provides a summary of Wolff-Parkinson-White syndrome. The introduction includes background information, pathophysiology, frequency, mortality, and gender and age factors. Clinical information includes patient history and physical characteristics, in addition to diagnostic differential links, electrocardiogram morphology, and additional presentation details. Treatment of atrial fibrillation and tachycardias, including profiles of commonly used antiarrhythmic agents, is provided.   http://www.eMedicine.com/emerg/topic644.htm

9.10 CONGENITAL HEART DISEASE (CHD)

GENERAL RESOURCES

Adult Congenital Heart Association   The Adult Congenital Heart Association is a national organization for adults and adolescents with congenital heart disease. The site provides information on recent association events, a newsletter, a message board, and a list of references. A listing of clinics for adults with congenital heart disease and links to chat rooms and support groups are provided. The site offers connections to general information about congestive heart disease, American and international organizations, professional organizations, and heart transplant resources.
http://www.achaheart.org

American Family Physician: Caring for Infants with Congenital Heart Disease and Their Families   Classifications of congenital heart defects and review of the most common acyanotic and cyanotic lesions are found at this online article, courtesy of the American Academy of Family Physicians. Detection of disease prenatally, women at risk, life-threatening symptoms in the newborn are discussed. A table outlining the most common congenital heart defects and their features is found, along with in-depth characteristic and intervention reviews. Health maintenance issues, categories of physical activity recommendations, and psychosocial issues are investigated, and an additional connection to a patient education handout is provided.
http://www.aafp.org/afp/990401ap/1857.html

CachNet   The site is the home of the Canadian Adult Congenital Heart Network, the Toronto Congenital Cardiac Centre for Adults, and the International Society for Adult Congenital Cardiac Disease. The goal of these organizations is to provide comprehensive care and information to adult patients with congenital heart disease and their healthcare providers. A restricted portion of the site, limited to physicians, is provided, and the full text of a consensus conference on adult congenital heart disease is offered, covering management issues for the most common congenital heart anomalies. Links to additional organizations, support groups and forums, a patient magazine, and other cardiology sites of interest, such as the American Heart Association, PediHeart, and the American College of Cardiology, are found. Forthcoming meeting details are offered. (some features fee-based) http://www.cachnet.org

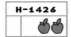

Children's Health Information Network: Congenital Heart Disease
The goal of this site is to provide resources and information to adults with congenital heart defects, families of children with congenital and acquired heart disease, and the professionals who care for them. Community resources offer patient educational materials and support forums, and the resource section contains publication listings and information on local and national events. An extensive collection of Internet links provides access to a wide variety of resources related to congenital heart disease.
http://www.tchin.org

CliniWeb International: Congenital Heart Defects
This index links the user to the latest research and preformatted PubMed query links on a variety of topics within the field of congenital heart disease. Topics are listed alphabetically and include aortic coarctation, arrhythmogenic right ventricular dysplasia, cor triatriatum, ductus arteriosus, Ebstein's anomaly, hypoplastic left heart syndrome, and truncus arteriosus.
http://www.ohsu.edu/cliniweb/C14/C14.240.400.html

Congenital Heart Defect Support Group
The Congenital Heart Defect Support Group seeks to support those affected by congenital heart defects. The site contains a message board, photos, and a chat room, as well as links to other support groups, a list of contacts, and a calendar of events. Several sections of the site are restricted to members and are available following a free registration.
(free registration) http://clubs.yahoo.com/clubs/congenitalheartdefectsupport

Congenital Heart Defects Resource Page
Designed for parents of children with congenital heart disease, this award-winning site features a publication listing and direct connection to Amazon.com. Links to online support groups, hospitals, newsgroups, personal and professional sites, transplant sites, and articles are found, in addition to a page of alphabetical links on syndromes and disorders. Information is offered courtesy of the American Heart Association, Congenital Heart Disease on the World Wide Web, and Heart Surgery Forum. http://www.csun.edu/~hcmth011/heart

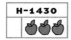

Congenital Heart Disease Online Handbook
This Web site is a resource for anyone with an interest in congenital heart disease. It contains a list of abbreviations and definitions of terms associated with congenital heart disease, with each term linked to several sites that provide in-depth information. Surgical procedures to correct congenital heart disease, including arterial switch, Fontan surgery, heart transplant, and stents, are reviewed, and each procedural

link offers further connections to related topical sites. Further sources of information on adult issues, medications, and diagnostic tests are provided.
http://www.execpc.com/~markc/congring.html

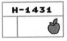

Gloria's Place of Hope   Gloria's Place of Hope was established to help children with congenital heart disease from around the world receive the surgery and medical care they need. The site contains details about children awaiting surgery, updates on children helped by the organization, fund donation, and related articles and news releases. Information is provided in several languages, including Chinese, French, German, Italian, Portuguese, and Spanish.
http://www.gloriasplaceofhope.org

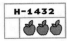

New York Online Access to Health (NOAH): Pregnancy and Congenital Heart Defects   From New York Online Access to Health comes this site linking visitors to public health information sheets from the March of Dimes. Congenital heart disease and pregnancy are covered, including background information on congenital heart defects, cardiovascular anatomy and physiology, how heart defects affect children, causes of congenital heart defects, treatment, prenatal tests and prevention, and current research.
http://www.noah-health.org/english/pregnancy/march_of_dimes/birth_defects/congnitl.html

University of Alabama: Congenital Heart Disease   Professionals can browse through links to Internet documents on congenital heart anomalies by subtopics that include aortic stenosis, atrial septal defect, patent ductus arteriosus, pulmonary stenosis, and ventricular septal defect. A link to "Congenital Heart Disease Patient/Family Resources" allows visitors to view educational materials categorized by the aforementioned subtopics.
http://www.slis.ua.edu/cdlp/unthsc/clinical/cardiology/congenital/index.htm

University of Iowa: Three-Dimensional Visualization of Congenital Heart Disease   This site provides an overview of three-dimensional magnetic resonance imaging of congenital heart disease. Patient scan protocols, case studies, and examples in the literature are offered, including right aortic arch, hypoplastic aorta, and vascular rings. Graphics and links to online moving images are found, along with links to related Web sites.
http://everest.radiology.uiowa.edu/nlm/app/cnjheart/cnjheart.html

University of Kansas Medical Center: Congenital Heart Defects   This directory of Internet resources related to congenital heart defects offers links to support groups, discussion networks, and professional associations. Connections include pages of the Texas Heart Institute, specific congenital heart defects, a pediatric surgery forum, and perinatal cardiology connections. "The Heart: An Online Exploration" offers review of the complexities of heart development and structure, and directories of genetic clinics, centers, and academic departments are provided.
http://www.kumc.edu/gec/support/conghart.html

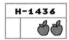

West Virginia Health Page: Types of Congenital Heart Defects More than a dozen congenital heart defects are reviewed at this site, with components of each condition briefly outlined. Diseases are categorized under obstruction, septal, and cyanotic defects.
http://www.wvhealth.wvu.edu/clinical/heart/contypes.htm

Absence of the Left Pericardium

Korean Society of Thoracic Radiology: Complete Unilateral Absence of the Left Pericardium The Korean Society of Thoracic Radiology and the Korean Radiological Society provide this case presentation from a 1998 meeting symposium of the relatively rare congenital disorder, absence of the pericardium. Theory as to its pathogenesis; occasional, associated conditions; and characterization of the condition on chest radiography are described.
http://kstr.radiology.or.kr/chest/Symphosium98/15/case15-dx.htm

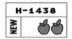

Royal Belgian Radiological Society: Congenital Absence of the Left Pericardium A case example is found at this site, describing the clinical history and radiological diagnosis of congenital absence of the left pericardium. Enlargeable images and a detailed discussion of the condition and its variants are provided.
http://www.rbrs.org/journal/volume80/page296.html

Aortic Stenosis

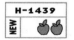

American Heart Association (AHA): Aortic Stenosis The AHA's online *Heart and Stroke Guide* provides readers with this discussion of abnormal formation of the aortic valve. Symptoms in children, treatment with balloon valvuloplasty, and the importance of good dental hygiene prior to and following surgery are emphasized.
http://216.185.112.5/presenter.jhtml?identifier=1659

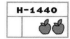

Mayo Adult Congenital Heart Disease Clinic Answers to frequently asked questions regarding aortic stenosis, such as what effect this disorder has on blood flow, are reviewed at this site of the Mayo Adult Congenital Heart Disease Clinic. Diagrams of the aortic valve, symptoms of the disorder, and three specific types are summarized, including aortic valve obstruction, subaortic obstruction, and supra-valvular obstruction. All variations are accompanied by labeled explanatory illustrations. Treatment for aortic stenosis, including observatory measures, valvotomy, balloon valvuloplasty, aortic valve replacement, and resection of subaortic and supra-aortic obstructions, is discussed.
http://www.mayo.edu/cv/wwwpg_cv/congenit/aorticst.htm

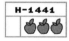

University of Alabama: Aortic Stenosis Aortic stenosis clinical resources from the University of Alabama include online textbook chapters, reference books, a page from the eMedicine database, and an assortment of professional management guidelines. Resources specific to pediatrics and genetics are found, in addition to basic health reviews for clinicians. Although most resources are free, some textbooks require an online subscription.

(some features fee-based)

http://www.slis.ua.edu/cdlp/uab/clinical/cardiology/congenital/as.html

Arrhythmogenic Right Ventricular Dysplasia (ARVD)

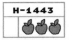

ARVD.net   Designed as a resource for information on research and treatment of arrhythmogenic right ventricular cardiomyopathy/dysplasia, this site includes clinical features, ARVD and sports, genetics, molecular genetics, epidemiology, therapy, and current ARVD research. Information about ARVD scientists, upcoming symposia on the disorder, and links to support groups are offered, in addition to a physician-oriented discussion forum.

http://telethon.bio.unipd.it/ARVDnet/

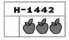

Johns Hopkins Hospital: ARVD.com   Devoted to the rare heart disease, arrhythmogenic right ventricular dysplasia (ARVD), this site contains a list of specialists in the United States and around the world. The archives section of the site provides links to updates, papers, books, news items, and clinical findings. A diagnosis section contains links to protocols and charts developed by international medical experts to assist doctors in diagnosing ARVD. The site also provides information about upcoming conferences and lectures and links to related Web sites.

http://www.arvd.com/

Atrial Septal Defect

American Heart Association (AHA): Atrial Septal Defect   Part of the AHA's collection of consumer-oriented publications, this information sheet describes the inefficiency that occurs with atrial septal defect and offers a connection to information on the normal function of the heart. The excellent outlook for those with this condition is noted.

http://216.185.112.5/presenter.jhtml?identifier=1664

eMedicine: Atrial Septal Defect, General Concepts   Developmental aspects of atrial septal defect are reviewed at this eMedicine resource, with a classic model of cardiac development described. Evidence in favor of the Van Praagh and Corsini model and four basic types of ASDs are examined. Left-to-right shunting of blood, related to the size of the defect, is discussed, along with demographics and clinical effects. The page describes possible causes and offers related eMedicine connections to differentials.

http://www.eMedicine.com/ped/topic171.htm

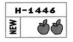

Loyola University: Atrial Septal Defect   The left-to-right shunting of blood that occurs with atrial septal defect is described at this page of the Neu-

robiology and Anatomy Department of Loyola University Medical Center. A right sagittal view and frontal cross section of the heart illustrate types of atrial septal defect, and a link to figures and descriptions of atrial partitioning is available.
http://www.meddean.luc.edu/lumen/
MedEd/GrossAnatomy/thorax0/Heart_Development/AtrialSeptalDefect.html

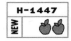

University of Minnesota: Cardiovascular Division   Embryology and occurrence of atrial septal defect are described at this page, maintained by the University of Minnesota Medical School. A table at the site outlines incidence, age at presentation, clinical effects, pulmonary vasculature, radiologic findings, associated findings, complications, and treatment. Additionally, the site offers five case presentations, including secundum type ASD, postoperative, and increased pulmonary vascularity radiographs and discussions.
http://www.med.umn.edu/radiology/cvrad/chd/asd.html

Atrioventricular (A-V) Canal Defect

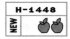

American Heart Association (AHA): Atrioventricular Canal Defect
Also known as endocardial cushion defect and atrioventricular septal defect, this discussion focuses on the abnormalities found with atrioventricular septal defect in both the lower and upper chambers of the heart. Information on fetal echocardiography can be accessed, and surgical repair of the atrioventricular canal and postsurgical care are reviewed.
http://216.185.112.5/presenter.jhtml?identifier=132

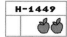

Virtual Children's Hospital: Atrioventricular Canal Defect   A discusson of the clinical presentation, pathophysiology, and imaging findings in atrioventricular canal defect is presented at this site of the Virtual Children's Hospital of the University of Iowa. The document is internally peer reviewed and makes the distinction between partial and complete endocardial cushion defect.
http://www.vh.org/Providers/TeachingFiles/PAP/CVDiseases/CAVC.html

Barth Syndrome (X-Linked Cardiomyopathy)

Kennedy Krieger Institute: Barth Syndrome   Resources devoted to Barth syndrome are provided at this site, including a detailed description of the syndrome, a publication synopsis from the Online Mendelian Inheritance in Man (OMIM) database, a bibliography of important publications with abstracts, and information on a family support group.
http://www.med.jhu.edu/CMSL/Barth_Syndrome.html

BICUSPID AORTIC VALVE

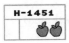

European Association for Cardio-Thoracic Surgery: Outcome of Bicuspid Aortic Valve Repair for Prolapsing Leaflet An abstract presents details of this clinical study, investigating the outcome of bicuspid aortic valve repair for prolapsing leaflet and the reasons for repair failure. Methods and results are summarized, and a graph presents numbers of patients free of reoperation within a nine-year period.
http://www.ctsnet.org/doc/2436

CARDIO-FACIO-CUTANEOUS (CFC) SYNDROME

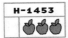

Family Village: Cardio-Facio-Cutaneous Syndrome Cardio-facio-cutaneous syndrome resources provided by this collection of links include fact sheets, contact details for a professional organization devoted to this disease, information on support groups, and connection to the related Online Mendelian Inheritance in Man (OMIM) entry.
http://www.familyvillage.wisc.edu/lib_cfcs.htm

CHARGE SYNDROME

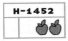

CHARGE Syndrome Foundation CHARGE (choanal atresia, posterior coloboma, heart defect, choanal atresia, retardation, genital and ear anomalies) syndrome, a rare and complex genetic disorder, is described at the home page of this organization. Each aspect of the syndrome is described, and information is available on causes, affected population, related disorders, therapies, and outcome. Additional resources include links to related sites, reference citations, membership details, and administrative resources.
http://www.chargesyndrome.org

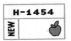

National Organization for Rare Disorders (NORD): CHARGE Syndrome A general discussion of CHARGE syndrome is found at this page, which defines the acronym and criteria for diagnosis. A listing of possible abnormalities in infants is offered, in addition to links to sites providing further information. Full-text disease reports can be ordered from NORD for a fee.
http://www.stepstn.com/cgi-win/nord.exe?proc=Redirect&type=rdb_sum&id=550.htm

COARCTATION OF THE AORTA

American Heart Association (AHA): Coarctation of the Aorta Development of congestive heart failure or high blood pressure in an infant with coarctation of the aorta is described at this page of the AHA. Information on surgical repair and postsurgical outlook is offered, and a discussion of normal heart anatomy and physiology is available.
http://216.185.112.5/presenter.jhtml?identifier=1667

eMedicine: Coarctation of the Aorta Examining the relatively common defect, coarctation of the aorta, this eMedicine site includes details on pathophysiology, early and late presentation, and a number of theories addressing causes of the condition. Several diagnostic differential links within the eMedicine database are available, and elements of medical, surgical, and dietary care are reviewed. Information on activity restrictions, pharmacologic agents in treatment, deterrence, and complications is introduced.
http://www.eMedicine.com/ped/topic2504.htm

Ochsner Clinic and Hospital: Coarctation of the Aorta An introduction to coarctation of the aorta, its clinical presentation in both neonates and young children, and primary surgical interventions are reviewed. Screening for coarctation and the common occurrence of undiagnosed infants are discussed.
http://www.ochsner.org/pcs/primarycare/pediatrics/SpecClinic/phi/phiAorta.phtml

Perfusion Line: Coarctation of the Aorta The deformity of the media of the aorta and additional defects found in coarctation of the aorta are reviewed at this site, which also summarizes the anatomy and pathophysiology of the condition. Left-to-right shunt and right-to-left shunt variations are differentiated, and five associated abnormalities are listed, including mitral valve malformation and congestive heart failure. Hemodynamics of the condition, clinical manifestations, medical management, and prognosis are presented.
http://perfline.com/student/coa.html

Congenital Heart Block

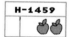

Neonatal Network: Complete Congenital Heart Block From an issue of *Neonatal Network,* this site provides a concise overview of complete congenital heart block, a rare disease of the newborn that carries significant morbidity and mortality.
http://www.neonatalnetwork.com/nn3/Abstracts/NN0499_4.htm

Cor Triatriatum

eMedicine: Cor Triatriatum A discussion of this disorder, also known as subdivided left atrium, is found at this site of the eMedicine online reference. Authored by Jeff L. Myers, M.D., Ph.D., of Duke University Medical Center, the article addresses pathophysiology, clinical presentation, and physical signs of disease. Several diagnostic differential links within the eMedicine database are available for convenient comparison. The diagnostic workup and information on clinical management are presented, with profiles of inotropes and diuretics, inpatient care, and prognostic details included.
http://www.eMedicine.com/ped/topic2507.htm

Coronary Artery Anomalies, General

Canadian Adult Congenital Heart Network: Coronary Anomalies
Three types of coronary anomalies are described at this page, including background information, diagnostic recommendations, and indications for interventions. Additional information on surgical and interventional options is found, as well as details regarding follow-up procedures.
http://www.cachnet.org/consensus/coros.htm

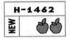

Cardiothoracic Surgery Notes: Coronary Artery Anomalies Normal coronary anatomy is described at this page, followed by descriptions of minor and major coronary anomalies. Details on hemodynamically significant defects and congenital arteriovenous fistulas are found, along with a general overview of signs and symptoms.
http://www.ctsnet.org/

eMedicine: Coronary Artery Anomalies Coronary artery malformations are the focus of this eMedicine site, which describes the normal coronary anatomy, variability in coronary circulation, and pathophysiologies involved. Tables at the site review incidence figures in adult patients with suspected arterial obstructive disease. Presentation in infancy is summarized, and an outline of anomalies of origination and course, of intrinsic coronary arterial anatomy, of coronary termination, and of collateral vessels is provided.
http://www.eMedicine.com/ped/topic2506.htm

Double Aortic Arch

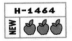

eMedicine: Vascular Ring, Double Aortic Arch The pediatric chapter of eMedicine includes this page outlining the background, pathophysiology, assessment, diagnosis, and management of double aortic arch. Associated syndromes and noncardiac conditions are discussed, and differential links and diagnostic images are included. Every MEDLINE abstract referenced in the article can be accessed from the site.
http://www.emedicine.com/ped/topic2541.htm

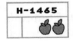

Vanderbilt Medical Center: Double Aortic Arch A technical description of double aortic arch is available from this fact sheet. Clinical manifestations, corrective surgery, diagnostic techniques, and general morbidity and mortality rates are discussed, with reference citations listed.
http://www.mc.vanderbilt.edu/peds/pidl/cardio/dblaort.htm

Double Outlet Right Ventricle

eMedicine: Double Outlet Right Ventricle, Normally Related Great Arteries The partial transposition of the great arteries is explained at the site,

with variations in pathophysiology examined. Variable histories by type of anatomy are reviewed, along with findings upon physical examination and embryology of the condition. Additional features of the page include complete review of diagnostic and therapeutic procedures, summary of overall goals of medical therapy, and several illustrative images.
http://www.eMedicine.com/ped/topic2509.htm

Double-Chambered Right Ventricle

eMedicine: Double-Chambered Right Ventricle A clinical discussion of this congenital heart defect is found at this site, examining the terminology surrounding the condition, its pathophysiology, and physical presentation. Imaging studies and management details are introduced, and captions at this site include a related ECG tracing and computed tomography images.
http://www.eMedicine.com/ped/topic612.htm

Down Syndrome and Congenital Heart Defects

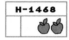

Down's Heart Group This nonprofit group is based in the United Kingdom and offers information and support resources to families affected by Down syndrome and congenital heart defects. The table of contents offers access to fact sheets related to surgical interventions, drug therapies, heart defects, medical terms, and other topics associated with Down syndrome and congenital heart disease. http://www.downs-heart.downsnet.org

Ebstein's Anomaly

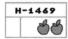

Ebstein's Anomaly Background information, unoperated history and management, an adequate diagnostic workup, and indications for intervention in the case of Ebstein's anomaly are provided at the site. Surgical and interventional options, with the intention of preservation of the native tricuspid valve, and regular follow-up management are summarized.
http://www.cachnet.org/consensus/ebstein.htm

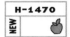

Mayo Foundation for Medical Education and Research: Ebstein's Anomaly The Mayo Adult Congenital Heart Disease Clinic at Rochester offers this page, defining the condition and reviewing treatment options. General considerations for patients to discuss with their physicians are offered, as well as reference citations.
http://www.mayo.edu/cv/wwwpg_cv/congenit/ebstein.htm

EISENMENGER SYNDROME

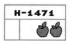

Clinical Cardiology: Thrombosed Pulmonary Arterial Aneurysm in Eisenmenger's Syndrome An aneurysmal dilatation of the right pulmonary artery and the pulmonary trunk, implying an intrinsic abnormality of the pulmonary arterial wall, is demonstrated in this discussion and radiographic image of an unusual case study of Eisenmenger syndrome. A computed tomography image is also displayed, courtesy of *Clinical Cardiology*.
http://clinical-cardiology.org/briefs/9902briefs/22-127.shtml

eMedicine: Eisenmenger Syndrome Pathophysiology, demographic details, and symptoms related to pulmonary hypertension are listed at this page, which also emphasizes cardiovascular and other signs present upon physical examination. Laboratory workup and imaging studies are reviewed, and goals of medical and surgical care for Eisenmenger syndrome are summarized. Several examples of diagnostic imaging are included in the presentation.
http://www.eMedicine.com/med/topic642.htm

HOLT-ORAM SYNDROME

eMedicine: Holt-Oram Syndrome A clinical discussion of Holt-Oram syndrome, also known as heart-hand syndrome, is presented at this site of the eMedicine database. Upper limb and cardiac involvement are described, and demographic information is included. Genetic causes of the disorder are outlined, and complete diagnostic workup details are presented. Several additional sections of the article provide treatment information, surgical care, and medical and legal pitfalls of management.
http://www.eMedicine.com/med/topic2940.htm

HealthlinkUSA: Holt-Oram Syndrome Several sites providing information related to Holt-Oran syndrome are accessible through links at this address. Support groups, fact sheets, discussion forums, and other consumer resources are included.
http://beta.healthlinkusa.com/152.html

HYPOPLASTIC LEFT HEART SYNDROME (HLHS)

eMedicine: Hypoplastic Left Heart Syndrome The complex pathophysiology of hypoplastic left heart syndrome is summarized at this page of the eMedicine database. The diagnosis, made by echocardiography, is discussed, as are the physical presentation and possible causes of the condition. Diagnostic differential links are found, and a complete outline of the imaging studies and laboratory tests commonly performed is presented. Reviews of cardiac catheterization procedures, a three-part surgical summary, and information on or-

thotopic cardiac transplantation are found. Ductal agents, diuretics, cardiac glycosides, and additional drug profiles are presented.
http://eMedicine.com/PED/topic1131.htm

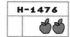

Left Heart Matters This Web site offers support and information for parents of children with hypoplastic left heart syndrome. The page provides news about the site, information about fundraising efforts and support groups, and a message board. An interesting feature allows parents to create Web sites for their children and submit articles about them. Links are provided to online booklets about different aspects of the disorders, sites about corrective surgery and transplantation, and additional research resources.
http://www.lhm.org.uk

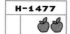

Perfusion Line: Hypoplastic Left Heart Syndrome General information and statistics on hypoplastic left heart syndrome are reviewed at this site, with sections included on the pathoanatomy and pathophysiology of the condition. Clinical manifestations, including hypoxemia and hypotension, are discussed, and a link to the Fontan procedure is provided.
http://www.perfline.com/student/lhh.html

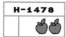

Virtual Hospital: Hypoplastic Left Heart Syndrome Virtual Hospital's teaching files offer this page on hypoplastic left heart syndrome, which provides an overview of the clinical presentation, the etiology and pathophysiology, imaging findings, and a list of differential diagnoses.
http://www.vh.org/Providers/TeachingFiles/PAP/CVDiseases/HLHS.html

IVEMARK SYNDROME (ASPLENIA)

Contact a Family: Ivemark Syndrome Ivemark syndrome, a condition characterized by a congenital absence of the spleen in conjunction with cardiac abnormalities, is described in this fact sheet. Common clinical presentation at birth is described, with a listing of several possible congenital heart anomalies.
http://www.cafamily.org.uk/Direct/i18.html

LONG QT SYNDROME (LQTS)

Canadian Sudden Arrhythmia Death Syndromes Foundation The Canadian Sudden Arrhythmia Death Syndromes Foundation was established to raise awareness and identify those at risk for preventable sudden death and treatable arrhythmia disorders. The site provides facts about sudden death and congenital long Q-T syndrome, as well as information about exercise for patients. Details regarding research and screening, a glossary of related terms, and links to related sites are included.
http://www.sadscanada.com

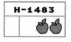

Vanderbilt Medical Center: Long Q-T Syndrome   This clinical summary of long Q-T syndrome, courtesy of Vanderbilt University, reviews congenital and acquired causes of the condition, as well as genetic patterns and mechanisms. The typical presentation of the syndrome, discussion of syncopal episodes due to torsade de pointes, and the disorder's common confusion with a neurological disorder are explained. Studies explore the genetic components of the disease, and beta blocker treatment and additional therapies are examined.
http://www.mc.vanderbilt.edu/peds/pidl/cardio/lqts.htm

MITRAL STENOSIS, SUPRAVALVULAR RING

eMedicine: Mitral Stenosis, Supravalvular Ring   Drawn from the pediatric chapter of eMedicine's online textbook, this page reviews the pathophysiology of this condition and its strong association with other, more common, congenital defects. Consequences of the supravalvular mitral membrane and comprehensive details on symptoms, assessment, diagnosis, and management are included. Relevant pharmacologic information and several interactive echocardiographic images are also presented.
http://www.eMedicine.com/ped/topic2516.htm

NOONAN SYNDROME

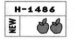

Noonan Syndrome Support Group   The Noonan Syndrome Support Group offers statistics related to this disease and a brief overview of the organization's activities at this home page. An order form for publications, membership details, research information, and annual meeting details are provided.
http://www.noonansyndrome.org/home.html

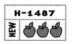

Pediatric Database (PEDBASE): Noonan Syndrome   Etiology and clinical features of Noonan syndrome are outlined at this site of the Pediatric Database. Craniofacial dysmorphism and organ malformations, including those of the heart, are introduced. Other manifestations, diagnostic investigations, and management are introduced.
http://www.icondata.com/health/pedbase/files/NOONANSY.HTM

PARTIAL ANOMALOUS PULMONARY VENOUS RETURN

eMedicine: Partial Anomalous Pulmonary Venous Connection   Factors in pathophysiology and review of the clinical disease presentation are found at this eMedicine reference site. Links to several diagnostic differentials provide opportunities for comparison of this and other congenital anomalies, and additional information on diagnostic testing is included.
http://www.eMedicine.com/ped/topic2522.htm

Kansas University Medical Center: Anomalous Pulmonary Venous Drainage Featuring a variety of pathologic images, this site includes chest radiographs, echocardiographic videos, still frame echocardiograms, and electrocardiograms for anomalous pulmonary venous drainage. More than 30 images are found and include normal hearts, an ECG electrophysiological interval diagram, areas of auscultation, and a variety of angiographic images, drawn from the *Multimedia Encyclopedia of Congenital Heart Disease* and the University of Kansas.
http://www.kumc.edu/kumcpeds/cardiology/apvddfct.html

University of Minnesota: Partial Anomalous Pulmonary Venous Return The table found at this site introduces three types of partial anomalous pulmonary venous return based on location of drainage. Incidence, age at presentation, clinical features, pulmonary vasculature, radiologic findings, and treatment are concisely reviewed.
http://www.med.umn.edu/radiology/cvrad/chd/papvr.html

Patent Ductus Arteriosus

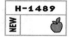

American Heart Association (AHA): Patent Ductus Arteriosus Failure of the ductus arteriosus to close in premature and full-term infants is the focus of this AHA Web site, which offers a connection to information on normal heart anatomy and physiology.
http://216.185.112.5/presenter.jhtml?identifier=1672

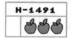

eMedicine: Patent Ductus Arteriosus This eMedicine review of patent ductus arteriosus includes the pathophysiology of the abnormality, demographic information on this common congenital defect, physical presentation, and an extensive listing of related diagnostic differential links within the eMedicine database. Diagnostic studies, emergency and surgical treatment, and drug profiles on prostaglandins and nonsteroidal anti-inflammatories (NSAIDs) are provided, in addition to a schematic diagram of the condition.
http://eMedicine.com/cgi-
bin/foxweb.exe/showsection@d:/em/ga?book=emerg&topicid=358

University of Alabama: Patent Ductus Arteriosus An assortment of links to clinical guidelines, textbook chapters, and pediatric resources is available at this site of the Clinical Digital Libraries Project of the University of Alabama. By clicking on any one of the document links, visitors are taken to information on diagnosis, management, and surgical protocol material for patent ductus arteriosus. The Pediatric Database (PEDBASE), Paediapaedia, hospital Web sites, and a host of additional, free references are provided. Some material may require an online subscription. (some features fee-based)
http://www.slis.ua.edu/cdlp/unthsc/clinical/cardiology/congenital/pda.html

University of Wisconsin Medical School: Patent Ductus Arteriosus An explanation of patent ductus arteriosus and what happens when blood trav-

els from the aorta to the lungs is presented at this site, with testing procedures in suspected disease and treatment modalities concisely reviewed. Answers to frequently asked questions about the condition are provided.
http://www2.medsch.wisc.edu/childrenshosp/parents_of_preemies/pda.html

PULMONARY ATRESIA

eMedicine: Pulmonary Atresia with Intact Ventricular Septum
Offering comprehensive information on this congenital heart defect, this eMedicine article describes variations in pathophysiology and necessities of management for patient survival. The physical presentation of infants with pulmonary atresia is outlined at the page, and details on diagnosis with echocardiography, angiocardiography, and plain film imaging are discussed. Treatment, including medical, surgical, and consultative management, is introduced, and cited MEDLINE reference abstracts can be accessed from the page.
http://www.eMedicine.com/ped/topic2526.htm

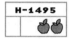

Perfusion Line: Pulmonary Atresia Pulmonary atresia is described in this clinical fact sheet, including pathology, hemodynamics, clinical manifestations, and surgical and medical interventions. Links are available to information on important terms.
http://www.perfline.com/student/pulm_atres.html

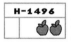

Rush Children's Heart Center: Pulmonary Atresia This consumer fact sheet provides an overview of pulmonary atresia, including a detailed definition, incidence, effects of the disorder, disease progression, treatment, and possible complications. Explanatory diagrams accompany the discussion.
http://www.rchc.rush.edu/rmawebfiles/chd%20for%20parents%20pa.htm

PULMONARY STENOSIS

American Heart Association (AHA): Pulmonary Stenosis This discussion of pulmonary stenosis includes symptoms in children and treatment for relief of the obstruction. Outlook after balloon valvuloplasty and follow-up information are included, as well as a link to information on the normal heart and how it works.
http://216.185.112.5/presenter.jhtml?identifier=1321

eMedicine: Pulmonic Valvular Stenosis The eMedicine database offers a comprehensive review of pulmonary valvular stenosis. Visitors will find an article relating to the pathophysiology, clinical and physical presentation, and management of the condition, as well as several diagnostic differential links, a diagnostic workup review, and surgical and medical management summaries. Complications, prognosis, and patient education are detailed.
http://eMedicine.com/cgi-bin/foxweb.exe/showsection@d:/em/ga?book=emerg&topicid=491

University of Alabama: Pulmonary Stenosis   The Clinical Digital Libraries Project of the University of Alabama offers this collection of resources on the Web specific to pulmonary stenosis. The *Merck Manual* chapter, eMedicine's online articles, and additional authoritative material may be accessed. Some resources may require an online subscription, but a wide variety of free professional references are available, ranging from documents of academic medical centers to genetic database information. (some features fee-based)
http://www.slis.ua.edu/cdlp/cchs/clinical/cardiology/congenital/ps.html

Septal Defects, General

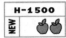
CliniWeb International: Heart Septal Defects   Including connections to information on endocardial cushion defects, atrial septal defects, and ventricular septal defects, this collection provides access to fact sheets from academic institutions, echocardiographic images, and preformatted PubMed queries, courtesy of Oregon Health Sciences University.
http://www.ohsu.edu/cliniweb/C14/C14.240.400.560.html

Texas Heart Institute: Ventricular and Septal Defects   Ventricular and atrial septal defects are described in this consumer fact sheet. Information on symptoms, surgical management, and general prognosis is available from the site.
http://texasheartinstitute.org/septal.html

Single Ventricle Anomalies, General

Annals of Thoracic Surgery: Staged Surgical Approach to Neonates with Aortic Obstruction and Single-Ventricle Physiology   This full-text clinical article offers an overview of the variable surgical management of neonatal systemic outflow obstruction and complex single ventricle pathology. A link is available to a discussion of the findings presented in this article, and contact details for reprints are provided. Reference citations are listed.
http://www.ctsnet.org/journal/ats/68/962

Cardiothoracic Surgery Notes: Single Ventricle Anomalies   Morphological subsets of single ventricle are outlined at this site, which also includes a summary of palliative treatment procedures, additional operations, and classifications and subsets of tricuspid atresia. Clinical diagnosis and features are reviewed, as well as characteristics of the ideal candidate for the Fontan procedure.   http://www.ctsnet.org/doc/4764

SINUS OF VALSALVA ANEURYSM

eMedicine: Sinus of Valsalva Aneurysm   First described by John Thurnman in 1840, this rare congenital defect is examined at this page. The deficiency of abnormal elastic tissue and other abnormal developments associated with the condition are reviewed, and several diagnostic differential links can be accessed. Additional assessment, diagnosis, and management information is found, offering a complete introduction to clinical care.
http://www.eMedicine.com/med/topic2133.htm

SUBAORTIC STENOSIS

eMedicine: Aortic Stenosis, Subaortic   Created to provide information to cardiologists and other interested clinicians, this eMedicine review examines the pathophysiology, symptoms, and physical presentation of children with subaortic stenosis. Possible causes, links to diagnostic differentials, and other problems to be considered are reviewed. Visitors will also find a complete guide to imaging studies and medical care. Diagnostic images of subaortic stenosis are found at the page.
http://www.eMedicine.com/ped/topic2485.htm

Heart Institute for Children: Subaortic Stenosis   The Heart Institute for Children offers a graphically illustrated presentation of subaortic stenosis at its site, with the basics of this valvular defect discussed.
http://www.thic.com/sub.htm

TETRALOGY OF FALLOT

American Heart Association (AHA): Tetralogy of Fallot   Major defects of tetralogy of Fallot are reviewed at this site, intended to provide a general overview of the condition. Components of corrective surgery are introduced, as well as information concerning lifelong management.
http://216.185.112.5/presenter.jhtml?identifier=1299

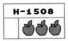

eMedicine: Tetralogy of Fallot   This eMedicine article offers a comprehensive clinical guide to the pathophysiology, diagnosis, and treatment of tetralogy of Fallot. The complex abnormalities are described, and the physical presentation is thoroughly reviewed. Clinicians will find access to several diagnostic differential links, discussion of possible causes, hematology and imaging studies, and emergency department treatment for hypercyanotic episodes. Analgesic and alpha-adrenergic agonist profiles are found, as well as a diagram depicting cardiac catheterization findings in tetralogy of Fallot.
http://www.eMedicine.com/emerg/topic575.htm

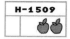

Hope for Henry This site is dedicated to educating the public about Fanconi anemia and tetralogy of Fallot, a genetic heart disease attributed to Fanconi anemia. The site contains information about the related defects in a young patient. A list of links is provided to additional information about Fanconi anemia and related medical sites, as well as to the Fanconi Anemia Research Fund, Fanconi Anemia Mutation Database, and MEDLINE.
http://www.hsg.org

PediHeart: Tetralogy of Fallot and Pulmonary Stenosis The Pedi-Heart Web site offers a comprehensive morphological review of tetralogy of Fallot and pulmonary stenosis at this site, with features of the abnormal outlet septum, interventricular communication, and variations of the clinical presentation. Associated lesions, central clinical features, and operative indications are reviewed. Reoperation information is found.
http://pediheart.org/practitioners/defects/ventriculoarterial/TOF_PS.htm

TOTAL ANOMALOUS PULMONARY VENOUS (P-V) CONNECTION

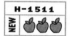

eMedicine: Total Anomalous Pulmonary Venous Connection A description of the abnormality of blood flow in total anomalous pulmonary venous connection is presented at this eMedicine site, and a complete review of embryology, pathophysiology, and clinical presentations is found. Additional problems to be considered in the newborn, infant, and older child are listed, as well as laboratory and imaging studies, treatment, and complications. Images are available at the page to illustrate the condition.
http://www.eMedicine.com/ped/topic2540.htm

Society of Thoracic Surgeons: Total Anomalous Pulmonary Venous Connection and Cor Triatriatum Topics discussed at this technical fact sheet devoted to total anomalous pulmonary venous connection (TAPVC) include embryology, TAPVC classification, anatomic factors, pathophysiology, diagnosis, management, operative technique, results, and risk factors. Cor triatriatum topics include morphology, clinical features, operative technique, and common clinical results. Highlighted terms provide links to explanatory illustrations. http://www.sts.org/resident/ctsn/archives/11frmtxt.html

TRANSPOSITION OF THE GREAT ARTERIES

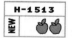

American Heart Association (AHA): Transposition of the Great Arteries Reversal of the major vessels in transposition of the great arteries is described at the consumer information site of the AHA. Situations in which survival is possible are discussed, and procedures used during heart catheterization to reduce cyanosis are introduced. The arterial switch and Mustard surgical procedures used to correct transposition are presented.
http://216.185.112.5/presenter.jhtml?identifier=1682

Don't type in long URLs – add the site number to the eMedguides URL: www.eMedguides.com/**G-1234**.

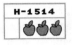

Canadian Cardiovascular Society: Congenitally Corrected Transposition of the Great Arteries   This article offers a discussion of congenitally corrected transposition of the great arteries. Technical background information is followed by discussions of unoperated/operated history and management, diagnostic recommendations, indications for intervention or reintervention, surgical/interventional options, surgical/interventional outcomes, and follow-up care. http://www.cachnet.org/consensus/ctga.htm

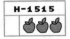

PediHeart: Transposition of the Great Vessels   At this PediHeart Web site location visitors can view an illustration of reversal of the great arteries and a description of the resulting separate circulations. Procedures necessary to infant survival and connections to the morphology and embryology of the development of this defect are found. Associated malformations, hemodynamics, clinical presentation and management, and the preferred surgical intervention are discussed.   http://www.pediheart.org/parents/defects/TGA.htm

Tricuspid Atresia

PediHeart: Tricuspid Atresia   This literature search, courtesy of PediHeart, provides the text of 15 investigation abstracts on tricuspid atresia. The *American Heart Journal,* the *Annals of Thoracic Surgery,* the *British Heart Journal,* and additional indexed publication abstracts may be viewed regarding such topics as the clinical status of patients after the Fontan procedure, assessment of risk factors associated with postoperative death, and embryologic abnormalities associated with abnormal cardiac development. http://www.pediheart.org/searches/topic/tri_atr.htm

Royal Children's Hospital: Tricuspid Atresia   This patient handout describes tricuspid atresia, the absence of connection between the right atrium and the right ventricle. Illustrative diagrams of the heart are included. http://www.rch.unimelb.edu.au/cardiology/ website/Library/Tricuspid_Atresia/tricuspid_atresia.html

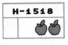

Virtual Children's Hospital: Tricuspid Atresia   This Virtual Children's Hospital page reviews the clinical presentation, pathophysiology, and imaging findings of tricuspid atresia in a condensed outline format. http://www.vh.org/Providers/TeachingFiles/PAP/CVDiseases/TriAtresia.html

Truncus Arteriosus

HeartPoint: Truncus Arteriosus   The distinction between normal heart anatomy and truncus arteriosus is illustrated at this HeartPoint Web site, with a comparison to transposition and the origin of the great vessels discussed. Eight links to similar presentations are found, for clear, concise differentiation of common congenital heart defects. http://www.heartpoint.com/congtruncus.html

PediHeart: Truncus Arteriosus PediHeart's professional reference offers a clinical discussion of the truncus arteriosus defect and the necessary surgical correction. An illustration at the site demonstrates the truncus arising from a ventricular septal defect, causing the singular artery defect and the resulting mixture of high- and low-oxygen blood. Further information on the disorder, such as morphology, associated cardiac conditions, hemodynamics, clinical presentation and workup, and medical and surgical management, may be accessed by clicking on the link at the bottom of the page.
http://pediheart.org/parents/defects/truncus.htm

TURNER'S SYNDROME

Pediatric Database (PEDBASE): Turner Syndrome A definition of this chromosomal disorder, its epidemiology, and its multisystem defects are reviewed at this site of the Pediatric Database. Pathogenesis, specific chromosomal abnormalities, and diagnostic investigations are outlined. Both congenital heart malformation and vascular abnormalities are presented.
http://www.icondata.com/health/pedbase/files/TURNERSY.HTM

VELO-CARDIO-FACIAL SYNDROME
(CAYLER SYNDROME, DIGEORGE SYNDROME)

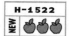

eMedicine: Velocardiofacial Syndrome Characteristics of this genetic condition are reviewed at this site of the eMedicine online journal. Historical clues to diagnosis, physical presentation, and links to diagnostic differentials are included. Laboratory, imaging, and other studies are listed, and a comprehensive introduction to appropriate medical and surgical care is presented. Captions at the site include a karyotype of a patient with the disorder.
http://www.eMedicine.com/ped/topic2395.htm

Velo-Cardio-Facial Syndrome Information on Velo-cardio-facial syndrome (VCFS), a common genetic disorder in humans, is found at this site. Professionals dealing with VCFS are provided with clinical information on the various problems and abnormalities associated with the disorder. By accessing the cardiac disorders link, visitors will find a listing of more than 10 associated congenital heart anomalies and connections to further information on tetralogy of Fallot. Links to support groups, related articles, and other Web resources are provided. A glossary of medical terms, a photo album, and speech samples are offered. http://www.crosslink.net/~marchett/vcfs/vcfs.shtml

VENTRICULAR SEPTAL DEFECT (VSD)

American Heart Association (AHA): Ventricular Septal Defect Symptoms occurring in children with ventricular septal defect are reviewed at

this fact sheet, courtesy of the AHA. The site introduces concepts behind the defect and the necessity of early repair. A link to information on normal heart anatomy and function is available.

http://216.185.112.5/presenter.jhtml?identifier=1306

PediHeart: Ventricular Septal Defect The morphology, pathophysiology and natural history, diagnosis, and operative closure of ventricular septal defect are reviewed at this site of the professional PediHeart Web reference. An enlargeable GIF image is provided.

http://pediheart.org/practitioners/defects/ventricular/VSD.htm

WILLIAMS SYNDROME

(SUPRA-AORTIC STENOSIS/PULMONARY STENOSIS)

Canadian Association for Williams Syndrome This site provides information about Williams syndrome. It includes a general overview of the disorder and details about diagnosis, physical characteristics, school-age characteristics, adolescent and adult characteristics, psychological characteristics, current medical research, and patient management. The site also provides news about association events and links to other articles and Web sites about the disorder.

http://www.bmts.com/~williams

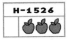

Williams Syndrome Association This source contains the latest information on Williams syndrome. It provides facts about the disorder, information about diagnosis, answers to frequently asked questions, and updated medical guidelines. A calendar of events, online newsletter, and details regarding camps and workshops are provided. Information on lifesaving surgeries for heart disease in Williams syndrome patients and links to additional information about the disorder, including the Lili Claire Foundation and the Association for Retarded Citizens, are provided.

http://www.williams-syndrome.org

9.11 CONNECTIVE TISSUE DISEASE

KAWASAKI SYNDROME

Health Gazette: Kawasaki Disease This site describes Kawasaki disease, a clinical illness that causes acquired heart disease in children. Information about epidemiology, etiology, symptoms, diagnosis, treatment, and complications is provided, and references are included.

http://www.freenet.scri.fsu.edu/HealthGazette/kawasaki.html

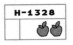

Kawasaki Families' Network The Kawasaki Families' Network is devoted to supporting those affected by the disease. The Web site is designed to share information on research and provide links to medical literature, including pages at the Imperial College School of Medicine at St. Mary's, the Pediatric Database, and Mosby Consumer Health. A link to a glossary of related medical terms is provided. http://ourworld.compuserve.com/homepages/kawasaki

MDchoice.com: Kawasaki Disease   Images and information about Kawasaki disease are found at this address, including photographs of affected children's hands, legs, and face. Details about diagnostic criteria, effects of the disease, and treatment are presented.
http://www.mdchoice.com/photo/ptod0024.asp

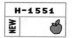

Pediatric Database (PEDBASE): Kawasaki's Syndrome   Provided by the Pediatric Database, this site provides clinical information about Kawasaki's syndrome. Information includes a definition of the disorder, disease epidemiology, pathogenesis, symptoms, stages, complications, investigations, and management.   http://www.icondata.com/health/pedbase/files/KAWASAKI.HTM

MARFAN SYNDROME

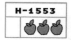

American Heart Association (AHA): Marfan Syndrome   Fundamental information on this connective tissue disorder is found at this site of the AHA consumer publication collection. In addition to physical characteristics of the disease, details on blood vessel and cardiac valve problems are examined. Treatment information and lifestyle change recommendations are introduced.
http://216.185.112.5/presenter.jhtml?identifier=4672

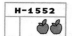

National Marfan Foundation: Early Heart Repair for Marfan Syndrome Patients   The careful monitoring required for individuals with Marfan syndrome is reviewed in this online article, which summarizes results of a recently published study in the *New England Journal of Medicine*. The general weakness of the aorta in Marfan syndrome and information on early diagnosis and proper management are discussed. The lead author of the study comments on the research, entailing a retrospective record examination, and concludes that many patients may increase survival significantly with aggressive, appropriate interventions.   http://www.marfan.org/pub/nejm.html

National Marfan Foundation: The Heart and the Blood Vessels   This subsite of the National Marfan Foundation offers diagrams that show normal aortic structure and function and the progressive aortic enlargement due to the connective tissue abnormalities of Marfan syndrome. By clicking on the link to the *Marfan Syndrome Resource Manual*, visitors will be brought to a table of contents, that provides access to similar articles on diagnosis of the disorder, and the role of genetics, as well as a complete listing of cardiac-related issues. Preventive measures to reduce aortic enlargement, surgical procedures, endocarditis prophylaxis, and extensive review on the use of beta-blockers in Marfan syndrome for promotion of injured arterial tissue, blood pressure reduction, and reduction in force and velocity of heart muscle contraction are provided.
http://www.marfan.org//pub/resourcebook/heartandblood.html

POLYARTERITIS NODOSA

American College of Rheumatology: Classification Criteria of Polyarteritis Nodosa The 1990 criteria for the classification of polyarteritis nodosa are presented at this site, with 10 requirements listed. Included are elevated systolic blood pressure value, arteriographic abnormality, and mononeuropathy or polyneuropathy.
http://www.rheumatology.org/research/classification/polyart.html

Johns Hopkins Vasculitis Center: Polyarteritis Nodosa Characterization of polyarteritis nodosa is offered at this Johns Hopkins site, which also provides enlargeable angiographic and skin biopsy images of the disease. A connection at the site offers readers a thorough discussion of polyarteritis nodosa, authored by David Hellmann, M.D. Onset of disease, diagnostic confirmation, treatment, and newly proposed regimens are included.
http://vasculitis.med.jhu.edu/pan.htm

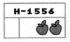

Polyarteritis Nodosa: Treatment Information and Self-Assessment
Provided by the Horus Global HealthNet, this site was designed to help people learn more about the signs and symptoms of polyarteritis nodosa to facilitate improved physician-patient communication. A self-assessment test is provided, and links to other sites about polyarteritis nodosa are found.
http://www.ibionet.com/rarediseases/polyarteritisnodosa.html

SYSTEMIC LUPUS ERYTHEMATOSUS

Lupus Foundation of America: Cardiopulmonary Disease and Lupus
Heart disease is the third most common cause of death in patients with systemic lupus erythematosus. This page, published by the Lupus Foundation of America, explains how lupus affects the pericardium, myocardium, endocardium, and coronary arteries. The discussion includes symptoms, diagnosis, drug therapy, and management of the disease. The site also gives information about the Lupus Foundation of America and provides a link to their Web site.
http://www.lupus.org/topics/cardi.html

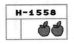

Lupus Foundation of America: Lupus and Vasculitis Produced by the Lupus Foundation of America, this site provides patient information about the disorder. Resources include a general overview, causes, associated diseases, symptoms, diagnosis, treatment, and prognosis of vasculitis. Details about the foundation are also available.
http://www.lupus.org/topics/vascul.html

TAKAYASU'S ARTERITIS

Johns Hopkins Vasculitis Center: Takayasu's Arteritis   A description of Takayasu's arteritis is provided at this page, as well as an example angiographic image of involved arteries. Other names for the disease, a profile of a typical patient, and classic symptoms and signs are reviewed. Clinical disease phases, including systemic and occlusive, are discussed, as well as disease causes, the difficulty of diagnosis, and its relation to the other vasculitides. Recent research conducted by the International Network for the Study of Systemic Vasculitides, providing hope for future diagnosis and treatment, is addressed.
http://vasculitis.med.jhu.edu/takayasu's.htm

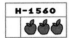

Takayasu's Arteritis Association   The Takayasu's Arteritis Association is a nonprofit organization serving patients, family members, health professionals, and the general public. The site contains information about the association, including membership and events; an overview of Takayasu's arteritis, including a discussion of symptoms, diagnosis, and treatment; and links to related Web sites. http://www.takayasus.com

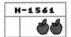

Takayasu's Arteritis Foundation International   Intended to be a resource for patients, friends, families, and healthcare providers, this site provides information about Takayasu's arteritis. The site presents a general overview of the disease, information about living with the disorder, and a discussion of treatment and therapy. Lists of physicians in the United States, Canada, Japan, the United Kingdom, India, and Mexico are found, in addition to personal stories and links to related sites.
http://www.takayasu.org

TEMPORAL ARTERITIS (GIANT CELL ARTERITIS)

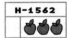

eMedicine: Temporal Arteritis   This inflammation of the temporal artery, also known as giant cell arteritis, is discussed in terms of its pathophysiology, clinical presentation, constitutional symptoms, and additional historical information. The physical examination, diagnostic differential links, and laboratory, imaging, and other diagnostic procedures are outlined. Commonly employed pharmacologic agents are profiled; complications are reviewed; and patient education material is presented.
http://eMedicine.com/cgi-bin/foxweb.exe/showsection@d:/em/ga?book=emerg&topicid=568

Johns Hopkins Vasculitis Center: Giant Cell Arteritis   Johns Hopkins offers this organized overview of giant cell arteritis, also known as temporal arteritis. A specimen showing the characteristic giant cells is displayed, and facts on symptoms, causes, and diagnosis are presented. A link at the page offers access to in-depth information about temporal artery biopsy and other diagnostic

possibilities. At the bottom of the page, readers will find a connection to a detailed clinical discussion of the disease addressing symptoms and management.
http://vasculitis.med.jhu.edu/gca.htm

Temporal Arteritis Temporal arteritis is reviewed at this online information sheet, as a service of Clinical Reference Systems. Information on the symptoms, diagnosis, and treatment of the disorder is provided.
http://ekhsin.morehead-st.edu/sha/sha/temparte.htm

Vasculitis, General Resources

Johns Hopkins Vasculitis Center This site was created by the Johns Hopkins Vasculitis Center as a patient resource and includes information about the center and updates on current research in vasculitis. General review of the symptoms, diagnosis, and different types of vasculitis is found, along with discussion of treatments and explanations of individual drug regimens. Answers to frequently asked questions and links to other organizations related to vasculitis are provided.
http://vasculitis.med.jhu.edu/welcome.htm

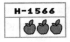

National Jewish Medical and Research Center: Vasculitis This article, written by a physician of the National Jewish Medical and Research Center, contains useful information about vasculitis. The disorder is categorized into four main types, including systemic necrotizing vasculitides and granulomatous vasculitides. The clinical challenge of diagnosis, immune mechanisms and pathogenesis, several treatment modalities, and specific drugs are discussed.
http://Library.NationalJewish.org/MSU/12n5MSU_Vasculitis.html

University of Western Sydney: Vasculitis This technical page instructs healthcare professionals and medical students about vasculitis and includes background disease information, etiology, pathology, clinical presentation, diagnosis, and treatment. Tables and references are provided, offering classifications of vasculitis and characteristics of the different types.
http://fohweb.macarthur.uws.edu.au/podiatry/vasculit.htm

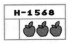

Vasculitis This site provides patient information about many types of vasculitis. It includes a general overview, a section on diagnosis, and information on the Churg-Strauss variant, giant-cell arteritis, Henoch-Schonlein purpura, leukocytoclastic vasculitis, microscopic polyangiitis, and overlapping syndromes. Discussions of polyarteritis nodosa and Takayasu's arteritis are found, and links are provided to patient and family resources.
http://www.blackandwhite.org/savvy/index.shtml

9.12 CORONARY ARTERY DISEASE (CAD)

GENERAL RESOURCES

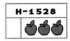

American Board of Family Practice: Coronary Artery Disease The American Board of Family Practice developed this reference guide as a component of the office record review portion of the recertification process. An in-depth overview is followed by details of physical examination, diagnostic procedures, management of acute myocardial infarction, and ambulatory management. Additional topics include postmyocardial infarction and angina pectoris drug therapies, physical rehabilitation, dietary control, control of risk factors, surgical therapy, patient and family education, and follow-up care.
http://www.familypractice.com/references/
referencesframe.htm?main=/references/ABFPGuides/Artery/artery.htm

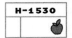

drkoop.com: Coronary Artery Disease Library Providing access to several cardiology resources, this page from Tallahassee Memorial HealthCare provides treatment and management information, an introduction to basic diagnostic tests in cardiology, a page discussing physical symptoms of coronary artery disease, and a wellness and prevention site. "All About Coronary Artery Disease" offers fundamental information on normal heart disease function and heart disease causes.
http://tmh.drkoop.com/conditions/coronary_artery_disease/toc.asp

ANGINA PECTORIS/MYOCARDIAL ISCHEMIA

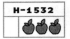

American Heart Association (AHA): Angina Pectoris Treatments Published by the AHA, this site details the treatment of angina pectoris, including a discussion of drugs, procedures, warning signs, and variant angina. Related topics within the guide are listed, including angioplasty and cardiac revascularization treatment, arteriography, atherectomy, and stent procedure, and can be accessed through the site's search engine.
http://216.185.112.5/presenter.jhtml?identifier=4496

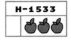

Doctor's Guide: Angina Links are available at this address to medical news and alerts, general information, discussion groups and newsgroups, and other Internet resources relevant to angina. Visitors can register for e-mail notification of site updates.
http://www.pslgroup.com/ANGINA.HTM

eMedicine: Angina This eMedicine article provides a detailed discussion of angina. Resources include general background information on the condition, pathophysiology, frequency, morbidity and mortality rates, and demographics related to sex and age. Clinical information includes details of clinical history in most patients suffering from stable, unstable, and variant angina; details of the physical signs associated with angina; and a discussion of causes. Descriptions of suggested laboratory and imaging studies are available, and treatment discussion includes information on prehospital care, emergency department care, and consultations. A table lists information on related medications, suggested adult and pediatric doses, contraindications, drug interactions, pregnancy safety, and precautions. Suggested follow-up inpatient and outpatient care procedures are described, including medications, transfer of patient, measures for prevention of recurrence, possible complications, prognosis, and important patient education concepts. http://www.eMedicine.com/emerg/topic31.htm

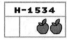

Hebrew University: Antianginal Therapy   These online lecture notes present a thorough overview of angina pectoris therapy. Pharmacologic agents are described in detail, including mechanism of action, therapeutic effects, pharmacokinetics, and possible side effects. Distinct types of angina are also discussed, including factors affecting myocardial oxygen requirements. http://www.md.huji.ac.il/mirrors/netpharm/angina.htm

Louisiana State University: Angina   Part of a larger group of patient education materials, this page is intended for use by healthcare professionals for patient distribution. A pamphlet about angina includes answers to commonly asked questions about the condition, including its duration, incidence, and treatment. The site explains the difference between an anginal attack and a heart attack. http://lib-sh.lsumc.edu/fammed/pted/angina.html

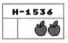

Merck Manual of Diagnosis and Therapy: Angina Pectoris   From the *Merck Manual of Diagnosis and Therapy,* this site presents the etiology, pathogenesis, symptoms and signs, diagnosis, prognosis, and treatment of angina pectoris. Discussions of unstable angina and variant angina are also provided. http://www.merck.com/pubs/mmanual/section16/chapter202/202c.htm

National Heart, Lung, and Blood Institute (NHLBI): Angina   Developed by the National Heart, Lung, and Blood Institute, this site provides a description of angina, its causes, and its relationship to heart attacks and other chest pain. It contains sections on diagnosis, treatment, medications, exercise, stable versus unstable angina, and other types of the disorder. There is also a list of other resources produced by the NHLBI. http://www.nhlbi.nih.gov/health/public/heart/other/angina.htm

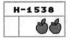

WellnessWeb: Angina Pectoris   Angina pectoris is described in nontechnical language at this address, including a definition and information on angina triggers, diagnosis, and treatment. The differences between stable and unstable angina are summarized, and information on other types of angina is available. http://www.wellnessweb.com/masterindex/cardio/aboutangina.htm

MYOCARDIAL INFARCTION (MI)

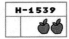

Complications of Myocardial Infarction A listing of eight post-myocardial infarction complications is provided at this site, with access to a complete module on myocardial infarction management.
http://medmic02.wnmeds.ac.nz/groups/rmo/mi/mi4.html

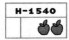

Heart Attacks General information about heart attacks is found at this site, which contains information about both modifiable and nonmodifiable risk factors. The heart attack treatments described include streptokinase thrombolytic therapy, balloon angioplasty, atherectomy, and stent. The site also describes the role of a physical therapist in preventing future occurrences of myocardial infarction. http://www.geocities.com/HotSprings/3049/human.htm

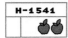

Infarct Combat Project The Infarct Combat Project is a nonprofit organization created to provide information related to diagnosis, prevention, and clinical therapeutics for myocardial infarction. The site contains current news updates related to the treatment of heart attacks. Included are journal articles about the use of cardiotonics, transmyocardial laser revascularization, survival advantages for heart attacks, hospitals and therapies, and the latest findings about ECG diagnosis. The site also contains a list of selected books, a library of electrocardiograms, information on funding, a list of supported projects, and discussion groups. http://www.infarctcombat.org

SpringNet: When Minutes Matter: Responding Quickly to Acute Myocardial Infarction Written for healthcare professionals, this article seeks to demonstrate how the latest research can improve patient care. The discussion begins with a review of the pathophysiology of myocardial infarction and goes on to describe treatment priorities. Diagnostic review, treating acute Q-wave MI, assessing reperfusion, and follow-up care information are provided. The site includes references and links to the National Heart Attack Alert Program and the American Heart Association.
http://www.springnet.com/ce/ccce.htm

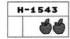

University of Alabama: Myocardial Infarction Visitors to this address will find links to Internet resources on myocardial infarction, including pages from the *Merck Manual;* CME articles; pathology images; clinical guidelines from the American Heart Association; and the National Heart, Lung, and Blood Institute; as well as an assortment of additional textbook chapters on myocardial infarction. Links are also available to directory listings of related disorders.
http://www.slis.ua.edu/cdlp/WebDLCore/clinical/cardiology/cardiovascular/mi.html

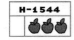

Virtual Hospital: Complications of Acute Myocardial Infarction The Virtual Hospital chapter on complications of acute MI includes outlines of both left and right ventricular dysfunction, tachyarrhythmias complicating acute MI, atrioventricular block types, left ventricular aneurysm, recurrent chest pain, and

Dressler's syndrome. Each post-MI disorder may include information on causes, symptoms, signs, and treatment.
http://www.vh.org/Providers/ClinRef/FPHandbook/Chapter02/03-2.html

Syndrome X (Microvascular Angina)

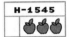

Hospital Practice: Cardiac Syndrome X This article provides an overview of the diagnostic and therapeutic challenges of cardiac syndrome X. Main clinical features are listed, and typical ECG findings during exercise-induced angina are reviewed. An in-depth discussion of proposed disease mechanisms, as well as information on prognosis, is provided by the author, who emphasizes a multidisciplinary approach to treatment.
http://www.hosppract.com/issues/2000/02/kaski.htm

Unstable Angina

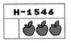

Diagnosing and Managing Unstable Angina Intended for doctors, this site provides extensive information on the care of patients with unstable angina. Topics discussed include initial evaluation and treatment, outpatient care, intensive medical care, nonintensive medical care, noninvasive testing, cardiac catheterization and myocardial revascularization, hospital discharge, and postdischarge care. The site provides an extensive bibliography of sources and links to tables and charts. http://www.medana.unibas.ch/eng/internt/angqtxt.htm

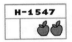

Stanford Interventional Cardiology: Unstable Angina The management of unstable angina is discussed in this article, including a historical perspective, clinical details of the syndrome, and current conventional management strategies. Results of recent relevant clinical trials are summarized, and reference citations are provided.
http://www-cvmed.stanford.edu/cvmfellowship/interventional/usa.htm

University of Texas at Houston: Unstable Angina Definitions of specific subtypes of unstable angina are provided by this fact sheet, followed by explanations of risk stratification. Information is presented in a concise outline format. http://www.uth.tmc.edu/~atonnese/utangus.html

Variant Angina (Prinzmetal's Angina)

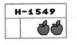

Clinical Cardiology: Prinzmetal's Variant Angina From *Clinical Cardiology,* this site contains an abstract of an article on Prinzmetal's variant angina, which discusses its prevalence, diagnosis, and long-term survival. Reprint information is provided.
http://clinical-cardiology.org/briefs/9804briefs/21-243.shtml

eMedicine: Coronary Artery Vasospasm Also known as vasospastic angina or Prinzmetal's angina, coronary artery vasospasm is discussed at this eMedicine page, created to provide medical education to clinicians. Chest pain, electrocardiographic findings, and other disease features are introduced, as well as pathophysiology, additional workup studies, and management considerations. Drug profiles for nitrates and calcium channel blockers are included, and the possibility of myocardial infarction and arrhythmias as complications of the condition is addressed.

http://www.eMedicine.com/med/topic447.htm

Vein Graft Aneurysms

eMedicine: Saphenous Vein Graft Aneurysms Presented in 11 parts, this eMedicine article discusses coronary artery revascularization with saphenous veins and variable pathophysiologies of aneurysms, including vein graft necrosis, hypertension, fibrosis, and other weaknesses and traumas. Clinical presentation and links to diagnostic differentials are included, along with imaging studies and a complete medical care review.

http://www.eMedicine.com/med/topic3145.htm

9.13 Diseases of the Aorta and Its Branches

General Resources

Merck Manual of Diagnosis and Therapy: Diseases of the Aorta and Its Branches The etiology, symptoms, and signs, diagnosis, and prognosis and treatment are offered for abdominal aortic; thoracic aortic; and popliteal, iliac, and femoral aneurysms at this page. Concise information on upper extremity, splanchnic artery, and intracranial aneurysms is provided, and links to similar information on additional diseases of the aorta and its branches can be accessed from the site. Separate chapters on aortic dissection, inflammation of the aorta, and occlusive disease are available.

http://www.merck.com/pubs/mmanual/section16/chapter211/211a.htm

Temple University: Diseases of the Aorta Aortic diseases are examined in this online review, providing reference to normal anatomy and function and several categories of aortic pathogenesis. Atherosclerotic aortic aneurysms, aortic dissection, annuloaortic ectasia, aortic arteritis syndromes, aortic trauma, aortic thromboembolic disease, and aortic infections are all reviewed in terms of their clinical presentations, diagnosis, and management. An illustration at the site reviews the distinctions between the DeBakey and Stanford classifications of aortic dissection.

http://blue.vm.temple.edu/~pathphys/cardiology/aortic_diseases.html

AORTIC ANEURYSM

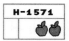

Aortic Aneurysm   Sponsored by the surgeons at Surgical Care Associates, this Web site provides general patient information about aortic aneurysm. The site describes the disorder, symptoms, risks, and treatment. There is a list of vascular surgical procedures, with detailed information given about carotid endarterectomy. The site also offers answers to frequently asked questions.
http://www.aorticaneurysm.com

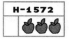

Merck Manual of Geriatrics: Aneurysms   The online *Merck Manual of Geriatrics* provides this comprehensive chapter on aneurysms of the aorta and its branches, including thoracic aortic aneurysms, abdominal aortic aneurysms, and popliteal, femoral, and carotid arterial aneurysms. Symptoms, signs, and diagnosis, as well as prognostic and treatment information, are provided. Symptoms and signs of aortic dissection of the proximal and distal varieties are discussed, and a table outlining the findings in aortic dissection is provided.
http://www.merck.com/pubs/mm_geriatrics/sec11/ch95.htm

University of Iowa: Aortic Aneurysms, 3-D Visualization and Measurement   A valuable tool for professionals, the site contains an overview of abdominal aortic aneurysm and its analysis with basic volumetric techniques, including oblique sectioning, region of interest analysis, geometric analysis of outer aortic boundaries and vessel tortuosity, volume rendering, and surface rendering. The site covers imaging techniques such as helical CT scanning, cine CT, conventional 2-D-CT interpretation, volumetric structural analysis (VSA), tortuosity analysis, and eccentricity analysis. The site features a collection of case studies with images involving abdominal aortic aneurysm (AAA), large saccular AAA, long fusiform arteriosclerotic AAA, dissecting aorta, and thoracic aneurysm. Abstracts of related literature are also included.
http://everest.radiology.uiowa.edu/nlm/app/aorta/aorta.html

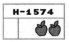

University of Pittsburgh: Bioengineering Studies of Abdominal Aortic Aneurysm   The site offers animations that demonstrate studies investigating the effects of increasing abdominal aortic aneurysm (AAA) diameter and asymmetry on wall stress distribution. An additional case study of a noninvasive computational stress analysis of AAA in-vivo may be found, for which illustrations are provided.
http://www.pitt.edu/~vorp

AORTIC DISSECTION

eMedicine: Aortic Dissection   This eMedicine article offers review of the pathophysiology of this catastrophe of the aorta. Anatomic classification by the Stanford and DeBakey systems is reviewed, in addition to descriptions of severe pain and other presenting symptoms. The site features links to several diagnostic differential links and offers review of diagnostic studies, drawbacks of angiography, urgent surgical intervention in type A dissections, and additional management measures. Radiographic, angiographic, and ECG tracing images are included. http://www.emedicine.com/emerg/topic28.htm

MCP Hahnemann University: Pathogenesis and Diagnosis of Aortic Dissection A CME activity is offered at this page, describing the pathophysiology, risk factors, and classification of aortic dissection. Chapters on clinical manifestations and diagnostic options are included, as well as directions on obtaining CME credit for the exercise. Enlargeable radiography, angiography, computed tomography, magnetic resonance, transthoracic echocardiography, transesophageal echocardiography, and intravascular ultrasound images are available. http://www.mcphu.edu/continuing/cme/medicine/v1n4/toc.html

Virtual Hospital: Aortic Dissection (Thoracic) The University of Iowa *Family Practice Handbook* includes this outline in emergency medicine, providing details on the diagnosis and treatment of aortic dissection. This externally peer reviewed site briefly describes symptoms and pharmacologic control of blood pressure.
http://www.vh.org/Providers/ClinRef/FPHandbook/Chapter01/17-1.html

Aortic Trauma

Eastern Association for the Surgery of Trauma: Guidelines for the Diagnosis and Management of Blunt Aortic Injury Recommendations addressing diagnosis and management for several levels of injury are stated at this site, which also includes information on prevalence of the problem and a review of literature. Common mechanisms of injury; information on angiography, radiography, and other diagnostic modalities; and recommendations for future investigations are included.
http://www.east.org/tpg/chap8body.html

Fibromuscular Dysplasia

Fibromuscular Dysplasia Authored by a medical student at the University of Queensland, this site answers many questions about fibromuscular dysplasia. Arteries affected are discussed, as well as prevalence, diagnosis, and management. An image of multifocal disease can be accessed. A listing of FAQs provides answers to questions about familial patterns and offers resources for further information on the disease and its prognosis.
http://student.uq.edu.au/~s012974/fibrodys.html

9.14 DRUG-INDUCED HEART DISEASE

ALCOHOL

eMedicine: Holiday Heart Syndrome   Also known as paroxysmal atrial fibrillation, alcohol-related heart disease, and acute cardiac alcohol toxicity, holiday heart syndrome is discussed at this electronic article. Background information on alcohol-induced cardiomyopathy and several mechanisms involved are reviewed. Readers will find a list of components of the physical presentation, as well as links to diagnostic differentials for convenient comparisons.
http://www.eMedicine.com/med/topic1024.htm

AMPHETAMINES

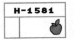

Methamphetamine Addiction   This fact sheet offers an overview of methamphetamine use and its effects on the body. Serious effects on the central nervous system and the cardiovascular system, as well as other physiological consequences, are described in detail. Additional information includes details of drug use, sources of the drug, and a brief historical perspective.
http://www.addiction2.com/faqmeth.htm

ANDROGENS

Testosterone   The effects of testosterone on the body are summarized in this fact sheet. The discussion focuses on the effects of androgens on post-menopausal women and the risks of heart disease due to androgen therapy.
http://www.midlife-passages.com/page52.html

CARBON MONOXIDE

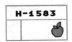

Carbon Monoxide   An overview of carbon monoxide is presented at this consumer fact sheet, provided by Paitson Heating and Air. Health effects resulting from exposure are listed, followed by information on preventing carbon monoxide poisoning in the home.
http://www.paitson.com/carbonmonoxide.htm

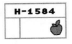

Carbon Monoxide (CO)   Information provided by this consumer fact sheet includes an overview of the effects of carbon monoxide on the body and suggestions on preventing carbon monoxide poisoning in the home.
http://www.nagd.com/carbon.htm

COCAINE

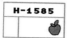

Good Drug Guide: Cocaine Triggers Heart Attacks within One Hour
Assessing the risk of heart attack, this article reviews research published in *Circulation* that supports the direct relationship between cocaine use and heart disease. Short-term effects of cocaine on the heart, several ways in which cocaine may trigger a heart attack, and the need for further research are discussed.
http://www.cocaine.org/health/

Medical College of Wisconsin: Cocaine and Heart Disease   This
general article describes the adverse effects of cocaine use on the heart. The mechanisms of heart damage are explained, and other long-term effects of cocaine use are listed.
http://healthlink.mcw.edu/article/921033839.html

NICOTINE

American Academy of Family Physicians (AAFP): Heart Disease and Smoking   Information on heart disease, smoking, and smoking cessation is
available in this fact sheet. Risks from cigarette smoke exposure, the addictive quality of cigarettes, smoking cessation strategies, nicotine replacement, and other pharmacologic aids are discussed.
http://familydoctor.org/handouts/289.html

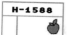

Bureau of Naval Personnel: Nicotine   An increased risk of heart disease
and certain cancers due to tobacco use is described in this consumer fact sheet. General statistics are available, and the addictive quality of nicotine is briefly described. Other harmful components of cigarette smoke are discussed.
http://navdweb.spawar.navy.mil/drugsofabuse/nicotine.htm

PHENTERMINE/FENFLURAMINE (PHEN/FEN)

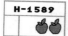

Doctor's Guide: No Change in Cardiovascular Clinical Status in Phen-Fen Patients   This article discusses recent research suggesting that no
statistically significant differences exist in the cardiovascular status of patients who had previously taken phentermine and fenfluramine and those who did not. Statistics on specific types of valvular diseases are available, demonstrating no increase in risk in phen/fen patients.
http://www.pslgroup.com/dg/eb636.htm

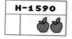

Research on Phen/Fen Heart Valve Controversy   This site offers links
to recent articles related to the controversy surrounding phen/fen weight-loss therapy and the risk of valvular heart disease. Articles from the *New England Journal of Medicine* and recent evidence from *Circulation: Journal of the*

American Heart Association are found, with current research suggesting that problems generated by use of the drug may be reversible and are not serious.
http://www.loop.net/~bkrentzman/meds/Phen.Fen/phen_fen_research.html

PSYCHOTROPIC DRUGS

American Heart Association (AHA): Cardiovascular Monitoring of Children and Adolescents Receiving Psychotropic Drugs Proper cardiovascular monitoring and important considerations in children and adolescents undergoing treatment with psychotropic drugs are discussed in this AHA Scientific Statement. Topics include potential mechanisms of sudden death, the effects of specific drugs, drug interactions, and official clinical recommendations. Reference citations are available.
http://circ.ahajournals.org/cgi/content/full/99/7/979

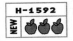

Pharmaceutical Journal: Drug-Induced Cardiovascular Disorders This issue of *The Pharmaceutical Journal* contains information on drugs known to cause adverse effects on the cardiovascular system. Drug-induced arrhythmias are discussed, in addition to their possible effects on the QT interval. Psychiatric drugs associated with torsade de pointes, cardiac conduction velocity, and QT interval prolongation; substances that may cause atrial fibrillation; agents associated with bradycardia; and drug causes of cardiac failure, hypertension, myocardial ischemia, thromboembolic disorders, and valvular disorders are included. A case study introduces management of potential interactions.
http://www.pharmj.com/Editorial/19990123/education/cardiovascular.html

9.15 HEART FAILURE

GENERAL RESOURCES

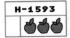

Heart Failure Online This online resource provides information on heart failure and related topics for consumers and patients. Normal heart function and heart failure are described, along with prevention and treatment. Additional resources include information on symptoms and living with heart failure, a FAQ listing, and a glossary. Links are also available to related sites.
http://www.heartfailure.org

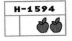

Heart Failure Society of America The Heart Failure Society of America is composed of heart failure professionals who seek to provide a forum for those interested in heart function, heart failure, and congestive heart failure research. The mission is to promote research, educate physicians, encourage preventive care, and enhance the quality and duration of life for individuals with heart failure. The site contains information about membership, corporate support for the organization, and developments within the field. Conference details are provided. http://www.hfsa.org

HeliosHealth.com: Heart Failure A detailed description of heart failure is available from this fact sheet, accompanied by discussions of causes, symptoms, diagnosis, and treatment. The site offers an appendix of drug details and a glossary of terms.
http://www.helioshealth.com/heart_health/heart_failure

University of Alabama: Congestive Heart Failure Clinical Resources
This site provides a comprehensive directory of links to heart failure documents on the Internet, including the *Merck Manual,* the eMedicine online textbook, and CliniWeb, courtesy of the University of Alabama. Access is also available to related resources from the American Board of Family Practice, the American Heart Association, the National Guideline Clearinghouse, WebMedLit, and HealthWeb, as well as to the Congestive Heart Failure Patient/Family Resources sites. http://www.slis.ua.edu/cdlp/unthsc/clinical/cardiology/cardiovascular/chf.html

ACUTE PULMONARY EDEMA

Initial Diagnostic Evaluation of Acute Pulmonary Edema A report of the American College of Cardiology and the American Heart Association Task Force on Practice Guidelines summarizes the evaluation and management of heart failure with acute pulmonary edema at this site. Class I, II, and III evaluations are listed, from initial physical examination to more extensive evaluations.
http://www.cl.spb.ru/cheelila/assPEng.html

Virtual Hospital: Acute Pulmonary Edema Peer reviewed by Mosby, this page of the University of Iowa *Family Practice Handbook* offers an outline of causes, diagnosis, treatment, and follow-up management for acute pulmonary edema. Diagnostic tests, oxygen administration, and pharmacologic measures of treatment are described.
http://www.vh.org/Providers/ClinRef/FPHandbook/Chapter02/09-2.html

CARDIOMYOPATHY

American Heart Association (AHA): Cardiomyopathy This fact sheet describes cardiomyopathy, including individual discussions of hypertrophic cardiomyopathy, dilated cardiomyopathy, and restrictive cardiomyopathy. Treatment options are discussed.
http://216.185.112.5/presenter.jhtml?identifier=4468

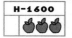

Cardiomyopathy Association The background, diagnosis, and treatment of cardiomyopathy are discussed in common medical terms at this site from the Cardiomyopathy Association. Information is provided on each of the four recognized conditions of cardiomyopathy, including dilated cardiomyopathy, hy-

pertrophic cardiomyopathy, and restrictive cardiomyopathy. Discussions include illustrations. The site also offers exercise guidelines, information about fundraising efforts, and links to related resources.
http://www.cardiomyopathy.org

eMedicine: Cardiomyopathy, Dilated Contributors to worsening heart failure in this common childhood condition are discussed at this page, as well as history, physical presentation, and factors identified as causes of myocardial damage. Laboratory studies, imaging workup, and other procedures for diagnosis are summarized, and a table at the site outlines several approaches to diagnosis, findings, and conclusions. Reviews of medical care, surgical care, and a multidisciplinary approach to management are presented.
http://www.eMedicine.com/ped/topic2502.htm

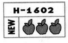

eMedicine: Cardiomyopathy, Hypertrophic Information on this inherited autosomal dominant disorder is provided at this page, which includes hallmarks of the disease, pathophysiology, and a review of associated signs and symptoms. Abnormal calcium kinetics, genetic causes, and other suggested causes are introduced, as well as complete diagnostic and management information. http://www.eMedicine.com/ped/topic1102.htm

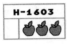

Hypertrophic Cardiomyopathy Association This informational organization offers membership details, general overview of hypertrophic cardiomyopathy (HCM), and detailed fact sheets related to this condition. Educational resources provide information on how HCM affects the heart, when the disease most often develops in an affected individual's life, symptoms, diagnosis, and treatments, including medications, surgical intervention, pacemakers, and automatic implantable defibrillators. Possible complications and illustrations of the heart in HCM, including patterns of muscle thickening, are provided.
http://www.kanter.com/hcm

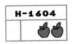

Johns Hopkins Cardiomyopathy and Heart Transplant Service: Heart Failure Web Clinical developments in the fight against cardiomyopathy and heart failure are described at this page. The site includes definitions, discussion of pressure-volume loops, and information about causes, patient evaluation, new treatments and procedures, and heart transplantation. A listing of heart failure studies is also available. Photographs of various types of cardiomyopathy and links to related sites are provided, in addition to information about the clinical faculty.
http://www.hopkinsmedicine.org/cardiology/heart/

CONGESTIVE HEART FAILURE

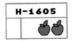

American Heart Association (AHA): Understanding Heart Failure
Published by the American Heart Association, this site contains useful information about congestive heart failure for consumer reference. It includes a discus-

sion of causes, diagnosis, treatment, and pharmacologic and other interventions. A description of heart failure classification is presented.
http://216.185.112.5/presenter.jhtml?identifier=1593

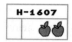

Doctor's Guide: Congestive Heart Failure The Doctor's Guide provides information and resources for congestive heart failure at this address. The information is intended to benefit consumers, offering up-to-date medical news and alerts, congestive heart failure information, links to discussion and news groups, and links to related sites.
http://www.docguide.com/news/content.nsf/
PatientResAllCateg/Congestive%20Heart%20Failure?OpenDocument

Medical College of Virginia: Congestive Heart Failure The Medical College of Virginia Hospitals offers patient information about congestive heart failure at this Web address. There are articles about acute pulmonary edema, medical therapies, current therapies, heart transplantation, and coronary artery bypass grafting. Information about the rising cost of care and participation in clinical trial protocols is offered.
http://views.vcu.edu/chf/congesti.htm

University of Alabama: Congestive Heart Failure Peer-reviewed congestive heart failure resources, courtesy of the Clinical Digital Libraries Project, are available from this online directory, including clinical fact sheets, CME articles, pathology images, clinical guidelines, consumer resources, and miscellaneous congestive heart failure resources. Links are available to directory listings of related disorders, as a service of the University of Alabama.
http://www.slis.ua.edu/cdlp/WebDLCore/clinical/cardiology/cardiovascular/chf.html

COR PULMONALE

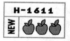

eMedicine: Cor Pulmonale A comprehensive article on right heart failure is found at this address, examining several pathophysiological disease mechanisms and generally nonspecific clinical manifestations. Physical findings and laboratory investigations to be considered are outlined at the article, which also includes a listing of useful imaging studies and medical care for acute and chronic conditions. http://www.eMedicine.com/med/topic449.htm

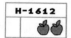

Family Practice Notebook.com: Cor Pulmonale A concise outline at this address offers a technical overview of cor pulmonale. Topics include pathophysiology, causes, symptoms, signs, differential diagnosis, appropriate laboratory tests and diagnostic imaging, and therapeutic management. Links are available to similar resources on related topics.
http://www.fpnotebook.com/CV124.htm

Merck Manual of Diagnosis and Therapy: Cor Pulmonale The etiology of both acute and chronic forms of cor pulmonale are described at this Merck reference. In addition to pathogenesis, symptoms, signs, and diagnosis,

the causes of primary pulmonary hypertension and its management are found, along with links to related chapters on heart failure.
http://www.merck.com/pubs/mmanual/section16/chapter203/203c.htm

LEFT VENTRICULAR FAILURE

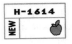

Virtual Hospital: Left Ventricular Failure Principles of treatment for left ventricular failure are concisely presented at this site, part of the "Hypertensive Emergencies" lectures at the University of Iowa. Links to further information on the drug of choice and other alternatives are found.
http://www.vh.org/Providers/Lectures/EmergencyMed/Hypertension/LVF.html

PRIMARY PULMONARY HYPERTENSION (PPH)

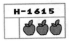

PHCentral: Pulmonary Hypertension The mission of PHCentral is to provide an Internet resource for pulmonary hypertension - related information for patients, caregivers, and medical professionals. The site offers clinical, emotional, and financial information regarding pulmonary hypertension. There are links to current scientific publications, as well as to the site's "Newsroom," which provides the latest updates on the treatment of pulmonary hypertension.
http://www.phcentral.org

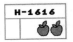

PPH Cure Foundation PPH Cure Foundation, a large, nongovernmental funding source of medical research into the causes and treatment of primary pulmonary hypertension, established this Web site to provide information to patients, researchers, and potential donors. The site contains information about PPH, the foundation, and current clinical trials.
http://www.pphcure.org

9.16 HYPERTENSION

GENERAL RESOURCES

American Society of Hypertension The American Society of Hypertension is dedicated solely to hypertension and related cardiovascular disease. The site contains information about the society, news, publications, and society membership. Review of the organization's scientific meeting is found, and access to articles of particular interest that have been adapted for the media is provided, courtesy of the *American Journal of Hypertension*.
http://www.ash-us.org/

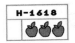

Heart Information Network: Hypertension Guide Created by the Heart Information Network, this site provides comprehensive patient information about hypertension. Information includes a description of hypertension, risk factors, symptoms, and the difference between primary and secondary hypertension. There is also information about screening, complications, treatment, and prevention along with links to related articles about hypertension, optimal blood pressure levels, and beneficial diets.

http://www.heartinfo.org/search/display.asp?Id=429&header=T_pat.gif&caller=458

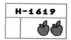

HeartPoint: High Blood Pressure This page contains comprehensive patient information about blood pressure, high blood pressure, and associated risks. The article discusses risk factors, secondary causes, treatment, medication, variation in blood pressure, and white coat syndrome. There are links to heart-healthy food, health tips, and commentary.

http://www.heartpoint.com/highbloodpage.html

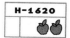

High Blood Pressure Foundation Established by the Department of Medicine at Western General Hospital in the United Kingdom, the High Blood Pressure Foundation seeks to improve understanding and treatment of the disorder. The site provides news from the field and information about treatment, research, donations, education, and fundraising.

http://www.hbpf.org.uk

Hypertension Network Bloodpressure.com, the official site of the Hypertension Network, provides educational materials, details on current research initiatives, and up-to-date information regarding hypertension management at this address. Visitors will find basic fact sheets with home monitoring device information, as well as an assessment tool that will ascertain blood pressure risk. Other resources, include a hypertension dictionary, hypertension treatment database that provides detailed prescription information; and online discussion group. Practitioners may add their name to an extensive network of physicians who specialize in the treatment of hypertension. Also available at this site are weekly research updates and reports on new medications.

http://www.bloodpressure.com

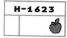

Hypertension-Info This site is dedicated to providing patients and healthcare professionals with up-to-date and accurate resources for the treatment of hypertension. The site contains multimedia educational activities and information about the latest advancements in hypertension diagnostics and therapeutics. There are links to related associations and organizations, as well as information about clinical trials and research.

http://www.hypertension-info.com

Inter-American Society of Hypertension This nonprofit professional organization is dedicated to understanding, preventing, and controlling hypertension and vascular diseases. The site contains information about the society, including its origin, objectives, challenges, committees, meetings, and newsletter. The site also provides links to related organizations and centers.

http://www.caduceus.com.pe/iash/iashe.htm

Life Extension Foundation: Hypertension Nearly 20 article abstracts presenting information on hypertension are available at this address. Article content includes studies of nutritional factors, physical activity, and other non-pharmacological approaches to the treatment of hypertension.
http://www.lef.org/protocols/abstracts/abstr-060.html

New York Online Access to Health (NOAH): High Blood Pressure
Part of New York Online Access to Health, this site provides comprehensive patient information about high blood pressure, including causes, occurrence, complications associated with the disorder, symptoms, diagnosis, testing, lifestyle changes, drug therapy, enzyme inhibitors, and hypertension in pregnancy. Links to recent literature and other resources are provided.
http://www.noah-health.org/english/illness/heart_disease/heartdisease.html#H

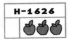

University of Alabama: Hypertension Clinical Resources This online directory provides links to valuable clinical sources of information on hypertension. General fact sheets, CME articles, pathology images, clinical guidelines and scientific statements, and other miscellaneous resources are listed, courtesy of the Digital Libraries Project of the University of Alabama. The online *Merck Manual* reference guide, the *Family Practice Handbook,* and the Versalius Image Archive are accessible, as well as National Guideline Clearinghouse search results and current governmental clinical trials.
http://www.slis.ua.edu/cdlp/WebDLCore/
clinical/cardiology/cardiovascular/hypertension.html

World Hypertension League The World Hypertension League is dedicated to the control of arterial hypertension in world populations. This site contains information about the organization, its goals and objectives, activities and projects, and history and membership. Patient resources include blood pressure measurement, links to both scientific and popular articles, and connections to the American Heart Association, the Hypertension Network, the Inter-American Society of Hypertension, and the National Heart, Lung, and Blood Institute. http://www.mco.edu/whl/index.html

COEXISTING CARDIOVASCULAR DISEASE

Hypertension in Patients with Coexisting Cardiovascular Disease
The importance of blood pressure control in the presence of heart disease is stressed at the Web site, with the benefits of reducing left ventricular hypertrophy and complications, such as heart failure and stroke. Antihypertensive agents, shown to reduce morbidity and mortality, are discussed, and special therapeutic considerations in heart failure are listed, courtesy of the Malaysian Society of Hypertension. The superior drug class for treatment of hypertension in left ventricular hypertrophy is mentioned, and cautionary guidelines regarding ACE inhibitors and beta blockers in peripheral vascular disease are pro-

vided. The gradual reduction of blood pressure in cerebrovascular accidents and overall blood pressure control to prevent future events are summarized.
http://www.msh.org.my/html/hyper_in_cvd.htm

DIABETES MELLITUS

American Diabetes Association: Treatment of Hypertension in Diabetes   The American Diabetes Association offers these practice recommendations concerning diabetes and hypertension complications. Seeking to answer questions related to epidemiology, pathophysiology, goals of therapy, and future research, the guideline provides a comprehensive tool for assessment, diagnosis, and treatment. Lifestyle modifications, the foundation of diabetic and hypertension management, are presented, as well as pharmacologic interventions. The importance of protecting renal function is emphasized.
http://www.diabetes.org/DiabetesCare/Supplement/s107.htm

Hypertension in Patients with Diabetes Mellitus   The increased risk of morbidity and mortality in patients with coexisting diabetes mellitus and hypertension is discussed at the Web address, with early detection and intervention emphasized. Nonpharmacological management, such as dietary considerations and optimal weight maintenance, is discussed, and important factors specific to pharmacological treatment are noted. Ensuing complications from poor hypertension control are summarized, and proper therapies, recommended for their renal protective properties, are mentioned, as a service of the Malaysian Society of Hypertension. Reduction of adverse events that affect metabolic function is of primary concern and is a major topic of discussion.
http://www.msh.org.my/html/hyper_diabetes mellitus.htm

GERIATRIC HYPERTENSION

American Family Physician: Hypertension Treatment and the Prevention of Coronary Heart Disease in the Elderly   Published by the American Academy of Family Physicians, this clinical opinion reviews the basis for treatment of systolic or systolic/diastolic hypertension in the elderly. Summaries of several research initiatives, the effects of therapy in older patients with hypertension, and general information on the prevention of congestive heart failure and progressive hypertension are included. The use of various pharmacologic agents in the geriatric population is addressed, and a complete treatment algorithm is found at the page.
http://www.aafp.org/afp/990301ap/1248,html

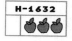

Hypertension in the Elderly   Provided as a service of the Malaysian Society of Hypertension, this site addresses the higher prevalence of associated cardiovascular risk factors in elderly patients with hypertension and the increasing importance of this public health concern. Early detection and intervention are

stressed, and special considerations in the elderly are mentioned, such as the importance of recognition of the cause of secondary hypertension and the use of positional blood pressure measurement, due to postural hypotension. Different blood pressure reduction goals are outlined, and topics such as patient compliance, adverse events in the elderly, and effective nonpharmacological and pharmacological management are emphasized.
http://www.msh.org.my/html/hypertension_in_elderly.htm

MALIGNANT HYPERTENSION

eMedicine: Hypertension, Malignant   The difference between hypertensive urgency and emergency is noted at this article, which offers a complete review of the pathogenesis, clinical presentation, and management of malignant hypertension. The differentials section of the site provides connection to several similar conditions in the eMedicine database for convenient comparisons. Additionally, the article contains pharmacologic profiles of vasodilators and adrenergic inhibitors, as well as enlargeable images of hypertensive retinopathy and papilledema. http://www.eMedicine.com/med/topic1107.htm

PEDIATRIC HYPERTENSION

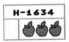

Hypertension in the Pediatric Patient   A discussion regarding differences in blood pressure measurement in children is found at the site, provided by the Malaysian Society of Hypertension. In addition to information regarding recognition of secondary causes of hypertension and treatment of underlying illness, antihypertensive drugs for the treatment of chronic and acute hypertension in children are outlined in table format, with dosage and dosing intervals listed. Blood pressure percentile charts for boys and girls for the 90th and 95th percentiles of blood pressure, according to age and percentiles of height, are provided, with a goal of reducing blood pressure below these values.
http://www.msh.org.my/html/hypertension_in_paediatric_patient.htm

PREGNANCY AND HYPERTENSION

Hypertension in Pregnancy   Hypertension in pregnancy, also known as preeclampsia or toxemia of pregnancy, is discussed at the Web site of the Malaysian Society of Hypertension, with significant complications and dangers to the fetus outlined. Diagnostic criteria and proper blood pressure measurement techniques in pregnancy are specified, as are the four special categories of hypertension. Hypertension with proteinuria, relevant laboratory tests, and the fetal monitoring procedures used are examined. Chronic hypertension, preeclampsia superimposed on chronic hypertension, and transient hypertension management discussions are offered. Drugs of choice, postpartum management, and careful consideration of both maternal and fetal health in regard to pregnancy continuation are stressed.

http://www.msh.org.my/html/hypertension_in_pregnancy.htm

Virtual Hospital: Hypertension in Pregnancy, Preeclampsia, and Eclampsia Produced by the University of Iowa, this page of the *Family Practice Handbook* offers definitions of pregnancy-induced hypertension, preeclampsia, and eclampsia, along with criteria for diagnosis. Risk factors, components of the evaluation, and management are reviewed, including ambulatory management, hospital care, and antihypertensive medications. Anticonvulsive treatment is summarized, as well as prevention and treatment of chronic hypertensive conditions.

http://www.vh.org/Providers/ClinRef/FPHandbook/Chapter08/10-8.html

9.17 HYPOTENSIVE DISORDERS/DYSAUTONOMIAS

CAROTID SINUS HYPERSENSITIVITY

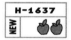

Annals of Long-Term Care: Carotid Sinus Syndrome: A Frequently Overlooked Cause of Falls and Syncope in Older Adults Published by MultiMedia Healthcare/Freedom, LLC, this article, adapted from a session of the 1999 American Geriatrics Society Annual Meeting, introduces the location of the carotid sinus and the consequences of carotid sinus hypersensitivity. Elicitation of the response, the connection of carotid sinus syndrome with syncope and falls, and successful management possibilities are explored.

http://www.mmhc.com/nhm/articles/NHM0007/kenny.html

eMedicine: Carotid Sinus Hypersensitivity Also known as hypersensitive carotid reflex or Weiss-Baker syndrome, the disorder is discussed at this page in terms of its role in blood pressure homeostasis. Possible causes, three types of the disorder, and symptoms and signs are reviewed. Protocol for diagnosis with carotid sinus massage is outlined, and the technique's clinical utility and predictive value are introduced. Management details, based on frequency and severity of symptoms, are presented, as well as several treatments used for patients with incapacitating disease.

http://www.eMedicine.com/med/topic299.htm

NEUROCARDIOGENIC SYNCOPE (VASOVAGAL SYNCOPE)

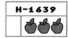

Annals of Internal Medicine: Diagnosing Syncope This position paper from the *Annals of Internal Medicine,* courtesy of the American College of Physicians and the American Society of Internal Medicine, reviews studies that were evaluated for their usefulness based on diagnostic yield. The article discusses the usefulness of history, physical examination, and electrocardiography;

the inability of neurological testing to be helpful in most circumstances; and the higher risk in suspected heart disease of adverse outcomes. Additional topics provide information on the cause of syncope in the elderly, important diagnostic testing in recurrent syncope without suspected heart disease, psychiatric evaluation, and indications for hospitalization in patients at high risk for cardiac syncope. http://www.acponline.org/journals/annals/15jun97/ppsyncop.htm

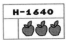

HeartWeb: Role of Cardiac Rhythm Disorders in the Etiology of Vasovagal Syncope
This article from HeartWeb discusses the relationship of arrhythmia pathology to circulatory syncope. Analysis of Holter monitoring of patients with vasovagal syncope is provided, yielding information on diagnosis, according to the Vasovagal International Study classification. No statistically significant relationship was observed between conduction disturbances and the occurrence of vasovagal syncope.
http://www.heartweb.org/heartweb/1196/ep0003.htm

ORTHOSTATIC HYPOTENSION

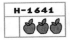

American Family Physician: Evaluation and Treatment of Orthostatic Hypotension
Courtesy of the American Academy of Family Physicians, this online article reviews nonneurogenic and neurogenic causes, the diagnostic evaluation, specific testing for autonomic function, and treatment directed at improving patient symptoms in orthostatic hypotension. Classifications and clinical features are reviewed, and nonneurogenic causes are outlined in table format. Nonpharmacologic and pharmacologic interventions are summarized by the authors.
http://www.aafp.org/afp/971001ap/engstrm.html

Case Western Reserve University: Instructions for Patients with Orthostatic Hypotension
This site provides patient information about orthostatic hypotension. After a general description of the disorder, the site offers simple measures of relief, including positional strategies; water jogging; eating small, frequent meals; and taking salt tablets.
http://mediswww.cwru.edu/dept/neurology/autonomic/orthostatic.html

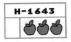

Johns Hopkins University: Neurally Mediated Hypotension
Produced by the Neurally Mediated Hypotension Working Group at Johns Hopkins Hospital, this brochure offers well-organized information about the disorder. Following a brief definition of the disease, the site answers frequently asked questions related to symptoms, posture, diagnosis, causes, treatment, and management. A sample high sodium diet, a sample high potassium diet, and information about drugs used to treat the disorder are provided.
http://ww2.med.jhu.edu/peds/cfs.html

Merck Manual of Diagnosis and Therapy: Orthostatic Hypotension
The etiology and pathophysiology of orthostatic hypotension are described at this page, including gravitational stress and impairment of the autonomic reflex

arc. Causes, including hypovolemia, drugs that impair autonomic reflex mechanisms, neurologic disorders affecting the autonomic nervous system, Shy-Drager syndrome, and idiopathic orthostatic hypotension, are examined. Cardiac etiologies and orthostatic hypotension in the elderly, criteria for diagnosis, and management are reviewed.

http://www.merck.com/pubs/mmanual/section16/chapter200/200a.htm

ORTHOSTATIC INTOLERANCE SYNDROMES, GENERAL

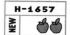

National Dysautonomia Research Foundation: Orthostatic Intolerance Syndromes Abnormal responses to changes in body position are the focus of this site, which discusses the history and three main categories used to describe orthostatic intolerance conditions. Similar symptoms for these conditions, new insight into the mechanisms of these disorders, management possibilities, and prognosis are reviewed.

http://www.ndrf.org/orthostat.htm

Vanderbilt Medical Center: Autonomic Dysfunction Center The Autonomic Dysfunction Center at Vanderbilt Medical Center presents this site, which addresses the symptoms of orthostatic intolerance and introduces several disorder names and their similar presentations. Demographics of the condition, long-term outlook for patients, and the need for further research into the causes of autonomic nervous system dysfunction are discussed.

http://www.mc.vanderbilt.edu/gcrc/adc/oi.html

POSTURAL ORTHOSTATIC TACHYCARDIA SYNDROME

New York Medical Center: Postural Orthostatic Tachycardia Syndrome General information on the orthostatic tachycardia syndrome is reviewed at this page, with illustrations of characteristic heart rate patterns and blood pressure abnormalities. A discussion of the literature, proposing several potential explanations of the disease, is found.

http://www.nymc.edu/fhp/centers/syncope/POTS.htm

Postural Orthostatic Tachycardia Syndrome Detailed information about postural orthostatic tachycardia syndrome (POTS) is provided at this site, where a patient diagnosed with POTS outlines an experience with the disease. A detailed explanation of POTS, its causes, symptoms, treatment, and current research are reviewed. Several studies list possible complications with use of certain drugs and offer prevalent theories about the disease. A link to the National Dysautonomia Research Foundation, which lists doctors qualified in the diagnosis and treatment of POTS, is offered, as well as a link to an abstract regarding the surgical treatment of POTS. A list of articles from medical journals and links to related sites are found.

http://home.att.net/~potsweb/POTS.html

9.18 METABOLIC DISORDERS AFFECTING THE HEART

ACID-BASE/ELECTROLYTE DISORDERS

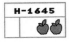

Acid-Base Disorders Acid-base disorders are described in outline form at this address of OutlineMed, Inc. An introduction, as well as details of interpretation, compensation, and effects on hemoglobin, is found. Additional information includes discussion of pH and other laboratory values, diagnosis, and etiologies. http://www.outlinemed.com/demo/nephrol/5596.htm

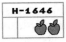

Virtual Hospital: Hematologic, Electrolyte, and Metabolic Disorders Details of metabolic acidosis and metabolic alkalosis are presented in outline form at this site of the University of Iowa. Metabolic acidosis topics include normal anion-gap acidosis and increased anion-gap acidosis. Information on metabolic alkalosis includes a basic definition, clinical findings, diagnosis, and treatment. Electrolyte and metabolic formulas are available through a link at this site. http://www.vh.org/Providers/ClinRef/FPHandbook/05.html

DIABETES AND HEART DISEASE

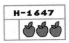

Dorothy Bullock Memorial National Diabetes Center This home page offers links to several articles discussing diabetes as a risk factor in cardiovascular disease, including treatment issues. Comprehensive resources on other diabetes issues are also provided through this site.
http://www.diabetes-mellitus.org

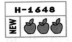

Endocrine Society: Diabetes and Cardiovascular Disease A Real Video version of an interview with Alan J. Garber, M.D., Ph.D., of Baylor College of Medicine is found at this site, intended to update professionals on the latest information in diabetes management. Five categories of assault on the vascular system in diabetes, including hyperglycemia, are introduced and explored at a series of online slides. Interventional trials examining glucose control, several other prevention trials, research on coronary events in diabetic patients, and details on reduction of recurring coronary events in those receiving pharmacologic intervention are presented. Data on treatment of LDL cholesterol and other management goals and treatment decisions are addressed at this recording of a live, interactive satellite broadcast.
http://www.meetingcast.com/dnm/garber.html

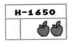

Your Family's Health: Diabetes and Heart Disease This consumer fact sheet offers a detailed discussion of diabetes and heart disease. Information includes overviews of type 1, type 2, and gestational diabetes; diagnosis and treatment details; and valuable suggestions on minimizing the risk of heart disease. http://www.yourfamilyshealth.com/cardiology/diabetes

HYPERLIPIDEMIA

American Heart Association (AHA): Hyperlipidemia   Presented in simple terms, this site defines hyperlipidemia and outlines several types. Related fact sheets of the AHA, including those on dietary needs and cholesterol-lowering drugs, can be accessed by using the AHA search engine.
http://216.185.112.5/presenter.jhtml?identifier=4600

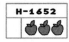

Atherogenesis and Dyslipidemia   Provided by the Preventive Health Center, this site offers information about atherogenesis and dyslipidemia. The discussion includes cholesterol and atherosclerosis, lipid metabolism, and atherogenesis. Information about modifiable and nonmodifiable risk factors, classifications of dyslipidemias, and secondary dyslipidemias is provided, as well as recent primary prevention and secondary prevention trials. The National Cholesterol Education Program Guidelines are found at the site, as well as sections on the pharmacologic and nonpharmacologic management of hypercholesterolemia and hypertriglyceridemia. Special considerations with regard to risk factors, treatment in the elderly, and concomitant hypertension are reviewed. http://www.md-phc.com/education/cholest.html

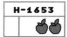

Doctor's Guide: Elevated Cholesterol   Medical news and alerts, general information sites, discussion groups and newsgroups, and other related sites devoted to elevated cholesterol reduction are found through links at this site. Visitors can register for e-mail notifications of Web page updates.
http://www.docguide.com/news/content.nsf/
PatientResAllCateg/Elevated%20Cholesterol?OpenDocument

THYROID DISORDERS AND HEART DISEASE

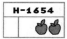

Thyroid Foundation of Canada: The Heart and the Thyroid Gland
Heart problems related to abnormal thyroid function are summarized in this fact sheet. The signs and symptoms, possible complications, and treatment of both hyperthyroidism and hypothyroidism are discussed in detail.
http://www.thyroid.ca/Articles/EngE6A.html

9.19 NONINFECTIVE ENDOCARDITIS

LIBMAN-SACKS LESIONS

eMedicine: Libman-Sacks Endocarditis   This characteristic cardiac manifestation of systemic lupus erythematosus is presented at this page, which includes discussion of its pathophysiology and cardiac manifestations. History, physical presentation, and causes are reviewed, and information on assessment, histologic findings, and treatment is included. An enlargeable image of a transesophageal view of Libman-Sacks endocarditis is displayed at the end of the article. http://www.eMedicine.com/med/topic1295.htm

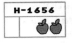

Merck Manual of Diagnosis and Therapy: Noninfective Endocarditis
The etiology and pathophysiology; symptoms, signs, and diagnosis; and prognosis and treatment of noninfective endocarditis are summarized in this online textbook chapter, courtesy of the *Merck Manual of Diagnosis and Therapy.* Links are available to related topic discussions.
http://www.merck.com/pubs/mmanual/section16/chapter208/208b.htm

9.20 PERICARDIAL DISEASE

GENERAL RESOURCES

American College of Cardiology (ACC): Guidelines for Echocardiography in Pericardial Disease From *Echocardiography*, this site provides guidelines from the American College of Cardiology and the American Heart Association for the clinical application of echocardiography in the diagnosis of pericardial disease. Types of pericardial diseases discussed include pericardial effusion, cardiac tamponade, increased pericardial thickness, pericardial tumors and cysts, constrictive pericarditis, and congenital absence of the pericardium.
http://www.acc.org/clinical/guidelines/echo

Pericardial Disease This site links visitors to summaries of a variety of pericardial diseases. The discussion includes an introduction and sections on anatomy, imaging technique, normal pericardium in MRI, congenital anomalies, effusive pericardial disease, pericardial thickening, constrictive pericarditis, and pericardial tumors.
http://imagerie-cv.univ-lyon1.fr/WEB_CARDIO/documents/Documents_references/pericarde/perica_c.htm

CARDIAC TAMPONADE

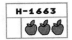

About.com: Cardiac Tamponade Definitions of tamponade, cardiac tamponade, and pericardial space are included at this site, which discusses the etiology, pathophysiology, clinical presentation, diagnosis, and treatment of the condition. Illustrative graphics and links to related Web sites are provided.
http://nursing.about.com/sitesearch.htm?terms=Cardiac+Tamponade&SUName=nursing&type=0&TopNode=3042&Action.x=10&Action.y=7

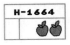

Clinical Reference Systems: Cardiac Tamponade Written by a physician, this site provides patient information about cardiac tamponade and offers a clear discussion of causes, symptoms, diagnosis, and treatment.
http://www.patienteducation.com/B3a.htm

PERICARDITIS, GENERAL

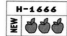

American Family Physician: Electrocardiographic Manifestations and Differential Diagnosis of Acute Pericarditis   Examining etiologies of acute pericarditis, this site of the American Academy of Family Physicians reviews infectious disease processes, as well as drug-related, immunonologic, rheumatologic, and neoplastic causes. An illustrative case, anatomy and physiology of the pericardium, electrocardiographic presentations, findings, and follow-up recommendations are summarized.
http://www.aafp.org/afp/980215ap/marinell.html

Cardiologychannel: Pericarditis   Provided by Cardiology World, this fact sheet on pericarditis addresses symptoms of the disease, several possible causes, and information on the physical examination and characteristic findings on electrocardiogram. Primary methods of treatment are summarized, including anti-inflammatory therapy and pericardiocentesis, when necessary.
http://www.cardiologychannel.com/pericarditis/

eMedicine: Pericarditis and Cardiac Tamponade   Clinical problems of pericarditis and cardiac tamponade are explored at this eMedicine article, which discusses common signs and symptoms and disease pathophysiology. Causes of acute and chronic conditions are listed, as well as laboratory diagnostics, imaging studies, and other assessment modalities. The traditional approach to pericardiocentesis is outlined, and recommendations for prehospital and emergency department care are included. In addition, the site offers pharmacologic profiles and enlargeable diagnostic images.
http://www.eMedicine.com/emerg/topic412.htm

Merck Manual of Diagnosis and Therapy: Pericarditis   The online *Merck Manual of Diagnosis and Therapy* presents this chapter on pericarditis, with review of the etiology and pathophysiology of acute pericarditis and chronic pericarditis, including both chronic restrictive and chronic effusive types. Signs and symptoms, cardiac tamponade review, diagnostic techniques, and treatment summaries are provided.
http://www.merck.com/pubs/mmanual/section16/chapter209/209b.htm

PERICARDITIS, CONSTRICTIVE

eMedicine: Pericarditis, Constrictive   The constrictive form of pericarditis is specifically considered at this eMedicine address. Diagnostic challenges are introduced, as well as pathophysiology and varied etiologies. A discussion of distinctions between this disease and restrictive cardiomyopathy is found, and differential links, diagnostic studies, and pharmacologic profiles are included in the presentation. http://www.eMedicine.com/med/topic1782.htm

9.21 PREGNANCY AND CARDIAC DISEASE

GENERAL RESOURCES

American Heart Association (AHA): Pregnancy and Heart Disease A concise fact sheet is found at this site, outlining the AHA recommendations regarding pregnancy and heart conditions. Important self-care measures are listed, as well as related publications of the AHA.
http://216.185.112.5/presenter.jhtml?identifier=4688

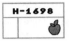

Cardiovascular Institute of the South: Pregnancy and Heart Disease
Authored by a physician at the Cardiovascular Institute of the South, this site provides general information about pregnancy and heart disease. A range of precautions for pregnant women with heart disease and details on peripartum dilated cardiomyopathy are included. Doctors' biographies, online articles, and external links related to cardiology may be accessed.
http://www.cardio.com/articles/preg-hrt.htm

HeartCenterOnline: Gestational Heart Related Problems A fact sheet found at this page offers summaries of a variety of pregnancy-related heart problems. Information on peripartum cardiomyopathy, pregnancy-induced hypertension, gestational diabetes, heart palpitations, varicose veins, and amniotic fluid embolism is provided. The warning signs of a gestational heart problem are outlined, and a printer-friendly version of the site is available.
http://www.heartcenteronline.com/myheartdr/common/articles.cfm?ARTID=109

AMNIOTIC FLUID EMBOLISM

Harbor UCLA Medical Center: Amniotic Fluid Embolism The overall incidence of amniotic fluid embolism and other statistical information is offered at this page, which also presents details on risk factors, phase I and II of the clinical presentation, and signs and symptoms noted in patients. Theories regarding etiology, diagnostic details, and management considerations are summarized. http://prl.humc.edu/obgyn/web/fellow/conferences/amniot.htm

PERIPARTUM CARDIOMYOPATHY

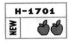

iVillage: Peripartum Cardiomyopathy A discussion of this rare form of congestive heart failure is found at this personal Web site, which includes overviews of symptoms, risk factors, diagnosis, and treatment. Links to related information and support on the World Wide Web are offered.
http://pages.ivillage.com/twins73/

MEDLINEplus Medical Encyclopedia: Peripartum Cardiomyopathy
Maintained by the National Library of Medicine, this encyclopedia entry includes an illustration of the condition and general information on causes, risks, symptoms, diagnosis, treatment, prognosis, and complications. MEDLINEplus encyclopedia sites include a variety of hyperlinks to related pages within the database. http://www.nlm.nih.gov/medlineplus/ency/article/000188.htm

PREGNANCY AND HYPERTENSION

Agency for Healthcare Research and Quality (AHRQ): Management of Chronic Hypertension during Pregnancy   An evidence report is offered at this site, intended to serve as a quality improvement tool in the delivery of healthcare services. Problems associated with chronic hypertension in pregnancy are reviewed, and key diagnostic and treatment considerations are addressed. Appropriate management, pharmacologic intervention, combination pharmacologic/nonpharmacologic treatment, and special monitoring techniques are examined. Other topics under review include the benefits of treating hypertension prior to conception and the adverse effects of antihypertensive agents. Future research directions are considered.
http://www.ahcpr.gov/clinic/pregsum.htm

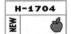

National Heart, Lung, and Blood Institute (NHLBI): High Blood Pressure in Pregnancy   Sponsored by the U.S. Department of Health and Human Services, this NHLBI site defines high blood pressure and offers information on its occurrence in pregnancy and preeclampsia. Additional consumer information includes details about those likely to develop the condition, facts about its detection, and information on related long-term heart and vessel problems. http://www.nhlbi.nih.gov/health/public/heart/hbp/hbp_preg.htm

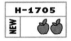

Preeclampsia (Hypertension in Pregnancy)   Created by the Allina Hospitals and Clinics, this guideline is intended to encourage high standards of care in cases of transient high blood pressure of pregnancy, preeclampsia, and eclampsia. Definitions, screening standards, and management issues are considered. Clinical manifestations of severe disease in women with gestational hypertension are summarized.
http://www2.allina.com/hnf/mpol.nsf/19bdeacd82b52379862567
f600745555/6f644ec79286064f86256866005bfde3?OpenDocument

RUBELLA (GERMAN MEASLES)

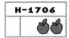

Physicians' Desk Reference Family Care Encyclopedia of Medical Care: German Measles   This site offers a description of the rubella virus, signs and symptoms of the disease, and suggested home care. The site describes symptoms requiring immediate medical attention and the danger of this virus to pregnant women.
http://www.healthsquare.com/ndfiles/nd0611.htm

Rubella Infection in Pregnancy The article found at this site, courtesy of *Communicable Diseases Intelligence,* offers a discussion of the devastating effects of the congenital rubella syndrome, despite its virtual elimination as a result of immunization practices. Four case studies present information on two cases of rubella infection and two cases of rubella primary infection occurring in pregnancy. The estimated risk of fetal damage in infection and the importance of monitoring antibody titres with each pregnancy are stressed.
http://www.dhac.gov.au/pubhlth/cdi/cdi2304/cdi2304a.htm

9.22 TRAUMATIC HEART DISEASE

eMedicine: Myocardial Rupture Myocardial rupture is described in this eMedicine publication. Background information on the condition is followed by a discussion of pathophysiology, frequency, mortality and morbidity, and demographics. Typical clinical history and physical findings, causes, differential links, suggested diagnostic procedures, and treatment details are listed. Profiles of therapeutic medications are listed, including drug name, dosage, contraindications, interactions, pregnancy safety, and important precautions. Suggested follow-up care and prognosis details are included, and images and reference citations are available.
http://www.eMedicine.com/med/topic1571.htm

Southern Medical Journal: Cardiac Rupture due to Blunt Trauma This article, courtesy of *Southern Medical Journal,* presents two case studies describing cardiac rupture due to blunt trauma. Statistics related to trauma are presented, followed by case reports and discussion of the clinical manifestations of cardiac rupture. The use of transthoracic echocardiogram, pericardiocentesis, and definitive treatment is reviewed, in addition to a discussion of the high mortality rate associated with blunt cardiac trauma.
http://www.sma.org/smj/97july17.htm

9.23 VALVULAR HEART DISEASE

GENERAL RESOURCES

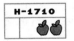

Internet Medical Education, Inc.: Valvular Disorders of the Heart Valvular disorders of the heart and related subjects are discussed in detail at this address. Specific topics include an overview of the valves of the heart, aortic regurgitation, aortic stenosis, mitral regurgitation, mitral stenosis, tricuspid regurgitation, tricuspid stenosis, pulmonic regurgitation, pulmonic stenosis, echocardiography, artificial valves, and anticoagulation. Discussion regarding diseased heart valves and prophylaxis for endocarditis is found.
http://www.med-edu.com/patient/valvular/valvular.html

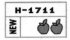

Medical Journal of Allina: Etiology of Valvular Heart Disease
Authored by Alan G. Rose, M.D., of the University of Minnesota Medical
School, this article explores the increase in incidence of acquired forms of valvular heart disease. Congenital conditions and a large variety of rare and more
common causes of valvular disease are explored, providing a basic diagnostic
tool for clinicians.
http://www.allina.com/Allina_Journal/Fall1996/rose.html

AORTIC REGURGITATION

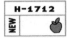

American Heart Association (AHA): Aortic Regurgitation A definition
of aortic regurgitation is provided at this AHA Web site, part of its online consumer publication collection. Causes of aortic regurgitation and an assortment
of related publications are listed, including both patient information sites and
Scientific Statements on valvular heart disease.
http://216.185.112.5/presenter.jhtml?identifier=4448

eMedicine: Aortic Regurgitation This eMedicine article provides a
discussion of aortic regurgitation, including background information on the
condition, pathophysiology, frequency, morbidity and mortality, and most
commonly affected age group. Clinical details of the condition, causes, differentials, diagnostic tools, treatment, and suggested follow-up care are also listed.
http://www.eMedicine.com/emerg/topic39.htm

AORTIC VALVE DISEASE, GENERAL

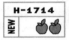

Cardiothoracic Surgery Notes: Aortic Valve Disease The morphology
of aortic valve disease and additional review of aortic valve incompetence,
symptoms, diagnosis, and natural history of aortic valve disease are found at
this page of the Cardiothoracic Surgery Notes domain. Information on associated coronary artery disease, treatment options, and selection of replacement
device is presented. Links throughout the text provide access to illustrations of
diseased valves.
http://www.ctsnet.org/residents/ctsn/archives/not42.html

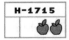

University of Alabama: Aortic Valve Disease Connections are available
at this address to a wide variety of resources on aortic valve disease. Resources
include pages of the online *Merck Manual*, CME articles, pathology images,
clinical guidelines, and consumer resources. Links are also available to directory
listings of related disorders.
http://www.slis.ua.edu/cdlp/WebDLCore/clinical/cardiology/valvular/aorticvalvedisease.html

Aortic Valve Stenosis

MedicineNet.com: Aortic Valve Stenosis MedicineNet.com offers this discussion on aortic valve stenosis, which reviews causes of the condition, its affect on the left ventricle pump, symptoms, and possible methods of diagnosis. Treatment details and related links within MedicineNet to information on diagnostic procedures and tests are available.
http://www.medicinenet.com/Script/Main/Art.asp?li=MNI&ArticleKey=279

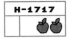

Royal Children's Hospital: Aortic Stenosis Produced by the Royal Children's Hospital in Melbourne, Australia, this site provides an overview of aortic stenosis and subaortic stenosis. The site discusses aortic valve replacement and the Ross operation, with hyperlinks to additional information on balloon valvuloplasty and the homograft valve replacement. The page also contains links to information on other heart defects, answers to frequently asked questions, a glossary of terms, and other related resources.
http://www.rch.unimelb.edu.au/cardiology/
website/Library/Aortic_Stenosis/aortic_stenosis.html

Mitral Valve Disease, General

MVPS Research and Support Dedicated to research and support for mitral valve prolapse syndrome (MVPS), offers a definition of MVPS and a discussion of complications, history, demographics, diagnosis, symptoms, and the condition in pregnancy. In a self-help section, practical methods for controlling symptoms are given and include relaxation, exercise, diet, attitude, education, medication, and quick tricks and tips. Links to support groups, information for family and friends, political action, and other resources are found, as are connections to the American Medical Association, HealthWorld Online, Stress.com, and the Health Resource Directory.
http://www.mvpsupport.com

University of Alabama: Mitral Valve Disease Resources on mitral valve disease are available through links in this online directory. Visitors can access the *Merck Manual,* CME articles, fact sheets, and clinical guidelines on mitral valve stenosis, mitral valve insufficiency, and mitral valve prolapse. Articles from eMedicine, clinical trial listings, and additional clinical resources for healthcare providers are found.
http://www.slis.ua.edu/cdlp/WebDLCore/clinical/cardiology/valvular/valve.html

Mitral Regurgitation

Cardiologychannel: Mitral Regurgitation Following a discussion of normal blood flow in the heart, this article offers readers information on symptoms associated with mitral regurgitation and the diagnostic workup. Details

concerning the decision to proceed with valve surgery, mitral valve surgical procedures, and long-term management are reviewed at the site.
http://www.cardiologychannel.com/mitralregurgitation/

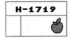

Mitral Regurgitation   Provided by the Cardiology Associates of Fort Lauderdale, this consumer fact sheet offers an overview of mitral regurgitation, including a definition and a discussion of causes, prevention, symptoms, diagnosis, and treatment.
http://cardiology-associates.com/faq/24.html

MITRAL VALVE PROLAPSE (MVP)

eMedicine: Mitral Valve Prolapse   This common anomaly of the mitral valve is described in its entirety at this page of the eMedicine database, which includes a history of the condition, its pathophysiology, physical presentation, causes, and differentials. Imaging studies and management information are provided at this comprehensive tutorial, as well as antibiotic regimens for those considered to be at risk for infective endocarditis. A chest radiograph of a child with mitral valve prolapse is displayed, and ECG tracings and both two- and three-dimensional echocardiographic images are shown.
http://www.eMedicine.com/ped/topic1465.htm

Physician and Sportsmedicine: Mitral Valve Prolapse in Active Patients   The article at this site presents information on pathophysiology and epidemiology, systemic symptoms, details regarding a multifactorial pathogenesis, key diagnostic findings, management and risk stratification, and exercise guidelines for mitral valve prolapse. Included is a table on evaluation and management of the disorder, which contains risk categories, echocardiogram evaluation guidelines, additional testing recommendations, and summaries of treatment. A section addressing complications of the disorder includes discussion of mitral regurgitation, infective endocarditis, cerebrovascular accidents, and sudden death.   http://www.physsportsmed.com/issues/jul_96/joy.htm

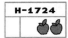

Texas Heart Institute: Mitral Valve Prolapse   Produced by the Texas Heart Institute, this site provides information about mitral valve prolapse, including a discussion of causes, risks, and treatment of the disease. A toll-free telephone information service and answers to frequently asked questions are provided, in addition to a heart health test for patients, a glossary of cardiovascular terms, and a handbook for heart health.
http://www.tmc.edu/thi/mvp.html

MITRAL VALVE STENOSIS

Clinical Reference Systems: Mitral Valve Stenosis   This fact sheet on mitral valve stenosis offers answers to several frequently asked questions about the condition. How it occurs, a listing of symptoms, methods of diagnosis, and

prophylactic treatment with antibiotics before dental work are reviewed. The page also lists several important self-care measures. http://ekhsin.morehead-st.edu/aha/crs/stenosis.htm

Virtual Hospital: Mitral Valve Stenosis Hosted by University of Iowa Health Care, this page offers a case presentation of mitral valve stenosis. An illustrative X-ray image is offered, with information on determining left ventricle enlargement concisely presented. http://www.vh.org/Providers/Lectures/icmrad/chest/parts/MVPLAE2.html

PULMONARY REGURGITATION

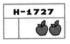

Internet Continuing Education Services: Pulmonic Regurgitation A description of an incompetent pulmonic valve and the pathophysiology and characterization of this murmur are reviewed, with connections found to a pulmonic regurgitation sound file and an illustration of proper stethoscope location. http://wices.com/PulmonicRegurgitation.htm

PULMONARY STENOSIS

American Heart Association (AHA): Pulmonary Stenosis A discussion of pulmonary stenosis includes symptoms in children and treatment for relief of the obstruction. Outlook after balloon valvuloplasty and follow-up information are included, as well as illustrations of normal and stenotic pulmonary valves. http://216.185.112.5/presenter.jhtml?identifier=1321

eMedicine: Pulmonic Valvular Stenosis The eMedicine database offers a comprehensive review of pulmonary valvular stenosis. Visitors will find an article relating to the pathophysiology, clinical and physical presentation, and management of the condition, as well as several diagnostic differential links, a diagnostic workup review, and surgical and medical management summaries. Complications, prognosis, and patient education are detailed. http://eMedicine.com/cgi-bin/foxweb.exe/showsection@d:/em/ga?book=emerg&topicid=491

University of Alabama: Pulmonary Stenosis The Clinical Digital Libraries Project of the University of Alabama offers this collection of resources on the Web specific to pulmonary stenosis. The *Merck Manual* chapter, eMedicine's online articles, and additional authoritative material may be accessed. Some resources may require an online subscription, but a wide variety of free professional references are available, ranging from documents of academic medical centers to genetic database information. (some features fee-based) http://www.slis.ua.edu/cdlp/cchs/clinical/cardiology/congenital/ps.html

TRICUSPID VALVE DISEASE, GENERAL

Merck Manual of Diagnosis and Therapy: Tricuspid Valve Disease
The *Merck Manual* online reference includes this chapter on tricuspid valve disease, addressing tricuspid insufficiency and tricuspid stenosis. Symptoms, signs, diagnosis, and management details are summarized. A link to further information on invasive diagnostic procedures is offered.
http://www.merck.com/pubs/mmanual/section16/chapter207/207d.htm

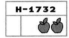

University of Alabama: Tricuspid Valve Disease   An online directory lists clinical Internet resources devoted to tricuspid valve disease. Sources include the *Merck Manual of Diagnosis and Therapy,* the American Heart Association, and the National Guideline Clearinghouse. Resources include clinical guidelines, clinical trials, and a variety of online textbook entries. Links are available to similar directories devoted to closely related topics.
http://www.slis.ua.edu/cdlp/WebDLCore/
clinical/cardiology/valvular/tricuspidvalvedisease.html

TRICUSPID REGURGITATION

Annals of Thoracic Surgery: Influence of Functional Tricuspid Regurgitation on Right Ventricular Function   This full-text article offers results of an investigation into the effect of functional tricuspid regurgitation on right ventricular function. Contact details for reprints and reference citations are available.
http://www.ctsnet.org/journal/ATS/66/2044

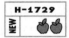

MEDLINEplus Medical Encyclopedia: Tricuspid Regurgitation
Maintained by the National Library of Medicine, this MEDLINEplus encyclopedia entry includes a variety of illustrations depicting tricuspid insufficiency. A definition of the condition, fundamental information about common causes and risks, and the importance of obtaining prompt treatment are summarized. Links to related pages of the MEDLINE database offer further details on symptoms, diagnostic tests, and possible complications.
http://www.nlm.nih.gov/medlineplus/ency/article/000169.htm

TRICUSPID STENOSIS

Internet Continuing Education Services: Tricuspid Stenosis   A description of the narrowing of tricuspid stenosis is found at this site, and information on its detection is offered. Proper stethoscope placement and different types of tricuspid stenosis murmurs are introduced. In addition, a related audio file of the murmur and a listing of causes are offered.
http://www.wices.com/TricuspidStenosis.htm

9.24 VASCULAR DISEASE

GENERAL RESOURCES

American Heart Association (AHA): Peripheral Vascular Disease The AHA introduces information on functional and organic peripheral vascular disease, including its causes, diagnosis, and treatment. An online brochure on peripheral vascular disease can be accessed from the site by connecting to a link of the Society of Cardiovascular and Interventional Radiology. Related AHA publications are listed, in addition to AHA Scientific Statements on diagnosis and treatment of these conditions.
http://216.185.112.5/presenter.jhtml?identifier=4692

Columbia University Home Medical Guide: Peripheral Blood Vessel Diseases This home medical guide, offered as a service of Columbia University, provides comprehensive information about peripheral blood vessel diseases. The diseases are divided into the two categories of peripheral arterial diseases and peripheral venous diseases. The site describes arteriosclerosis obliterans, Buerger's disease, and Raynaud's disease and phenomenon. For each disease, there is a definition as well as information about causes, diagnosis, treatment, prevention, and gender specificity.
http://cpmcnet.columbia.edu/texts/guide/hmg16_0005.html

International Society on Thrombosis and Haemostasis This nonprofit organization has more than two thousand members from more than 50 countries. The site provides information about the organization and membership, fellowship programs, upcoming meetings and conferences, and committees. The site contains links to relevant registries and databases, working groups and liaison reports, and a variety of related sites.
http://www.med.unc.edu/isth/welcome

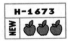

Postgraduate Medicine: Peripheral Vascular Disease An introduction to a three-article symposium on peripheral vascular disease is found at the September 1999 issue of *Postgraduate Medicine,* with all chapters accessible from the page. The first article introduces noninvasive diagnostics of patients with suspected or known disease and offers information on nonsurgical treatment methods. Diagnostic approaches are the focus of the second article, which discusses appropriate use of both catheter-based diagnostic and treatment options. Surgical management of peripheral vascular disease is the subject of the third article, providing insight into the risks and benefits of various surgical techniques. http://www.postgradmed.com/issues/1999/09_99/symp_int.htm

ACROCYANOSIS

Merck Manual of Diagnosis and Therapy: Acrocyanosis Acrocyanosis is described briefly in this online chapter of the *Merck Manual of Diagnosis*

and Therapy. Links are available to information on related peripheral vascular disorders. http://www.merck.com/pubs/mmanual/section16/chapter212/212e.htm

ARTERIOVENOUS FISTULA

CliniWeb International: Arteriovenous Malformations Links are available in this directory to research articles and other resources devoted to arteriovenous fistula and related arteriovenous malformations. Access is provided to discussions of multimodality treatment, as well as to preformatted query links at the National Library of Medicine's PubMed database.
http://www.ohsu.edu/cliniweb/C16/C16.131.240.150.html

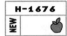

Merck Manual of Diagnosis and Therapy: Arteriovenous Fistula A description of the abnormal communication between an artery and a vein involved in this disease process is found at this page. Details on variants of the condition and additional information concerning symptoms, signs, and conservative management are included.
http://www.merck.com/pubs/mmanual/section16/chapter212/212i.htm

CAROTID ARTERY DISEASE

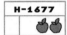

BrighamRAD: Carotid Artery Stenosis This teaching case file, created by Brigham and Women's Hospital and Harvard University, contains information about carotid artery stenosis. Nine diagnostic images are included, accompanied by a discussion of differential diagnosis.
http://www.brighamrad.harvard.edu/Cases/bwh/hcache/6/full.html

ERYTHROMELALGIA

eMedicine: Erythromelalgia This eMedicine entry provides nearly a dozen sections on erythromelalgia, including pathophysiology, a classic description of the condition, and details on the physical examination and causes. Diagnostic differential links within the eMedicine database can be accessed, and information on the diagnostic workup is included. Additional details on medical care are provided, as well as a figure illustrating cardinal symptoms.
http://www.emedicine.com/med/topic730.htm

Merck Manual of Diagnosis and Therapy: Erythromelalgia The *Merck Manual of Diagnosis and Therapy* reference offers this chapter on the specific peripheral vascular disorder erythromelalgia. This rare condition of paroxysmal vasodilation combined with burning and increased skin temperature is further characterized at the site, with diagnostic information and differentiation between primary and secondary types discussed. Methods of attack avoidance are outlined, and links to related, indexed peripheral vascular disorders may be accessed directly from the site.
http://www.merck.com/pubs/mmanual/section16/chapter212/212f.htm

Klippel-Trenaunay-Weber Syndrome
(Lymphedema/Venous Thrombosis)

Klippel-Trenaunay Syndrome Support Group   Designed as a resource for families, adults with Klippel-Trenaunay syndrome, and healthcare professionals, this site offers background information about the disease and the Klippel-Trenaunay Syndrome Support Group. It provides a description of the disorder, including its association with a variety of peripheral vascular symptoms, its etiology, treatment, and associated terminology. A summary chapter about the disease, authored by a professor of pediatric cardiology at the Mayo Clinic, is found, and information about the group is provided, including upcoming meetings, activities, and goals and objectives.
http://www.k-t.org

Lipedema

Merck Manual of Diagnosis and Therapy: Lipedema   A brief description of this peripheral vascular disorder is available at this online chapter of the *Merck Manual of Diagnosis and Therapy*. Otherwise referred to as painful fat syndrome, an overall characterization of the condition and general recommendations are made. Links are provided to information on related conditions.
http://www.merck.com/pubs/mmanual/section16/chapter212/212k.htm

Lymphedema

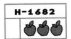

National Lymphedema Network   The National Lymphedema Network spreads information on the prevention and management of primary and secondary lymphedema to patients, healthcare professionals, and the general public. Information on lymphedema treatment centers and support groups, the quarterly newsletter, and the biennial conference is available from the site. Other resources include a discussion of lymphedema, contact details for local support groups, suggestions on choosing a lymphedema therapist, treatment and diagnostic center directories, a catalog of publications, and information on legislation activities.
http://www.lymphnet.org

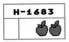

University of Pittsburgh: Lymphedema Family Study   The Lymphedema Family Study hopes to identify the gene or genes resulting in primary lymphedema, leading to improved methods of early detection and treatment of this condition. This site offers discussions of the genetics of primary lymphedema, prior investigations of the disorder, and current research at the University of Pittsburgh. Frequently asked questions about lymphedema are answered at the site.   http://www.pitt.edu/~genetics/lymph

RAYNAUD'S DISEASE/PHENOMENON

Life Extension Foundation: Raynaud's Syndrome Comprehensive in its treatment of Raynaud's syndrome, this site provides a brief overview, history, and definition of the disease. There is extensive information about the symptoms and physical effects of the disorder, in addition to behavioral strategies for preventing attacks and physical therapies for arresting an attack in progress. The site discusses specific pharmacologic therapies, such as calcium channel blockers, vasodilators and pentoxifylline, antiplatelet agents, nitroglycerine cream, and new drugs. A discussion of vitamins and minerals used to manage the condition and several journal abstracts related to Raynaud's syndrome may be accessed.
http://www.lef.org/protocols/prtcl-128.shtml

National Heart, Lung, and Blood Institute (NHLBI): Raynaud's Syndrome As a service of the National Institutes of Health, this site offers information about symptoms, causes, incidence, and diagnosis of Raynaud's disease. A discussion outlining the difference between primary and secondary stages of the disease is found.
http://www.nhlbi.nih.gov/health/public/blood/other/raynaud.htm

Raynaud's Foundation This nonprofit organization promotes education and research on Raynaud's phenomenon and related diseases, including autoimmune and non-autoimmune varieties. Resources at this site include general information about the disease, information on biofeedback training, research projects, and details regarding the foundation and its membership. A collection of links to related sites may be viewed.
http://members.aol.com/raynauds

TELANGIECTASIAS

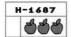

American College of Phlebology: Technique for Treating Telangiectasias and Reticular Veins This online treatment primer, courtesy of the American College of Phlebology, offers practitioners information on the major principles involved in treatment of telangiectasias, including maximizing therapeutic efficacy and the incidence of side effects. Materials for sclerotherapy, presclerotherapy compression and photographic documentation, and technique alternatives are reviewed.
http://www.phlebology.org/syllabus6.htm

THROMBOANGIITIS OBLITERANS (BUERGER'S DISEASE)

HealthCentral: Thromboangiitis Obliterans This informative site provides an overview of thromboangiitis obliterans. Alternative names for the

disease and discussions on causes, incidence, risk factors, prevention, symptoms, signs and tests, treatment, prognosis, and complications are found.
http://www.healthcentral.com/peds/top/000172.cfm

National Organization for Rare Disorders (NORD): Buerger's Disease In addition to synonyms for Buerger's disease, this NORD entry includes a general discussion on the symptoms and possible causes for the disorder. Resources for additional information are available, and the opportunity to order the full-text report for a fee is offered.
http://www.rarediseases.org/cgi-bin/nord/abstrfly?id=NqFIWi7a&mv_arg=RDB%2d712&mv_pc=66

Varicose Veins

MEDLINEplus Health Information: Varicose Veins The National Library of Medicine has organized an extensive collection of Web links at this site, intended for a variety of audiences. General overviews on varicose veins and their treatment; clinical trial connections; a self-care flowchart from the American Academy of Family Physicians; and an interactive tutorial on sclerotherapy from the Patient Education Institute are available.
http://www.nlm.nih.gov/medlineplus/varicoseveins.html

VEINSonline.com VEINSonline is an Internet-based organization of doctors seeking to inform the general public about vein problems and treatments. Their site provides varicose vein information and provider referrals. Lists of specialists in the United States, Australia, and Canada are found, and the site answers frequently asked questions on the condition. Before and after treatment photographs and information for physicians about upcoming meetings and medical products for sale are offered. http://www.veinsonline.com/index.html

Venous Thrombosis

American College of Phlebology The American College of Phlebology (ACP) was founded in 1985 to improve the standards of practice and patient care related to venous disorders. The site contains information about the ACP's founders, history, workshops, courses, publications, meetings, and membership. A phlebology primer provides current guidelines in the evaluation and management of patients with varicose veins, thrombosis, thrombophlebitis, and venous leg ulcers. The site also contains a patient brochure, a member database, and links to additional sites related to phlebology.
http://www.phlebology.org

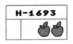

Boston University Medical Center: Phlebitis This site provides a general definition of phlebitis and its causes. A discussion of the symptoms and complications associated with the disease is found, and information about treatment for pain and itching is offered.
http://web.bu.edu/cohis/cardvasc/vessel/vein/phlebtis.htm

Boston University Medical Center: Venous Thrombosis A product of the Community Outreach Health Information System, this site provides comprehensive patient information about thrombosis. It contains sections on causes, diagnosis, and treatment. A discussion of deep venous thrombosis contains graphics and hyperlinks, and a list of drugs used to treat the disorder is found. Links to discussions of related problems, including chronic venous insufficiency, phlebitis, pulmonary embolism, varicose veins, and problems with the arteries, are accessible.
http://web.bu.edu/cohis/cardvasc/vessel/vein/thrombos.htm

Sol Sherry Thrombosis Research Center Part of Temple University School of Medicine, the Sol Sherry Thrombosis Research Center provides information about the disorder to patients and professionals alike. Answers to frequently asked questions are found, as well as details regarding genetic clotting disorders and deep venous thrombosis. Physician references include links to the Thrombosis Interest Group, the Online Mendelian Inheritance in Man (OMIM) database, and the National Center for Biotechnology Information. Connections to information on potential therapeutic agents and development of diagnostics are provided, as well as direct access to scientific, peer-reviewed journals in hemostasis and thrombosis. Related research centers, such as the Mount Sinai Thrombosis Research Center, are accessible.
http://www.temple.edu/sstrc/generalinfo.html

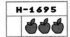

Thrombosis Interest Group of Canada The mission of the Thrombosis Interest Group of Canada is to promote education and research in the prevention and treatment of thrombosis. The Web site contains links to treatment guidelines divided into adult and pediatric patients, long-term therapy, acute therapy and diagnosis, and monitoring and testing sections. Patients taking anticoagulant medication may access information about the drug they are using. The site also contains links to other Web resources in the categories of societies, research groups, images, journal searches, treatment information, and medical links. http://www.tigc.org/english.htm

VON HIPPEL-LINDAU DISEASE

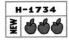

Von Hippel-Lindau (VHL) Family Alliance The VHL Family Alliance is dedicated to improving diagnosis, treatment, and quality of life for patients with von Hippel-Lindau disease. The site provides information in seven languages, including answers to frequently asked questions; details regarding meetings, donations, and membership; news about the society; and current headlines about the disease. An online reference handbook offers information about contraction, detection, possible manifestations, pregnancy and VHL, diagnosis, treatment, research, and living with the disease. An extensive reference section containing a glossary is available, and links to related sites are provided.
http://www.vhl.org

GENERAL MEDICAL WEB RESOURCES

REFERENCE INFORMATION AND NEWS SOURCES

10.1 GENERAL MEDICAL SUPERSITES

Visitors interested in medical supersites may also find similar information under the medical search engine section.

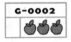

American Medical Association (AMA) The AMA develops and promotes standards in medical practice, research, and education; acts as advocate on behalf of patients and physicians; and provides discourse on matters important to public health in America. General information is available at the site about the organization; journals and newsletters; policy, advocacy, activities, and ethics; education; and accreditation services. AMA news and consumer health information are also found at the site. Resources for physicians include membership details; information on the AMA's current procedural terminology (CPT) information services, the resource-based relative value scale (RBVS), and electronic medical systems; information on the AMA Alliance (a national organization of physicians' spouses); descriptions of additional AMA products and services; a discussion of legal issues for physicians; and information on AMA's global activities. Information for consumers includes medical news; detailed information on a wide range of conditions; family health resources for children, adolescents, men, and women; interactive health calculators; healthy recipes; and general safety tips. Specific pages are devoted to comprehensive resources related to HIV/AIDS, asthma, migraines, and women's health.

http://www.ama-assn.org

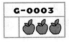

BioSites BioSites is a comprehensive catalog of selected Internet resources in the medical and biomedical sciences. The sites were selected as part of a project by staff members of Resource Libraries within the Pacific Southwest Region of the National Network of Libraries of Medicine. Sites are organized by medical topic or specialty field, and users can also search the site by keyword. Featured Web sites are listed by title; details are provided within each hyperlink.

http://www.library.ucsf.edu/biosites

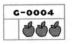

Doctor's Guide The Doctor's Guide to the Internet, provided by PSL Consulting Group, Inc., contains a professional edition for healthcare professionals and a section directed at patients. Information of medical and professional interest includes medical news and alerts, new drugs or indications, medical conferences, the Congress Resource Center, a medical bookstore, and Internet medical resources. Patient resources are organized by specific diseases or condition. Users can search the World Wide Web through Excite, InfoSeek, McKinley, and Alta Vista search engines or can search the Doctor's Guide medical news and conference database.

(free registration) http://www.docguide.com

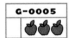

Emory University: MedWeb   Maintained by the library staff of Emory University, MedWeb offers more than 100 subjects encompassing a comprehensive catalog of thousands of biomedical and health-related sites. Visitors can perform a keyword search or browse through categories such as biological and physical sciences, clinical practice, consumer health, diseases and conditions, drugs, healthcare, institutions, mental health, publications, and specialties. A subject index is available to browse the entire catalog.

http://www.medweb.emory.edu/Medweb/

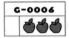

Galaxy: Medicine   Intended primarily for consumer reference, Galaxy Health provides topic-specific search engines in over 30 health-related areas. Categories include diseases, fitness, mental health, weight loss, and dentistry. Each topic contains links to online articles, discussion groups, periodicals, and organizations. http://health.galaxy.com

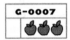

Hardin MD   Hosted by the Hardin Library for the Health Sciences at the University of Iowa, this site features a meta-directory of Internet health sites. More than 40 subjects are listed in the directory such as AIDS, cancer, dermatology, neurology, pregnancy, and pediatrics. The directory contains thousands of sites. By clicking on a subject, visitors will find lists of Internet sites compiled from other Web pages. Each list is ranked according to depth of content. In addition to the meta-directory, links are provided to an array of news sources, medical libraries, free journals online, and consumer-oriented sites.

http://www.lib.uiowa.edu/hardin/md/

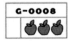

Health On the Net (HON) Foundation   The Health On the Net Foundation site offers an engine that searches the Internet as well as the foundation's database for medical sites, hospitals, and support communities. HON also provides a dossier with in-depth information on topics such as mother and child, allergy, vision and eye care, smoking cessation, hepatitis B, rare diseases, and aging. A media gallery contains a database of medical images and videos from various sources. The site also features articles from a daily news archive, a conference locator, and surveys of health trends. Users can select a target group, such as healthcare providers, medical professionals, or patients and other individuals, to receive more tailored search results.

http://www.hon.ch

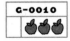

HealthWeb   With support from a National Library of Medicine grant, this collaborative effort of over 20 health sciences libraries offers a meta-directory of health-related, noncommercial Web sites. The sites are categorized into approximately 70 different subject areas such as AIDS, anatomy, dermatology, hematology, and toxicology. Within each subject, sites are further classified by clinical resources, academic institutes, statistics, conferences, consumer health resources, online publications, and organizations. For each site listed, there is a brief description of its contents.

http://healthweb.org/index.cfm

Karolinska Institutet: Diseases, Disorders and Related Topics

Karolinska Institutet, a medical university, offers ample resources for both professionals and the general public at this collection. Covering every major field of medicine, the site provides a database of fact sheets and Web sites on individual diseases, pathology databases, clinical guidelines, research, and anatomy and other medical tutorials. Databases for biological sciences, bioethics, medical images, and medical news are also available, as well as "Ask the Doctor" and second-opinion services. Visitors can locate information via an alphabetical list of diseases or through more than 20 directories in a particular field of medicine. Other resources of the Karolinska Institutet include MEDLINE access, electronic journals, and a Medical Subject Headings (MeSH) tree tool for finding references and links to other resources.

http://micf.mic.ki.se/Diseases

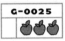

Martindale's Health Science Guide: Virtual Medical Center

The Virtual Medical Center claims to have more than 61,500 teaching files, 129,800 medical cases, 1,155 courses/textbooks, 1,580 tutorials, 4,100 databases, and thousands of movies. The information is listed in categories on the home page such as biomechanics, cancer, immunology, microbiology, sports medicine, and toxicology. Separate sections contain information on public health, environmental health, and travel warnings. The site also provides resources such as a physician finder, clinical trials, CME, medical codes, laboratory diagnostics, blood-related information, hospitals worldwide, medical auctions, and medical dictionaries in eight languages.

http://www-sci.lib.uci.edu/~martindale/Medical.html

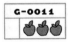

MedExplorer

Created by a Canadian paramedic, MedExplorer provides a database of Web sites covering a wide array of health topics for health professionals and the public. Links to an enormous number of sites, along with brief descriptions of site contents, are categorized into nearly 30 health-related topics such as allied health, alternative medicine, education, employment, government, laboratory, medical imaging, research, and specialty medicine. There are also discussion forums, an employment center, and health news headlines. Health centers of resources for women, men, children, and seniors are also included, as well as a nutrition database, an online health exam, access to MEDLINE, and more than 250 health newsgroups.

http://www.medexplorer.com/

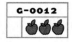

Medical Matrix Medical Matrix offers a list of directories categorized into specialties, diseases, clinical practice resources, literature, education, healthcare and professional resources, medical computing, Internet and technology, and marketplace resources containing classifieds and employment opportunities. Additional features include a site search engine; access to MEDLINE, clinical searches, and links to symposia on the Web; medical textbook resources; patient education materials; CME information; news; and online journals. Free registration is necessary to access the site.

(free registration) http://www.medmatrix.org

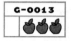

Medicine Online Offering a broad range of medical information, this site contains resources of interest to both physicians and patients. The reference section features a medical dictionary, fact sheets on diseases and treatments, and a drug index. Visitors will also find comprehensive listings of Internet resources in categories such as diseases and conditions, medicine, public health, women's health, and allied health. Unique to the site are "Bid for Surgery" and "Bid for Rx" centers where consumers enter their requirements for cosmetic procedures or prescriptions and physicians or pharmacists respond with their qualifications, location, and price. Directories of physicians, hospitals, and vendors are provided, and a link to MOL.net takes the visitor to a portal offering a customizable home page for professionals with access to "Bid for surgery," reference information, message boards, and information on laboratory management. By accessing the "Health Topics" menu, viewers are taken to large selections of general resources and links for the chosen topic.

(free registration) http://www.medicineonline.net/

MedicineNet.com Described as "100 percent doctor-produced healthcare information," this Web page offers fact sheets written in laymen's terms on a variety of health-related topics. Areas covered include allergies, arthritis, asthma, cancer, cholesterol, depression, diabetes, digestion, high blood pressure, HIV, thyroid, and women's health. Alphabetized indices on diseases and conditions, procedures and tests, medications, and healthy living (nutrition and fitness) are also available, as well as a medical dictionary and an online drugstore. The home page features news, updates, and information on commonly requested conditions such as acne, asthma, cancer, and diabetes. Also on the home page is quick reference information such as first aid, poison control, and product recalls. http://www.medicinenet.com/Script/Main/hp.asp

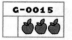

MEDLINEplus Sponsored by the National Library of Medicine, the world's largest medical library, and the National Institutes of Health, this site provides up-to-date, high-quality healthcare information. Resources on this Web page cover an array of health information for professionals and consumers. The "Health Topics" section offers more than 30 broad topics, each with several subsections leading to additional links to information such as overviews, clinical trials, diagnosis and symptoms, specific conditions, policy, organizations, statistics, and Spanish publications. The site also features drug information, with a guide to more than 9,000 prescription and over-the-counter medications. There

are several medical dictionaries, along with directories of physicians and hospitals. Information found under the "Other Resources" section includes organizations, libraries, publications, databases, and access to MEDLINE.
http://www.medlineplus.gov/

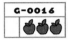

MedMark: Medical Bookmarks Designed by a physician, this Web page is a comprehensive directory of thousands of health-related sites with information for both the professional and consumer. Sites are categorized under more than 30 specialties such as endocrinology, immunology, and pediatrics. Clicking on a specialty brings up a list of Internet sites organized in categories such as associations, centers, departments, education and training, consumer information, guidelines, journals, and programs. There are also links for free access to MEDLINE (registration required), as well as a list of related sites that contain large directories of resources. At the top of the site, there is a link for sites in Korea.
http://members.kr.inter.net/medmark/

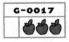

MedNets This international research site uses proprietary search engines for accessing information on specialties in medicine. Users select from one of four areas including a research engine and communities geared toward professionals, patients, and the health industry. The community for professionals covers nearly 50 topics of interest to clinicians, including anesthesiology, family medicine, managed care, pathology, practice guidelines, and telemedicine. Within each topic are links to associations, clinical information, centers of excellence, and news and research.
http://www.mednets.com

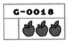

Medscape Medscape offers a directory of Web sites that provide information on a wide range of medical specialties. Information in each specialty includes news items, conference summaries and schedules, treatment updates, practice guidelines, articles, and patient resources. Medscape also offers resources for medical students, medical office managers, nurses, and pharmacists.
(free registration) http://www.medscape.com

Medscout The Medscout Web page offers a directory of health-related Web sites. More than 50 broad topics are listed such as clinical alerts, CME, diseases, employment, guidelines, hospitals, informatics, journals, medical supplies, and telemedicine, and each topic is broken down into further subtopics with hyperlinks. The site also includes extensive information on the Health Insurance Portability and Accountability Act (HIPAA), as well as several fee-based tools for securely connecting healthcare professionals to payers, pharmacies, and each other. (some features fee-based) http://www.medscout.com/

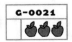

Megasite Project: A Metasite Comparing Health Information Megasites and Search Engines The Megasite Project, created by librarians at Northwestern University, the University of Michigan, and Pennsylvania State University, evaluates and provides direct links to 25 of the largest health information Internet sites. Criteria for evaluation and comparison include administration and quality control, content, and design. Users can access results of site

evaluations, tips for successful site searches, unique features of particular sites, lists of the best general and health information search engines reviewed, and site comparisons listed by evaluation criteria. A bibliography of articles on Web design and Internet resource evaluation is found at the address, as well as descriptions of other aspects of the project.
http://www.lib.umich.edu/megasite/toc.html

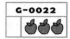

National Library of Medicine (NLM)   The National Library of Medicine, the world's largest medical library, collects materials in all areas of biomedicine and healthcare and focuses on biomedical aspects of technology; the humanities; and the physical, life, and social sciences. This site contains links to government medical databases, including MEDLINE and MEDLINEplus, information on funding opportunities at the National Library of Medicine and other federal agencies, and details of services, training, and outreach programs offered by NLM. Users can access NLM's catalog of resources (LOCATORPlus), as well as NLM publications, including fact sheets, published reports, and staff publications. NLM research programs discussed at the site include topics in computational molecular biology, medical informatics, and other related subjects. The Web site features 15 databases, covering journal searches via MEDLINE; AIDS information via AIDSLINE, AIDSDRUGS, and AIDSTRIALS; bioethics via BIOETHICSLINE; and numerous other important topics. The NLM Gateway—a master search engine—searches MEDLINE using the user-friendly retrieval engine called PubMed. There are over 11-million citations in MEDLINE and PreMEDLINE and the other related databases. Additionally, the NLM provides sources of health statistics, serials programs, and services maintained through a system called SERHOLD.
http://www.nlm.nih.gov

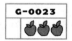

New York Online Access to Health (NOAH): Health Topics and Resources   The entire NOAH Web page is available in English and Spanish and offers a broad array of health information. Visitors can browse by subject or alphabetically. The home page features more than 30 health topics such as AIDS, arthritis, cancer, kidney diseases, and nutrition. By clicking on a topic, a long list of links appears for in-depth information such as a description of the disease or condition along with diagnosis, symptoms, and treatment. There is also a resource section for more information including patient rights, medications, support groups, and New York City and county healthcare and community services resources.
http://www.noah-health.org/english/qksearch.html

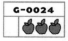

University of Iowa: Virtual Hospital   A service of the University of Iowa Health Care system, this Web page features the Virtual Hospital, a digital library with more than 350 peer-reviewed books and booklets. Separate sections are available for healthcare providers and patients. The provider section is organized by categories such as specialty, department, organ system, and by type of information, including multimedia, textbooks, journals, and guidelines. The patient section contains categories such as problem, department, organ system, and FAQs. The "Common Problems" link provides a comprehensive alphabetical list of the site's contents, with separate professional and patient links. The home page also features a link to the Virtual Children's Hospital, as well as CME online courses.

http://www.vh.org

WebMDHealth High-quality consumer health information and resources are available at this address. Consumer resources include information on conditions, treatments, and drugs; medical news and articles; a forum for obtaining answers to health questions; online chat events with medical experts; and articles and expert advice on general health topics. Consumers can also join a "community" for more personalized information and forums. A section for health teachers offers lesson guides and teacher supports for improving school-based health education. Physician services, available for a fee, include access to medical news, online journals, and reference databases; online insurance verification and referrals; e-mail, voice mail, fax, and conference call capabilities; practice management tools; online trading; financial services; and other resources. The site offers a preview tour of the service for interested professionals.

(some features fee-based) http://www.webmd.com

10.2 ABBREVIATIONS

Acronym and Abbreviation List This site offers a database of acronyms and abbreviations. Visitors can search for an acronym and see what it means, or search for a word and its related acronym.

http://www.ucc.ie/info/net/acronyms/index.html

Common Medical Abbreviations Several hundred major medical abbreviations are defined in an alphabetical listing at this educational information site.

http://courses.smsu.edu/jas188f/690/medslpterm.html

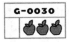

How to Read a Prescription A guide to interpreting a prescription is offered on this Web page, directed to consumers. More than 20 common abbreviations are listed along with their interpretation.

http://www.oag.state.md.us/Consumer/ibt1.htm

National Council for Emergency Medicine Informatics The National Council for Emergency Medicine Informatics provides a database for medical abbreviations and acronyms. By clicking on "Abbreviation Translator" and entering the letters to be identified, single or multiple definitions will be returned.

http://www.ncemi.org

10.3 ABSTRACT, CITATION, AND FULL-TEXT SEARCH TOOLS

EMBASE: Medical Abstracts Database Produced by Elsevier Science, the EMBASE database contains more than 13-million citations from the biomedical and pharmacological literature. Entries from 1974 to the present also contain abstracts. A distinction noted from the site asserts that EMBASE is "renowned for its comprehensive international coverage." The database is updated daily, and a free demo is available from this site.

(fee-based) http://www.embase.com/

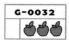

Infomine: Scholarly Internet Resources Infomine offers biological, agricultural, and medical Internet Web site collections, primarily consisting of university-level research and education. There are close to 20,000 links, including databases, electronic journals, textbooks, and conference proceedings. Web sites can be browsed by author, title, subject, or keyword. Recently added sites are stored in a separate section. The site also offers links to additional Internet medical resources.

http://infomine.ucr.edu/search/bioagsearch.phtml

InfoTrieve: Article Finder A database of more than 20 million citations drawn from over 30,000 scientific, technical, and medical journals can be searched on this site, dating back to 1966. Users can order reprints of articles through the site for a fee.

(some features fee-based) http://www4.infotrieve.com/search/databases/newsearch.asp

National Cancer Institute (NCI): Literature and Bibliographic Database of Cancer Information The NCI offers this Web page with links to a broad array of cancer literature. Visitors can search CancerLit, NCI's bibliographic database with more than 1.5 million citations and abstracts. NCI publications for professionals and the public are available online; categories include types of cancer, treatment options, clinical trials, genetics, coping with cancer, testing for cancer, and risk factors. A general category encompasses clinical research and statistics. Peer-reviewed summaries on treatment, screening, prevention, genetics, and supportive care are available through a link to PDQ, NCI's cancer database. There are separate sections for professionals and patient information in PDQ, as well as directories of physicians and cancer care organizations. The *Journal of the National Cancer Institute* is available online to subscribers. In addition, there are links to other cancer literature Internet sites.

(some features fee-based) http://cnetdb.nci.nih.gov/cancerlit.html

National Library of Medicine (NLM): Online Databases This site offers links to and descriptions of the databases and electronic information sources provided by the National Library of Medicine. Topics covered include bioethics, biotechnology, cancer information, clinical trials, consumer information, HIV/AIDS resources, history of medicine, population information, and toxicology and environmental health information. Links provided include MEDLINE via PubMed; MCA/MR; a multiple congenital anomaly/mental retardation database; and MEDLINEplus, information for consumers. Hyperlinks on each topic offer further information on the resources available and how to access them.

http://www.nlm.nih.gov/databases/databases.html

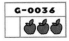
G-0036

National Library of Medicine (NLM): PubMed PubMed is a free MEDLINE search service, from the National Library of Medicine, providing access to over 11-million citations with links to the full text of articles from more than 4,000 biomedical journals. Probably the most heavily used and reputable free MEDLINE site, PubMed permits advanced searching by subject, author, journal title, and many other fields. It includes an easy-to-use "citation matcher" for completing and identifying references, and its PreMEDLINE database provides journal citations before they are indexed, making this version of MEDLINE more up-to-date than most.
http://www.ncbi.nlm.nih.gov/PubMed

G-0034
NEW

National Library of Medicine Gateway Designed as a "one-stop shopping" portal for Internet users seeking information in the extensive National Library of Medicine collections, the NLM Gateway offers an extremely convenient and powerful search tool to simultaneously search multiple retrieval systems at NLM. Information for both professionals and consumers is drawn from MEDLINE, a bibliographic database containing more than 11 million journal citations from 1966 to the present; OLDMEDLINE, journal citations from 1958 to 1965; MEDLINEplus, consumer health information on more than 400 topics; and MEDLINEplus drug information covering more than 9,000 drugs. Additional resources at NLM include LOCATORPlus, a catalog of records for books, serials, and audiovisual materials; DIRLINE, a directory of health organizations, research resources, projects, and databases; meeting abstracts from AIDS meetings and health services research (HSR) meetings; as well as information on HSR projects in progress. Links on the site direct visitors to information on ordering documents, clinical trials, clinical alerts, TOXNET (a toxicology database), and the health services/technology assessment text (HSTAT) database. http://gateway.nlm.nih.gov/gw/Cmd

10.4 FEDERAL HEALTH AGENCIES

GENERAL RESOURCES

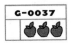
G-0037

Federal Web Locator This is a useful search engine for links to federal government sites and information on the World Wide Web. The locator maintains separate sections of latest additions, quick jumps, and Web servers. Users can also search by agency name.
http://www.infoctr.edu/fwl

HEALTH AND HUMAN SERVICES

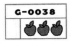
G-0038

Department of Health and Human Services This site lists Department of Health and Human Services (HHS) agencies and provides links to the individual agency sites. It offers news, press releases, and information on accessing

HHS records and contacting HHS officials. It also provides a search engine for all federal HHS agencies and access to HealthFinder.
http://www.os.dhhs.gov

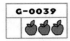

Administration for Children and Families This site provides descriptions of, resources for, and links to ACF programs and services. These sites detail programs and services that relate to areas such as welfare and family assistance, child support, foster care and adoption, Head Start, and support for Native Americans, refugees, and the developmentally disabled. Updated news and information are provided as well.
http://www.acf.dhhs.gov

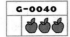

Administration on Aging (AOA) This site provides resources for seniors, practitioners, and caregivers. Resources include news on aging, links to Web sites on aging, statistics about older people, consumer fact sheets, retirement and financial planning information, and help finding community assistance for seniors. http://www.aoa.dhhs.gov

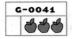

Agency for Healthcare Research and Quality (AHRQ) The Agency for Healthcare Research and Quality (AHRQ) site offers healthcare professionals clinical information, research findings, quality assessment, and information on funding opportunities. In the clinical information section there are evidence-based practice reports, outcomes research findings, technology assessments, preventive services, and clinical practice guidelines. Users may also access data and surveys such as the medical expenditure panel survey and an interactive tool for hospital statistics, a publications catalog, and an electronic reading room. A section of the site is dedicated to consumers and offers fact sheets on health conditions, health plans, prescriptions, prevention, quality of care, smoking cessation, and surgery. Some fact sheets are available in Spanish.
http://www.ahrq.gov/

Agency for Toxic Substances and Disease Registry The mission of this agency is "to prevent exposure and adverse human health effects and diminished quality of life associated with exposure to hazardous substances from waste sites, unplanned releases, and other sources of pollution present in the environment." To this end, the site posts national alerts and health advisories. It provides answers to frequently asked questions about hazardous substances and lists the minimal risk levels for each of them. The site offers the HazDat database, developed to provide access to information on the release of hazardous substances from Superfund sites or from emergency events as well as to information on the effects of hazardous substances on the health of human populations. The quarterly *Hazardous Substances and Public Health Newsletter* is available at the site, as are additional resources for children, parents, and teachers. http://www.atsdr.cdc.gov/atsdrhome.html

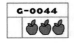

Centers for Medicare & Medicaid Services Information on Medicare, Medicaid, and child health insurance programs is provided at this site of the Centers for Medicare & Medicaid Services, formerly the Health Care Financing

Administration. Statistical data on enrollment in the various programs as well as analysis of recent trends in healthcare spending, employment, and pricing is also provided. The site offers consumer publications and program forms which are available for download.

http://www.hcfa.gov

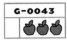

Food and Drug Administration (FDA)   The FDA is one of the oldest consumer protection agencies in the United States, monitoring the manufacture, import, transport, storage, and sale of about $1-trillion worth of products each year. This comprehensive site provides information on the safety of foods, human and animal drugs, blood products, cosmetics, and medical devices. The site also contains details of field operations, current regulations, toxicology research, medical products reporting procedures, and answers to frequently asked questions. Users can search the site by keyword and find specific information targeted to consumers, industry, health professionals, patients, state and local officials, women, and children.

http://www.fda.gov

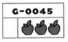

Indian Health Service   The Indian Health Service provides federal health services to American Indians and Alaskan Natives. Information of interest to physicians is primarily contained in the "About the IHS" section. This section offers access to the Native Health Research bibliographic database, with some entries containing full-text articles. There is also a Native Health History database covering the years 1652-1970. Clinical practice guideline information is provided, including IHS patient education protocols. Also within this section is an IHS facility locator. The site also describes their programs under the "Medical Programs" section, relating to such topics as AIDS, child health, diabetes, and elder care. In addition, there is information on health professional jobs, scholarships, and office locations.

http://www.ihs.gov

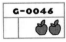

National Center for Toxicological Research   Charged with supporting the U.S. Food and Drug Administration's regulatory needs by researching the effects of toxicity and improving human exposure and risk assessment methods, the National Center for Toxicological Research describes their activities on this site. Under the "Science" section, there are descriptions of NCTR research projects, a bibliography of related NCTR publications, and the full text of the report on each year's activities.

http://www.fda.gov/nctr/index.html

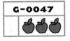

National Guideline Clearinghouse (NGC)   The National Guideline Clearinghouse (NGC) is a database of evidence-based clinical practice guidelines and related documents produced by the Agency for Healthcare Research and Quality, in partnership with the American Medical Association and the American Association of Health Plans. Users can search the database by keyword or browse by disease category.

http://www.guidelines.gov/index.asp

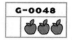

Public Health Service The Public Health Service is an umbrella organization consisting of many health service agencies and programs. Their site offers links to public health service agencies such as the National Institutes of Health, the Centers for Disease Control and Prevention, and the U.S. Food and Drug Administration. Links to offices dedicated to public health include the Office of Minority Health and the Office of Women's Health. In addition, Health and Human Services' vacancy announcements are available at the site. The site is linked directly to the Office of the Surgeon General, providing transcripts of speeches and reports, a biography of the current Surgeon General, and a history and summary of duties associated with the position.
http://www.hhs.gov/phs/

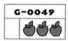

Substance Abuse and Mental Health Services Administration Examining substance abuse and mental illness, the Substance Abuse and Mental Health Services Administration site offers resources dedicated to the prevention, treatment, and rehabilitation of these conditions. The site features SAMHSA programs and centers, namely the Center for Mental Health Services, the Center for Substance Abuse Prevention, and the Center for Substance Abuse Treatment. Information clearinghouses on the site feature online booklets, fact sheets, and conference proceedings from these three centers. There is also information on their managed care initiative, including reports on quality improvement, policy studies, and technical assistance and training. Grant opportunities, along with data and statistics on substance abuse and mental illness, are included. A public information section offers easy-to-understand publications as well as directories of service providers. http://www.samhsa.gov

NATIONAL INSTITUTES OF HEALTH

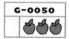

National Institutes of Health (NIH) The NIH is one of eight health agencies of the Public Health Service which, in turn, is part of the U.S. Department of Health and Human Services. The NIH mission is to uncover new knowledge that will lead to better health for everyone. NIH works toward that mission by conducting research in its own laboratories; supporting the research of non-federal scientists in universities, medical schools, hospitals, and research institutions throughout the country and abroad; helping in the training of research investigators; and fostering communication of biomedical information. The site provides employment and summer internship program information, science education program details, and a history of the NIH. A site search engine and links to the home pages of all NIH institutes and centers are available.
http://www.nih.gov

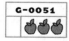

Center for Information Technology The Center for Information Technology incorporates the power of modern computers into the biomedical programs and administrative procedures of the NIH by conducting computational biosciences research, developing computer systems, and providing computer facilities.

The site provides information on the activities and organization of the center, as well as links to many useful information technology sites.
http://www.cit.nih.gov/home.asp

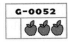

Center for Scientific Review The Center for Scientific Review is the focal point at NIH for the conduct of initial peer review, the foundation of the NIH grant and award process. The center carries out a peer review of the majority of research and research training applications submitted to the NIH. The center also serves as the central receipt point for all Public Health Service applications and makes referrals to scientific review groups for scientific and technical merit review of applications and to funding components for potential award. To this end, the center develops and implements innovative, flexible ways to conduct referral and review for all aspects of science. The site contains transcripts of public commentary panel discussions, news and events listings, grant applications, peer review notes, and links to additional biomedical and government sites.
http://www.drg.nih.gov

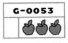

Fogarty International Center The Fogarty International Center for Advanced Study in the Health Sciences leads NIH efforts to advance the health of the American public and citizens of all nations through international cooperation on global health threats. Resources at the site include the center's publications, regional information on programs and contacts, research and training opportunities, a description of the center's Multilateral Initiative on Malaria (MIM), details of the NIH Visiting Program for Foreign Scientists, and news and vacancy announcements.
http://www.nih.gov/fic

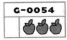

National Cancer Institute (NCI) The National Cancer Institute (NCI) leads a national effort to reduce the burden of cancer morbidity and mortality, ultimately to prevent the disease. Through basic and clinical biomedical research and training, the NCI conducts and supports programs to understand the causes of cancer; prevent, detect, diagnose, treat, and control cancer; and disseminate information to the practitioner, patient, and public. The site provides visitors with many informational resources related to cancer, including Cancer-Trials for clinical trials resources and CancerNet for information on cancer tailored to the needs of health professionals, patients, and the general public. Additional resources relate to funding opportunities as well as to events and research at NCI.
http://www.nci.nih.gov

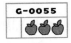

National Center for Biotechnology Information A comprehensive site that provides a wide array of biotechnology resources, the center includes sources such as a genetic sequence database (GenBank); links to related sites, a newsletter, and genetic sequence search engines; information on programs, activities, and research projects; seminar and exhibit schedules; and database services. Databases available through this site include PubMed for free access to

MEDLINE searches and the Online Mendelian Inheritance in Man (OMIM) for an extensive catalog of human genes and genetic disorders.
http://www.ncbi.nlm.nih.gov

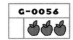

National Center for Complementary and Alternative Medicine (NCCAM)   The National Center for Complementary and Alternative Medicine identifies and evaluates unconventional healthcare practices; supports, coordinates, and conducts research and research training on these practices; and disseminates information. The site describes specific program areas; answers common questions about alternative therapies; and offers news, research grants information, and a calendar of events. Information resources include a citation index related to alternative medicine obtained from MEDLINE; a bibliography of publications; the NCCAM clearinghouse of information for the public, media, and healthcare professionals; and a link to the National Women's Health Information Center.   http://nccam.nih.gov

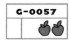

National Center for Research Resources   The National Center for Research Resources creates, develops, and provides a comprehensive range of human, animal, technological, and other resources to support biomedical research advances. The center's areas of concentration are biomedical technology, clinical research, comparative medicine, and research infrastructure. The site offers specific information on each of these research areas, grants information, news, current events, press releases, publications, and research resources.
http://www.ncrr.nih.gov

National Eye Institute (NEI)   The National Eye Institute (NEI) conducts and supports research, training, health information dissemination, and other programs with respect to blinding eye diseases, visual disorders, mechanisms of visual function, preservation of sight, and the special health problems and requirements of the visually impaired. Information at the site is tailored to the needs of researchers, health professionals, the general public and patients, educators, and the media. Resources include a clinical trials database, intramural research information, funding, grants, a news and events calendar, publications, and an overview of the NEI offices, divisions, branches, and laboratories.
http://www.nei.nih.gov

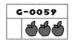

National Heart, Lung, and Blood Institute (NHLBI)   The National Heart, Lung, and Blood Institute (NHLBI) provides leadership for a national research program in diseases of the heart, blood vessels, lungs, and blood, and in transfusion medicine through support of innovative basic, clinical, and population-based health education research. The site provides health information; scientific resources; research funding information; news and press releases; details of committees, meetings, and events; clinical guidelines; notices of studies seeking patient participation; links to laboratories at the NHLBI; and technology transfer resources. Highlights of the site include cholesterol, weight, and asthma management resources.
http://www.nhlbi.nih.gov

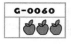

National Human Genome Research Institute The National Human Genome Research Institute supports the NIH component of the Human Genome Project, a worldwide research effort designed to analyze the structure of human DNA and determine the location of the estimated 50,000-100,000 human genes. The NHGRI Intramural Research Program develops and implements technology for understanding, diagnosing, and treating genetic diseases. The site provides information about NHGRI, the Human Genome Project, grants, intramural research, policy and public affairs, workshops and conferences, and news items. Resources include links to the institute's Ethical, Legal, and Social Implications Program and the Center for Inherited Disease Research, genomic and genetic resources for investigators, and a glossary of genetic terms.
http://www.nhgri.nih.gov

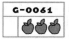

National Institute of Allergy and Infectious Diseases (NIAID) The National Institute of Allergy and Infectious Diseases provides support for scientists conducting research aimed at developing better ways to diagnose, treat, and prevent the many infectious, immunologic, and allergic diseases that afflict people worldwide. This site provides NIAID news releases, a calendar of events, links to related sites, a clinical trials database, grants and technology transfer information, and current research information including meetings, publications, and research resources. Fact sheets are available for different immunological disorders, allergies, asthma, and infectious diseases.
http://www.niaid.nih.gov

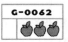

National Institute of Arthritis and Musculoskeletal and Skin Diseases (NIAMS) NIAMS conducts and supports a broad spectrum of research on normal structure and function of bones, muscles, and skin, as well as the numerous and disparate diseases that affect these tissues. NIAMS also conducts research training and epidemiologic studies in addition to disseminating information. The site provides details of research programs at the institute and offers personnel and employment listings, news, and an events calendar. Health information is provided in the form of fact sheets, brochures, health statistics, and other resources. Scientific resources include bibliographies of publications, consensus conference reports, grants and contracts applications, grant program announcements, and links to scientific research databases. Information on current clinical studies and transcripts of NIAMS advisory council, congressional, and conference reports are also available at the site.
http://www.nih.gov/niams

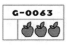

National Institute of Child Health and Human Development (NICHD) The institute conducts and supports laboratory, clinical, and epidemiological research on the reproductive, neurobiologic, developmental, and behavioral processes that determine and maintain the health of children, adults, families, and populations. Research in the areas of fertility, pregnancy, growth, development, and medical rehabilitation strives to ensure that every child is born healthy and wanted and grows up free from disease and disability. The site provides general information about the institute; funding and intramural research details; information about the Division of Epidemiology, Statistics, and Prevention Research; a publications bibliography; fact sheets; reports; employment and fellowship listings; and research resources. http://www.nichd.nih.gov

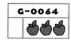

National Institute of Dental and Craniofacial Research (NIDCR) The National Institute of Dental and Craniofacial Research (NIDCR) provides leadership for a national research program designed to understand, treat, and ultimately prevent the infectious and inherited craniofacial-oral-dental diseases and disorders that compromise millions of human lives. General information about the institute, news and health information, details of research activities, and NIDCR employment opportunities are all found at the site.
http://www.nidr.nih.gov

National Institute of Diabetes and Digestive and Kidney Diseases (NIDDK) The National Institute of Diabetes and Digestive and Kidney Diseases conducts and supports basic and applied research and also provides leadership for a national program in diabetes, endocrinology, and metabolic diseases; in digestive diseases and nutrition; and in kidney, urologic, and hematologic diseases. Information at the site includes a mission statement, history, organization description, and employment listing. Additional resources include news; a database for health information; clinical trials information, including a patient recruitment section; and information on extramural funding and intramural research at the institute.
http://www.niddk.nih.gov

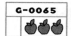

National Institute of Environmental Health Sciences (NIEHS) The National Institute of Environmental Health Sciences (NIEHS) reduces the burden of human illness and dysfunction from environmental causes by defining how environmental exposures, genetic susceptibility, and age interact to affect an individual's health. News and institute events, research information, grant and contract details, fact sheets, employment and training notices, teacher support, and an online resource for kids are all found at this site. Library resources include a book catalog, electronic journals, database searching, NIEHS publications, and reference resources. Visitors can use search engines at the site to find environmental health information and news, publications, available grants and contracts, and library resources.
http://www.niehs.nih.gov

National Institute of General Medical Sciences (NIGMS) The National Institute of General Medical Sciences (NIGMS) supports basic biomedical research that is not targeted to specific diseases but that increases the understanding of life processes and lays the foundation for advances in disease diagnosis, treatment, and prevention. Among the most significant results of this research has been the development of recombinant DNA technology, which forms the basis for the biotechnology industry. The site provides information about NIGMS research and funding programs, information for visitors, news, a publi-

cations list, reports, grant databases, employment listings, and links to additional biomedical resources.
http://www.nigms.nih.gov/

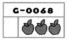

National Institute of Mental Health (NIMH) The National Institute of Mental Health (NIMH) provides national leadership dedicated to understanding, treating, and preventing mental illnesses through basic research on the brain and behavior as well as through clinical, epidemiological, and services research. Resources available at the site include information for visitors to the campus, employment opportunities, NIMH history, and publications from activities of the National Advisory Mental Health Council and Peer Review Committees. News, a calendar of events, information on clinical trials, funding opportunities, and intramural research are also provided. Pages tailored specifically for the public, health practitioners, and researchers contain mental disorder information, research fact sheets, statistics, science education materials, news, links to NIMH research sites, and patient education materials.
http://www.nimh.nih.gov

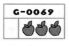

National Institute of Neurological Disorders and Stroke (NINDS)
The National Institute of Neurological Disorders and Stroke supports and conducts research and research training on the normal structure and function of the nervous system and on the causes, prevention, diagnosis, and treatment of more than 600 nervous system disorders including stroke, epilepsy, multiple sclerosis, Parkinson's disease, head and spinal cord injury, Alzheimer's disease, and brain tumors. The site provides visitors with an organizational diagram, links to advisory groups, the mission and history of NINDS, employment and training opportunities, and information on research at NINDS. Information is available for patients, clinicians, and scientists. It includes publications, details of current clinical trials, links to other health organizations, and research funding information. http://www.ninds.nih.gov

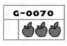

National Institute of Nursing Research (NINR) The National Institute of Nursing Research (NINR) supports clinical and basic research to establish a scientific basis for the care of individuals across the life span, from management of patients during illness and recovery to the reduction of risks for disease and disability and the promotion of healthy lifestyles. NINR accomplishes its mission by supporting grants to universities and other research organizations as well as by conducting research intramurally. Visitors to this site can find the NINR mission statement and history, employment listings, news, conference details, publications, speech transcripts, answers to frequently asked questions, information concerning legislative activities, research program and funding details, health information, highlights and outcomes of current nursing research, and links to additional Web resources.
http://www.nih.gov/ninr

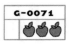

National Institute on Aging (NIA) The National Institute on Aging (NIA) leads a national program of research on the biomedical, social, and behavioral aspects of the aging process. The goals of the institute include the prevention of age-related diseases and disabilities and the promotion of a better quality of life for all older Americans. The site presents recent announcements and upcoming events, employment opportunities, press releases, and media advisories of significant findings. Research resources include news from the National Advisory Council on Aging, links to extramural aging research conducted throughout the United States, and funding and training information. Health professionals and the general public can access publications on health and aging topics or order materials online.

http://www.nih.gov/nia

National Institute on Alcohol Abuse and Alcoholism (NIAAA) The National Institute on Alcohol Abuse and Alcoholism (NIAAA) conducts research focused on improving the treatment and prevention of alcoholism and alcohol-related problems to reduce the enormous health, social, and economic consequences of this disease. General resources at the site include an introduction to the institute, extramural and intramural research information, an organizational flowchart, details of legislative activities, Advisory Council roster and minutes, information on scientific review groups associated with the institute, and employment announcements. Institute publications, data tables, press releases, conferences and events calendars, answers to frequently asked questions on the subject of alcohol abuse and dependence, and links to related sites are also available. The ETOH Database, an online bibliographic database containing over 100,000 records on alcohol abuse and alcoholism, can be accessed from the site, as can the National Library of Medicine's MEDLINE database.

http://www.niaaa.nih.gov:80

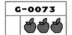

National Institute on Deafness and Other Communication Disorders (NIDCD) The National Institute on Deafness and Other Communication Disorders (NIDCD) conducts and supports biomedical research and research training in the normal and disordered processes of hearing, balance, smell, taste, voice, speech, and language. The institute also conducts and supports research and research training related to disease prevention and health promotion; addresses special biomedical and behavioral problems associated with people who have communication impairments or disorders; and supports efforts to create devices that substitute for lost and impaired sensory and communication function. The site provides visitors with fact sheets and other information resources on hearing and balance; smell and taste; voice, speech, and language; hearing aids; otosclerosis; vocal abuse and misuse; and vocal cord paralysis. Other resources include a directory of organizations related to hearing, balance, smell, taste, voice, speech, and language; a glossary of terms; an online newsletter; information for children and teachers; and clinical trials details. Information on research funding and intramural research activities, a news and events calendar, and general information about NIDCD are also available.

http://www.nidcd.nih.gov

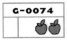

National Institute on Drug Abuse (NIDA) The National Institute on Drug Abuse (NIDA) site offers resources for healthcare professionals, featuring news, events, research updates, and special NIDA Web sites covering common drugs of abuse, such as steroids and club drugs. There are also sections on drug abuse research and prevention, grant funding, international opportunities, and legislative issues. The publications section offers online publications as well as items for purchase. Research training at NIDA, as well as the proceedings from their scientific meetings, can also be found. A comprehensive list of related resources is provided.

http://www.nida.nih.gov/

National Library of Medicine (NLM) The National Library of Medicine (NLM), the world's largest medical library, collects materials in all areas of biomedicine and healthcare and focuses on biomedical aspects of technology; the humanities; and the physical, life, and social sciences. This site contains links to government medical databases, including MEDLINE and MEDLINEplus; information on funding opportunities at the NLM and other federal agencies; and details of services, training, and outreach programs offered by NLM. Users can access NLM's catalog of resources (LOCATORPlus), as well as NLM publications, including fact sheets, published reports, and staff publications. NLM research programs discussed at the site include topics in computational molecular biology, medical informatics, and other related subjects. The Web site features 15 searchable databases, covering journal searches via MEDLINE; AIDS information via AIDSLINE, AIDSDRUGS, and AIDSTRIALS; bioethics via BIOETHICSLINE; and numerous other important topics. The NLM Gateway—a master search engine—searches MEDLINE using the user-friendly retrieval engine called PubMed. There are more than 11 million citations in MEDLINE and PreMEDLINE and the other related databases. Additionally, the NLM provides sources of health statistics, serials programs, and services maintained through a system called SERHOLD.

http://www.nlm.nih.gov

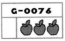

Warren Grant Magnuson Clinical Center The Warren Grant Magnuson Clinical Center is the clinical research facility of the National Institutes of Health, supporting clinical investigations conducted by the NIH. The clinical center was designed to bring patient-care facilities close to research laboratories, allowing findings of basic and clinical scientists to move quickly from the laboratory to the treatment of patients. The site provides visitors with news, events, details of current clinical research studies, patient recruitment resources, links to departmental Web sites, and information resources for NIH staff, patients, physicians, and scientists. Topics discussed in the center's Medicine for the Public Lecture Series and resources in medical and scientific education offered by the center are included at the site.

http://www.cc.nih.gov:80

CENTERS FOR DISEASE CONTROL AND PREVENTION (CDC)

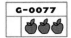

Centers for Disease Control and Prevention (CDC)   The mission of the Centers for Disease Control and Prevention is to promote health and quality of life by preventing and controlling disease, injury, and disability. The site provides users with links to nearly a dozen associated centers, institutes, and offices; a Web page devoted to travelers' health; publications, software, and other products; data and statistics; training and employment opportunities; and subscription registration forms for online CDC publications. Highlighted publications include the *Emerging Infectious Disease Journal* and the *Morbidity and Mortality Weekly Report,* both of which can be received by e-mail on a regular basis. The CDC offers a comprehensive, alphabetical list of general and specific health topics as well as links to additional CDC resources and state and local agencies concerned with public health issues. Visitors can also search the site by keyword and read spotlights on current research and information.
http://www.cdc.gov

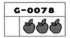

Epidemiology Program Office   Information and resources on public health surveillance are provided by the Epidemiology Program Office at this Web address. Publications and software related to epidemiology are available for download. Updated news, events, and international bulletins are also featured at the site.   http://www.cdc.gov/epo/index.htm

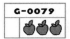

National Center for Chronic Disease Prevention and Health Promotion   Maintained by the CDC, this site focuses on many different aspects of chronic disease prevention. Intended for healthcare professionals, the site provides facts on the economic burden of chronic disease, risk prevention, and comprehensive approaches to prevention. Resources available in the chronic diseases section include information on the center's programs; reports; and fact sheets for arthritis, cancer, cardiovascular disease, diabetes, epilepsy, and oral diseases. Additional links provide information on specific populations such as pregnant women and minorities.
http://www.cdc.gov/nccdphp/index.htm

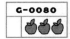

National Center for Environmental Health   The National Center for Environmental Health Web page offers information on the center's programs and activities related to the prevention of health problems from environmental hazards. The health topics section offers an A-to-Z listing of topics covered on the site, including such issues as the prevention of birth defects by the use of folic acid. The publications section offers fact sheets, brochures, and scientific publications on issues such as lead poisoning and the indoor use of pesticides. There is also an index of articles from the *Morbidity and Mortality Weekly Report*. In addition, the site offers current employment opportunities and information on training programs. Spanish and child-oriented versions of the NCEH site are also available.
http://www.cdc.gov/nceh/default.htm

National Center for Health Statistics The National Center for Health Statistics Web page features health data and statistics on a broad array of topics including AIDS, chickenpox, divorce, and obstetrical procedures. Visitors can read descriptions of the NCHS survey and data collection systems; healthcare professionals can learn how to include their patients in the surveys. A "Data Warehouse" section offers tabulated data on the national and state level, as well as an international classification of diseases. A link to FASTATS A to Z provides national statistics, along with links for more comprehensive data. There is also information on NCHS research and development.
http://www.cdc.gov/nchs/default.htm

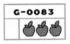

National Center for HIV, STD, and TB Prevention Part of the CDC, the National Center for HIV, STD, and TB Prevention offers general information for professionals and the public on the control and prevention of HIV/AIDS, sexually transmitted diseases, and tuberculosis. The home page highlights news and CDC updates. Information of interest to professionals is accessed by clicking on the link for "Site Highlights" in the sidebar menu; among the highlights is a link to the National Prevention Information Network, which offers information on HIV/AIDS, STD, and TB and the connections between them. By clicking on a disease, visitors will find resources, related links, a bulletin board, distance learning, publications, and FAQs. The site also features a database of organizations that provide HIV/AIDS, STD, and TB prevention, education, healthcare, and social services. CDC laboratory research is accessible including disease information and reports, and the top of the home page has a link for funding opportunities. http://www.cdc.gov/nchstp/od/nchstp.html

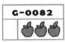

National Center for Infectious Diseases Dedicated to the study of infectious diseases, the National Center for Infectious Diseases Web page provides an A-to-Z listing of disease information with links to fact sheets, laboratory assistance information, and related articles. Visitors can access the NCID online journal, *Emerging Infectious Diseases,* with full-text articles. There are also articles, booklets, and a video on preventing emerging infectious diseases. Data and reports on diseases can also be found under "Surveillance Resources." A link to "DPDx" features reviews on parasites and parasitic diseases, diagnostic procedures, diagnostic assistance, and an image library. A travel section covers region-specific issues, diseases, recommended vaccinations, and tips. In addition, the publications section offers many free online brochures. A short list of related links is provided.
http://www.cdc.gov/ncidod/index.htm

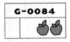

National Center for Injury Prevention and Control Healthcare professionals and the public will find a broad array of information on injury prevention on this Web page. The site offers fact sheets on injuries and safety such as child passenger safety, fireworks injury prevention, suicide, and fall prevention programs for seniors. The data section features WISQARS, an interactive database of injury-related mortality data. There is also a list of publications, viewable online, as well as information on research funding. Facts and

data in categories such as injury care, violence, and unintentional injury are also available. Consumers can click on the SafeUSA link to access safety tips.
http://www.cdc.gov/ncipc/ncipchm.htm

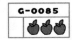

National Immunization Program The National Immunization Program of the CDC offers a wide range of immunization information resources directed to healthcare professionals and consumers. The site features clinical information in categories such as vaccine recommendations; advances in immunization; educational resources, including training for professionals, and vaccine safety. Information on grants and funding, as well as data and statistics. Under the category of "Subsites," visitors can find information on the development of immunization registries, along with downloadable clinical assessment software (CASA) to track immunization practices within an office. Links at the top of the page are provided to publications for both the professional and consumers and to the Web site's Dictionary of Immunization Terms.
http://www.cdc.gov/nip/

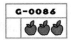

National Institute for Occupational Safety and Health (NIOSH) Created to conduct research on work-related illnesses and injuries, the National Institute for Occupational Safety and Health (NIOSH) describes the organization's activities and recommendations on this site. A topic index provides articles and guidelines on issues such as chemical safety, indoor air quality, and latex. The publications section features fact sheets, brochures, and bulletins, with some available online. In addition, there is information on NIOSH research activities, funding opportunities, and training.
http://www.cdc.gov/niosh/homepage.html

National Prevention Information Network Designed to provide information on HIV/AIDS, STDs, and TB, the CDC's National Prevention Information Network site offers useful resources for the healthcare professional and consumer. A bulletin board, distance learning, FAQs, mortality and morbidity reports, and related links are provided in each disease category. A large list of publications is found, along with a database of organizations. Information on the CDC's prevention research is also available with links to numerous reports and journal articles.
http://www.cdcnpin.org/

OTHER HEALTH AGENCIES

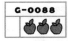

Center for Nutrition Policy and Promotion The Center for Nutrition Policy and Promotion, within the U.S. Department of Agriculture (USDA), conducts research on the nutritional needs of Americans and disseminates their findings. The center's site provides statistical information and resources for educators, contains dietary guidelines for Americans, and offers official USDA food plans. A database on the nutrient content of the U.S. food supply (on a per cap-

ita basis) is provided. In addition, there is a 76-page booklet available that offers recipes and tips for healthy meals.
http://www.usda.gov/cnpp

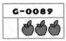

Food and Nutrition Service   The Food and Nutrition Service (FNS) of the U.S. Department of Agriculture "reduces hunger and food insecurity in partnership with cooperating organizations by providing children and needy families access to food, a healthful diet, and nutrition education in a manner that supports American agriculture and inspires public confidence." The site provides details of FNS nutrition assistance programs such as food stamps, WIC, and child nutrition. Research, in the form of published studies and reports, is also available at the site.
http://www.fns.usda.gov/fns

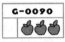

Food Safety and Inspection Service   The Food Safety and Inspection Service, part of the U.S. Department of Agriculture, is dedicated to food safety. Its site offers news, recall notification on meat and poultry products, a newsletter, and related links. A consumer education section offers fact sheets on the safe handling and cooking of meat, poultry, and eggs. Technical publications and a video library can be accessed under the publications section. Also of interest to professionals is a fellowship program related to food safety, which can be found in the drop-down menu under "Featured Topics." In addition, information on distance learning at the Food Safety Virtual University is provided.
http://www.fsis.usda.gov

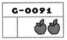

National Bioethics Advisory Commission   The National Bioethics Advisory Commission (NBAC) studies bioethical issues related to genetics and the protection of humans as research subjects and directs their reports to the National Science and Technology Council. The NBAC also advises on the applications of their research, including clinical applications. This site lists meeting dates, full-text transcripts of meetings, and news. Reports they have produced are available for such topics as ethical issues in human stem cell research, research involving persons with mental disorders, and cloning human beings. A list of links to related sites is provided.
http://bioethics.georgetown.edu/nbac/

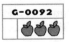

National Science Foundation (NSF): Directorate for Biological Sciences   The Division of Integrative Biology and Neuroscience (IBN), part of the National Science Foundation (NSF), supports research aimed at understanding the living organism—plant, animal, or microbe—as a unit of biological organization. Current scientific emphases include biotechnology, biomolecular materials, environmental biology, global change, biodiversity, molecular evolution, plant science, microbial biology, and computational biology, including modeling. Research projects support the education and training of future scientists, including doctoral dissertation research, research conferences, workshops, symposia, Undergraduate Mentoring in Environmental Biology (UMEB), and a variety of NSF-wide activities. This site describes in detail the activities and divisions of IBN and offers award listings and deadline dates for funding applications. http://www.nsf.gov/bio/ibn/start.htm

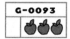

Office of National Drug Control Policy   This site states the missions and goals of the ONDCP. It has a clearinghouse of drug policy information with a staff that will respond to the needs of the general public, providing statistical data, topical fact sheets, and information packets. There is information on related science, medicine, and technology. There are also resources on prevention, education, and treatment programs. Information on the enforcement of the policies is provided for the national, state, and local levels.
http://www.whitehousedrugpolicy.gov

10.5   FULL-TEXT ARTICLES

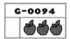

Amedeo   Amedeo is a free medical literature service that allows users to select topics and journals in specific areas of interest. Visitors can browse among more than 20 health-related topics for new articles and preselected recommended journals. For each article, links are provided to its abstract and to related articles in PubMed. The service also offers a weekly e-mail with an overview of new articles reflecting specifications indicated by the user, with the option to create a personal home page with abstracts of relevant articles. The site allows registered users to access a network center, which facilitates literature exchange among users with similar interests. This service is supported through educational grants by numerous pharmaceutical companies.
(free registration) http://www.amedeo.com

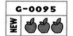

BioMed Central: Online Journals   Produced by the commercial publisher, Current Science Group, BioMed Central makes full-text peer-reviewed articles available on this Web page. The site's content is grouped by subject into journals published by BMC including *BMC Cancer, BMC Infectious Diseases, BMC Surgery,* and *BMC Pediatrics.* Each journal's articles are available for download in PDF format.
http://www.biomedcentral.com/browse/medicine/

CatchWord   There are more than 1,100 journals on a variety of subjects available on this Web page. Visitors can view the journal's table of contents and abstracts, then purchase full-text articles online. Institutions can utilize the services of CatchWord to provide a single interface to their online journal collections. Approximately 20 specialties of medicine are found, including cardiology, oncology, and psychiatry.
(some features fee-based) http://www.catchword.co.uk/

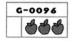

EurekAlert   This site allows professionals and consumers to search the archives for the latest articles, press releases, news items, events, awards, and grants in broad areas of science, including chemistry and physics. The "Medicine and Health" section covers nearly 70 topics including Alzheimer's disease,

diabetes, fertility, and sleep disorders. Under each heading, press releases are categorized by date and provide the source and contact information.
http://www.eurekalert.org

Free Medical Journals.com: Full-Text Articles Healthcare professionals will find more than 550 free medical journals on this site with access to full-text articles. The site organizes the journals into categories that indicate whether the journal is free, free one to six months after publication, free one year after publication, or free two years after publication. However, the home page only shows a fraction of what is available; visitors should click on "Journals Sorted by Specialty" on the left side of the page to view all of the journals. Specialties include AIDS, cardiology, dermatology, hematology, oncology, infectious diseases, psychiatry, rheumatology, and pediatrics. Some journals are available in other languages. Visitors can register for an alert service that will e-mail information on new free online journals as they become available.
http://www.freemedicaljournals.com/

HighWire Press: Full-Text Articles Stanford University's HighWire Press, developer of the Web versions of many important biomedical journals, maintains this extensive listing of links to full-text journal archives. A list of journals offering free access is provided at this site, with a notation indicating whether a title is free, free for a trial period, or free for back issues. More than 100 journals are listed, and a link on the left side of the page brings up a list of full-text science archives on the Web.
http://highwire.stanford.edu/lists/freeart.dtl

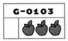

Ingenta This enormous database of medical and nonscientific journals' tables of contents permits searching by keyword, journal title, or author. Full articles can be obtained by fax or e-mail for a fee. As the result of a merger between Ingenta and UnCover, an integrated service provides tables of contents for specific journals as they are published and added to the database. Ingenta UnCover users can log in to Ingenta using their UnCover profile ID and password.
(some features fee-based) http://www.ingenta.com

Journal Watch Online Subscribers to the Journal Watch service can access summaries, written by physicians, of the most recent clinical research literature for many subspecialties at this Web site. Produced by the Massachusetts Medical Society, publishers of the *New England Journal of Medicine,* Journal Watch updates its summaries four times a week in the areas of dermatology, cardiology, psychiatry, women's health, infectious diseases, neurology, and gastroenterology. Research summaries and commentary are drawn from approximately 50 journals, including general medical and specialty journals, to provide a broad range of coverage. Sample summaries are also available.
(fee-based) http://www.jwatch.org/

MD Consult Physicians can access the full text of nearly 40 major medical textbooks and nearly 50 core medical journals on this Web site. Journals available on the site include *Arthritis and Rheumatism,* the *Cancer Journal, Chest,*

and the *Journal of the American Academy of Dermatology.* The site also offers the ability to search MEDLINE and other key databases simultaneously in order to locate full-text articles. Other features include clinical practice guidelines, CME modules, patient education handouts, and prescription information. A 10-day free trial of full site access is available for physicians.
(fee-based) http://www.mdconsult.com/

MedBioWorld: Medical Journals Main Index Visitors to this address will find comprehensive listings of online journals, categorized by specialty topic. Major broad-coverage medical journals, nursing journals, science journals, and books on medical writing are also listed through the site, as well as links to many publishers' Web sites.
http://www.medbioworld.com/journals/medicine/med-bio.html

MEDLINE Journal Links to Publishers Through the National Library of Medicine, MEDLINE provides direct access to hundreds of medical journals in all fields, listed alphabetically by name, with direct links to their respective publishers. Upon accessing an individual publication, the reader can view the current issue table of contents and abstracts for the articles. Some articles are available without charge while others require a fee. Each page explains the available information and the conditions for access since policies vary by publisher and journal. http://www.ncbi.nlm.nih.gov/entrez/journals/loftext_noprov.html

Medscape Visitors to this site can access more than 25,000 full-text articles from more than 40 journals and medical news periodicals. Medical journals include *Chest, American Heart Journal,* and *Southern Medical Journal.* The site also features "Journal Scan," clinical summaries of the latest literature for specialties such as cardiology, dermatology, infectious diseases, psychiatry, and respiratory care. There are also several online textbooks available. (free registration)
http://www.medscape.com/Home/
Topics/multispecialty/directories/dir-MULT.JournalRoom.html

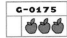

PubList: Health and Medical Sciences This site contains a list of links to thousands of medical journals, divided by subject areas. Information such as frequency, publisher, and format is included for each publication, as well as links to the publication. A search engine can be used to identify titles of interest.
http://www.publist.com/indexes/health.html

PubMed Central: Full-Text Articles PubMed Central is a digital library with archives of life sciences literature. It was developed and is managed by the National Center for Biotechnology Information and the National Library of Medicine. Currently, eight journals with full-text articles and archives are found on the site with 10 more slated for addition in the future. Available journals include all BioMedCentral journals (see separate write-up of this site), *Arthritis Research, Breast Cancer Research,* and the *British Medical Journal.* Many of these journals delay release of their full-text content to this site, with the most current content available at their own sites on a subscription basis.
http://www.pubmedcentral.nih.gov/

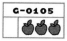

University of Georgia: Science Library An A-to-Z listing of science journals available on the Internet is provided on this site. The list can be navigated by clicking on the appropriate letter at the bottom of the site. Some journals can only be accessed by faculty and students at the University of Georgia.
http://www.libs.uga.edu/science/fullalph.html

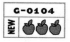

WebMedLit WebMedLit provides access to the latest medical literature on the Web by indexing medical Web sites daily and presenting articles from each site organized by subject categories. All WebMedLit article links are from the original source document at the publisher's Web site, and most articles are available in full text.
http://webmedlit.silverplatter.com/index.html

10.6 GOVERNMENT INFORMATION DATABASES

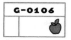

Agency for Healthcare Research and Quality (AHRQ): Search Tool
This site offers a search tool to find information located on the Agency for Healthcare Research and Quality Web page. There is information appropriate to professionals and the public.
http://www.ahcpr.gov/query/query.htm

Centers for Disease Control and Prevention (CDC): Web Search
Both healthcare professionals and consumers can find useful information using the search tool provided on the CDC site. Visitors have the opportunity to search all CDC Web sites by keyword and to search state health departments. By checking the box next to the state health department of interest, one can search one or more of them or all of them at once.
http://www.cdc.gov/search.htm

Combined Health Information Database Designed as a bibliographic database, the Combined Health Information Database (CHID) draws upon health information from health-related federal agencies. The database is categorized under nearly 20 health topics such as Alzheimer's, cancer, diabetes, and weight control. Searches can be limited to individual subtopics, or the database can be searched in its entirety. Access to information is only available through a keyword search, which can be done with a simple or detailed search. Results include health promotion and educational materials aimed at consumers and not indexed elsewhere.
http://chid.nih.gov/

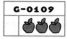

CRISP: Computer Retrieval of Information on Scientific Projects
Funded by the NIH, CRISP is a database of federally funded biomedical research projects conducted at universities, hospitals, and other research institutions. Users, including the public, can use CRISP to search for scientific concepts, emerging trends, and techniques or to identify specific projects and/or investigators. http://www-commons.cit.nih.gov/crisp

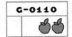

Department of Energy: Comprehensive Epidemiologic Data Resource Compiled by the U.S. Department of Energy, this site features a collection of resources on health and radiation exposure data related to DOE installations. Included are data from epidemiologic studies performed by DOE-funded investigators on health and mortality, classic radiation, and dose reconstruction. The site also covers studies of populations living near DOE installations and other studies on radiation effects, such as those on atomic bomb survivors. http://cedr.lbl.gov/

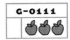

FedWorld Information Network Information from many federal agencies can be accessed through this Web page. By clicking on the database section at the top of the page, visitors will find links to 20 databases encompassing a variety of information such as Supreme Court decisions, EPA Clean Air Act data, and U.S. Customs Headquarter's rulings. The home page features search tools for the entire FedWorld network, U.S. government reports, and U.S. government Web sites. (some features fee-based) http://www.fedworld.gov/

Government Databases in Health Maintained by St. Mary's University of San Antonio, Texas, this site features a list of more than 25 selected government sites dealing with health and medicine. Sites covered include those on clinical trials, Congressional Research Service reports, food composition data, and MEDLINE; each site listed has a description of its contents. (free registration) http://library.stmarytx.edu/acadlib/doc/electronic/dbhealth.htm

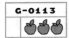

Government Information Locator Service Visitors to this site can search for government information across several federal agencies, such as the Department of Health and Human Services and the Environmental Protection Agency, at the same time. The agencies listed on the site have compiled their public information on the same server for easy access to a wide variety of information. http://www.access.gpo.gov/su_docs/gils/index.html

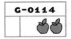

Healthfinder Healthfinder provides links to public medical or health sciences libraries on the Internet. Directories of libraries are also available to find local facilities, library organizations, and research and reference resources. http://www.healthfinder.gov/scripts/SearchContext.asp?topic=14332&section=5

MEDLINEplus A comprehensive database of health and medical information, MEDLINEplus serves a different purpose from its sister service, MEDLINE, which is a bibliographic search engine to locate citations and abstracts in medical journals and reports. MEDLINEplus offers the ability to search by topic and obtain full information rather than citations. One can search body systems, disorders and diseases, treatments and therapies, diagnostic procedures, side effects, and numerous other important topics related to personal health and the field of medicine in general. http://www.nlm.nih.gov/medlineplus/medlineplus.html

10.7 HEALTH AND MEDICAL HOTLINES

Toll-Free Health Hotlines A categorized list of hundreds of toll-free health information hotlines is provided by this site. Each hotline provides educational materials for patients.
http://www.health.gov/nhic/NHICScripts/
Hitlist.cfm?Keyword=Toll%2DFree%20Information%20Services

10.8 HEALTH INSURANCE PLANS

HealthPlanDirectory.com Produced by a commercial marketing company, DoctorDirectory.com, this site contains a directory of health insurance plans, listed by state. Contact information for each plan is provided.
http://www.doctordirectory.com/healthplans/directory/default.asp

10.9 HEALTHCARE LEGISLATION AND ADVOCACY

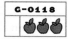

American Medical Association (AMA): AMA in Washington The purpose of this site is to encourage physicians around the country to get involved in the AMA's grassroots lobbying efforts. It covers information on legislation relevant to the medical profession, the AMA's congressional agenda, and educational programs available through the AMA on political activism for physicians. The Web site is updated regularly with the latest news on medical issues in the government.
http://www.ama-assn.org/ama/pub/category/4015.html

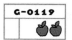

American Medical Group Association: Public Policy and Political Affairs The AMGA provides legislative advocacy to medical groups, addressing current political debates in the medical community. Updated legislative and media alerts, an electronic newsletter for members, and comments and testimony on several subjects affecting healthcare providers are offered. Relevant Web sites of interest are accessible. (some features fee-based)
http://www.amga.org/AMGA2000/PublicPolicy/index_publicPolicy.htm

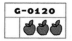

American Medical Student Association: Health Policy AMSA is an organization that attempts to improve healthcare and medical education. Its "Health Policy" department contains news of legislation that affects medical education, educational information on how to be a health policy activist, and a listing of printable documents concerning relevant health policy issues such as gene patents and prescription drug coverage.
http://www.amsa.org/hp/hpindex.cfm

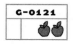

American Medical Women's Association AMWA promotes issues related to women's health and professional development for female physicians. The

site's advocacy and actions sections contain articles on news and legislation that are relevant to these issues and also give advice on how to get involved.
http://www.amwa-doc.org/index.html

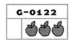

THOMAS: U.S. Congress on the Internet   Within THOMAS, one can find information on bills, laws, reports, or any current U.S. federal legislation. *Congressional Record*, the official record of the proceedings of the U.S. Congress, and committee information are also available. The site's search engine can be used to find current congressional bills by keyword or bill number.
http://thomas.loc.gov

10.10   HOSPITAL RESOURCES

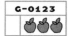

American Hospital Association   An extremely broad range of resources pertaining to hospitals is available either at this site or at a link from this site, including advocacy, health insurance, hospital information, research and education, health statistics, and valuable links to the National Information Center for Health Services Administration as well as other organizations and resources.
http://www.aha.org

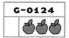

HospitalDirectory.com   This useful site provides a listing of states and territories, each of which is a direct link to a further listing of cities in the state or territory. By clicking on a city, the database provides a listing of hospitals in that area including name, address, and telephone numbers. The site also offers other links pertaining to health plans, doctors, health news, insurance, and medical products for physicians.
http://www.doctordirectory.com/hospitals/directory

HospitalWeb   This site is a guide to hospitals throughout the world that have sites established on the World Wide Web. Under each country, the names of a number of hospitals in that country are listed. By clicking on the hospital name, the user is taken to the hospital's Web site which provides further information.
http://neuro-www2.mgh.harvard.edu/hospitalwebworld.html

10.11   INTERNET MEDICAL NEWSGROUPS

General Medical Topic Newsgroups

Internet newsgroups are places where individuals can post messages on a common site for others to read. Many newsgroups are devoted to medical topics, and these groups are listed below. To access these groups you can either use a newsreader program (often part of an e-mail program) or search and browse using a popular Web site, groups.google.com

On the Google site, visitors can look for one of the newsgroup names listed below, such as sci.med, by either browsing the list of newsgroups or searching by the group name. Once there, the forum appears as a bulletin board with a posting on a particular topic, followed by responses to it. One can navigate the discussion by clicking on the postings of interest or post a reply.

Since newsgroups are mostly unmoderated, there is no editorial process or restrictions on postings. The information at these groups is therefore neither authoritative nor based on any set of standards.

sci.med	sci.med.nutrition	sci.med.vision
sci.engr.biomed	sci.med.occupational	alt.image.medical
sci.med.aids	sci.med.orthopedics	alt.med
sci.med.cardiology	sci.med.pathology	alt.med.allergy
sci.med.dentistry	sci.med.pharmacy	alt.med.cfs
sci.med.diseases.cancer	sci.med.physics	alt.med.ems
sci.med.diseases.hepatitis	sci.med.prostate.bph	alt.med.equipment
sci.med.diseases.lyme	sci.med.prostate.cancer	alt.med.fibromyalgia
sci.med.diseases.viral	sci.med.prostate.prostatitis	alt.med.outpat.clinic
sci.med.immunology	sci.med.psychobiology	alt.med.phys-assts
sci.med.informatics	sci.med.radiology	alt.med.urum-outcomes
sci.med.laboratory	sci.med.telemedicine	alt.med.veterinary
sci.med.nursing	sci.med.transcription	alt.med.vision.improve

10.12 LOCATING A PHYSICIAN

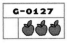

American Medical Association (AMA): Physician Select Online Doctor Finder The AMA is the primary "umbrella" professional association of physicians and medical students in the United States. The AMA Physician Select system provides information on virtually every licensed physician, including more than 690,000 physicians and doctors of osteopathy. According to the site, physician credentials have been certified for accuracy and authenticated by accrediting agencies, medical schools, residency programs, licensing and certifying boards, and other data sources. The user can search for physicians by name or by medical specialty.
http://www.ama-assn.org/aps/amahg.htm

DoctorDirectory.com This commercial site contains a directory of physicians, organized by specialty. Within the specialties, visitors can click on the state and city of interest. Results include the physician's name, gender, graduation year, specialties, and address.
http://www.doctordirectory.com/doctors/directory/default.asp?newSession=true

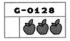

HealthPages This search tool allows visitors to locate doctors in their area by specialty and location. Over 500,000 physicians and 120,000 dentists are listed. Doctors may update their profiles for free. Local provider choices are displayed to consumers in a comparative format. They can access charts that compare the training, office services, and fees of local physicians; the provider networks and quality measures of area managed care plans; and the size, services, and fees of local hospitals. Patients can post ratings and comments about their doctors. http://www.thehealthpages.com

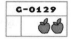

Physicians' Practice   This site allows the user to search for doctors in many specialty areas. Searches are performed by specialty and zip code. Physicians must pay a fee to be listed but enjoy benefits such as referrals, Internet presence, and a newsletter.
http://www.physicianpractice.com

10.13   MEDICAL AND HEALTH SCIENCES LIBRARIES

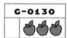

Medical Libraries at Universities, Hospitals, Foundations, and Research Centers   This site includes an up-to-date listing of libraries that can be accessed through links produced by staff members of the Hardin Library at the University of Iowa. Libraries are listed by state, enabling easy access to hundreds of library Web sites. Numerous foreign medical library links are also provided. http://www.lib.uiowa.edu/hardin-www/hslibs.html

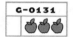

National Institutes of Health (NIH): Library Online   Information on the NIH Library is presented on this site, including current exhibits, hours, materials available to NIH personnel and the general public, current job vacancies, maps for visitors, and answers to frequently asked questions about the library. Users can search the library's catalog of books, journals, and other periodicals; access public and academic medical databases; and find seminar and tutorial information as well as links to related sites.
http://nihlibrary.nih.gov

National Library of Medicine (NLM)   The National Library of Medicine, the world's largest medical library, collects materials in all areas of biomedicine and healthcare and works on biomedical aspects of technology, the humanities, and the physical, life, and social sciences. This site contains links to government medical databases, including MEDLINE and MEDLINEplus; information on funding opportunities at the National Library of Medicine and other federal agencies; and details of services, training, and outreach programs offered by NLM. Users can access NLM's catalog of resources (LOCATORPlus), as well as NLM publications, including fact sheets, published reports, and staff publications. NLM research programs discussed at the site include topics in computational molecular biology, medical informatics, and other related subjects. The Web site features 15 searchable databases, covering journal searches via MEDLINE; AIDS information via AIDSLINE, AIDSDRUGS, and AIDSTRIALS; bioethics via BIOETHICSLINE; and numerous other important topics. The NLM Gateway, a master search engine, searches MEDLINE using the retrieval engine called PubMed. It is very user-friendly. There are over 11 million citations in MEDLINE and PreMEDLINE and the other related databases. Additionally, the NLM provides sources of health statistics, serials programs, and services maintained through a system called SERHOLD. http://www.nlm.nih.gov

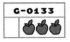

National Network of Libraries of Medicine   Composed of eight regional libraries, the NN/LM provides access to numerous other health science libraries in each region, located at universities, hospitals, and institutes. The Web site enables the user to link directly to each of the libraries in any region of the United States. These libraries have access to the NLM's SERHOLD system database of machine-readable holdings for biomedical serial titles. There are approximately 89,000 serial titles that are accessible through SERHOLD-participating libraries. http://nnlm.gov/

10.14 MEDICAL CONFERENCES AND MEETINGS

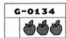

Doctor's Guide: Medical Conferences and Meetings   This address lists several hundred conferences and meetings, including continuing medical education programs worldwide, organized by date, meeting site, and subject. Location and other details are provided. http://www.docguide.com/crc.nsf/web-byspec

EventOnline.org   Sponsored by Excerpta Medica, this site offers a comprehensive database of medical, biotechnical, and scientific events. Search results yield contact information, as well as a basic description of the event. Some events have links to the sponsor's Web page. In addition, there are links for weather, hotels, and maps to assist in planning a visit. http://www.eventonline.org/

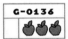

Medical Conferences.com   A broad range of medical conference listings is covered on this site, including meetings related to many different areas of healthcare, such as pharmaceuticals and hospital supplies, as well as the clinical medical specialties. An easy-to-use search mechanism provides access to the numerous listings, each of which links to details concerning each conference. The site is updated daily, providing details on over 7,000 forthcoming conferences. http://www.medicalconferences.com

MediConf Online   This site categorizes conferences by medical subject and provides information on conference dates, location, and organizer, mostly covering meetings to be held in the next month or two. The listings include research conferences, seminars, annual meetings of professional societies, medical technology trade shows, and opportunities for CME credits. The information provided free on the Internet is only a small percentage of the complete fee-based database, which includes more than 60,000 listings of meetings to be held through 2014 and is available through the information vendors, Ovid or Dialog. (some features fee-based) http://www.mediconf.com/online.html

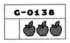

Medscape: Multispecialty Conference Schedules   Medical conference schedules are posted on this Web page, courtesy of Medscape. The schedules are listed chronologically and categorized by specialties such as family medicine,

pediatrics, nursing, and radiology. Conference dates, addresses, Web site links, and contact information are provided.
http://www.medscape.com/Home/Topics/multispecialty/directories/dir-MULT.ConfSchedules.html

Physician's Guide to the Internet Dates and locations for major national medical meetings are listed alphabetically by association at this site. There are also hyperlinks to association pages for additional information.
http://www.physiciansguide.com/meetings.html

Princeton Medicon: The Medical Conference Resource Details regarding worldwide major medical conferences of interest to medical specialists and primary care professionals are featured on this site. It is also periodically published in printed form. Access to lists of meetings is provided through a search engine that permits searching by specialty, year, and geographic region.
http://www.medicon.com.au

10.15 MEDICAL DATABASE SERVICES

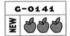

American Chemical Society: SciFinder This site provides information on the SciFinder research database, designed for scientists to use for searching Chemical Abstracts and MEDLINE. The database system contains more than 16 million abstracts, with links to full-text articles. Users can search by company name, chemical reactions, substructure, or keyword. Subscription information for research organizations is provided.
(fee-based) http://www.cas.org/SCIFINDER/scicover2.html

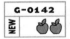

Cambridge Scientific Abstracts: Internet Database Service More than 50 bibliographic databases and electronic journals can be searched through this site. Databases include MEDLINE, TOXLINE, and other science/technology databases such as Biotechnology & Bioengineering. CSA-published electronic collections of abstracts, called "journals," such as *Genetics Abstracts, Medical & Pharmaceutical Biotechnology Abstracts,* and *Virology and AIDS Abstracts,* are also included.
(fee-based) http://www.csa.com/csa/ids/ids-main.shtml

Cochrane Library An international working group of experts has developed the Cochrane Library database with evidence-based medicine reviews by specialty and a bibliography of controlled trials. Searching, browsing, and displaying of abstracts is available free of charge; full access is available only to subscribers. (fee-based) http://www.cochranelibrary.com/enter/

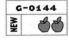

Database of Abstracts of Reviews of Effectiveness Quality-assessed reviews of the literature are compiled in the DARE database of evidence-based medicine, courtesy of the University of York. Reviews included have been assessed and selected for their high methodological value. Searches return structured abstracts that state the author's objective, intervention, participants in-

cluded, and outcomes assessed. Additional information includes the sources searched, methods by which data was extracted, and results. A complete guide to searching the DARE database is provided.
http://agatha.york.ac.uk/darehp.htm

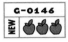

EBSCO Information Services   EBSCO information services provides subscription services for biomedical libraries plus access to numerous electronic journals and databases, some with full-text articles, such as Alternative Medicine, CancerLit, International Pharmaceutical Abstracts, and MEDLINE.
(fee-based) http://www.epnet.com/database.html

Electric Library   The Electric Library is an online database containing full-text articles from more than 150 newspapers; hundreds of magazines; national and international news wires; 2,000 books; photos; maps; television, radio, and government transcripts; and a free, complete encyclopedia. There is a 10-day free trial period.
(fee-based) http://wwws.elibrary.com

Information Quest   IQ seeks to link publishers, libraries, and the research audience electronically. The database is divided into libraries including life sciences, medicine, and physical sciences. Each library offers access to hundreds of journals and their abstracts; some have full-text articles.
(fee-based) http://www.informationquest.com/

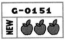

Institute for Scientific Information   A list of the bibliographic databases and research information available to ISI subscribers is provided on this site. Database topics include biotechnology, clinical medicine, and neuroscience. In addition, many of these databases provide citation searching capabilities through the ISI search tool, Web of Science, the unique search feature for which ISI is known. Users can find all of the published materials that have cited a particular work, regardless of discipline.
(fee-based) http://www.isinet.com/isi/products/index.html

International Digital Electronic Access Library   IDEAL offers users access to the full text of journals published by Academic Press, Churchill Livingstone, W. B. Saunders, Bailliere Tindall, and Mosby. There are also full-text reference encyclopedias related to immunology, human nutrition, virology, food microbiology, spectroscopy and spectrometry, and forensic sciences. Subscriptions are available for libraries; individuals can access articles on a pay-per-view basis. (fee-based) http://www.idealibrary.com

LINK: Online Library: Medicine   The LINK online library, dedicated to medicine, lists more than 100 journals, many containing full-text articles. The site can be searched and abstracts viewed free of charge; access to full-text articles requires a subscription.
(some features fee-based) http://link.springer.de/ol/medol/index.htm

Manual, Alternative, and Natural Therapy (MANTIS) Database The MANTIS database contains citations and abstracts for healthcare disciplines such as acupuncture, alternative medicine, chiropractic, herbal medicine, homeopathy, naturopathy, osteopathic medicine, physical therapy, and traditional Chinese medicine. The database covers domestic and international sources for more than 1,000 journals.

(fee-based) http://www.healthindex.com/MANTIS.asp

Ovid Medical Databases Bibliographic databases available through Ovid include MEDLINE and EMBASE for medicine and allied health, CINAHL for nursing, and BIOSIS for bioscience. Ovid's clinical products include resources on evidence-based medicine and drug information as well as decision support reference texts and journals. In total, there are more than 80 commercial bibliographic databases available. The Ovid interface offers many advanced search features, including links to full-text articles, and for most databases it incorporates database-specific thesauri to promote retrieval of relevant results.

(fee-based) http://www.ovid.com/products/databases/index.cfm

ScienceDirect Described as the "largest online full-text platform for scientific, technical, and medical information," the ScienceDirect database offers more than one million full-text articles from more than 1,200 journals, most published by Elsevier Science. Subject areas include biochemistry, clinical medicine, microbiology and immunology, pharmacology and toxicology, and neurosciences. Subscriptions are available only to libraries.

(fee-based)

http://www.sciencedirect.com/science/page/static/scidir/static_scidir_splash_about.html

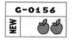

SilverLinker A new service from SilverPlatter.com, SilverLinker offers more than 2.5 million Internet links to over 6,500 journals and 2 million articles from more than 90 SilverPlatter databases. The SilverLinker database Internet links take visitors directly from citations to full-text articles.

(fee-based) http://www.silverplatter.com/silverlinker/index.htm

SilverPlatter: Medical and Pharmaceutical Collection Full-text access to research, clinical findings, policy issues, and practice is available through this collection of databases. The databases include MEDLINE, EMBASE, International Pharmaceutical Abstracts, Patient Education Library, Biological Abstracts, and Drug Information Fulltext.

(fee-based) http://www.silverplatter.com/hlthsci.htm

STNEasy This site provides subscribers with a user-friendly interface for searching a variety of databases covering bioscience, health, medicine, and pharmacology. More than 30 databases are listed under "Medicine." A new feature called eScience provides relevant Web content by automatically entering the user's search terms into the Google or Chemindustry.com search engines. Users are charged by the length of time spent searching for information.

(fee-based) http://stneasy.fiz-karlsruhe.de/html/english/login1.html

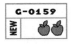

SwetsnetNavigator   More than 5,000 journals related to medicine are found in the SwetsnetNavigator database, some with access to full-text articles. This tool is designed to help institutions organize access to the tables of contents and full text for the titles to which they subscribe. Journals published by major bio-medical publishers, such as Academic Press, Elsevier, and Kluwer, are included. (fee-based) http://www.swetsnet.nl/cgi-bin/SB_main

10.16   MEDICAL EQUIPMENT AND MANUFACTURERS

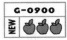

Medical Equipment and Pharmaceutical Companies   An A-to-Z listing of medical equipment and pharmaceutical manufacturers is provided on this site, courtesy of the Andrews School of Medical Transcription. The list is comprehensive with hyperlinks to hundreds of companies.
http://www.mtdesk.com/mfg.shtml

10.17   MEDICAL GLOSSARIES

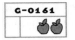

Boston University: Pharmacology Glossary   Provided by the Boston University School of Medicine, this Web page features a glossary of terms and symbols used in pharmacology. Each word has a definition and related terms.
http://www.bumc.bu.edu/www/busm/pharmacology/Programmed/framedGlossary.html

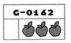

CancerWEB: Online Medical Dictionary   This site offers a comprehensive medical dictionary online for clinical, medical student, and patient audiences. It is a convenient source for a quick definition of an unfamiliar term.
http://www.graylab.ac.uk/omd/index.html

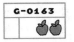

drkoop.com: Insurance   This site provides descriptions of both terms and phrases relating to health insurance. Terms are listed alphabetically.
http://www.drkoop.com/hcr/insurance/glossary.asp

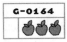

HealthAnswers: Disease Finder   A wide range of diseases is listed in this alphabetical directory of information for patients and consumers. Visitors can search by keyword or browse the directory for information. Details include alternative names, definitions, causes, incidence, risk factors, prevention, symptoms, signs and tests, treatment, prognosis, and complications. Many helpful diagrams or representative photographs related to the condition are also provided. http://www.healthanswers.com/Library/library_fset.asp

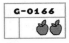

Immunology Glossary   A glossary of immunology is featured on this Web page, courtesy of the University of Leicester, Department of Microbiology and Immunology, in the United Kingdom. The entire glossary can be browsed at once since it is all located on this one page.
http://www-micro.msb.le.ac.uk/MBChB/ImmGloss.html

Don't type in long URLs – add the site number to the eMedguides URL: www.eMedguides.com/**G-1234**.

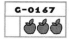

InteliHealth: Vitamin and Nutrition Resource Center InteliHealth offers this comprehensive glossary of vitamins and minerals, listed under fat-soluble vitamins, water-soluble vitamins, and minerals. Information provided under each entry includes important facts about the vitamin or mineral, daily intake recommendations for men and women, benefits, food sources, amounts of the substance present in various food sources, and cautions in terms of health consequences of the overuse or deficiency of the substance.
http://www.intelihealth.com/IH/ihtIH/WSIHW000/325/20932.html

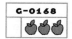

MedicineNet.com: Medications An index of medications is featured on this Web page, produced by MedicineNet. Of interest to both professionals and consumers, the index consists of an A-to-Z listing of prescription and over-the-counter drugs. Each drug has information such as its generic name, brand names, drug class and mechanism, storage, reasons for use, dosing, drug interaction, and side effects. In addition, each drug has links to further information such as related diseases, medications, and health facts.
http://www.medicinenet.com/Script/Main/AlphaIdx.asp?li=MNI&p=A_PHARM

MedicineNet.com: Procedures and Tests Index By clicking on "Procedures and Tests" at the top of the MedicineNet.com Web page, visitors will find a comprehensive, user-friendly index to common and not-so-common diagnostic tests and treatment procedures. Each diagnostic and treatment mini-forum contains a main article for general information, outlining the purpose and safety of the procedure, related diseases and treatments, articles written by physicians on related topics of interest, and interesting related consumer health facts. http://www.medicinenet.com

National Human Genome Research Institute: Genetics Glossary The National Human Genome Research Institute has developed this online glossary of genetic terms. The glossary can be browsed alphabetically or searched by keyword. Each term comes with a definition, an audio clip explaining the term, and a list of related terms.
http://www.nhgri.nih.gov/DIR/VIP/Glossary/

Spellex Development: Medical Spell Spellex Medical and Spellex Pharmaceutical online spelling verification allows visitors to check the spelling of medical terms. The search returns possible correct spellings if the word entered was not found.
http://www.spellex.com/speller.htm

Stedman's Shorter Medical Dictionary (1943): Poisons and Antidotes Posted as an item of historical interest only, this site features poisons and their antidotes from *Stedman's Shorter Medical Dictionary* (1943). An alphabetical listing of poisons is provided; each has a description of symptoms and appropriate treatment.
http://www.botanical.com/botanical/steapois/poisonix.html

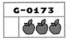

University of Texas: Life Science Dictionary   This free online dictionary designed for the public and professionals contains terms that deal with biochemistry, biotechnology, botany, cell biology, and genetics. The dictionary also contains some terms relating to ecology, limnology, pharmacology, toxicology, and medicine. The search engine allows the user to search by a specific term or by a term contained within a definition.
http://biotech.icmb.utexas.edu/search/dict-search.html

10.18   MEDICAL JOURNAL PUBLISHERS

Academic Press   This site lists a variety of journals published by Academic Press, a Harcourt Science and Technology Company. By clicking on "Biomedical Sciences" in the "Subject Categories" drop-down box, a listing of journals is presented including *Epilepsy and Behavior, Experimental Neurology, Seminars in Cancer Biology,* and *Virology.* A table of contents, along with abstracts, is available at no charge. Full-text articles can be purchased individually online or viewed by subscribers.
(some features fee-based)   http://www.academicpress.com/journals/

Annual Reviews: Biomedical Sciences   Volumes of the *Annual Reviews* for biomedical sciences are listed on this site; each review offers in-depth analysis and commentary on current topics from the previous year. Subjects include genomics and human genetics, immunology, and medicine. Visitors can access abstracts of articles from the current and past volumes. Full-text articles are available online to subscribers.
(some features fee-based)   http://arjournals.annualreviews.org/biomedicalhome.dtl

Ashley Publications Ltd.   The Ashley publishing group offers journals related to pharmacology, including *Expert Opinions* on biological therapy, pharmacotherapy, emerging drugs, investigational drugs, therapeutic patents, and therapeutic targets. In addition to free sample issues, visitors can access tables of contents and abstracts from back issues of each journal. Subscribers can access full-text articles.
(some features fee-based)   http://www.ashley-pub.com/html/journals.asp

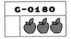

Blackwell Science   This site offers online access to information regarding over 200 Blackwell Science publications. Journals are sorted alphabetically by title and are available in all major fields of science and medicine. Blackwell Science provides a good general overview regarding the content and aim of each of its journals. Tables of contents are available for current and back issues of each title. Access to abstracts and articles requires a fee.
(some features fee-based)   http://www.blackwell-science.com/uk/journals.htm

Brookwood Medical Publications of PJB Publications   Five journals related to clinical research are described on this site: the *Journal of Drug Assessment,* the *Journal of Clinical Research,* the *Journal of Outcomes Research, Good Clinical Practices Journal,* and the *Journal of Medical Economics.* Abstracts of selected articles are available on the site. There is also a link to PharmaProjects, a leading pharmaceutical intelligence database available only on a subscription basis.

http://www.pjbpubs.com/brookwood/index.html

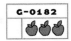

Cambridge University Press Journal titles available from Cambridge University Press are listed at this address. Topics encompass all subject areas, but many are devoted to medical specialties. The journals can be browsed alphabetically, by subject, and by online availability; tables of contents are provided. Visitors can browse both current and archived issues and journals can be ordered online.

http://www.cup.org/journal/

Carden Jennings Publishing Co, Ltd. The Carden Jennings medical multimedia publishing division offers journals, online publications, CD-ROMs, and books. Abstracts and free full-text articles (in Adobe Acrobat PDF format) are available online for journals including the *Biology of Blood and Marrow Transplantation, Laboratory Hematology,* and the *Heart Surgery Forum.*

http://www.cjp.com/stories/storyReader$6

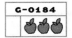

Elsevier Science Covering all Reed-Elsevier publications related to medicine, this site includes a subject index for access to individual journals in a variety of specialties including cardiology, obstetrics and gynecology, and psychiatry. Free sample copies of the journals are available online. Information is also included on Elsevier's books, CD-ROMs, and related products.

http://www.elsevier.com

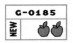

Gordon and Breach Publishing Group This section of the Gordon and Breach Web page offers books, journals, and magazines related to medical and life sciences. Journals are available in anesthesiology, cardiology, general medicine, hematology, nuclear medicine, oncology, pediatrics, and surgery. Tables of contents are available for current and past issues. Some journals have a link to online full-text articles for subscribers.

(some features fee-based) http://www.gbhap-us.com/medical.htm

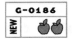

Guilford Press A publisher of psychology, psychiatry, and behavioral health publications, Guilford Press offers PDF samples of each of its journals. Information includes a list of titles available online and ordering details.

http://www.guilford.com/cartscript.cgi?page=home.html&cart_id=202303.24572

Hanley & Belfus A list of over 10 medical journals published by Hanley & Belfus is provided on this site. Titles include *Academic Medicine, Journal of Cancer Education,* and *Prehospital Emergency Care.* Tables of contents and article abstracts are available online. Subscribers can read full-text articles.

(some features fee-based) http://www.hanleyandbelfus.com/browse.asp?category=5

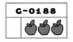

Harcourt Health Sciences Information on journals published by the Harcourt Health Sciences group, which includes Churchill Livingstone, IMNG,

JEMS Communications, Mosby, and W. B. Saunders, is presented on this site. By clicking on "Find a Journal by Specialty," visitors can access journals related to topics such as cardiology, endocrinology, and oncology. Tables of contents and subscription information are provided.

http://www.harcourthealth.com/scripts/om.dll/serve?action=home

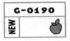

Harcourt International International medical journals published by Harcourt are provided on this site, sorted into more than 75 specialties. Topics covered include clinical cancer, gastroenterology, midwifery, and surgery. Visitors can access the tables of contents and abstracts to current and back issues of the journals. Full-text articles are available for a fee.

(some features fee-based) http://www.harcourt-international.com/journals/jsbrowse.cfm

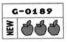

Haworth Medical Press Information on the Haworth Medical Press, an imprint of the Haworth Press, is provided at this site including a listing of its 15 medical journals. The online catalog provides additional information on the journals, including a section for reader reviews.

http://www.haworthpressinc.com/imprints/details.asp?ID=HMP

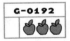

HighWire Press HighWire Press presents a list of its biomedical journals, organized alphabetically or by subject, including detailed information regarding the features available at no charge for each title. For each journal there is a link to its home page, where tables of contents and abstracts are available. The full text of entire journals or back issues is available for many titles.

http://highwire.stanford.edu

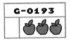

Karger Medical journals published by Karger are listed alphabetically on this site. The abstracts and tables of contents of current and back issues are available online. Subscribers can access full-text articles. A free sample copy of each journal is available online.

(some features fee-based) http://www.karger.com/journals/index.htm

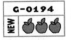

Kluwer Academic Publishers Journals of interest in medicine and related subjects are listed on this page. Journal categories include cardiology, internal medicine, neurology, oncology, and urology. Visitors can browse through the table of contents of each publication for current and archived issues or conduct searches by keyword for returns of specific articles.

http://kapis.www.wkap.nl/jrnlsubject.htm/E+0+0+0

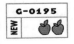

Lippincott Williams & Wilkins Medical and scientific journals published by Lippincott Williams & Wilkins can be browsed by specialty on this site. There are more than 80 specialties and subspecialties represented. A table of contents, abstracts, and subscription information are provided for each journal, including full-text access options and links. http://www.lww.com/periodicals.htm

Marcel Dekker Scientific, technical, and medical journals published by Marcel Dekker are listed on this site. By clicking on "Medicine," journals and other types of publications can be searched. There are more than a dozen journals related to medicine, including the *Journal of Toxicology, Immunopharmacology and Immunotoxicology,* and the *Journal of Asthma.* The tables of contents and abstracts are free. Many full-text articles are available online to subscribers. (some features fee-based) http://www.dekker.com/index.jsp

Mary Ann Liebert, Inc. This site offers more than 50 journals and 25 books published by Mary Ann Liebert, Inc., in the field of biotechnology. Journal titles include *AIDS Patient Care and STDs, Microbial Drug Resistance,* and *Thyroid.* General information on each journal is provided, as well as the table of contents for current and archived issues, and a free sample copy.
http://www.liebertpub.com/journals/default1.asp

Medical Economics Company The Medical Economics Company site offers healthcare professionals journals and newsletters related to the diagnosis and treatment of disease. Journals include *Contemporary OB/GYN, Contemporary Urology, Contemporary Pediatrics,* and the *Journal of the American Academy of Physician Assistants.* Journals have their own Web sites and some include full-text articles. In addition, there are clinical newsletters.
(some features fee-based) http://www.medec.com/

Munksgaard New titles, along with an alphabetical index of more than 70 scientific, technical, and medical journals, are provided on this site, which also allows visitors to view journals by subject. The journals are international in scope. General information on each journal is provided, along with a sample issue. Subscribers can access some of the journals online.
(some features fee-based) http://journals.munksgaard.dk/

Nature Publishing Group of Macmillan Publishers, Ltd. An alphabetical list of more than 25 specialist medical journals is provided on this Web site, along with the *Nature* scientific specialty journals. Titles include the *European Journal of Human Genetics, Leukemia,* and the *Hematology Journal.* Tables of contents and abstracts are available online. There is also an online sample copy. Full-text articles are available only to subscribers.
(some features fee-based) http://www.naturesj.com/sj/journals/journals_index.html

Oxford University Press Medical journals from Oxford University Press are listed on this site. There are over 20 journals listed; each publication offers tables of contents and abstracts. Subscribers can access full-text articles. A free e-mail alert service is available to receive, in advance, the table of contents for new issues. (some features fee-based) http://www.oup.co.uk/medicine/journals/

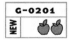

Parthenon Publishing Group Links to more than a dozen journals published by Parthenon are featured on this Web page. Titles include *Gynecological Endocrinology,* the *Aging Male,* the *Journal of Drug Evaluation,* and the *Journal of Maternal-Fetal Medicine.* The table of contents from the most recent issue of each journal is posted. In addition, a catalog of the group's books, slides, videos, and CD-ROMs is provided.
http://www.parthpub.com/journal.html

Pulsus Group The Pulsus Group offers information at this site on journals published by the group for specialties such as plastic surgery, cardiology, gastroenterology, infectious diseases, and pediatrics. Visitors can access abstracts and full-text articles in some of the journals. http://www.pulsus.com/

SLACK Inc. In addition to journals, this site lists books, Internet resources, and symposia on the Web for a variety of medical specialties, allied health, and nursing subspecialties. A sample table of contents along with general information about each journal is provided. Visitors must scroll down the page to view the entire index of publications.
http://www.slackinc.com/areas.asp

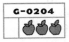

Springer Covering the large list of journals published by Springer-Verlag, this site primarily contains abstracts rather than full-text articles. Full-text articles are available for individuals or institutions who maintain print subscriptions. The site covers a broad range of biomedical titles, all of which provide tables of contents from the most recent years.
(some features fee-based) http://link.springer.de/ol/medol/index.htm

Swets & Zeitlinger The journal catalog of Swets & Zeitlinger is featured on this Web site. Journals related to health can be found under life sciences, neuroscience, ophthalmology, and psychology. The list of journals includes *Pharmaceutical Biology, Neuro-Ophthalmology,* and the *Clinical Neuropsychologist.* Tables of contents and abstracts for the current issue, as well as back issues, of each journal are available.
http://www.swets.nl/sps/journals/jhome.html

Taylor & Francis Group Journals are listed by subject on this site and include the behavioral sciences, biomedical sciences, and biosciences. The journals are international in nature. Although the table of contents is free, access to the articles is by subscription only.
(some features fee-based) http://www.tandf.co.uk/journals/sublist.html

Thieme There are over 30 medical journals listed on this Web page published by the German publisher Thieme. Topics covered include pediatric surgery, reproductive medicine, liver disease, and perinatology. Selected article citations are provided. http://www.thieme.com/SID1997012758581/journals/index.html

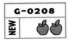

VSP: International Science Publishers A listing of more than 40 VSP journals is offered on this site. The journals cover a broad array of sciences; titles of interest to healthcare professionals include *Gene Therapy and Regulation, Haematologia, Inflammopharmacology,* and *Trauma Quarterly.* The tables of contents from previous issues are online. A free sample issue of any journal can be requested through the Web site.
http://www.vsppub.com/journals/index.html

Wiley Interscience This site is maintained by John Wiley and Sons, Inc., and provides a subject index to all Wiley journals. More than 90 journals are listed

under the "Life and Medical Sciences" section. Free registration allows access to tables of contents and abstracts published within the last 12 months. Full-text access is available via registration to both individual and institutional subscribers of the print counterparts of the Wiley online journals.

(some features fee-based) http://www3.interscience.wiley.com/journalfinder.html

10.19 MEDICAL NEWS

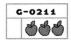

American Medical Association (AMA): American Medical News
Published by the American Medical Association, *American Medical News* is "the newspaper for America's physicians." The site offers free access to the latest issue online, with each electronic publication providing coverage of top stories, legislative updates, and professional issues. Business information and the ability to read a mobile edition on any handheld device are provided, as well as archived issues and e-mail headline alerts.

http://www.ama-assn.org/public/journals/amnews/amnews.htm

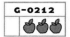

CNN: Health News Health News from CNN is produced in association with WebMDHealth. Specific articles are available in featured topics, ethics matters, research, and home remedies, and an allergy report is also provided. National and international health news is presented, and users can access specific articles on AIDS, aging, alternative medicine, cancer, children's health, diet and fitness, men's health, and women's health. Visitors can also access patient questions and answers from doctors, chat forums, and special community resources available through WebMD. Information and articles are also offered by Mayo Clinic and AccentHealth.com.

http://www.cnn.com/HEALTH

Doctor's Guide: Medical and Other News This site provides current medical news and information for health professionals. Visitors can search the Doctor's Guide medical news database and access medical news Webcasts within the past week or the past month. News items organized by subject, first-hand conference communiques, and journal club reviews are also available at this informative news site.

http://www.pslgroup.com/MEDNEWS.HTM

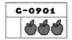

MDLinx MDLinx offers daily medical journal articles organized by subspecialty. There are nearly 25 medical fields as well as areas in allied health represented in the menu at this home page. Each field is further categorized into subspecialties, providing articles in each area. Article selections are updated daily to reflect the release of new issues of monthly journals.

http://www.mdlinx.com

Medical Breakthroughs Daily news updates are posted and can be delivered to individual e-mail addresses from this site. Visitors can also search archived articles by keyword, read weekly general interest articles, find links to related sites, and watch videos related to current health issues. The site is sponsored by

Ivanhoe Broadcast News, Inc., a medical news gathering organization providing stories to television stations nationwide.
(free registration) http://www.ivanhoe.com/#reports

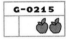

Reuters Health The Reuters Health Web page provides breaking medical news, updated daily, as well as a subscription-based database of the news archives of reuters news service. Visitors can access MEDLINE and a database of drug information from the site.
(some features fee-based) http://www.reutershealth.com

UniSci: Daily University Science News This site offers current articles related to all branches of science, including medicine. Many medical articles are available, and special archives offer additional medical resources. Users can access news from the past 10 days and perform searches for archived material.
http://unisci.com

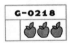

USA Today: Health *USA Today's* feature stories and headline archives are directly accessible at this Web site where visitors can view some of the best in nationwide medical news coverage. Articles are listed by topic, including addiction, AIDS, allergies, alternative medicine, arthritis, cancer, diabetes, genetics, hepatitis, mental health, surgery, and vision. Visitors will also find the latest in medical and pharmacotherapeutic research.
http://www.usatoday.com/life/health/archive.htm

Yahoo!: Health Headlines Updated several times throughout the day, "Health Headlines" at Yahoo offers full news coverage and Reuters news with health headlines from around the globe. Earlier daily and archived stories may be accessed, and the site's search engine allows viewers to browse, with full color, the latest in photographic coverage of news and events.
http://dailynews.yahoo.com/headlines/hl

10.20 MEDICAL SEARCH ENGINES

Similar information can be found under the medical supersites section.

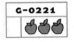

Achoo Healthcare Online A directory of Web sites in three main categories—human health and disease, business of health, and organizations and sources—is featured on this Web page. Extensive subcategories and short descriptions are provided for each site. Daily health news of interest to patients, the public, and medical professionals is available at the site, as well as links to journals, databases, employment directories, and discussion groups.
http://www.achoo.com

All the Web Visitors can search the Web in more than 25 languages using this search tool. The option to search for pictures, videos, MP3 files, or FTP files is also featured. http://www.alltheweb.com

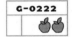

Biocrawler: The Life Science Search Engine   Described as a life science search engine, this Web page contains a large directory with thousands of Internet sites. The directory can be searched by keyword or by clicking on a particular topic such as anthropology, biotechnology, genetics, bioinformatics, and biomedicine. There is also a directory of biology-related jobs that have been posted on the Internet. http://www.biocrawler.com/

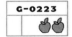

Citeline.com Search Tool   The search tool on this Web page allows visitors to search the Web by keyword and, if desired, to limit the search to any or all of the following categories: disease and treatment, organizations, news and journals, and research and trials.
(free registration) http://www.citeline.com/C1SE/search

CliniWeb International   CliniWeb, a service of Oregon Health Sciences University, provides an index and table of contents for clinical resources available on the World Wide Web. Information found at the site is of particular interest to healthcare professional students and practitioners. Search terms can be entered in five different languages: English, German, French, Spanish, and Portuguese. The site offers links to additional search resources and is linked directly to MEDLINE. http://www.ohsu.edu/cliniweb

Galen II: The Digital Library of the University of California, San Francisco (UCSF)   This online library directory includes UCSF and UC resources and services, links to the AMA Directory, Drug Info Fulltext, Harrison's Online (requires a password), the *Merck Manual,* Consumer Health, and a database of additional resources and publications including electronic journals. Visitors can search the Galen II database or the World Wide Web using a variety of search engines.
http://galen.library.ucsf.edu

Google   Google offers a comprehensive search tool, integrating resources from several smaller search engines. Several subject areas are available for more specific queries, including health and related subtopics. Visitors can enter a search term, view Google results, and try the same query through AltaVista, Excite, HotBot, Infoseek, Lycos, and Yahoo through the site.
http://www.google.com

Health On the Net (HON) Foundation: MedHunt   The Health On the Net Foundation provides several widely used medical search engines including MedHunt, HONselect, and MEDLINE. Users can access databases containing information on newsgroups, LISTSERVs, medical images and movies, upcoming and past healthcare-related conferences, and daily news stories on health-related topics. Topical searches yield brief site descriptions, which are ranked by relevance. http://www.hon.ch/MedHunt

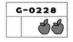

InfoMedical.com: Medical Search Engine   This site features a directory with hundreds of medical sites categorized as companies, distributors, products, organizations, services, and Web resources. The directory can be searched or

browsed by category. Of interest to physicians, the Web resources section contains clinical trial postings, job postings, online libraries, online medical discussions, and online medical multimedia. Each site has a company profile and a list of their products and services. http://www.infomedical.com/

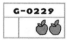

MDchoice.com   MDchoice.com is a privately held company founded by academic physicians with the goal of making access to health and medical information on the Internet as efficient and reliable as possible. The site features an UltraWeb search with all content selected by board-certified physicians. In addition, users have access to MEDLINE, drug information, health news, and a variety of clinical calculators. Also offered are several interactive educational exercises, online journals and text books, and employment opportunities.
http://www.mdchoice.com

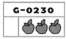

Med411.com: Medical Research Portal   This site offers separate links to a variety of comprehensive search tools, allowing users to search medical libraries, professional associations, online health manuals, peer-reviewed journals, health services, images, and clinical trials. Linked institutions include the National Library of Medicine, the Combined Health Information Database (CHID), CancerNet, the National Institute of Diabetes and Digestive and Kidney Diseases, HealthFinder, and WebPath.
http://www.med411.com/resources.html

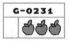

MedExplorer   MedExplorer is a comprehensive medical and health directory. Short descriptions of each site are provided. The site also lists related newsgroups and has information on conferences and employment.
http://www.medexplorer.com

Medscape   Medscape provides several databases from which users can search the Web. Resources that can be accessed include articles, news, information for patients, MEDLINE, AIDSLINE, TOXLINE, drug information, a dictionary, a bookstore, the Dow Jones Library, and medical images. There is a wealth of additional information provided including articles, case reports, conference schedules and summaries, CME resources, job listings, journals, news, patient information, practice guidelines, treatment updates, and links to medical specialty sites. Access requires free online registration.
(free registration) http://www.medscape.com

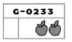

Metacrawler   At the Metacrawler site users can search for Web resources through a directory or a search engine. The search engine offers extensive coverage in the field of medicine. http://www.metacrawler.com

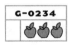

Search Taxi.com: Health   A directory dedicated to health is featured on this site. There are thousands of sites listed under categories such as alternative medicine, conditions and diseases, medicine, and mental health. These categories are broken down further into topics such as employment, health insurance, men's health, and substance abuse.
http://www.searchtaxi.com/dir/Health/

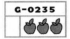

Stanford University: MedBot   Offered by Stanford University, this site allows users to search medical and health resources on the Web using major general and medical search engines. More specific searches can be performed within topics such as education and learning, news and information, and medical images, as well as multimedia resources.
http://www-med.stanford.edu/medworld/medbot

Yahoo!   Yahoo offers visitors the opportunity to search the Web and browse sites listed in multiple categories including health and science. Within each category are more specific subcategories that indicate the number of entries available. Most sites are suggested by users. Additionally, Yahoo offers a wealth of services such as free e-mail, shopping, people search, news, travel, weather, and stock reports. http://www.yahoo.com/health

10.21   MEDICAL STATISTICS

Centers for Disease Control and Prevention (CDC): Biostatistics/Statistics   This address provides visitors with links to sources of national and regional statistics. Resources include federal, county, and city data, as well as statistics related to labor, current population, public health, economics, trade, and business. Sources for mathematics and software information are also found through this site.
http://www.cdc.gov/niosh/biostat.html

Health Sciences Library System: Health Statistics   The University of Pittsburgh's Falk Library of the Health Sciences developed this site to provide information on obtaining statistical health data from Internet and library sources. Resources include details on obtaining statistical data from U.S. population databases, government agencies collecting statistics, organizations and associations collecting statistics, and other Web sites providing statistical information. The site explains specific Internet and library tools for locating health statistics and offers a glossary of terms used in statistics.
http://www.hsls.pitt.edu/intres/guides/statcbw.html

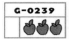

National Center for Health Statistics   The National Center for Health Statistics, part of the Centers for Disease Control and Prevention, provides an extensive array of health and medical statistics for the medical, research, and consumer communities. This site provides express links to numerous surveys and statistical sources at the NCHS.
http://www.cdc.gov/nchs/default.htm

University of Michigan: Statistical Resources on the Web: Health   Online sources for health statistics are cataloged at this site, including comprehensive health statistics resources and sources for statistics by topic. Topics include abortion, accidents, births, deaths, disability, disease experimentation, hazardous substances, health insurance, HMOs, hospitals, mental health, nutrition, occupational safety, pregnancy, prescription drugs, risk behaviors, sleep, smoking, substance abuse, surgery, transplants, and vital statistics. Users can also access an alphabetical directory of sites in the database and a search engine for locating more specific resources.

http://www.lib.umich.edu/libhome/Documents.center/sthealth.html

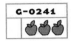

World Health Organization (WHO): Statistical Information System
The Statistical Information System of the WHO is intended to provide access to both statistical and epidemiological data and information from this international agency in electronic form. The site provides health statistics, disease information, mortality statistics, AIDS/HIV data, immunization coverage and incidence of communicable diseases, and links to statistics from other countries as well as links to the Centers for Disease Control and Prevention. This site is the premier resource for statistics on diseases worldwide. The WHO main site, http://www.who.int, provides additional disease-related statistics.

http://www.who.int/whosis

10.22 ONLINE TEXTS AND TUTORIALS

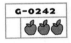

eMedicine: World Medical Library A medical library is featured on this Web page, with online textbooks for professionals and consumers, courtesy of eMedicine. Professionals can read *Emergency Medicine,* and they have access to Gold Standard Multimedia online books. The Gold Standard books focus on basic science such as clinical pharmacology, human anatomy, and immunology. A Gold Standard link provides access to their Web site, where specific books can be selected from a drop-down menu. Books for consumers include *Consumer Treatment Guidelines* and *Wilderness Emergencies.*

(free registration) http://www.emedicine.com/

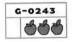

Harrison's Online Directed to physicians, this Web page features the online text of *Harrison's Principles of Medicine.* Each chapter includes information such as diagnosis, prevalence, pathogenesis, clinical features, treatment, complications, and a bibliography. Links are also provided on each topic for related sites, updates, clinical trial information, and self-assessment quizzes.

(fee-based) http://www.harrisonsonline.com/

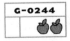

Medical Textbooks Online Professionals will find a directory of links to online medical textbooks on this Web page maintained by medic8.com. Close to 30 specialties are represented, including geriatric medicine, neurosurgery, microbiology, and pediatrics.

http://www.medic8.com/MedicalTextbooksOnline.htm

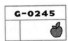

Medical Texts on the Internet This list of medical texts, arranged by specialty, includes access to a variety of medical papers and articles in over 25 areas. Links to documents in cardiology, dermatology, oncology, and urology are included, with each listing a series of related tutorials and texts.

http://members.tripod.com/gustavo_01/textmed.html

Merck Manual of Diagnosis and Therapy   Hosted by Merck, this site features the *Merck Manual of Diagnosis and Therapy*. Primarily of interest to healthcare professionals, the site offers a table of contents with links to a broad range of disorders categorized in sections such as nutritional disorders, gastro-intestinal disorders, pulmonary disorders, and pediatrics. In total, there are 23 sections with 308 chapters. Typical chapters provide a detailed clinical discussion of the disorder including an overview, etiology, symptoms and signs, and treatment information. Within the chapter, links are provided to related topics.
http://www.merck.com/pubs/mmanual/sections.htm

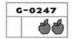

University of Illinois: Atlases and Other Medical Texts   Maintained by the University of Illinois at Urbana-Champaign, this Web page features more than 50 links for atlases and online medical textbooks. At the bottom of the page, there are hyperlinks to general medical information and medical education sites. http://alexia.lis.uiuc.edu/~buenker/atlases.html

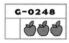

University of Iowa: Family Practice Handbook   The *University of Iowa Family Practice Handbook* is featured on this Web page, primarily of interest to physicians. This searchable textbook has 20 chapters covering topics such as cardiology, pulmonary medicine, gynecology, pediatrics, and dermatology. Chapters typically cover diseases and conditions by providing an overview, along with causes, diagnosis, and treatment information. In addition to disorders, office and hospital procedures, as well as drug doses of commonly prescribed medications, are covered.
http://www.vh.org/Providers/ClinRef/FPHandbook/FPContents.html

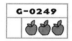

Virtual Hospital: Multimedia Textbooks   Intended for healthcare providers, a list of multimedia textbooks is featured on this Web page, hosted by the University of Iowa Virtual Hospital. All textbooks listed are drawn from the Virtual Hospital and include more than 40 topics such as anatomy, dermatology, pediatrics, the human brain, and pathology. Along with text, there are also video clips, photomicrographs and photographs, and radiographic images.
http://www.vh.org/Providers/Textbooks/MultimediaTextbooks.html

10.23 PHARMACEUTICAL INFORMATION

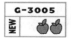

CenterWatch: Newly Approved Drug Therapies   For many researchers and physicians, information about FDA drug approvals is of central concern. A concise summary of such approvals by medical specialty and condition from 1995 to the present is featured on this Web page.
http://www.centerwatch.com/patient/drugs/druglist.html

Doctor's Guide: New Drugs and Indications   The Doctor's Guide provides an ongoing source of new drug information, including FDA approvals and drug indications. Drug articles are presented in order of article datelines, with the most current stories listed first. Information for drug releases for the past 12 months is provided.   http://www.pslgroup.com/NEWDRUGS.HTM

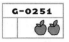

drkoop.com: Drug Interactions Search   Visitors can enter drug names into a search tool for general information as well as access to Drug Checker information on warnings, side effects, pharmacology, lactation, and pregnancy. The Drug Checker also provides information on interactions between two or more drugs.
http://www.drugchecker.drkoop.com/apps/drugchecker/DrugMain?cob=drkoop

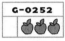

Drug InfoNet   Information and links to areas on the Web concerning healthcare and pharmaceutical-related topics are available at this site. The drug information is available by brand name, generic name, manufacturer, and therapeutic class. Visitors can also obtain pharmaceutical manufacturer information.
http://www.druginfonet.com/phrminfo.htm

DrugFacts.com Library   Described as the "most comprehensive source of free and premium drug, interaction, and herbal information on the Internet," this site offers information drawn from *Drug Facts,* courtesy of the Wolters Kluwer International Health and Science companies. An "A to Z Drug Facts" section offers more than 4,500 drugs, along with information such as action, indication/contraindication, dosage, interactions, adverse reactions, precautions, and patient education tips. An abridged version for professionals is available after a free registration process. Other highlights include information drawn from *Drug Interaction Facts* and from a guide to 125 herbal products. Patients can access "Med Facts" for easy-to-read information on more than 4,000 drugs.
http://www.drugfacts.com/DrugFacts/tabs/library.jhtml?pf=&ps=&cr=&si=#druginfo

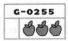

Food and Drug Administration (FDA): Approved Drug Products
The U.S. Food and Drug Administration's *Electronic Orange Book* for approved drug products is posted on this Web site. The book can be searched by active ingredient, proprietary name, applicant holder, or application number. The results for a search provide all of this information as well as the dosage form, route, and strength.
http://www.fda.gov/cder/ob/default.htm

Food and Drug Administration (FDA): Center for Drug Evaluation and Research   The Center for Drug Evaluation and Research provides information on prescription, consumer, and over-the-counter drugs at this address. Resources include alphabetical lists of new and generic drug approvals, new drugs approved for cancer indications, the *Electronic Orange Book* listing all FDA-approved prescription drugs, a national drug code directory, labeling notices, patient information, and alerts of new indications. Links are available to many resources related to drug safety and side effects, public health alerts and warnings, and pages offering information on major drugs. Reports and publications, special projects and programs, and cancer clinical trials information are also found through this address.
http://www.fda.gov/cder/drug/default.htm

MedicineNet.com: Medications Index   This pharmacological database from MedicineNet provides a mini-forum for each prescription and nonprescription medication, including a brief main article pertaining to the medication, related medications, related news and updates, diseases associated with the medication, and a listing of articles pertinent to the pharmacological agent's usage. http://www.medicinenet.com/Script/Main/AlphaIdx.asp?li=MNI&d=51&p=A_PHARM

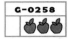

MedWatch: The FDA Medical Products Reporting Program MedWatch, the FDA Safety Information and Adverse Event Reporting Program, is designed to educate health professionals about the importance of being aware of, monitoring for, and reporting adverse events and problems to the FDA and/or the product manufacturer. The program is also intended to disseminate new safety information rapidly within the medical community, thereby improving patient care. To these ends, the site includes an adverse event reporting form and instructions as well as safety information for health professionals, including "Dear Health Professional" letters and notifications related to drug safety. It also includes relevant full-text continuing education articles and reports regarding drug and medical device safety issues.
http://www.fda.gov/medwatch

PDR.net PDR.net publishes health-related articles geared toward specific groups including physicians, pharmacists, physician assistants, oncologists, nurse practitioners, nurses, and consumers. Sections dedicated to each type of audience present articles from sources that include professional journals, CenterWatch, MEDLINE, Cancerfacts.com, the Centers for Disease Control and Prevention, the Government Clinical Trial Website, and the Mayo Health Clinic Oasis. Physicians can access "PDR Online" and obtain extensive information on drugs, herbal medicine, multidrug interactions, and drug pricing. Online CME materials are also provided for physicians, nurses, pharmacists, and veterinarians. (free registration) http://www.pdr.net

Pharmaceutical Research and Manufacturers of America This association Web site includes a "New Medicines in Development" database; a publications section containing reports relating to the pharmaceutical industry; various links for facts and figures on pharmaceutical research and innovation; and an issues and policies section covering many current topics of interest to pharmaceutical companies, such as genetics research and healthcare liability reform. http://www.phrma.org

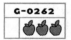

RxList: The Internet Drug Index This site allows users to search for drug information by name, imprint code, or keyword. The top 200 prescribed drugs for the previous six years are listed alphabetically or by rank. Patient monographs are available for a wide range of drugs, and one section is devoted to alternative medicine information and answers to frequently asked questions. The site also provides a forum for drug-specific discussions.
http://www.rxlist.com

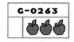

Virtual Library Pharmacy This library of pharmacy information contains resources for professionals in all medical areas. The site provides information on pharmacy schools, associations, companies, journals and books, Internet data-

bases relating to pharmaceutical topics, conferences, hospital sites, government sites, pharmacy LISTSERVs, and news groups. Hundreds of site links are provided for the above areas.
http://www.pharmacy.org

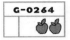 **World Standard Drug Database** Information on pharmaceutical products at this address includes ingredients, dosage, routes of administration, and products with the same ingredients and/or strengths. Visitors can search for relevant information by drug, ingredient, indications, contraindications, or side effects.
http://209.235.4.229/drugcgic.cgi/START

10.24 PHYSICIAN BACKGROUND

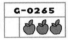 **American Board of Medical Specialties** This verification service contains the names of all physicians certified by an American Board of Medical Specialties (ABMS) member board. It permits the public to verify the credentials and certification status of any physician, searching by name, city, state, and specialty within the 24 member board specialty areas. There is no fee for this service.
http://www.abms.org

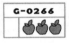 **Healthgrades.com** This resource specializes in healthcare ratings, providing hospital ratings by procedure or diagnosis, physician ratings by specialty and geographic area, and ratings of health plans. Directories of hospitals, physicians, health plans, mammography facilities, fertility clinics, assisted-living facilities, home health agencies, hospice programs, cancer centers, dentists, and chiropractors are also available. Visitors can access tips on choosing a hospital, physician, or health plan, as well as a glossary of terms and health news articles. http://www.healthgrades.com

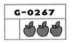 **Physician Background Information Service** Searchpointe.com offers background information on doctors and chiropractors licensed in the United States, such as name of medical school and year of graduation, residency training record, ABMS certifications, states where certified, and records of sanctions or disciplinary actions. There is a fee for license and sanction reports.
(some features fee-based) http://www.searchpointe.com

10.25 STATE HEALTH DEPARTMENTS

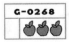 **State Health Departments** A list of links to U.S. state health departments is featured on this site maintained by the Centers for Disease Control and Prevention. A search tool enables the visitor to search state health departments for certain information. In addition, links to related international resources can be found on the left side of the page, such as the Pan American Health Organization and the World Health Organization.
http://www.cdc.gov/mmwr/international/relres.html

PROFESSIONAL TOPICS AND CLINICAL PRACTICE

11.1 ANATOMY AND PHYSIOLOGY

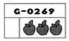

American Medical Association (AMA): Atlas of the Body   The Atlas of the Body is a site offered by the American Medical Association that provides detailed information and labeled illustrations of the various systems and organs of the human body. The site also provides descriptions of disorders that affect these systems and organs.
http://www.ama-assn.org/insight/gen_hlth/atlas/atlas.htm

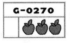

Health On the Net (HON) Foundation: Medical Images   Part of a larger Health On the Net Foundation Web page, this site features a medical image and video library on anatomy. There are more than 750 images related to topics such as the cardiovascular system, digestive system, musculoskeletal system, and nervous system. In addition to organ systems, other categories include organisms, diseases, chemicals and drugs, techniques, and biological sciences. Each image has a hyperlink to its source for additional information.
http://www.hon.ch/Media/anatomy.html

Karolinska Institutet: Anatomy and Histology   Resources available on this site directed to physicians include more than 50 links on anatomy and nearly 20 on histology. Many of the sites contain numerous illustrations and photographs, and some have video. The sites are drawn primarily from universities around the world.
http://www.mic.ki.se/Anatomy.html

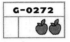

Martindale's Health Science Guide: Virtual Medical Center: Anatomy and Histology Center   This "Virtual Medical Center" offers links to examinations, tutorials, and associations. It lists numerous atlases and sites with anatomical images, including some on embryology and developmental anatomy. The center which also provides links to general medical dictionaries, glossaries, and encyclopedias, as well as sites containing information on metabolic pathways and genetic maps.
http://www-sci.lib.uci.edu/HSG/MedicalAnatomy.html

MedBioWorld: Anatomy and Physiology Journals   More than 65 journals related to anatomy and physiology are listed on this Web page. Hyperlinks are provided to the online versions of the journals; some are for subscribers only. http://www.medbioworld.com/journals/medicine/anatomy.html

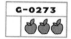

MedNets: Anatomy Dedicated to anatomy, this site features links for information such as associations, databases, and journals. Some journals are for subscribers only. General resources include information on specific parts of the anatomy, as well as 3-D anatomy for students.
(some features fee-based) http://www.mednets.com/anatomy.htm

Purdue University: Anatomy Links A list of links on human anatomy and resources for medical students is featured on this Web page, courtesy of Purdue University. The links are accessed in a sidebar menu where there are more than a dozen categories including cardiology, clinical information, embryology, histology, gross anatomy, lumen, neuroscience, ophthalmology, radiology, the reproductive system, sports medicine, and surgery. Medical students will find a section dedicated to them with links for general resources.
http://www.vet.purdue.edu/bms/ai/frames/intlink_00.htm

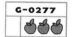

University of Arkansas for Medical Sciences: Anatomy Tables Maintained at the University of Arkansas for Medical Sciences, this site features anatomy tables. The tables are organized by system such as arteries or bones and by region of the body. Each table includes the proper name of the anatomical part and a description.
http://anatomy.uams.edu/HTMLpages/anatomyhtml/medcharts.html

Whole Brain Atlas Administered by the Harvard Medical School, this site shows imaging of the brain using magnetic resonance imaging (MRI), roentgen-ray computed tomography (CT), and nuclear medicine technologies. Structures within the images are labeled. Normal brain images are provided, as well as images of brains subjected to cerebrovascular disease, neoplastic disease, degenerative disease, and inflammatory or infectious disease. The entire atlas is available free of charge online or can be ordered on CD-ROM for a fee.
http://www.med.harvard.edu/AANLIB/home.html

11.2 BIOMEDICAL ETHICS

American Society of Bioethics and Humanities The American Society of Bioethics and Humanities is an organization that promotes scholarship, research, teaching, policy development, and professional development in the field of bioethics. The site offers information on the society, the annual meeting, position papers, and awards. There is also a large list of resource links covering academic centers, education, ethics and philosophy, law, medicine and the humanities, online texts, organizations, and science and technology.
http://www.asbh.org

American Society of Law, Medicine, and Ethics This site offers information on the American Society of Law, Medicine, and Ethics; the *Journal*

of Law, Medicine, and Ethics; and the *American Journal of Law and Medicine.* Also provided are details on research projects; a news section that gives updates on recent developments in law, medicine, and ethics; and information on future and past conferences held by the society. A comprehensive listing of related resources is also provided in categories such as bioethics, cancer, genetics, geriatrics, health law, managed care, and nursing.

http://www.aslme.org

Bioethics Discussion Pages   This page is a discussion forum for people to share their views on selected topics in the field of biomedical ethics. There are also polls and articles on ethical issues.

http://www-hsc.usc.edu/~mbernste/#Welcome

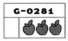

Bioethics.net   Produced by the Center for Bioethics of the University of Pennsylvania and hosted by the *American Journal of Bioethics Online,* Bioethics.net contains a host of resources pertaining to biomedical ethics. Included are sections on cloning and genetics, emergency room bioethics, surveys for pay, and assisted suicide. The site also provides news updates, book reviews, articles, and tables of contents of other journals. "Bioethics for Beginners" contains material that is meant to educate the general public and people interested in the field about bioethics, its meaning, and its applications. At this beginner's site, there are resources for students and educators, including a list of biomedical ethics associations.

http://www.med.upenn.edu/bioethics/index.shtml

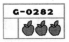

Human Genome Project: Ethical, Legal, and Social Issues (ELSI)   With funding from the U.S. Department of Energy and the National Institutes of Health, this site describes and explores the ethical, legal, and social issues surrounding availability of genetic information. A link to "Privacy and Legislation" gives more detail on who should have access to genetic information and how it can be used. Gene testing and gene therapy links feature the risks and limits of genetic technology, as well as the implementation of standards. A section on behavioral genetics examines conceptual and philosophical implications. In addition, a section on patenting covers who owns genes and other pieces of DNA.

http://www.ornl.gov/hgmis/elsi/elsi.html

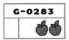

Medical Ethics: Where Do You Draw the Line?   Interactive scenarios on ethical decisions are featured on this site. Visitors can answer multiple choice questions about living with cancer, understanding cloning, or handling headaches. The site also provides a summary of visitors' responses. Links at the end of each section lead to an ethics forum, a bulletin board discussion, and related sites on cancer, cloning, and headaches.

http://www.learner.org/exhibits/medicalethics

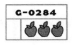

National Bioethics Advisory Commission   In addition to providing information on current research trends in the biotechnology industry, the commission explores the ethical implications of technological advances. The site acts as a forum for the ethical concerns of the public regarding rapidly advancing technology. Transcripts from its meetings are available on the site, as well as reports on topics such as ethical issues in human stem cell research and cloning human beings. A short list of bioethics-related links is provided.

http://bioethics.gov/cgi-bin/bioeth_counter.pl

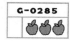

National Reference Center for Bioethics Literature Linked to the Kennedy Institute of Ethics at Georgetown University, this center holds a large collection of literature on biomedical ethics. Serving as a resource for both the public and scholars of ethics, the site also provides access to free searching of the world's literature in bioethics using BIOETHICSLINE or the Ethics and Human Genetics Database. Other relevant links are provided in the areas of educational and teaching resources, the center's library, bibliographies, and Internet resources for bioethics.

http://www.georgetown.edu/research/nrcbl

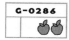

The Hastings Center The Hastings Center is a major center for the study of biomedical ethics. Its Web site provides information about current research activities in medicine and biomedical research, values and biotechnology, healthcare policy and healthcare systems, and humans and nature. Other resources include information on educational opportunities at the center, a catalog of publications, and a list of related links.

http://www.thehastingscenter.org

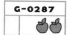

UNESCO: International Bioethics Committee The International Bioethics Committee of the United Nations Educational, Scientific, and Cultural Organization (UNESCO) created this Web site to inform the public of their work on human rights in relation to advances made in genetics and molecular biology. The site outlines their activities, along with proceedings from their meetings. The Universal Declaration on the Human Genome and Human Rights resolution is available on the site. Under the "Ethical Issues" section, visitors can read IBC reports on subjects such as the teaching of bioethics, neuroscience, the human genome, bioethics and human rights, and genetics. The site can also be viewed in French.

http://www.unesco.org/ibc

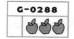

University of Buffalo Center for Clinical Ethics and Humanities in Health Care Information about the center, news and events notices, a library of bioethics and medical humanities documents, and the Ethics Committee Core Curriculum are available at this address. Links are presented to Internet resources on featured topics including bioethics education, hospice and palliative care, advance directives, philosophy of mind, medical record privacy, genetics, and ethics.

http://wings.buffalo.edu/faculty/research/bioethics/nav.html

11.3 BIOTECHNOLOGY

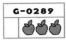

Bio Online   Bio Online is a comprehensive Web site for the life sciences and the biotechnology industry. This site provides general information, current news, an industry guide, academic and government links, and an extensive career center. It is an informative resource for seeking information on the biotechnology industry and related sciences.
http://www.bio.com

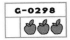

Biofind.com   Biofind.com provides insight into the biotechnology industry and is a resource for general information, news, and developments in emerging technologies. The site also contains a job search database, a chat room, the "Biotech Rumor Mill" for anonymous public discussion of current events in the field, an events database, a secure "Innovations" database for posting projects needing venture capital or corporate funding, and press releases from biotechnology companies. A subscription service, available for a fee, provides daily e-mail updates on jobs, candidates, business opportunities, innovations, and press releases. http://www.biofind.com

BioInfoSeek.com   Infobiotech is a collaboration of government, academic, and private sector resources. This Canadian-based site provides general information, resources, and links to both North American and international. In addition, it offers career information, events, and a large list of related sites providing current information on advances in the biotechnology industry.
http://www.cisti.nrc.ca/ibc/home.html

BioPortfolio.com   A database of biotechnology companies, technology, and products worldwide is featured on this Web site. More than 11,000 companies are included in the database. Some have detailed profiles, as well as hyperlinks for investor information and news. Subscribers can search the database by keyword, category, organization name, or region. The site allows a limited search on a free trial basis.
(fee-based) http://www.bioportfolio.com/bio/

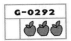

Bioresearch Online   Bioresearch Online is a virtual community, forum, and marketplace for biotechnology professionals. Users have access to the latest headlines, product information, and industry analyses, as well as career information. There are also specific pages devoted to pharmaceutical research and laboratory science.
http://www.bioresearchonline.com/content/homepage

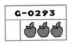

Biotechnology Industry Organization   This industry-sponsored Web site provides weekly news updates on developing technology and world news. The site also offers general information, links to corporate Web sites, an online library, and a number of other educational resources.
http://www.bio.org/welcome.html

Biotechnology: An Information Resource   Dedicated to providing current information in all areas of biotechnology, this site is a subsidiary of the National Agricultural Library and the U.S. Department of Agriculture. The site catalogs press releases and offers an exhaustive listing of links to other Web-based resources from around the world, especially in the area of agricultural biotechnology.   http://www.nal.usda.gov/bic

BioWorld Online   BioWorld Online tracks the growth of the biotechnology market. In addition to providing stock and financial information, the site provides access to current industry headlines, job search resources, forums, and news worldwide.

http://www.bioworld.com

CorpTech Database   This comprehensive database provides details on companies involved in high-tech industries, including biotechnology and pharmaceutical companies. Basic information such as each company's description, annual sales, and CEO name is available free; however, more in-depth financial and business data is only accessible to fee-paying subscribers. Searches for products or names of company officers are also available, with some information provided at no cost.

(some features fee-based)   http://www.corptech.com

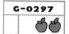

Enzyme Nomenclature Database   The database at this Web site provides access to enzyme information by Enzyme Commission (EC) number, enzyme class, description, chemical compound, and cofactor. There is also an accompanying user manual for the enzyme database, report forms for new enzyme entry, and links to resources on biochemical pathways and protein databases.

http://www.expasy.ch/enzyme

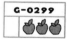

International Food Information Council   The International Food Information Council (IFIC)collects and disseminates scientific information on food safety, nutrition, and health by working with experts to help translate research findings into understandable and useful language for opinion leaders and consumers. This site provides information and news on food safety and nutrition in categories such as functional foods, agriculture and food production, and food biotechnology. The site also offers publications including IFIC's journal *Food Insight*, recent news articles, government guidelines and regulations, and links to other resources on the Internet.

http://ificinfo.health.org

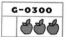

MedWebPlus: Biotechnology   MedWebPlus contains an extensive guide to online resources in biotechnology, organized alphabetically and in focused subsets, cataloging hundreds of Internet resources containing many forms of information. Links are provided to journals, online publications, and recent articles of interest.

http://www.medwebplus.com/subject/Biotechnology.html

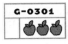

National Center for Biotechnology Information   A collaborative effort produced by the National Library of Medicine and the National Institutes of Health, NCBI is a national resource for molecular biology information. The center creates public databases, conducts research in computational biology, develops software tools for analyzing genome data, and disseminates information in an effort to improve the understanding of molecular processes affecting human health and disease. In addition to conducting and cataloging its own research, NCBI tracks the progress of important research projects worldwide. The site provides access to public molecular databases containing genetic sequences, structures, and taxonomy; literature databases; catalogs of whole genomes; tools for mining genetic data; teaching resources and online tutorials; and data and software available to download. Research performed at NCBI is also discussed at the site.
http://www.ncbi.nlm.nih.gov

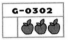

Recombinant Capital   ReCap acts as a "centralized industry 'filing cabinet'" for public resources relevant to biotechnology, serving as a database for biotechnology executives and investors. *Signals,* the online magazine, provides analysis of the biotechnology industry and is particularly appropriate for those seeking to invest in companies on the forefront of this rapidly growing industry. Although much of the information presented is from a financial perspective, the site gives an overview of the entire industry and provides daily news updates.
http://www.recap.com

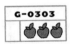

World Wide Web Virtual Library: Biotechnology   A directory of sites in the field of biotechnology is featured on this Web page. This site catalogs hundreds of reviewed links including publications, educational resources, products, genomics, software, pharmaceutical companies, clinical trials and regulatory affairs, and government links. There is also a rating system used by the editor of the site to point out links of specific importance.
http://www.cato.com/biotech

11.4 CLINICAL PRACTICE MANAGEMENT

GENERAL RESOURCES

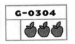

Cut to the Chase   This site offers information for healthcare management in the form of a list of over 30 categories relevant to a variety of work settings. Topics covered include accreditation, billing, career development, health policy, legal issues, medical records, practice management, and telemedicine. Within each category are subheadings containing articles, abstracts, and additional links. http://www.cuttothechase.com

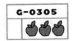

Guide to Clinical Preventive Services   This guide is a comprehensive online reference source covering recommendations for clinical practice on more

than 150 preventive interventions, including screening tests, counseling interventions, immunizations, chemoprophylactic regimens, and other preventive medical tools. Approximately 60 target conditions are discussed in the report.
http://cpmcnet.columbia.edu/texts/gcps/gcps0000.html

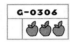

Health Services/Technology Assessment Text   This electronic resource provides access to consumer brochures, evidence reports, reference guides for clinicians, clinical practice guidelines, and other full-text documents useful in making healthcare decisions. Users can download documents from the site, access general information about the system, and browse links to additional sources for information. Searches can be comprehensive or limited to specific databases within the HSTAT system, and users can also search by keyword.
http://text.nlm.nih.gov

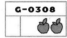

Medsite.com   Described as an e-services portal for the medical community, this site offers books, medical software, and supplies at discounted prices; financial resources; a scheduling tool geared for medical professionals; and free e-mail accounts. Also available are daily health news updates, interactive grand rounds and other online courses, and links to medical textbooks and journals. Some areas require registration or subscription.
(some features fee-based) http://www.medsite.com

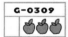

PDR.net   PDR.net is a medical and healthcare Web site created by the Medical Economics Company, publisher of healthcare magazines and directories including the *Physicians' Desk Reference*. The site has specific areas and content for physicians, pharmacists, physician assistants, nurses, and consumers. Access to the full-text reference book is free for U.S.-based M.D.s, D.O.s, and P.A.s in full-time practice. There is a fee for other users of this service, but most of the site's features are free.
(some features fee-based) http://www.PDR.net

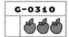

Physician's Guide to the Internet   A directory of Web sites for physicians is offered on this site. Features include physician lifestyle resources, such as sites offering suggestions on stress relief; news items; clinical practice resources, including access to medical databases and patient education resources; and postgraduate education and new physician resources. Other resources include links to sites selling medical books, products, and services for physicians; links to Internet search tools; and Internet tutorials.
http://www.physiciansguide.com

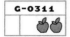

State Medical Boards Directory   This directory provides the names, addresses, telephone numbers, and e-mail or Web site information for each of the state medical boards. Physicians can contact a board for information on licensing in that state or for other information regarding medical regulation or standards.   http://www.fsmb.org/members.htm

CLINICAL CALCULATORS

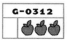

MedCalc 3000 Medical Calculator MedCalc 3000 offers several hundred online medical calculator tools at this site. It combines various equations, clinical criteria scores, and decision trees used in healthcare. In addition, there is a quick converter to convert value units easily and a math calculator. Alphabetical lists of the medical equations and clinical criteria topics are presented, with links to the actual calculators.

http://calc.med.edu/

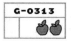

Medical Tools, Calculators and Scores Medic8.com provides clinicians with 60 medical calculators to measure blood oxygen content, body mass, opioid drug dosage, and numerous other factors. Scores such as coronary disease probability, the geriatric depression scale, the Glasgow coma scale, and the TWEAK alcoholism score are also included. A sidebar menu offers links to reference information on medical subjects, specialties, medical news, books, software, and services.

http://www.medic8.com/MedicalTools.htm

EVIDENCE-BASED MEDICINE

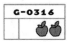

Cochrane Collaboration The Cochrane Collaboration is an international working group of experts who catalog and maintain information on evidence-based medicine by specialty. The site explains the history of the collaboration, along with a link to the Cochrane library site, which contains a database of systematic reviews and a controlled trials register. Abstracts are available free of charge at this address; full access is available only to subscribers.

(some features fee-based) http://www.cochrane.org/

Evidence-Based Medicine Resources offered on the New York Academy of Medicine's evidence-based medicine site may be useful to both teaching and practicing physicians. There are links to databases, publications, teaching tools, education resources, and tips on searching for evidence-based medicine. The "Practicing" section includes clinical guidelines, clinical trials, and systematic reviews. There are also organizations, glossaries, journals, LISTSERV discussion groups, and related links.

(some features fee-based) http://www.ebmny.org/thecentr2.html

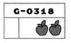

Medscout: Evidence-Based Medicine Guidelines Targeted to physicians, this site offers a comprehensive list of evidence-based medicine guidelines available on the Internet. There are more than 30 sites drawn mostly from universities and journals around the world.

http://www.medscout.com/guidelines/evidence_based/index.htm

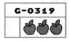

New York Online Access to Health (NOAH): Evidence Patients seeking information on evidence-based medicine (EBM) will find this site from

NOAH very useful. There are more than 55 sites listed offering information on types of evidence, research methods, statistical terms in EBM, and a basic overview of EBM. http://www.noah-health.org/english/ebhc/ebhc.html

MEDICAL ETHICS

American Medical Association (AMA): Ethics Standards Reports of the Council on Ethical and Judicial Affairs, an organization that sets ethics policy for the AMA, are accessible from this site. Visitors can access an online policy finder, which can be browsed alphabetically, or get answers to frequently asked questions about the role of the council, the Code of Medical Ethics, and the End-of-Life Care Project. The Institute for Ethics at the AMA, functioning as an independent research organization, provides news from its task force and information about the E-Force program. Other AMA ethics Web sites and pages of professional standards are available.
http://www.ama-assn.org/ama/pub/category/2416.html#ethics

American Society of Law, Medicine, and Ethics The search engine at this site allows visitors to access a variety of educational information related to law, medicine, and ethics. Details about the organization's peer-reviewed journals, access to research projects on pain undertreatment, and a news section offering up-to-date information on recent developments in the field are offered. A multimedia educational link connects visitors to more than 50 streaming audio presentations in the fields of genetics, health law, and end-of-life decision making. http://www.aslme.org/

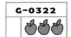

Medical Ethics A comprehensive listing of more than 100 links related to ethics is offered on this Web page. The links are categorized as bioethics, professional ethics, institutional ethics, scientific misconduct, humanism, and morals. The sites are drawn from Internet sources around the world.
http://www.mic.ki.se/Diseases/k1.316.html

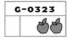

Medscout: Medical Ethics Over 100 medical ethics resources are presented at this site from Medscout. Examples of resources are the American Society of Bioethics and Humanities, the Center for Ethics and Professionalism, the Center for Clinical Ethics and Humanities in Health Care, and the National Human Genome Research Institute. Visitors to this site will also find topical links to resources in areas such as diseases, government, immunizations, journals, and health policy. http://www.medscout.com/ethics/

The Hastings Center This independent, interdisciplinary research and education center explores the ethical issues surrounding health, medicine, and the environment. Examination of the moral issues arising from advances in medicine can be found at the site's project pages on medicine and biomedical research, values and biotechnology, and health policy. Several relevant online resources for bioethics-related information are offered.
http://www.thehastingscenter.org/

MEDICAL INFORMATICS

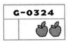

Agency for Healthcare Research and Quality (AHRQ): Healthcare Informatics   Healthcare informatics is featured on this Web site, courtesy of the Agency for Healthcare Research and Quality (AHRQ). The site provides data and survey reports covering public health, standard activities for federal agencies, medical informatics and health services research data, and the use of computers to advance healthcare. In addition, there are links to research findings, funding opportunities, consumer health, clinical information, and medical news.   http://www.ahcpr.gov/data/infoix.htm

American Health Information Management Association   Directed to health information managers, the American Health Information Management Association Web page offers details about the association and the field. "Hot Topics" in health information management covers more than a dozen areas such as accreditation, data quality management, and information security. Within each category are articles, position statements, seminars/events, and research and benchmarks. A resource center for patients includes information on accessing and protecting personal medical records.
(some features fee-based)   http://www.ahima.org/

American Medical Informatics Association   With the proliferation of medical information, the growth of medical research, the development of medical information systems, and the creation of management systems for computerized patient data, the medical informatics field has grown substantially. Major themes of the association are privacy and confidentiality of medical records, public policy development for legislation in the field, conferences of medical informatics professionals, and the issuance of papers and publications covering various aspects of the medical information field. The site features publications, including the *Journal of the American Medical Informatics Association,* and related reports and videos. Other resources include information on the various working and special interest groups, a job bank, and links to related sites.   http://www.amia.org

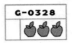

American Telemedicine Association   Dedicated to promoting access to medical care for consumers and professionals through the use of telecommunications technology, the American Telemedicine Association promotes education, research, and advocacy in the field. Visitors to the site can learn more about the association, its member groups, and meetings. Information under the "News and Resources" section includes bulletin boards, a comprehensive list of related links, and a job bank. In the same section is a library containing a member directory, telemedicine news updates, and proceedings from their annual meetings.   (some features fee-based)   http://www.atmeda.org

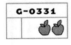

Galaxy: Medical Informatics Resources   This site provides links to more than 20 U.S. and international centers and medical departments dealing with medical informatics. Included in this list are centers at Oregon Health Sciences

University, Stanford University, Columbia University, and European institutions. There are also articles, directories, and discussion group links for further resources on medical informatics.

http://www.galaxy.com/cgi-bin/dirlist?node=25091

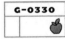

International Medical Informatics Association The International Medical Informatics Association's (IMIA) Web site features the association newsletter, along with information on IMIA working groups and member societies. A report on the recommendations of the IMIA on education in health and medical informatics is provided. There is also an extensive list of related resources that includes institutions and organizations, medical resources, and health informatics resources.

http://www.imia.org

Medscout: Medical Informatics For those interested in medical informatics, this Web page contains a comprehensive list of Internet resources. The sites are categorized as national information associations, newsletters and journals, and medical informatics on the Internet. In total, there are more than 85 sites from both domestic and international sources.

http://www.medscout.com/informatics/index.htm

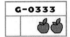

Telemedicine More than 20 telemedicine resources are provided at this site from Galaxy, a medical portal. Featured resources include the Center for Telemedicine Law, Cyberspace Telemedical Office, MediaStation 5000, and telemedicine initiatives by state. Links are provided to access remote consultation, telepathology, and teleradiology resources.

http://www.galaxy.com/galaxy/Medicine/Medical-Informatics/Telemedicine.html

MEDICAL LAW

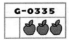

American Medical Association (AMA): Legal Issues for Physicians Healthcare providers can access information regarding legal issues in the areas of business and management, patient-physician relationships, and compliance at this Web site, maintained by the AMA. Various medical case summaries are provided, as well as a Compliance Interactive Tutorial System offering online assistance with fraud and abuse regulations for members of the association.

(some features fee-based) http://www.ama-assn.org/ama/pub/category/4541.html

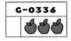

MedNets: Medical Law Links to more than 30 medical law resources, including the American Bar Association Health Law Section, AMA Statements on Advanced Directives, Expert Witness Net, the Health Care Liability Alliance, Medical Care Law, the U.S. States Abortion Laws, and the Law and Legislative Center are offered at this site from MedNets. Visitors can also access medical law databases, health law journals, news, and resources related to medical ethics through this site.

http://www.mednets.com/medlaw.htm

MEDICAL LICENSURE

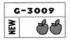

Administrators in Medicine: Association of State Medical Board Executive Directors   A list of participating state licensing authorities is compiled at this page, maintained by DocFinder. The list is not exhaustive but contains many connections to state medical examiners' home pages and tools that allow visitors to search for physicians by name or license number.
http://www.docboard.org/

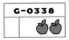

Federation of State Medical Boards   The Federation of State Medical Boards (FSMB) site provides visitors with policy documents, details on post-licensure assessment, a credentials verification service, and state medical board information. A publications catalog is provided, which includes the *Journal of Medical Licensure and Discipline* and the *FSMB Handbook*. The FSMB library is accessible to members of the organization. There is also information on their database of board actions taken against physicians.
(some features fee-based) http://www.fsmb.org/

PRACTICE GUIDELINES AND CONSENSUS STATEMENTS

Medscout: Medical Specialty Guidelines   Sponsored by Medscout, this Web page offers a comprehensive listing of more than 50 clinical guidelines plus links to other guidelines sites available on the Internet. The guidelines are drawn primarily from American and Canadian sources.
http://www.medscout.com/guidelines/medical_specialty/

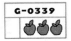

National Guideline Clearinghouse (NGC)   The National Guideline Clearinghouse is a comprehensive database of evidence-based clinical practice guidelines and related documents produced by the Agency for Healthcare Research and Quality, in partnership with the American Medical Association and the American Association of Health Plans. The guidelines can be searched by keyword or browsed by category such as disease and condition, treatment and intervention, and issuing organization. Each guideline has a brief summary and information for obtaining the full text. A useful tool on the site is the "Compare Guidelines," feature which allows users to add guidelines on a specific topic to their collection and then select a comparison button to produce a report that compares them. In addition, there are guideline syntheses on certain topics such as asthma treatment and childhood immunizations in which all the guidelines written on the topic are combined into one report.
http://www.guideline.gov/index.asp

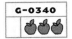

Primary Care Clinical Practice Guidelines   Clinical practice guidelines for primary care providers are offered on this Web page, courtesy of the University of California San Francisco. The guidelines can be searched by keyword, browsed alphabetically, or selected through clinical content categories such as mental disorders, cardiovascular system, and pregnancy. Each category has many subtopics listed, along with hyperlinks to the appropriate guideline. Also of interest is the resources section, which offers an enormous list of online textbooks, journals, superlists of links, and other related resources.

(some features fee-based) http://medicine.ucsf.edu/resources/guidelines/

PRACTICE MANAGEMENT TOOLS

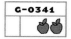

Medical Group Management Association   Primarily targeted to healthcare administrators, the Medical Group Management Association focuses on practice management solutions and tools. The site contains information on the association's research activities and on policy issues, as well as a job bank and career services. A catalog of survey reports features medical group practice performance data.

(some features fee-based) http://www.mgma.com/

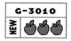

Medscape: The Journal of Medical Practice Management   Abstracts and full-text articles are available to registered users at this online journal site of Medscape. Available content includes current feature articles and archived issues that address software systems, managed care, economic trends in healthcare delivery, and billing and coding topics.

(free registration) http://managedcare.medscape.com/JMPM/public/JMPM-journal.html

11.5   CLINICAL TRIALS

CenterWatch   This clinical trials listing service offers both patient and professional resources. Patient resources include a listing of clinical trials by disease category, a notification and matching service, links to current NIH trials, drug directories including a clinical trials results database and drugs currently in clinical research, listings of new FDA drug therapy approvals, and current research headlines. Background information on clinical research is also available to patients unfamiliar with the clinical trials process. Industry professional resources include research center profiles, industry provider profiles, industry news, and career and educational opportunities. Links to related sites of interest to patients and professionals are also available.

http://www.centerwatch.com/main.htm

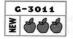

ClinicalTrials.gov   The National Institutes of Health and the National Library of Medicine provide access to information about clinical trials through ClinicalTrials.gov. Visitors can search the database by entering keywords or phrases into the search engine; by using a focused search by disease, location, treatment, or sponsor; or by browsing alphabetical listings of thousands of conditions and sponsors. Links to information on studies recruiting patients offer additional details on study purpose, protocol, and researcher contact.

http://clinicaltrials.gov/ct/gui/c/b

11.6 DISSERTATION ABSTRACTS

Dissertation Abstracts Database   A database of more than 1.6 million citations and abstracts from doctoral dissertations and master's theses is provided on this site. Visitors are offered free access to the most current two years of citations, which includes an abstract and a 24-page preview. Subscriber institutions are able to download the entire dissertation in PDF format for the years 1997 to the present. Subscribers can also search for citations dating back to 1861. (some features fee-based) http://wwwlib.umi.com/dissertations/about_pqdd

11.7 ENVIRONMENTAL HEALTH

Agency for Toxic Substances and Disease Registry   Environmental and occupational public health hazards and risks are the focus of this division of the U.S. Department of Health and Human Services. A variety of resources can be accessed, including national alerts, health advisories, answers to frequently asked questions about hazardous substances, and relevant legislation. Databases available from the site provide information on specific hazardous waste sites, as well as information on those exposed to such substances. Scientific papers published by the agency, sites addressing issues specific to children, and a calendar of events are included.
http://www.atsdr.cdc.gov/atsdrhome.html

New York Online Access to Health (NOAH): Environmental Health
This NOAH site features a directory of environmental health links available on the Internet. There are more than 55 links categorized under environmental health topics such as air quality, chemical sensitivities, toxins and pesticides, and water quality. More than 45 sites are found under a resources section that includes advocacy, governmental agencies, and legal resources. The site can also be accessed in Spanish.
http://www.noah-health.org/english/illness/environment/environ.html

11.8 GENETICS AND GENOMICS

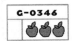

GeneClinics   Funded by the National Institutes of Health and developed by the University of Washington, GeneClinics is a knowledge base of expert-authored, up-to-date information relating genetic testing to the diagnosis, management, and counseling of individuals and families with inherited disorders. Directed at healthcare professionals, the site contains textbook-type genetic testing and counseling information on a large number of diseases. The disease profiles are peer reviewed and continuously updated.
http://www.geneclinics.org

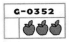

Genetics Jump Station   This site provides a comprehensive listing of Web-based resources for geneticists. Sites indexed here are technical in nature and in-

tended for investigators. Resources include links to molecular biology, microbiology, and genetics jump sites, which contain catalogs of links; sites containing protocols on laboratory techniques; journals and other online publications; news groups and mail lists; institutes and organizations; conferences and meetings announcements; commercial sites; and sources for ordering technical books. The site is sponsored by Beckman, Horizon Scientific Press, the *Journal of Molecular Microbiology and Biotechnology,* and MWG-Biotech.
http://www.horizonpress.com/gateway/genetics.html

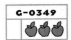

Genetics Virtual Library   A comprehensive listing of links to major Web sites on specific topics in genetics is featured on this site. Links are subdivided by organism, from yeast to humans, and by topic, including genetic testing, cloning, and pharmacogenomics. A list of human chromosomes by number is also provided, with links to information on gene markers, lineage maps, and animal models. The main site also features links to genome projects in a variety of organisms. http://www.ornl.gov/TechResources/Human_Genome/genetics.html

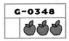

Genomics Lexicon   Part of a larger genomics site produced by the Pharmaceutical Research and Manufacturers of America and the Foundation for Genetic Medicine, Inc., this site features "Lexicon," a glossary of genomic terms. The glossary can be browsed alphabetically or by an index. Reference sources for the glossary are listed along with hyperlinks to the original source. The site also features *Genomics Today*, a collection of links to genomics news at other Web sites; news is posted daily and an archive is available.
http://genomics.phrma.org/lexicon/r.html

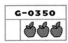

Genomics: A Global Resource   Presented by the Pharmaceutical Research and Manufacturers of America, this Web page offers a broad array of resources related to genomics and bioinformatics. Drawn from around the world and updated daily, the most recent news stories can be found in the "News & Tools" section. Also within this section are links to journals as well as education resources such as online textbooks, organizations, academic programs, and grants. "Lexicon" offers a glossary of terms. There are also links for legislative issues, controversial issues such as cloning, and biodiversity. A therapeutics section covers medical testing and bioethics. In addition, bioinformatic databases for microbials, plants, invertebrates, vertebrates, and humans can be accessed.
(some features fee-based) http://genomics.phrma.org/

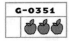

Kyoto Encyclopedia of Genomes and Genetics   The Kyoto Encyclopedia of Genes and Genomes attempts to computerize current knowledge of molecular and cellular biology in terms of information pathways consisting of interacting molecules or genes. The site also provides links to gene catalogs produced by genome sequencing projects. Information indexed at this site ranges from basic genetic information to technical descriptions of molecular pathways. Also provided is a listing of links to other major Internet sites containing information relevant to genetic research.
http://www.genome.ad.jp/kegg

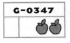

MedBioWorld: Genetics, Genomics, and Biotechnology Journals
This site offers a comprehensive list of genetics, genomics, and biotechnology journals. There are more than 100 links to journals from the United States and abroad. http://www.medbioworld.com/journals/genetics.html

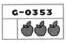

National Center for Biotechnology Information: Online Mendelian Inheritance in Man (OMIM)
Dr. Victor A. McKusick, a researcher at Johns Hopkins University, and his colleagues have authored this database of human genes and genetic disorders. The database was developed for the World Wide Web by the center. Reference information, texts, and images are found, as well as links to the Entrez database of MEDLINE articles and sequence information. Visitors can search the OMIM Database, OMIM Gene Map, and OMIM Morbid Map (a catalog of cytogenetic map locations organized by disease). Information on the OMIM numbering system, details on creating links to OMIM, site updates, OMIM statistics, information on citing OMIM in literature, and the OMIM gene list are all available. The site also hosts links to allied resources, and the complete text of OMIM and gene maps can be downloaded from the site. http://www.ncbi.nlm.nih.gov/Omim

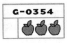

National Human Genome Research Institute
The National Human Genome Research Institute supports the NIH component of the Human Genome Project, a worldwide research effort designed to analyze the structure of the human genome and determine the location of the estimated 50,000 to 100,000 human genes. The NHGRI Intramural Research Program develops and implements technology for understanding, diagnosing, and treating genetic diseases. The site provides information about NHGRI, the Human Genome Project, grants, intramural research, policy and public affairs, workshops and conferences, and news items. Resources include links to the institute's Ethical, Legal, and Social Implications Program and to the Center for Inherited Disease Research. The site also provides genetic resources for investigators and a glossary of genetic terms.
http://www.nhgri.nih.gov

Office of Genetics and Disease Prevention
Created by the Centers for Disease Control and Prevention, this site offers access to current information on the impact of human genetic research and the Human Genome Project on public health and disease prevention. The site provides general information, indexes recent articles, lists events and training opportunities, and offers an extensive listing of links to other resources. Users can search the site by keyword and access the Human Genome Epidemiology Network (HuGENet), a global collaboration of individuals and organizations committed to the development and dissemination of population-based epidemiologic information on the human genome. http://www.cdc.gov/genetics

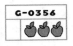

Primer on Molecular Genetics
The U.S. Department of Energy presents a comprehensive resource for those seeking basic background information on genetics and genetic research at this site. Discussions include an introduction to

genetics, DNA, genes, chromosomes, and the process of mapping the human genome. Mapping strategies, genetic linkage maps, and various physical maps are available, as well as links to mapping and sequence databases and a glossary of terms. The site also summarizes the predicted impact of the Human Genome Project on medical practice and biological research.
http://www.ornl.gov/hgmis/publicat/primer/intro.html

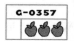

The Institute for Genomic Research (TIGR)   The Institute for Genomic Research is a not-for-profit research institute with interests in structural, functional, and comparative analysis of genomes and gene products in viruses, eubacteria, archaea, and eukaryotes. Information on recent advances in genetics and continuing research projects in the area of human genomics, an extensive database of previous research, and links to other genome centers worldwide are available at this site.
http://www.tigr.org

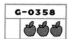

University of Kansas Medical Center: Genetics Education Center
Links are available at this address to Internet resources for educators interested in human genetics and the Human Genome Project. Sites are listed by topic, including the Human Genome Project, education resources, networking, genetic conditions, genetics programs and resources, and glossaries. Lesson plans are offered by the University of Kansas and other sources at the site. A description of different careers in genetics is also available. This site provides access to useful genetics Internet resources for nonprofessionals and educators.
http://www.kumc.edu/gec

11.9 GERIATRIC MEDICINE

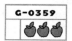

American Geriatrics Society   A national nonprofit association of geriatrics health professionals, research scientists, and other concerned individuals, the American Geriatrics Society is dedicated to "improving the health, independence, and quality of life for all older people." The site offers a description of the society, adult immunization information, AGS news, conference and events notices, legislation news, career opportunities, directories of geriatrics healthcare services in managed care, position statements, practice guidelines, awards information, and other professional education resources. Patient education resources, a selected bibliography in geriatrics, links to related organizations and government sites, and surveys are also found at this address.
(some features fee-based) http://www.americangeriatrics.org

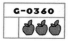

ElderWeb   Designed as a research source for consumers and professionals, this Web page offers a broad array of resources related to the care of the elderly. In the "Finance and Law" section, more than 20 topics are listed such as drug costs, elder law, and Medicaid. Each topic lists resources that can be found on the site, in their newsletter, and on the Internet. Resources are listed in the same way under sections such as living arrangements and body and soul. There are also a regional directory of sites related to living arrangements, finance, and law; a list of association; and an eldercare locator that covers domestic and international sites. Visitors can access news on the home page or register for a free newsletter. (free registration) http://www.elderweb.com/

Hardin MD: Geriatrics and Senior Health The Hardin Meta Directory on this site features geriatrics and senior health. Categorized as large, medium, and small lists, there are links to Web pages that contain relevant Internet resources. The lists are drawn from both domestic and international sources and cover hundreds of sites. There are also links to additional directories of lists on Alzheimer's and Parkinson's disease.
http://www.lib.uiowa.edu/hardin/md/ger.html

MedBioWorld: Geriatrics and Gerontology Journals A listing of geriatrics and gerontology journals available on the Internet is found on this site. There are more than 75 journals listed, some with full-text articles.
http://www.medbioworld.com/journals/medicine/geriatrics.html

Medscout: Geriatric Medicine Resources on geriatric medicine can be found on this Web site maintained by Medscout. More than 60 sites are listed and categorized as geriatric news, associations, geriatric education, hospitals and medical centers, and geriatrics on the Internet.
http://www.medscout.com/specialties/geriatrics/

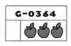

Merck Manual of Geriatrics The full text of the *Merck Manual of Geriatrics* is featured on this Web page. Sixteen chapters are provided for topics such as the basics of geriatric care; falls, fractures, and injury; surgery and rehabilitation; psychiatric disorders; neurologic disorders; and musculoskeletal disorders. In addition, disorders related to endocrinology, hematology/oncology, pulmonology, cardiology, urology/nephrology, infectious disease, dermatology, and gastroenterology are found. Each chapter contains numerous diseases and disorders with information on etiology, pathophysiology, symptoms, diagnosis, and treatment.
http://www.merck.com/pubs/mm_geriatrics/contents.htm

Resource Directory for Older People The National Institute on Aging and the Administration on Aging have compiled this directory of resources, serving older people and their families, health and legal professionals, social service providers, librarians, researchers, and others interested in the field of aging. The directory includes names of organizations and contact information. Visitors can search the directory by keyword or browse categories such as diseases and conditions, nutrition and fitness, and long-term-care planning from the table of contents.
http://www.aoa.dhhs.gov/directory/default.htm

11.10 GRANTS AND FUNDING SOURCES

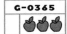

Foundation Center The Foundation Center provides direct links to thousands of grant-making organizations, including foundations, corporations, and public charities, along with a search engine to enable the user to locate sources of funding in specific fields. In addition, the site provides listings of the largest private foundations, corporate grant makers, and community foundations. Other resources include information on funding trends, a newsletter, and grant-seeker orientation material. More than 900 grant-making organizations are accessible through this site.
http://fdncenter.org

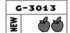

GrantSelect More than 10,000 funding opportunities are contained in the GrantSelect database for a variety of disciplines including biomedical and healthcare. The database is available to subscribers only; a free 30-day trial period is offered on the site. Subscribers can also receive an e-mail alert service for new additions to the database.
(fee-based) http://www.grantselect.com

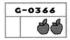

Mental Health Net: Grants and Funding Opportunities Part of a larger Mental Health Net Web page, this site features grant funding opportunities related to mental health and biomedicine in general that are available online. There are close to 20 sites listed with descriptions and ratings. The sites are categorized as Web resources; mailing lists; journals, publications, and research papers; professional organizations and centers; and other resources.
http://mentalhelp.net/guide/pro28.htm

National Institutes of Health (NIH): Funding Opportunities Funding opportunities for research, scholarship, and training are extensive within the federal government. At this site for the National Institutes of Health, there is a grants page with information about NIH grants and fellowship programs, information on research contracts containing information on requests for proposals (RFPs), research training opportunities in biomedical areas, and an NIH guide for grants and contracts. The latter is the official document for announcing the availability of NIH funds for biomedical and behavioral research and research training policies. Links are provided to major divisions of the NIH that have additional information on specialized grant opportunities.
http://grants.nih.gov/grants

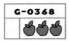

National Science Foundation (NSF): Grants and Awards Approximately 20 percent of the federal support to academic institutions for basic research comes from the National Science Foundation, making this site an important source of information for award opportunities, programs, application procedures, and other vital information. Forms and agreements may be downloaded as well, and regulations and policy guidelines are set forth clearly.
http://www.nsf.gov/home/grants.htm

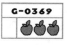

Society of Research Administrators: GrantsWeb The Society of Research Administrators has created this extremely useful grant information site with extensive links to government resources, general resources, private funding, and policy and regulation sites. The section devoted to U.S., Canadian, and other international resources provides links to government agency funding sources, the *Commerce Business Daily,* the Catalog of Federal Domestic Assistance, scientific agencies, research councils, and resources in individual fields, such as health, education, and business. Grant application procedures, regulations, and guidelines are provided throughout the site, and extensive legal information is provided through links to patent, intellectual property, and copyright offices. Associations providing funding and grant information are also listed, with direct links.

http://interchange.org/nsagislist/NL08249809.html

11.11 MEDICAL IMAGING AND RADIOLOGY

CT Is Us The CT (computed tomography) site offers information on medical imaging with a specific focus on spiral CT and 3-D imaging. Images of the body and various medical conditions are organized by region, and information on CME courses, teaching files, medical illustrations, and a 3-D vascular atlas are all available. The site also features protocols for multidetector CT and pediatric imaging, as well as teaching files and a gallery of medical illustrations.

http://www.ctisus.org

Health On the Net (HON) Foundation This site provides links to radiological and surgical images on the Internet. Images are available of the abdomen, ankle, arm, full body, brain, elbow, eye, foot, hand, head, heart, hilum, hip, kidney, knee, leg, liver, lung, muscle, neck, pancreas, pelvis, shoulder, skin, skull, teeth, thorax, trachea, blood vessels, and wrist. The site can also be viewed in French.

http://www.hon.ch/Media/anatomy.html

Medical Imaging Resources on the Internet Supported by the University of Leeds School of Computing in the United Kingdom, this Web page offers comprehensive resource lists for medical imaging. Visitors can view the list by geographic location, represented by the headings of Europe, North America, Asia, and Australasia. Within each region are subcategories such as universities, hospitals, research organizations, and the commercial sector. The list can also be viewed by content such as exhibits and publications, teaching aids, software, and general resources. There are also links for newsgroups, funding sources by region, and search engines.

http://www.comp.leeds.ac.uk/comir/resources/links.html

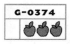

MedMark: Radiology The professional resources provided on this site focus on the field of radiology. Hundreds of sites are listed in categories such as associations, centers, departments, education, imaging, journals, lists of resources,

MRI/NMR, nuclear medicine, other organizations, PET, programs, research, and ultrasound. The sites are drawn from sources around the world and can be browsed in order or by using a drop-down menu to access the topic of interest. (some features fee-based) http://medmark.org/rad/rad2.html

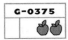

MultiDimensional Imaging   This Web site provides examples and applications of different techniques used in biomedical imaging. Multidimensional, multimodality, and multisensor applications are described in detail with methodology and specific examples of medical applications, along with discussions of new developments in this growing field.
http://www.expasy.ch/LFMI

Neurosciences on the Internet: Images   Hundreds of Internet sites are found through this address offering resources relating to human neuroanatomy and neuropathology, neuroscience images and methods, medical imaging centers, medical illustration, medical imaging indexes, and neuroanatomy atlases of animals.   http://www.neuroguide.com/neuroimg.html

Pediatric Radiology and Pediatric Imaging   Developed by Michael P. D'Alessandro, M.D., this Web page features a pediatric radiology digital library. The library contains common pediatric clinical problems with over 400 diseases represented by over 1,800 cases. There is a section on imaging approaches to common problems, as well as a section on performing common pediatric radiology procedures. Nearly 30 procedures are covered in a patient education section. There is also a link to pediatric radiology normal measurements and to musculoskeletal radiology of fractures. In addition to the library, the site lists hundreds of related links in categories such as textbooks, anatomy atlases, embryology, lectures, and patient education.
http://pediatricradiology.com/

University of Nebraska: Medical Images on the Web   A list of more than a dozen links is available at this address to Internet sources for medical images, maintained by the University of Nebraska Medical Center. Web pages listed include *Anatomy of the Human Body* by Henry Gray, a dermatology image library, a digital atlas of ophthalmology, the public health image library, the visible human project from the National Library of Medicine, and the whole brain atlas. All links are accompanied by short descriptions of resources at the site.   http://www.unmc.edu/library/eresources/medimage.html

11.12   MEDICAL SOFTWARE

Medical Software Reviews   The monthly newsletter found at this site publishes evaluations of medical software products for use by physicians and other health professionals. The contents of each issue are described, and information on Internet access for subscribers is provided. Categories of software include coding, databases, diagnosis, drug interactions, medical records, patient education, practice management, scheduling, and statistics. The table of contents for current and previous months can be viewed from the site's links; full reviews require a subscription. Subscriber information can be accessed by clicking on "Medical Software Reviews" at the bottom of the page. (fee-based) http://www.crihealthcarepubs.com/msrmain.html

11.13 PAIN MANAGEMENT

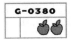

American Academy of Pain Management This site provides information about the academy and its activities, resources for finding a professional program in pain management, accreditation and continuing medical education resources, and a membership directory for locating a pain management professional. It also provides general information on pain management and a listing of relevant links. Access to the National Pain Data Bank is available at the site, containing statistics on various pain management therapies based on an outcomes measurement system. The site is divided into two sections with information tailored to the needs of both patients and healthcare professionals. http://www.aapainmanage.org

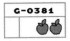

American Academy of Pain Medicine This site contains information about the academy's annual meeting, a member directory, FAQs, and related resources. Visitors can access an online newsletter, as well as a catalog of publications such as the academy's journal, *Pain Medicine,* pocket guides, and position papers. http://www.painmed.org/

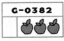

American Pain Foundation The American Pain Foundation is dedicated to education and advocacy for patients and their families coping with pain. A patient information section features fact sheets on a variety of conditions such as arthritis and digestive diseases, as well as information in general on pain management and medication. There is also a section on policy and legislative issues, with links provided to related sites. On the home page, icons at the bottom lead visitors to the "Pain Care Bill of Rights" which outlines patient rights. The "You are Not Alone" section provides information on support groups, and personal stories can be read under the "Voices of People in Pain" section. In addition, there is a pain action guide and a section on finding help that contains both emotional and financial resources. http://www.painfoundation.org/

American Pain Society The American Pain Society is a multidisciplinary, scientific organization that offers information on publications, advocacy, career opportunities, and upcoming events. A pain facility database allows the user to search for facilities by classifications, and additional resources for both patients and professionals provide contact information for related organizations. The American Pain Society site provides a search engine for abstracts in their database of pain-related topics. http://www.ampainsoc.org/

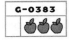

New York Online Access to Health (NOAH): Pain   Information on pain can be found through this large consumer health directory of Internet sites, maintained by the New York Online Access to Health project. The directory contains more than 100 sites categorized as the basics, types of pain, basic care, body-specific therapies, types of therapy, pain in children, and information resources.   http://www.noah-health.org/english/illness/pain/pain.html

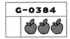

Pain.com   This site is a comprehensive resource for seeking information on pain and pain management, with separate sections available for health professionals and consumers. For clinicians, information on meetings, free online CME courses, pain management standards, and full-text articles from pain journals are provided. Pages specifically addressing perioperative pain, cancer pain, interventional pain management, migraine and headache pain, and regional anesthesia are found and include information on related CME and discussion forums. Consumers can locate both a list of support groups and a directory of pain clinics.
http://www.pain.com/index.cfm

11.14 PATENT SEARCHES

The following sites provide access to patent information for medical researchers and healthcare professionals interested in learning about the latest techniques, therapies, products, and drugs.

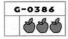

Intellectual Property Network   A spin-off of IBM, Delphion, Inc., provides this patent site which is ideal for physicians and researchers with an interest in patents. This service offers a database of patent information, titles and abstracts, and inventors and companies. The database displays patents on any topic, along with inventor information, dates of filing, application numbers, and an abstract of the patent. Users can search patent applications in the United States and Europe. The site also features a gallery of obscure patents.
(some features fee-based) http://www.delphion.com

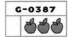

U.S. Patent and Trademark Office   Access to the database of the U.S. Patent and Trademark Office is available through this site for detailed searching of patents by number, inventor, and topic. There are both a full-text database and a bibliographic database.
http://www.uspto.gov/patft/index.html

11.15 PATHOLOGY AND LABORATORY MEDICINE

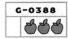

Hardin MD: Pathology and Laboratory Medicine Resources   Part of the Hardin Meta Directory from the University of Iowa, this site provides nearly 20 links to sites that each contain a list of other sites related to pathology and laboratory medicine. The sites are categorized as large, medium, or small lists.
http://www.lib.uiowa.edu/hardin/md/path.html

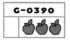

Indiana University: Pathology Image Library An image library for pathology is featured on this Web page, maintained by Indiana University. The library is categorized by organ system such as bone and soft tissue, cardiovascular, gastrointestinal, endocrine, hepatobiliary, genitourinary, pulmonary, and renal. There is also a section for gross pathology observations. The library can be searched by keyword.
http://erl.pathology.iupui.edu/c604/Default.htm

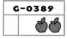

MedBioWorld: Laboratory Science, Forensic Science, and Pathology Journals Visitors to this Web page will find a listing of laboratory science, forensic science, and pathology journals available on the Internet. There are over 75 journals listed alphabetically.
http://www.medbioworld.com/journals/medicine/pathology.html

Pathology Images Developed by a group of physicians, this site features the "Lightning Hypertext of Disease," a database of pathology images with captions. The database is free to nonmembers but query results are limited to 30 images. Membership provides access to an alternate site where queries are returned with unlimited results. The results can be viewed in English, German, or Spanish. Other features include a spelling page for pathology terms, a precancer terminology page, and an abbreviations and acronyms page. There is also a section to help professionals study for their anatomic pathology and pathology specialty boards via a quiz that randomly selects questions from 6,000 multiple choice questions. (some features fee-based) http://www.pathinfo.com/

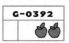

Tulane University: Pathology Educational Resources Primarily for healthcare professionals, this site offers a listing of links related to pathology. More than 30 sites are listed under topics such as catalogs of pathology links, laboratory resources and images, and other Web resources. The sites are drawn mostly from American universities.
http://www.tmc.tulane.edu/classware/
pathology/medical_pathology/New_for_98/Resources.html

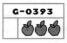

University of Illinois: The Urbana Atlas of Pathology The site provides a comprehensive collection of pathology images sectioned into general, cardiovascular, endocrine, pulmonary, and renal pathology. The general pathology section includes images of the kidney, heart, spleen, thyroid, testis, cervix, small intestine, lung, artery, pancreas, liver, lymph nodes, brain, colon, skin, mesentery, joints, uterus, and peritoneal cavity. Each image has an explanatory caption. http://www.med.uiuc.edu/PathAtlasf/titlepage.html

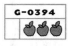

University of Michigan: Internet Resources for Pathology and Laboratory Medicine Hundreds of sites related to pathology and laboratory medicine are listed on this Web page, hosted by the University of Michigan Medical School Department of Pathology. The sites are listed in categories such as pathology departments (domestic and international), LISTSERVs, e-mail resources, databases and multimedia exhibits, regulatory and accreditation agencies, Usenet groups, job banks, organizations, and journals. There are also anatomic pathology and laboratory medicine resources. The entire list can be browsed or accessed quickly through a table of contents that lists the categories as well as subspecialty resources.

http://www.pathology.med.umich.edu/links

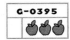

University of Utah: Pathology Image Library   Intended for students and healthcare professionals, this site offers a pathology image library with more than 1,900 images. Maintained by the Department of Pathology at the University of Utah, the library is organized as general pathology and organ system pathology. There are also special sections with images and tutorials dedicated to AIDS pathology and anatomy/histology. A section on laboratory exercises offers case studies with images and questions. In addition, practice exams drawn from a bank of more than 1,600 questions are found. Mini-tutorials on a variety of conditions such as breast cancer, inflammatory bowel diseases, and tuberculosis are also provided.

http://medstat.med.utah.edu/WebPath/webpath.html

11.16 PREVENTIVE MEDICINE

MedMark: Preventive Medicine   Dedicated to preventive medicine, this site features a comprehensive listing of Internet resources. Hundreds of sites are found in categories such as associations, centers, departments, education, consumer resources, general, government, and guidelines. There are also journals, lists of resources, and programs. The site can be browsed in order or through hyperlinks found in the table of contents presented in a sidebar menu.

http://members.kr.inter.net/medmark/prevent/

11.17 PUBLIC HEALTH

American Public Health Association   Health professionals may find the American Public Health Association site to be of interest. The site offers public health reports, abstracts from the *American Journal of Public Health,* and access to full-text articles from their newspaper, *The Nation's Health.* The site also has information on continuing education, legislative issues, and a publications catalog. Members will find funding opportunities under the "Programs/Projects & Practice" section. In addition, there are links for state public health associations, the World Federation of Public Health, and related public health resources.

(some features fee-based) http://www.apha.org/

National Health Service Corps   After accessing the introductory page, visitors are taken to the table of contents for the National Health Service Corps Web site. General information is provided about the organization's public health mission in assisting underserved populations. Details on opportunities available to health professionals and a site on community assistance services are also

available. Upcoming events and important dates, as well as other news items of the organization, are found.
http://www.bphc.hrsa.dhhs.gov/nhsc/

World Health Organization (WHO)   A site index and search tool assist in navigation of this site, which is available for viewing in English, Spanish, or French. World Health Organization press releases are displayed at the main page, and connections to information resources, a press media center, and disease outbreak information are provided. Information on current emergencies by country is addressed, and a traveler's health advisory is found.
http://www.who.int/home-page/

MEDICAL STUDENT RESOURCES

12.1 GENERAL RESOURCES

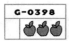

American Medical Association (AMA): Medical Student Section The Medical Student Section of the AMA is dedicated to representing medical students, improving medical education, developing leadership, and promoting activism for the health of America. The site offers information about current issues and advocacy activities, meetings, chapter information, and leadership news. A community service link provides information on policy promotion, grant application, organ and tissue donation, and ideas for community service projects. http://amaMedstudent.org

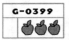

American Medical Student Association Containing many useful resources for medical students, this site features daily health and medical news, legislative and policy issues, and LISTSERVs for special populations. A menu of topics lists issues such as community and public health, global health issues, health policy, humanistic medicine, and medical education, along with resources to get involved. This section also provides resources for positions, internships, and fellowships; leadership training information; and a list of related Internet sites. The "Resource Center" provides links for financial resources; interest groups in areas such as death and dying, psychiatry, and bioethics; and strategic priorities including diversity in medicine and medical student well-being. Additional resources include information on personal data assistants (PDAs), residency selection, and an AMSA catalog that offers many free online publications. Members can register for the career development program online and apply for financial resources such as loans and grants.
(some features fee-based) http://www.amsa.org/

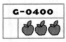

American Medical Women's Association A national association, AMWA provides information and services to women physicians and women medical students, as well as promoting women's health and the professional development of women physicians. Resources include news, discussions of current issues, events, conferences, online publications, fellowship and residency information accessed through the Fellowship and Residency Electronic Interactive Database Access system (FRIEDA), general information and developments from AMWA staff members, advocacy activities, a listing of AMWA continuing edu-

cation programs, and links to sites of interest. A variety of topics related to women's health are discussed at the site.
http://www.amwa-doc.org

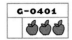

Association of American Medical Colleges   This nonprofit association committed to the advancement of academic medicine consists of American and Canadian medical schools, teaching hospitals and health systems, academic and professional societies, and medical students and residents. News, membership details, publications, meeting and conference calendars, medical education Internet resources, research findings, and discussions related to healthcare are all found at the site. Employment opportunities at the AAMC are also listed.
http://www.aamc.org

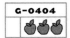

Integrated Medical Curriculum   This Web page integrates of major medical school courses, especially the first two years, with basic science and clinical program departments containing explanatory text, images, and cross-referenced hyperlinks. Anatomy is stressed, as well as basic clinical skills, clinical musculoskeletal pathology, and ethics. Other resources include a testing center with practice quizzes, a virtual student lounge, a faculty lounge, and related message boards.
(some features fee-based) http://www.imc.gsm.com

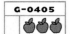

Internet Resources for Medical Students   A comprehensive listing of links is offered on this Web page, courtesy of Lviv State Medical University, Ukraine. More than 150 links are found in categories such as associations, general sites, education, study help, multimedia, grants and funding, humor, and other resources. The sites are drawn from around the world; some are in Russian.   http://www.meduniv.lviv.ua/inform/studlinks.html

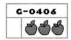

MedicalStudent.com   This site contains an extensive medical textbook section organized by discipline. Features of the site included patient simulations, consumer health information, access to MEDLINE and medical journals online, continuing education sources, board examination information, medical organizations, and Internet medical directories.
http://www.medicalstudent.com

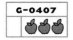

Stanford University: MedWorld   MedWorld, sponsored by the Stanford Medical Alumni Association, offers information for students, patients, physicians, and the healthcare community. Resources include case reports and global rounds, links to quality medical sites and MEDLINE, doctor diaries and medical news, and newsgroups and discussion forums. Visitors can access Stanford's medical search engine, MEDBOT, to utilize several Internet medical search engines simultaneously.
http://medworld.stanford.edu/home

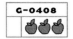

Student Doctor Network   Hosted by the Student Doctor Network, this Web page offers medical students a broad array of resources. The SDN student forums offer discussion boards for medical and premedical students. There are

also medical student diaries, where five medical students post their thoughts and experiences as they go through medical school. "The Links Resource" features more than 740 links to information such as academic success, career choices, finance, dental resources, osteopathic resources, and medical resources. In addition, there is information on getting in and getting through medical school, osteopathic medicine, and getting into dental school.

(free registration) http://www.studentdoctor.net/

12.2 FELLOWSHIPS AND RESIDENCIES

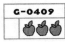

Accreditation Council for Graduate Medical Education The Accreditation Council for Graduate Medical Education (ACGME) reviews and accredits residency programs, establishes standards of performance, and provides a process to consider complaints and possible investigations by the council. The ACGME publishes standards on resident duty hours, citation statistics, and a moonlighting policy. The site also offers information about meetings, workshops, institutional reviews, program requirements, links to residency review committees, and a listing of accredited programs.

http://www.acgme.org

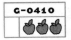

American Medical Association (AMA): Fellowship and Residency Electronic Interactive Database Access (FREIDA) Online System Operated as a service of the AMA, the FREIDA system provides online access to a comprehensive database of information on approximately 7,500 graduate medical educational programs accredited by the Accreditation Council for Graduate Medical Education (ACGME). FREIDA enables the user to search this comprehensive database and offers physician workforce statistics as reported by practicing physicians in a variety of subspecialties.

http://www.ama-assn.org/ama/pub/category/2997.html

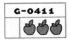

Educational Commission for Foreign Medical Graduates Through its certification program, the commission "assesses the readiness of graduates of foreign medical schools to enter residency or fellowship programs in the United States that are accredited by the Accreditation Council for Graduate Medical Education." The site provides information for foreign students on testing and examination dates, clinical skills required, medical education credentials, visa sponsorship, and certification verification.

http://www.ecfmg.org

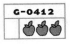

Electronic Residency Application Service The Association of American Medical Colleges (AAMC) provides this application service for students. It transmits residency applications, recommendation letters, deans' letters, transcripts, and other supporting credentials from medical schools to residency program directors via the Internet. At present, the service covers anesthesiology, dermatology, emergency medicine, family practice, internal medicine, nuclear medicine, obstetrics and gynecology, pathology, pediatrics, physical medicine and rehabilitation, psychiatry, radiology, radiation oncology, and surgery (general, orthopedic, and plastic). The system allows tracking of an application 24 hours a day via a special document tracking system.

(some features fee-based) http://www.aamc.org/eras/news/start.htm

---

G-0413

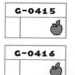

National Residency Matching Program The NRMP is a mechanism for the matching of applicants to programs according to the preferences expressed by both parties. Last year this service placed over 20,000 applicants for postgraduate medical training positions into nearly 4,000 residency programs at 700 teaching hospitals in the United States. The applicants and residency programs evaluate and rank each other, producing a computerized pairing of applicants to programs, in ranked order. This process provides applicants and program directors with a uniform date of appointment to positions in March, eliminating decision pressure when options are unknown. The site offers information about the service, publications, and forms for registration. Prospective residents can register with the service for a fee and access the directory of programs.

http://nrmp.aamc.org/nrmp

G-0414

ResidencySite.com ResidencySite.com provides an online listing of medical residencies organized by specialty, with links to residency program home pages. Program directors can access resumes of residency applicants, and prospective residents can review documents related to residency matching programs and publications offering advice on obtaining a position.

http://www.residencysite.com

12.3 MEDICAL SCHOOL WEB SITES

G-0415

American Universities All American university home pages are listed at this site. http://www.clas.ufl.edu/CLAS/american-universities.html

---

G-0416

Gradschools.com Sponsored by several universities and other teaching institutions, Gradschools.com offers a listing of graduate programs nationwide. Programs are found by indicating a specific area of study. A directory of distance learning programs is also available.

http://www.gradschools.com/noformsearch.html

G-0417

Medical Education Accredited medical schools are listed, with links, at this site. http://www.meducation.com/schools.html

---

G-0419

NEW

MedicalSchoolDirectory.com A directory of medical schools, organized by state, is provided on this site. Contact information and a hyperlink to each school's Web site is offered.

http://www.doctordirectory.com/medicalschools/directory/default.asp

---

13

PATIENT EDUCATION AND PLANNING

13.1 EXERCISE AND PHYSICAL FITNESS

MEDLINEplus Health Information: Exercise/Physical Fitness
Resources on exercise and physical fitness are provided on this Web page, maintained by the National Library of Medicine. The site provides links for overviews on exercise, nutrition for workouts, preventing injuries, specific conditions, organizations, and statistics. Much of the information comes from government agencies or scientific associations, such as the American Heart Association or the American Academy of Family Physicians. Specific aspects of fitness such as tips on buying exercise equipment, stretching, and walking are covered. Information for specific populations is also included with sections for men, women, teenagers, seniors, and children. Some publications are available in Spanish. http://www.nlm.nih.gov/medlineplus/exercisephysicalfitness.html

MedNets: Fitness This Web page presents a listing of links on fitness, sponsored by MedNets.com. More than 45 sites are listed in categories including journals and organizations, newsletters, and topics such as weight loss and stretching. http://www.mednets.com/fitness.htm

Medscout: Physical Fitness This Web page features a listing of links related to physical fitness for both patients and professionals. More than 100 sites are listed covering associations, nutrition guidelines, exercise guides, and a variety of sports and activities.
http://www.medscout.com/physical_fitness/

President's Council on Physical Fitness and Sports Resources provided at this site include a fitness guide, which details the benefits of physical activity and outlines solutions to common problems interfering with physical fitness. News about physical fitness, an online reading room, scientific research reports on physical activity topics, and resources for coaches and fitness professionals are offered. Details about the national President's Challenge and other programs for physical fitness are presented.
http://www.fitness.gov/

Prevention.com: Weight Loss and Fitness Targeted to consumers, this site from *Prevention* magazine offers information and support for losing weight

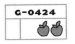

and exercising in the form of nutrition news and health articles. A fitness assessment section offers quizzes on topics such as heart health, hiking, and weight. The site also hosts message forums covering a variety of topics, including an online walking club for information and support.

(free registration) http://www.healthyideas.com/weight/

13.2 FOOD AND NUTRITION

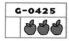

American Dietetic Association The American Dietetic Association (ADA) presents this informative site for consumers, students, and dietetic professionals. This site has information on nutrition resources, careers in dietetics, meetings and events, government affairs, current issues, and publications. The "Healthy Lifestyles" section has nutrition tips, fact sheets, and dieting guidelines. The "ADA Press Room" offers an extensive list of resources, including information on ADA campaigns, a link to the *Journal of the ADA*, position papers, and a reading list of consumer publications. There are also links to consumer education and public policy sites; dietetic associations and networking groups; dietetic practice groups; food service and culinary organizations; and medical, health, and other professional organizations.

http://www.eatright.org

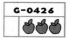

Arbor Nutrition Guide The Arbor Nutrition Guide covers all areas of nutrition including applied and clinical nutrition. The site provides links to information on dietary guidelines, special diets, sports nutrition, individual vitamins and minerals, and cultural nutrition. There are also links relating to food science, such as food labeling in other countries, food regulation, food additives, science journals, phytochemistry, and other related topics. Each link listed is accompanied by a brief description of the site. Arbor also provides links to journals and organizations.

http://www.netspace.net.au/%7Ehelmant/search.htm

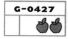

Department of Agriculture: Nutrient Values Visitors can utilize the search engine housed at this site to find the recommended daily allowance (RDA) nutrient values of over 5,000 food items for three different serving sizes for men averaging 174 pounds and for women averaging 138 pounds. The RDAs are calculated for individuals between the ages of 25 and 50.

http://www.rahul.net/cgi-bin/fatfree/usda/usda.cgi

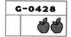

Food and Drug Administration (FDA): Selected Non-FDA Sources of Food and Nutrition Information A list of non-FDA sources of food and nutrition information is featured on this Web page, part of the Food and Drug Administration's Center for Food Safety and Applied Nutrition site. The list contains more than 75 sites categorized as U.S. government sources, non-U.S. government sources, and nutrition journals. There are also links for related LISTSERVs and commercial sites.

(some features fee-based) http://vm.cfsan.fda.gov/~dms/nutrlist.html

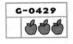

Food and Nutrition Information Center Links to hundreds of Web sites are provided through the A-to-Z food and nutrition listing on this site, maintained by the USDA's Food and Nutrition Information Center. Topics in the listing include food allergies, breastfeeding, child nutrition, eating disorders, and food labeling. Additional sections include resource lists and information on dietary supplements, food composition, dietary guidelines, the food guide pyramid, and FNIC databases. Frequently requested topics are listed in the "Consumer Corner."

http://www.nalusda.gov/fnic/

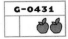

Food Science and Nutrition Journals Visitors to this site will find an alphabetical listing of over 100 food science and nutrition journals. Some provide full-text articles.

(some features fee-based) http://www.sciencekomm.at/journals/food.html

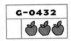

International Food Information Council The International Food Information Council (IFIC)presents resources at this site including current issues, up-to-date information for the media, food safety and nutrition facts, and extensive links to government affairs and agencies. The IFIC library provides an archive of publications geared toward educators, journalists, professionals, students, government officials, and consumers. Also featured is a glossary of food-related terms and *Food Insight*, the council's newsletter.

http://ificinfo.health.org

National Institutes of Health (NIH): Office of Dietary Supplements
The International Bibliographic Information on Dietary Supplements (IBIDS) database is featured on this Web site, courtesy of the NIH. Of interest to consumers and professionals, the IBIDS database contains more than 460,000 citations and abstracts on dietary supplements. The database can be searched via the consumer version, a full version, or peer-reviewed citations only. A journal list is provided to order full-text articles directly from the publisher. In addition, the home page contains links for grant information, a list of publications, and related resources.

http://ods.od.nih.gov/databases/ibids.html

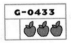

Nutrition and Healthy Eating Advice A broad array of nutrition resources is presented on this Web page. Hundreds of links are offered in categories such as healthy recipes, aging, child nutrition, cultural foods, diet analysis, diseases and conditions, and eating advice. Fad diets, food products including fast food nutrition, food safety, food science, guidelines, and organic foods are also covered. Links to related directories of sites are found as well as a question and answer forum and a free e-mail newsletter.

http://nutrition.about.com/health/nutrition/

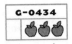

Science Reference Internet Guide to Food Science and Nutrition
Healthcare professionals and consumers may find the listing of food science and nutrition Internet sites on this Web page useful. Maintained by Michigan State University Libraries, the listing covers more than 100 resources. Categories in-

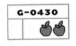

clude associations, comprehensive food and nutrition sites, business and industry resources, composition and nutrient analysis databases, safety and handling, human nutrition and health, and online journal abstracts and publications. (some features fee-based) http://www.lib.msu.edu/science/food.htm

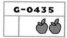

Tufts University: Nutrition Navigator Presented by the Center on Nutrition Communication in the School of Nutrition Science and Policy at Tufts University, this site offers an up-to-date, rated guide to other nutrition sites. It provides breaking and archived news stories related to nutrition policy and trends as well as information on general nutrition and special dietary needs. There are also sections with sites specifically targeted to parents, children, women, health professionals, educators, and journalists.
http://navigator.tufts.edu

13.3 GRIEF AND BEREAVEMENT

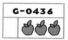

American College of Physicians Part of a larger *Home Care Guide to Advanced Cancer,* this site features the chapter on grieving. The chapter provides an overview of the grieving process and covers when to get help, self-help issues, common obstacles, and carrying out and adjusting a personal grieving plan. There are also links to related information.
http://www.acponline.org/public/h_care/10-griev.htm

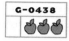

CancerNet: Loss, Grief, and Bereavement Designed for healthcare professionals, this Physician Data Query (PDQ) from the National Cancer Institute offers guidelines for helping patients cope with loss, grief, and bereavement. A model of life-threatening illness is provided to aid in understanding of the patient's psychological needs. Other topics covered include end-of-life decisions, patterns of dying, and phases of grief. General aspects of grief therapy are described, as well as complicated grief, children and grief, and cross-cultural responses to grief. A bibliography is included, and a link is provided to a patient version of this PDQ.
http://cancernet.nci.nih.gov/cgi-bin/srchcgi.exe?DBID=pdq&
TYPE=search&SFMT=pdq_statement/1/0/0&Z208=208_06750H

G-0438 **MEDLINEplus Health Information: Bereavement** Bereavement is the focus of this Web page produced by the National Library of Medicine. The site includes overviews on bereavement and grief as well as specific information for dealing with loss due to AIDS, sudden infant death syndrome, stillbirth, and suicide. Tips on helping children, teenagers, and seniors in the grieving process are also included. Some publications are available in Spanish.
http://www.nlm.nih.gov/medlineplus/bereavement.html

13.4 MEDICAL PLANNING

BLOOD BANK INFORMATION

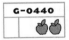

America's Blood Centers   America's Blood Centers (ABC) are found in 45 states and collect almost half of the U.S. blood supply. The site provides position papers; *ABC Blood News*, a quarterly awareness publication; and *ABC Blood Bulletin*, a publication written by the ABC Scientific Medical and Technical Committee about current issues in blood banking.
http://www.americasblood.org

American Association of Blood Banks   This site provides a contact list for each state on locating and arranging blood donation, including information on storing blood for an anticipated surgery or emergency (autologous blood transfusion). The association's regulatory affairs, legislative, and legal programs monitor and report on government, congressional, and legal issues affecting the blood banking and transfusion medicine communities. Resources for professionals in these areas include audio conferences, a virtual library, and certification programs. The education department sponsors conferences, workshops, and distance learning programs. Links are also available to AABB's journal *Transfusion*, news magazines, bulletins, and updates.
http://www.aabb.org

CAREGIVER RESOURCES

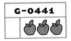

Family Caregiver Alliance   Information on long-term care is featured on the Family Caregiver Alliance (FCA) Web page. Highlights of the site include dealing with hot weather and communicating with your doctor, as well as links to the alliance newsletter, webcasts, and research studies. The "Resource Center" section of the site offers an online support group, FAQs, a discussion forum, and fact sheets regarding issues in long-term care, work, and eldercare. The "Clearinghouse" section contains fact sheets on diseases and disorders, reading lists, and a "News Bureau" to help reporters with background material and interviews. The site also provides information on policy issues, FCA position papers, and a list of related resources.
http://www.caregiver.org/

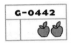

National Family Caregivers Association   The National Family Caregivers Association offers education, information, support, public awareness campaigns, and advocacy to caregivers of chronically ill, aged, or disabled loved ones. The address discusses care giving and provides statistics, a survey report, news, an informational pamphlet, a reading list, care giving tips, and contact details. Caregivers will find this site a source of support, encouragement, and information.   http://www.nfcacares.org

CHRONIC AND TERMINAL CARE PLANNING

Organ Donation This government site answers frequently asked questions, dispels myths, and presents facts about organ donation. The site also posts information on public affairs and legislative updates, a list of resources on grant applications, and links to related organizations and Web sites. Visitors can also download and print a donor card.
http://www.organdonor.gov

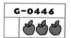

U.S. Living Will Registry This free service electronically stores advance directives and makes them available directly to hospitals by telephone. Registration materials are available to download online or by calling 1-800-LIV-WILL.
http://www.uslivingwillregistry.com

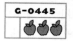

USAhomecare.com USAhomecare.com is a consumer-oriented home care (home health and hospice) site. The site provides answers to common questions, reviews considerations in implementing home care, and discusses the rights and responsibilities of clients and of the elderly population. The site also has an agency locator for the United States, a bookstore, links to related sites, and news. http://www.USAhomecare.com

DIRECTING HEALTHCARE CONCERNS AND COMPLAINTS

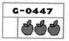

Congress.org This site offers a Capital directory, including members of Congress, the Supreme Court, state governors, and the White House. Users can also find comments on members of Congress by associations and advocacy groups, determine a bill's status through the site's search engine, send messages to Congress members, and find local congressional representatives.
http://congress.org/

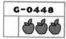

Families USA Families USA is a national, nonprofit, nonpartisan organization dedicated to the achievement of high-quality, affordable healthcare and long-term care for all Americans. The site offers a clearinghouse of information on Medicaid, Medicare, managed care, children's health, and the uninsured. Also included are news and analysis of current issues in healthcare policy. Within the site, at www.familiesusa.org/medicaid/state.htm, a state-specific healthcare information guide is provided, with state-specific issues and contacts for state officials involved with healthcare and/or insurance.
http://www.familiesusa.org

Joint Commission of Accreditation of Healthcare Organizations This independent, nonprofit organization offers an outlet for patients, their families, and caregivers to express concerns about the quality of care at accredited healthcare organizations by mail, fax, or e-mail. Complaints are addressed on issues such as patient rights, patient care, safety, infection control, medication use, and security. The commission may review and investigate warranted

complaints that cannot be resolved by the parties involved using its Quality Incident Review Criteria, also posted online here.
http://www.jcaho.org/compl_frm.html

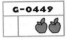

Medicare Rights Center   The Medicare Rights Center (MRC) is a national, nonprofit organization dedicated to ensuring that seniors and people with disabilities on Medicare have access to quality, affordable healthcare. Specific MRC programs include direct assistance through telephone hotlines, education and training, public policy, and communication to ensure public awareness. Publications available cover topics such as Medicare basics, home health and hospice, and Medicare bills.
(some features fee-based) http://www.medicarerights.org/Index.html

State Insurance Commissioners   Deloitte and Touche Financial Counseling Services offers the addresses and phone numbers of each state's insurance commissioner at this site.
http://www.dtonline.com/insur/inlistng.htm

ELDER AND EXTENDED CARE

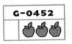

Administration on Aging (AOA)   Dedicated to providing information on older persons and services for the elderly, the Administration on Aging offers a broad array of resources. Information on the site is divided into sections such as older persons and their families, healthcare professionals, and researchers and students. The older persons section offers a comprehensive listing of Internet resources including an AOA guide for caregivers, an eldercare locator, booklets on health topics, and fact sheets on issues such as age discrimination, longevity, and pensions. Professional resources include information on legal issues, general resources, statistics, and specific program resources such as managed care. A section entitled the "Aging Network" offers a list of general resources, and the research section emphasizes statistics.
http://www.aoa.dhhs.gov

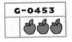

American Association for Retired Persons   This nonprofit group is dedicated to the needs and rights of elderly Americans. Topics discussed at the site include caregiver support, community and volunteer organizations, Medicare, Medicaid, help with home care, finances, health and wellness, independent living, computers and the Internet, and housing options. Benefits and discounts provided to members are described, reference and research materials are available, and users can search the site by keyword.
http://www.aarp.org

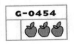

American Association of Homes and Services for the Aging   This association represents nonprofit organizations providing healthcare, housing, and services to the elderly. The site offers tips for consumers and family caregivers on choosing facilities and services, notices of upcoming events, press re-

leases, fact sheets, an online bookstore, and links to sponsors, business partners, an international program, and other relevant sites.
http://www.aahsa.org

Eldercare Locator The Eldercare Locator is a nationwide directory assistance service designed to help older persons and caregivers locate local support resources for aging Americans. This site helps senior citizens find community assistance and Medicaid information. Interested parties can also contact the Eldercare Locator toll free at 1-800-677-1116.
http://www.aoa.dhhs.gov/aoa/pages/loctrnew.html

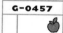

Extendedcare.com This site offers a wide variety of resources related to senior citizens, including information on choosing an extended care provider, a "Senior Health Library" of information resources on health and aging, a glossary of terms related to extended care, and information on over 70,000 care providers searchable by type of care and zip code. Of particular interest, the "Informed Living" section provides in-depth articles on many relevant topics including home adaptation for Alzheimer's sufferers, financial planning, nutrition, exercise, and information on commonly prescribed drugs. Visitors may also participate in online chats with healthcare professionals or with other seniors and caregivers, subscribe to an e-mail newsletter, and read archived newsletters and press releases. A tool for assessing an individual's care needs is also available. A professional section is available to users associated with registered hospitals.
(some features fee-based) http://www.elderconnect.com/asp/default.asp

Insure.com: Answers to Seniors' Health Insurance Questions (on Medicare and Medicaid) This site provides individual state phone numbers for the State Health Insurance Advisory Program (SHIP). SHIP, a federally funded program found in all states under different names, helps elderly and disabled Medicare and Medicaid recipients understand their rights and options for healthcare. Services include assistance with bills, advice on buying supplement policies, explanation of rights, help with payment denials or appeals, and assistance in choosing a Medicare health plan.
http://www.insure.com/health/ship.html

END-OF-LIFE DECISIONS

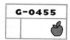

American Medical Association (AMA): Education for Physicians on End Supported by a grant from the Robert Wood Johnson Foundation, EPEC is a program designed to educate physicians nationwide on "the essential clinical competencies in end-of-life care." Visitors will find an overview of the project's purpose, design, and scope; a call for EPEC training conference applications; previous conference details; a mailing list; and an annotated list of educational resource materials. EPEC resources such as the *Participant's Handbook*, a guide to end-of-life care, can be downloaded from the site.
http://www.epec.net

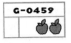

Before I Die   The Web companion to a public television program exploring the medical, ethical, and social issues associated with end-of-life care in the United States is featured at this address. Personal stories, a bulletin board, a glossary of terms, contact details for important support sources and organizations, and suggestions on forming a discussion group are available at the site. A program description, viewer's guide, outreach efforts and materials, and credits for the program are also provided.
http://www.pbs.org/wnet/bid

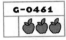

End of Life: Exploring Death in America   National Public Radio's "All Things Considered" presents transcripts of a recent series on death and dying and other resources at this informative site. Contact information and links to organizations and other support sources; a bibliography of important publications; texts related to death, dying, and healing; and a forum for presenting personal stories are found at this address.
http://www.npr.org/programs/death

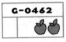

Last Acts   Designed to improve end-of-life care, Last Acts seeks to "bring end-of-life issues out in the open and to help individuals and organizations pursue the search for better ways to care for the dying." The site presents information on Last Acts activities, a newsletter, press releases, and discussion forums. Links are available to details of recent news headlines, sites offering additional information resources, grant-making organizations, and a directory of Robert Wood Johnson Foundation end-of-life grantees.
http://www.lastacts.org

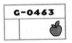

Living Wills   A brief description of a living will is offered on this Web site, written by attorney Michelle M. Arostegui. The purpose of the living will is described along with when it is used and what options may be included, such as "Do Not Resuscitate" and removal of nutrition and hydration.
http://estateplanning.about.com/library/weekly/aa080401a.htm?rnk=r3&terms=living+will

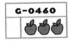

Partnership for Caring: America's Voices for the Dying   Partnership for Caring is a national nonprofit organization dedicated to improving the way society cares for dying people and their loved ones. The organization promotes communication by hosting live chats and moderated discussions. Resources at the site include a glossary of terms, fact sheets, and articles on topics related to end-of-life issues as well as downloads for state-specific documents on advance directives. Visitors may also access news, press releases, and *Voices*, the organization's newsletter.
http://www.partnershipforcaring.org/HomePage/

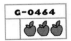

Project on Death in America: Transforming the Culture of Dying
The Project on Death in America supports initiatives in research, scholarship, the humanities, and the arts in transforming the American culture in the experience of dying and bereavement. The PDIA also promotes innovations in care, public education, professional education, and public policy. Information is presented on the project's Faculty Scholars Program, as well as on various other

funding initiatives, past and present, in such areas as nursing, social work, arts and humanities, public policy, legal issues, and community-based issues. Other resources described at the site include Grantmakers Concerned with Care at the End of Life, media resources, and other publications offered by the PDIA.
http://www.soros.org/death

HOSPICE AND HOME CARE

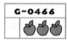

American Academy of Hospice and Palliative Medicine This national nonprofit organization is composed of physicians "dedicated to the advancement of hospice/palliative medicines, its practice, research, and education." Academy details, news, press releases, position statements, events and meetings notices, employment listings, and links to related sites are found at this address. Publications, CME opportunities, and conference tapes are also available.
http://www.aahpm.org

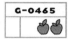

Hospice Association of America Serving the needs of the most seriously ill patients suffering from cancer and other diseases, the HAA offers a full menu of information about the field of hospice care including fact sheets and statistics for consumers; legislative, regulatory, research, and legal updates; hospice publications; and education programs offered at conferences.
http://www.hospice-america.org

Hospice Foundation of America The Hospice Foundation of America offers a range of books and training services for hospice professionals and the general public. The Web site provides information on hospices, patients and staff, services and expenses, myths and facts, and volunteering. There is also a reading list, with descriptions, and links related to organizations and resources for both the healthcare provider and the patient are also available.
http://www.hospicefoundation.org

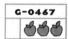

Hospice Net Hospice Net is dedicated to helping patients and families facing life-threatening illnesses. The site contains a listing of useful articles, FAQ sheets, caregiver information, and a listing of select links to other major Web resources. Information is categorized as services, patients, caregivers, and bereavement. Topics and resources covered include finding a local hospice, pain control, the Family and Medical Leave Act, and dealing with grief.
http://www.hospicenet.org

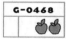

HospiceWeb This site contains general information, a list of frequently asked questions, a discussion board, a hospice locator, and an extensive list of links to related sites. Links to other hospice organizations are categorized by state. http://www.hospiceweb.com/index.htm

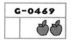

National Association for Home Care The National Association for Home Care (NAHC) is a trade association representing more than 6,000 home care agencies, hospices, and home care aide organizations and medical equip-

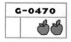

ment suppliers. General information offered includes news and association announcements, a newsletter on pediatric home care, and links to affiliates. Departments within NAHC cover legislative and regulatory information, meetings and conferences, statistics and technical papers, and directories of related state associations. Visitors can access a home care and hospice search tool for finding local service providers, as well as a consumer section offering information on choosing a home care provider. This section includes descriptions of agencies providing home care; tips for finding information about agencies; and discussions of services, payment, patients' rights, accrediting agencies, and state resources. One section is restricted to members.

(some features fee-based) http://www.nahc.org

National Hospice and Palliative Care Organization   The National Hospice and Palliative Care organization offers a comprehensive site providing information on all aspects of hospice care for the seriously and terminally ill. Areas covered include communicating end-of-life wishes, the Medicare hospice benefit, and details on the organization's public engagement campaign. Other site features include a career center, conference listings, news, and a state-by-state and city-by-city guide to hospice organizations in the United States.

http://www.nhpco.org

MEDICAL INSURANCE AND MANAGED CARE

Agency for Healthcare Research and Quality (AHRQ): Checkup On Health Insurance Choices   This discussion of health insurance choices informs consumers on topics such as why individuals need insurance, sources of health insurance, group and individual insurance, making a decision of coverage, and managed care. Types of insurance described at the site include fee-for-service and "customary" fees, health maintenance organizations, preferred provider organizations, Medicaid, Medicare, disability insurance, hospital indemnity insurance, and long-term-care insurance. The site also includes a checklist and worksheet to determine features important to an individual when choosing insurance. A glossary of terms is available for reference.

http://www.ahcpr.gov/consumer/insuranc.htm

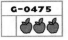

American Association of Health Plans   Located in Washington, D.C., the American Association of Health Plans represents more than 1,000 HMOs, PPOs, and other network-based plans. Geared toward professionals, the site's "Patient Care" section provides information on clinical practice guidelines, health plan operations, news, conferences, grants and awards, care delivery and disease management, prevention, public health, accreditation, industry standards, and performance measurement. The site also offers resources on government and advocacy activities, public relations materials, reports and statistics, selected bibliographies listed by subject, information on services and products, conference details, and training program information. Consumer resources in-

clude information on choosing a health plan, descriptions of different types of health plans, women's health resources, and fact sheets about health plans.
http://www.aahp.org

drkoop.com: Insurance Center   Part of drkoop.com, this site features an insurance library covering areas such as disability, workers' compensation, and long-term care. A glossary of insurance terms and health insurance news updates are also featured at the site.
http://www.drkoop.com/hcr/insurance

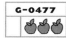

Employer Quality Partnership   The Employer Quality Partnership (EQP) is a volunteer coalition of employer organizations interested in promoting positive change in the healthcare marketplace and in educating employees regarding their employer-based healthcare plans. This site offers a guide for employees on selecting and understanding healthcare plans, assistance for employers in evaluating healthcare plans, and guides for employers on ways to improve the quality of their health plans.
http://www.eqp.org

Healthcare Financing Administration   This federal site provides a wealth of information on Medicare, Medicaid, and the State Children's Health Insurance Program (SCHIP) for both patients and healthcare professionals. It covers the basic features of each program and discusses laws, regulations, and statistics about federal healthcare programs. Information is also provided at the state level (state Medicaid), providing a list of sites with important state information.
http://www.hcfa.gov

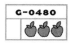

Joint Commission of Accreditation of Healthcare Organizations   The Joint Commission of Accreditation of Healthcare Organizations evaluates and accredits nearly 19,000 healthcare organizations and programs. "Quality Check," a service offered by the commission, allows consumers to check ratings and evaluations of accredited organizations at the site. Information is available for the general public, employers, healthcare purchasers, and unions; the international community; and healthcare professionals and organizations. The site also contains information on filing complaints, career opportunities, news, and links to related sites.
http://www.jcaho.org

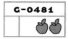

Managed Care Glossary   Designed to be used for professional training purposes or as a general information source, this managed care glossary contains a continuously updated compilation of new terminology related to managed care, with additional items in the field of information technology continuously being added. Physicians and other healthcare professionals may want to bookmark this site to ensure a more complete understanding of modern health maintenance and preferred provider organization structure and service delivery.
http://www.mentalhelp.net/poc/view_index.php/idx/34/collection/Managed%20Care

Medical Insurance Resources This site offers a large index of medical insurance resources on the Internet. Links are provided to major insurance companies and other related sites. Each link is accompanied by a brief explanation of the resources that can be found at that particular site.
http://www.nerdworld.com/trees/nw1654.html

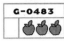

Medicare The Health Care Financing Administration (HCFA) administers Medicare, the nation's largest health insurance program, which covers nearly 40 million Americans. This site answers Medicare questions regarding eligibility, additional insurance, Medicare amounts, and enrollment. Consumer information includes answers to frequently asked questions on Medicare and help regarding health plan options. Those interested in additional information can call 1-800-MEDICARE to receive help in organizing Medicare health options.
http://www.medicare.gov

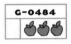

National Committee for Quality Assurance The National Committee for Quality Assurance (NCQA) is a private, nonprofit organization dedicated to assessing and reporting on the quality of managed healthcare plans. These activities are accomplished through accreditation and performance measurement of participating plans. Almost half the HMOs in the nation, covering three-quarters of all HMO enrollees, are involved in the NCQA accreditation process. A set of more than 50 standardized performance measures, called the Health Plan Employer Data and Information Set (HEDIS), is used to evaluate and compare health plans. The NCQA Web site allows the user to search the accreditation status list; results returned include the accreditation status designation and a summary report of the strengths and weaknesses of the plan. NCQA accreditation results allow users to evaluate healthcare plans in such key areas as quality of care, member satisfaction, access, and service.
http://www.ncqa.org

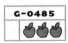

U.S. News Online: America's Top HMOs This site helps consumers to rate their managed care plan by ranking HMOs by state. Other useful tools include an HMO glossary, a medical dictionary, a best-hospitals finder, and a list of the 40 highest-rated HMOs in the United States. Fitness tips, articles related to HMOs, and an ask-the-doctor forum are all found at this site.
http://www.usnews.com/usnews/nycu/health/hetophmo.htm

13.5 ONLINE DRUG STORES

Accurate Pharmacy.com Accuate Pharmacy provides home care services to referred patients, supplying medical equipment, infusion products, oxygen and respiratory therapy products, and pharmaceuticals. The company also offers a 24-hour answering service, discharge assistance, and patient assessment. Patients may complete a Medication Profile to help pharmacists monitor their medications. http://www.accuratepharmacy.com

Caremark Therapeutic Services   Caremark provides pharmacy benefit services and therapeutic pharmaceutical services, specializing in the management of chronic or genetic disorders. The company covers over a dozen chronic conditions including cystic fibrosis, multiple sclerosis, and rheumatoid arthritis. Each condition is linked to an information sheet on the disorder, services offered by Caremark, and related links. Users may also freely access a drug database for information on drug indications and contraindications, dosages, interactions, and side effects. Caremark's online pharmacy services are available only to patients enrolled in participating healthcare organizations.
http://www.rxrequest.com

ClickPharmacy.com   ClickPharmacy seeks to enhance communication between patients, physicians, and independent pharmacies through services at their Web site. ClickPharmacy offers both personal products and prescription products. Prescriptions ordered online may be received by mail or picked up at a local independent pharmacy. Patients may also submit questions to a pharmacist online. http://www.clickpharmacy.com

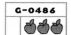

CVS Pharmacy   Consumers can order prescription and nonprescription drugs, along with other pharmacy items, on this Web page. The prescription section offers an extensive description of the purpose of the drug, side effects, precautions, drug interactions, and other prescribing information. Nonprescription drugs, vitamins, first aid, home care, and personal care items are also available. http://www.cvs.com

DrugEmporium.com   Powered by WebRx, DrugEmporium.com offers personal care products, prescription and over-the-counter medications, vitamins, and contact lenses for home delivery with online ordering. The site also features products in their "Specialty Store" such as home test kits, air purifiers for allergy sufferers, and diabetes test strips. Patients using the DrugEmporium.com pharmacy may view their prescription request history and check on the status of their prescriptions. The site also features an index of drug prices and an interaction checker.
http://www.drugemporium.com

Drugstore.com   As one of the first online drugstores, drugstore.com has developed an extensive and informative site that provides prescription and nonprescription medicine, personal care products, vitamins, and other products. There are also articles on solutions to health and beauty problems, an opportunity to ask a drugstore.com pharmacist questions, and opinions on products from customers.
http://www.drugstore.com

Eckerd.com   In addition to providing vitamins, beauty products, and health products, this online service allows visitors to place an order online and pick it up at their local store. A drug information and pricing database, home delivery, and "Ask the Pharmacist" departments are available.
http://www.eckerd.com

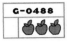

Familymeds.com   Familymeds is a prescription retailer with "brick and mortar" pharmacies as well as a Web address. This online drugstore can be used for both prescription and nonprescription needs. A personal health section features the latest news for topics such as asthma, diabetes, infant health, and women's health. A nutrition section offers fact sheets on vitamins, minerals, and herbal remedies, as well as on therapies such as acupuncture and yoga. For information and clinical recommendations on more than 200 common health concerns, the "Health Clinics" section provides fact sheets that cover causes, symptoms, natural remedies, and prescription remedies. Visitors have the option to view the entire site in Spanish. http://www.familymeds.com/familymeds

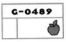

HomePharmacy.com   At Home Pharmacy visitors can perform a site-specific search for products or browse an A-to-Z listing of shopping categories. Popular products are displayed at the home page of this online drugstore, which provides a variety of healthcare products and several price specials.
http://www.homepharmacy.com

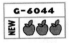

Merck-Medco   This Web site offers an online pharmacy where patients can order, refill, and renew prescriptions and purchase over-the-counter medications and personal care products. Patients can also access drug information and view their 12-month prescription history. In addition, the Merck-Medco site offers a wealth of health-related information directed to consumers. The "Health and Wellness" section contains a listing of health topics such as allergies, mental health, and skin disorders, as well as focused centers for arthritis, cardiovascular health, digestive health, respiratory health, wellness and prevention, and women's health. Each health center contains its own list of topics with articles, audio clips, practical tips, and drug information. "Health and Wellness" also offers health news, product alerts, and a variety of tools such as a health journal, allergy alerts, and a health profile calculator.
(free registration) http://www.merckmedco.com

OnlineDrugstore.com   The online pharmacy at this Web site allows patients to fill, refill, and transfer prescriptions; pose questions to a pharmacist; check drug interactions; and view an A-to-Z list of drug prices and information. The site has sections for over-the-counter medications and vitamins, as well as for pet medications. OnlineDrugstore.com also features a health center powered by MedicineNet.com, where consumers may link to articles on a variety of conditions, get first aid tips for injuries, read doctors' views on healthcare and prevention, and access health news and a medical dictionary.
http://www.onlinedrugstore.com/

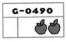

PRESCRIPTIONOnline.com   After registering, visitors can shop for prescriptions on this Web page. When requesting a medication, a close-up photo of the medication appears along with drug information and price. Pharmacists are available through an online chat room or by e-mail, phone, or fax. The site contains a list of state licenses, as well as health plans accepted.
http://prescriptiononline.com/

SafeWeb Medical SafeWeb Medical is unique in offering patients the ability to consult online with SafeWeb physicians to obtain nonessential medications, sometimes called "embarrassment" drugs. Patients participate in an anonymous, secure, online professional consultation in cases in which a physical exam may not be required. Medications available include Viagra, Xenical, Zyben, Valtrex, Retin-A, Vioxx, and Propecia.
http://www.safewebmedical.com/

Savon.com Sav-on is a retail outlet offering consumer products and prescription drugs. The site features the "Health Shopper," which provides premade shopping lists for over 40 health conditions including cataracts, fibromyalgia, hypoglycemia, and ulcerative colitis. The online pharmacy fills prescriptions and hosts an "Ask the Pharmacist" forum, as well as providing drug pricing and interactions links. In addition, a "Health" section offers tools, assessments, and health information covering dozens of health topics in more than 15 categories such as emotional health, men's health, skin health, and women's health.
(free registration) http://www.sav-ondrugs.com/default.asp

Tel-Drug Rx Tel-Drug Rx is a mail order pharmacy program focusing on medications prescribed for periods of 30 days or longer in the treatment of chronic conditions. Pharmacy services are available only to patients participating in the CIGNA HealthCare managed pharmacy program.
http://www.cigna.com/consumer/services/pharmacy/tel_drug.html

Verified Internet Pharmacy Practice Sites Program The Verified Internet Pharmacy Practice Sites (VIPPS) Program of the National Association of Boards of Pharmacy was developed in 1999 out of public concern for the safety of pharmacy practices on the Internet. This site contains a menu with links providing information on the criteria for VIPPS certification; a VIPPS list (which includes the pharmacy name and Web site address); VIPPS definitions; and links to Web sites of state boards of pharmacy, state medical boards, federal agencies, and professional organizations.
http://www.nabp.net/vipps/intro.asp

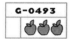

VitaRx.com Physicians can use the VitaRx.com site to order prescriptions or injectable drugs for their patients. Patients can refill their prescription online or place orders for over-the-counter medications. A disease support center provides patients with fact sheets on diseases such as Crohn's disease and rheumatoid arthritis, as well as directions on self-injection. There are also "Ask a Pharmacist" and "Ask a Nurse" services where answers are posted online.
http://vitarx.com/

Walgreens Walgreens allows patients to fill and refill prescriptions online, as well as offering an automatic refill service. Patients can view and print prescription records and histories and keep a health history online. The site also features immunization recommendations, customized e-mail reminders, and an online pharmacist who fields consumer questions. Additionally, the Walgreens

Specialty Pharmacy provides disease-specific care for patients with HIV/AIDS, multiple sclerosis, cystic fibrosis, growth hormone deficiency, and hepatitis. (free registration) http://www.walgreens.com/

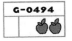

WebRx This Web site offers customers a wide variety of products, including over-the-counter medicine, personal care items, vitamins, electronics, and prescription medicine. New patients must register by filling out an online form and provide a way to contact their doctors for prescription information. Prescriptions are processed by a registered pharmacist. News and information on more than 90 health topics are included at this resource.
http://www.webrx.com

13.6 PATIENT EDUCATION

GENERAL RESOURCES

Patient information regarding various medical conditions and health issues can be obtained at any of the general medical search engines that are included. Below are listings of health Web sites accessible through the well-known search engines, as well as other sites that cover wide-ranging topics of interest to patients.

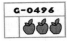

American Academy of Family Physicians (AAFP): Health Information for the Whole Family Directed toward consumers, this site provides a collection of fact sheets on a variety of conditions that can be searched by keyword, population group, or region of the body. The fact sheets can also be browsed alphabetically under the "Health Information Handouts" section. Advice on topics such as lowering cholesterol, preventing flus and colds, and pain relief for lower back pain can be found under the family health facts section. Self-care flowcharts for health concerns covering symptoms, diagnosis, self-care, and when to see a doctor are also provided. In addition, there are databases for conventional drug information, herbal and alternative drugs, and drug interactions that explain proper use, side effects, and reactions. A national directory of family doctors is found, and the site can be translated into Spanish.
http://familydoctor.org

Columbia University College of Physicians and Surgeons: Complete Home Medical Guide Patients will find this site to be a comprehensive resource for healthcare information. Topics include receiving proper medical care, the correct use of medications, first aid and safety, preventative medicine, and good nutrition. Chapters containing more specific information on health concerns for men, women, and children; disorders; infectious diseases; mental and emotional health; and substance abuse are also available.
http://cpmcnet.columbia.edu/texts/guide

DiscoveryHealth.com From the producers of the Discovery Channel, this site offers consumer health resources for all groups. News items, feature articles

and reports, links to health reference materials, chat forums, a forum for asking health questions, and descriptions of recent research advances are all found at this site. Visitors can access information specific to men, women, senior citizens, children, mental health, and health in the workplace. Nutrition, fitness, and weight management tools are also available at this site.
http://health.discovery.com/

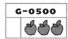

Federal Health Agencies   Consumers will find a list of links to federal health agencies on this Web site, part of a larger Patient Rights.com Web page. Each link is preceded by a short explanation of what the federal agency does. On the same page, there are links to elected officials, state health organizations, state insurance commissions, and state medical boards. Visitors can also research medical conditions through a list of links on conditions.
http://www.patientrights.com/links/links4.htm

HealthAnswers   This site provides consumers with informational resources on a wide range of health topics including senior health, pregnancy, cancer, and STDs in the form of articles, news, and streaming videos. The site also hosts a library with encyclopedia articles that can be searched or browsed on topics such as diseases and conditions, drugs, laboratory tests, nutrition, surgeries and procedures, and symptoms.
http://www.healthanswers.com

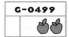

HealthTalk Interactive   Consumers will find articles, interviews, audio clips, and live interactive events with health experts on a variety of health topics on this site. Information on specific diseases can be accessed through the section titled "Disease Education Networks." Diseases covered include asthma, breast cancer, diabetes, lymphoma, menopause, multiple sclerosis, and rheumatoid arthritis. http://www.healthtalk.com/

InteliHealth   This comprehensive site offers consumers tips on healthy living, information and other resources on specific conditions, health news by topic, special reports, an online newsletter, pharmaceutical drug information, and an online store offering health items for the home. Other features include interactive diaries for specific health conditions, free e-mails on nearly 20 health topics, health assessments, and a medical dictionary. Conditions and health topics discussed at the site include allergy, arthritis, asthma, diabetes, mental health, pregnancy, nutrition, and weight management. Links are available to other sites offering consumer health resources. The site obtains its information from various sources, including the Harvard Medical School and the University of Pennsylvania School of Dental Medicine.
(free registration) http://www.intelihealth.com

MayoClinic.com   Visitors to this informative site will find answers to patient questions, news and articles on featured topics, registration details for e-mail alerts of site updates, and site search engines for health information and prescription drug information. Specific information centers are devoted to allergy and asthma, Alzheimer's disease, cancer, children's health, digestive health, and

heart health; the site also features an A-to-Z index of diseases and conditions. A library of answers to health questions, a glossary of medical terms, and a forum for asking specific questions are also available at the site.
http://www.mayohealth.org/home

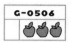

MDAdvice.com   Information on a broad array of health topics is featured on this Web page, targeted for consumers. The "Health Center" section offers a health library with patient fact sheets covering symptoms, conditions, medical tests, and surgeries; a drug information database; an ask-the-expert forum; and in-depth articles under the "Informative Material" link. A section titled "Condition Centers" features a center on cancer and one on heart disease. Each center offers fact sheets, support groups, clinical trial information, and expert advice. There are also community message boards and live chats.
http://www.mdadvice.com

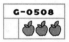

Med Help International   Visitors will find resources on a broad array of health topics on this consumer-oriented site. A comprehensive consumer health information library can be searched by keyword or browsed alphabetically and covers topics such as asthma, Hodgkin's disease, and diabetes. Each topic contains articles, a medical glossary, related questions and answers from an ask-the-expert forum, support groups, treatment options, and clinical trials. The site also features a patient-to-patient network designed to serve as an online support group, along with medical and health news updates.
http://www.medhelp.org

Medical Library   Of interest to consumers and professionals, the Medem site features a medical library, with information drawn from medical societies such as the American Academy of Pediatrics and the American Medical Association. The library is separated into four categories: life stages, diseases and conditions, therapies and health strategies, and health and society. Information in the library is further categorized into subtopics with links to articles, news, journals, and professional resources. In addition to the library, under the "Products and Services" section, physicians can develop their own Web site with secure e-mail messaging to patients. The site also offers a physician finder.
http://www.medem.com/MedLB/medlib_entry.cfm/

MedicineNet.com   An efficient and thorough source of information on hundreds of diseases and medical conditions, MedicineNet enables the user to click on subjects in an alphabetical list of diseases and conditions. The site's medical content is produced by board-certified physicians and allied health professionals. Other topics include procedures and tests, a pharmacy section, a medical dictionary, first aid information, and a list of poison control centers.
http://www.medicinenet.com

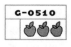

MEDLINEplus   A service of the National Library of Medicine, this consumer health site offers a wide variety of information categorized as health topics, drug information, dictionaries, directories, organizations, and publications. Under "Health Topics," there are hundreds of diseases and disorders, such as asthma, AIDS, epilepsy, and sickle cell anemia. Each condition contains links for more information such as overviews, symptoms, treatment, diagnostic tests, and research. The "Drug Information" section contains a guide to more than 9,000 prescription and over-the-counter medications. Also notable is a link to MED-LINE, the National Library of Medicine's bibliographic database of more than 11 million articles.

http://www.medlineplus.gov

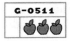

NetWellness NetWellness is a Web-based health information service with a large group of medical and health experts available to answer consumer questions online. Developed by the University of Cincinnati Medical Center, the Ohio State University, and Case Western Reserve University, the site has nearly 200 health faculty available to answer questions on over 40 topics. Responses are usually provided within two to three days. Visitors can also browse and search archives of articles listed under "Health Topics" or use the site's library which provides encyclopedias, patient education materials, handbooks, and magazines. (some features fee-based) http://www.netwellness.org

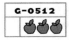

New York Online Access to Health (NOAH): Health Topics and Resources This site is offered as a public resource by many providers, including hospitals, institutes, foundations, research centers, and city and state agencies. Users can access information concerning over 40 health topics including diseases, mental health, and nutrition, with links provided to patient resources. A health information database containing abstracts and articles from selected health-related periodicals is only available to users accessing the site from specific institutions, including the New York Public Library branches.

http://www.noah-health.org/english/qksearch.html

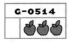

Quackwatch Quackwatch is a nonprofit corporation combating "health-related frauds, myths, fads, and fallacies." The group investigates questionable health claims, answers consumer inquiries, distributes publications, reports illegal marketing, generates consumer-protection lawsuits, works to improve the quality of health information on the Internet, and attacks misleading Internet advertising. Operation costs are generated solely from the sales of publications and individual donations. Sister sites, Chirobase and MLM Watch, offer a consumer's guide to chiropractors and a skeptical guide to multilevel marketing. Information for cancer patients includes alerts of questionable alternative health treatments, a discussion of how questionable practices may harm cancer patients, and other related discussions. Visitors to the site can purchase publications, read general information about questionable medical practices, and view details about specific questionable products and services. Links to government agencies and other sites providing information about health fraud are available at this site, which can be translated into several foreign languages.

http://www.quackwatch.com

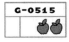

Virtual Hospital: Common Problems in Adults The Virtual Hospital Web page offers consumers and professionals resources for information on

common medical problems in adults. Provided by the University of Iowa, the site contains a table of links, with separate professional and patient sections. It covers more than 45 problems such as abdominal pain, arthritis, cancer, diabetes, pregnancy, and stroke. A link is provided to a similar site for pediatrics.
http://www.vh.org/CommonProblems/CommonProblems.html#Art

ADOLESCENT HEALTH

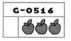

Adolescent Health Resources for Professionals   Provided by the Leadership Institute on Adolescent Health, this Web site offers a listing of more than 35 sites that provide adolescent health resources for professionals. The listing includes subject guides about adolescents, general subject guides, lists of resources from associations, adolescent health programs, and special topics such as accidents, drug abuse, and teen pregnancy. There are also professional organizations, philanthropic organizations, databases, and statistics, as well as pages from the federal government.
http://corc.oclc.org/WebZ/XPathfinderQuery?sessionid=0:term=196:xid=UMM

Centers for Disease Control and Prevention (CDC): Adolescent and School Health   Hosted by the CDC, this site focuses on adolescent and school health. Healthcare professionals and consumers may find the resources on the site of interest. A report on adolescent health is featured that covers pregnancy, sexually transmitted diseases, and risk behaviors among adolescents. The report offers statistics, state profiles, and trend information. The site also has information on grant funding, along with publications. School health initiatives are described, as well as ongoing research.
http://www.cdc.gov/nccdphp/dash/ahson/ahson.htm

Medscout: Adolescent Health   Dedicated to adolescent health, this site offers a comprehensive listing of Internet resources. There are more than 50 sites listed drawn from both domestic and international sources. Links are provided to many organizations dealing with adolescent health-related issues.
http://www.medscout.com/health/adolescent/

Society for Adolescent Medicine   Directed to professionals, the home page of the Society for Adolescent Medicine (SAM) offers information on special interest groups for adolescent healthcare professionals, the SAM newsletter, and a list of fellowships in adolescent medicine. Several position papers can be found in the "Activities" section. Of interest to consumers and professionals, there is a list of more than 50 related links covering eating disorders, gay and lesbian teens, adolescent health, sexuality, social development, substance abuse, and violence.
http://www3.uchc.edu/~sam/samfinal/introduction-low.html

INFANT AND CHILDREN'S HEALTH

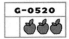

Centers for Disease Control and Prevention (CDC): Infants and Children Parents will find more than 65 fact sheets on infants' and children's health on this Web page, part of a larger CDC site. The fact sheets cover a variety of topics such as air bags, breastfeeding, child abuse, dog bites, fifth disease, immunizations, and swimming pool safety. Some Spanish-language articles are available. http://www.cdc.gov/health/nfantsmenu.htm

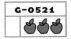

KidsGrowth.com This site offers a wealth of resources on parenting and child development. A section on parenting offers hundreds of articles and answers from experts on a variety of topics, including discipline, parent skills, and school health. Articles and answers can be found in a child development section, categorized by age group. A section on growth milestones offers parental guidance on development, with related articles arranged chronologically from the prenatal visit to the 10-year-old child. Also available are a free weekly e-mail newsletter, growth tables, an interactive car seat selector, and parent guides for vomiting, fever, coughing, and diarrhea. In addition, the site posts book reviews, poison control resources, and information on product recalls. http://www.kidsgrowth.com/index2.cfm

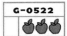

KidsHealth.org This site, created by the Nemours Foundation Center for Children's Health Media, provides expert health information about children from the prenatal period through adolescence. Specific sections target children, teens, and parents, with age-appropriate information and language. Within each section are categories containing a large number of links to articles on specific topics. Categories in the "Parents" section include emotions and behavior, positive parenting, and the healthcare system. http://kidshealth.org

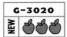

Medem Medical Library: Children's Health Provided by the American Academy of Pediatrics, information at this page includes coverage of more than 35 child-related health topics. The directory of subjects can be browsed by category and includes topics ranging from asthma to youth violence. Medical news and a site-specific search engine are provided. http://www.medem.com/MedLB/bufferpage_aap.cfm

Medscout: Children's Health A comprehensive listing of more than 100 links related to children's health are provided on this Web page, courtesy of Medscout. The sites are appropriate for both consumers and professionals and cover a broad range of topics relating to infants and children. http://www.medscout.com/health/childrens/

Virtual Children's Hospital: Common Problems in Pediatrics Parents and professionals will find information on common health problems in children on this Web page, courtesy of the Virtual Children's Hospital. More than 45 health topics are covered such as asthma, behavior problems, diabetes, and sleep

problems. Resources for consumers and health providers are in different sections of the table of resources.
http://www.vh.org/VCH/CommonProblems/CommonProblems.html#An

MEN'S HEALTH

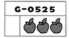

MEDLINEplus Health Information: Men's Health Topics Information on a variety of men's health topics is provided on this Web page, maintained by the National Library of Medicine. Topics include circumcision, STDs, infertility, and prostate diseases. Each topic has links for additional information categorized as an overview, clinical trials, diagnosis/symptoms, prevention, specific aspects, and related organizations.
http://www.nlm.nih.gov/medlineplus/menshealth.html

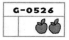

Men's Health Network Dedicated to education and advocacy on behalf of men's health, the Men's Health Network produces this Web page to provide information on their activities including education, advocacy, and health screening efforts. A library section contains links such as data and statistics on men's high-risk-job injuries, along with resources on prostate disease issues, stroke, diabetes, STDs, and parenting. The "Men's Links" section offers a long list of links covering health resources, workplace safety, domestic violence, and suicide, as well as journals and organizations.
http://www.menshealthnetwork.org/

New York Online Access to Health (NOAH): Men's Health Directed at consumers, more than 35 links related to men's health are offered on this site, maintained by the New York Online Access to Health project. The links cover basic information, such as anatomy and primary care for men; specific issues, such as fertility, impotence, prostate diseases, and testicular diseases; and information resources, including the Mayo Clinic.
http://www.noah-health.org/english/wellness/healthyliving/menshealth.html

MINORITY HEALTH

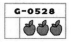

Department of Health and Human Services: Office of Minority Health Located within the U.S. Department of Health and Human Services, the Office of Minority Health focuses on public health issues affecting minorities. Their Web page offers information on conferences, a list of online publications from federal and nonfederal sources, data and statistics, and related links. There is also a section on federal clearinghouses that can be searched by topic. The "What's New" section covers legislation and funding announcements. Visitors can also learn more about the office's initiatives, programs, and work on health disparities. A resource center offers publications, funding information, and databases of organizations, programs, and documents related to minority health. http://www.omhrc.gov/

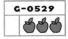

Health Information for Minority Women The National Women's Health Information Center has provided this Web site dedicated to health information for minority women. In addition to an overview of minority health, there are sections of the site dedicated to health information specific to African Americans, Asian/Pacific Islanders, American Indian/Alaskan Natives, and Hispanic/Latinas. Each minority section contains fact sheets on a variety of health topics such as asthma, cancer, and diabetes. Each fact sheet also offers links to publications and related organizations. In addition, there is a link for a list of federal minority offices. A fact sheet on leading causes of death among minority women, as well as a link to the Office on Women's Health site that describes that office's activities to promote minority health, is provided.
http://www.4woman.gov/minority/index.cfm

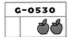

HealthWeb: Minority Health Examining minority health, this Web page offers a directory with hundreds of sites of interest to both professionals and the public. The sites are accessed by clicking on topics in the table of contents, which include general resources, education and training opportunities, African Americans, Asian Americans, Hispanic Americans, Native Americans, and research in minority health.
http://healthweb.org/browse.cfm?subjectid=53

SENIOR HEALTH

American Association for Retired Persons (AARP) The feature finder at this site connects visitors to a variety of services of the American Association for Retired Persons (AARP), including guides to health and wellness, life transitions, and legislative issues of interest to older Americans. The Web edition of the *AARP Bulletin* offers stories for those entering their middle and later years, and a department on making educated healthcare choices is provided. An online discussion center, links to local AARP chapters, and the current online edition of *Modern Maturity* are also found.
http://www.aarp.org/

Hardin MD: Geriatrics and Senior Health The Hardin Meta Directory on this site features geriatrics and senior health. Categorized as large and medium lists, there are links to Web pages that contain lists of relevant Internet resources. The lists are drawn from both domestic and international sources and cover hundreds of sites. There are also links to additional directories of lists on Alzheimer's and Parkinson's disease.
http://www.lib.uiowa.edu/hardin/md/ger.html

National Institute on Aging (NIA) The NIA, a division of the National Institutes of Health, leads the research effort to extend healthy lives and better understand the processes associated with aging. News and events about the division, a publications and resource list, and details of their research programs can be located from the site's links. The Alzheimer's Disease Education and Referral

(ADEAR), a service of the NIA, offers additional information on Alzheimer's disease and related conditions. The site also provides press releases, funding opportunities, and conference information.
http://www.nih.gov/nia

WOMEN'S HEALTH

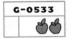

African American Women's Health   Visitors will find a variety of resources dedicated to the health of African American women. There is an A-to-Z listing of health topics such as alcohol addiction, diabetes, and fibroids; each topic has a fact sheet with references and resource links. There are also fact sheets in sections categorized as nutrition and fitness, spiritual and mental health, and finances. In addition, there are a discussion forum and a business directory. Physicians can add their names to a physician locator service.
http://www.blackwomenshealth.com/

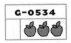

allHealth.com   Primarily directed toward female consumers, a variety of health resources are found at this iVillage Web page. The site offers "Health Tools," where visitors can take quizzes to test their knowledge of breast cancer or learn the difference between allergies and colds. The site also offers educational modules on managing conditions such as asthma, diabetes, and hypertension. Access to MEDLINE and related health databases is provided, as are articles, expert advice, and message boards on specific health concerns. Health topics can be browsed under an A-to-Z directory of conditions or researched in an illustrated medical encyclopedia.   http://www.allhealth.com

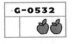

Department of Health and Human Services: National Women's Health Information Center   Focused on women's health, the National Women's Health Information Center offers resources for professionals and the public. The site can be searched by health topic or by keyword. Information on programs such as breastfeeding, violence against women, and healthy pregnancy is provided; each has consumer materials, publications, and a list of related links. A health professionals section offers links to medical journals, clinical trials, publications, and patient fact sheets. Also available are a media section with facts and statistics on women's health, a directory of residential and fellowship programs, and information on funding opportunities. Some areas of the site can also be viewed in Spanish.   http://www.4woman.org/index.htm

iVillageHealth   Primarily for consumers, the iVillageHealth site offers information on a variety of women's health topics. Visitors can access articles and fact sheets related to topics such as allergies, breast cancer, heart disease, pregnancy, and sexual dysfunction. A "tool kit" on the home page offers interactive tools such as quizzes, a health calculator, and access to MEDLINE. An ask-the-expert section is available on a variety of health topics. Chats, message boards, and support groups are also available.
http://www.ivillagehealth.com/

Don't type in long URLs – add the site number to the eMedguides URL: www.eMedguides.com/**G-1234**.

Medscape: Women's Health A variety of clinical information related to women's health is featured on this Web page, primarily for professionals. Resources on this site include the latest news, treatment updates, clinical management, and practice guidelines. There is also CME information with some online CME courses. A resource center provides condition-specific information. In addition, there are journals, related links, and an "Exam Room" with interactive case studies. Consumers can find disease information under a patient resources section. (free registration)
http://www.medscape.com/Home/Topics/WomensHealth/WomensHealth.html

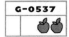

University of Maryland: Women's Health Web Sites Resources on women's health are featured on this site, maintained by the University of Maryland. The site contains a listing of links to more than 70 women's health Web pages. A short description of each site is provided.
http://research.umbc.edu/~korenman/wmst/links_hlth.html

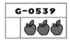

Women's Health A comprehensive consumer-oriented directory of links related to women's health is offered on this Web site. The site offers an A-to-Z listing of health topics, along with commonly referenced topics such as birth control, dieting, menopause, and STDs. Each section lists Internet resources with a description of site content. Also available are a physician locator, a section on surgical procedures, and a calculator/tools section with interactive quizzes on risk factors for disease.
http://womenshealth.about.com/health/womenshealth/library/blaward.htm

13.7 SUPPORT GROUPS

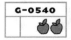

Genetic Alliance: Member Directory The Genetic Alliance, formerly the Alliance of Genetic Support Groups, offers their membership directory of support groups on this site. The directory can be searched by genetic condition, organization name, or services offered. Alternatively, one can browse the entire directory. A resources section contains links to disease information and genetic issues. http://www.geneticalliance.org/diseaseinfo/search.html

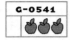

New York Online Access to Health (NOAH): Support Groups This directory of Web resources includes links to other directories, general health sites, toll-free telephone numbers, face-to-face support groups, support organizations, newsgroups, mailing lists, chat forums, and other online support resources. Visitors can browse listings by type of resource or by specific medical conditions. http://www.noah-health.org/english/support.html

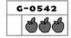

SupportPath.com SupportPath.com allows people with health, personal, and relationship issues to share their experiences through bulletin boards and online chats and also provides links to support-related information on the Internet. The A-to-Z listing offers hundreds of connections to areas such as disease-related support, bereavement assistance, marriage and family issue groups,

and women's/men's issues. The "Message Board Tracker" lists the most recent messages and provides a complete cross-reference of topics.
http://www.supportpath.com

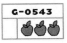

G-0543

University of Kansas Medical Center: Genetic and Rare Conditions

Organized by the Medical Genetics Department of the University of Kansas Medical Center, this site offers a comprehensive listing of links on genetics and rare conditions. The home page features an A-to-Z listing of rare diseases and conditions. Hyperlinks at the top of the site lead to hundreds of resources categorized as national and international organizations, specific conditions, genetic counselors, children and teens, and advocacy. Information on support groups can be found in the national and international organizations section.
http://www.kumc.edu/gec/support/groups.html

Web Site and Topical Index

C

O

PRAVACHOL®
(pravastatin sodium) Tablets

Rx only

DESCRIPTION

PRAVACHOL® (pravastatin sodium) is one of a new class of lipid-lowering compounds, the HMG-CoA reductase inhibitors, which reduce cholesterol biosynthesis. These agents are competitive inhibitors of 3-hydroxy-3-methylglutaryl-coenzyme A (HMG-CoA) reductase, the enzyme catalyzing the early rate-limiting step in cholesterol biosynthesis, conversion of HMG-CoA to mevalonate.

Pravastatin sodium is designated chemically as 1-Naphthalene-heptanoic acid, 1,2,6,7,8,8a-hexahydro-β,δ,6-trihydroxy-2-methyl-8-(2-methyl-1-oxo-butoxy)-, monosodium salt, [1S-[1α(βS*,δS*),2α,6α, 8β(R*),8aα]]-. Structural formula:

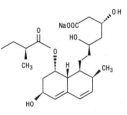

$$C_{23} H_{35} NaO_7 \quad MW\ 446.52$$

Pravastatin sodium is an odorless, white to off-white, fine or crystalline powder. It is a relatively polar hydrophilic compound with a partition coefficient (octanol/water) of 0.59 at a pH of 7.0. It is soluble in methanol and water (>300 mg/mL), slightly soluble in isopropanol, and practically insoluble in acetone, acetonitrile, chloroform, and ether.

PRAVACHOL is available for oral administration as 10 mg, 20 mg and 40 mg tablets. Inactive ingredients include: croscarmellose sodium, lactose, magnesium oxide, magnesium stearate, microcrystalline cellulose, and povidone. The 10 mg tablet also contains Red Ferric Oxide, the 20 mg tablet also contains Yellow Ferric Oxide, and the 40 mg tablet also contains Green Lake Blend (mixture of D&C Yellow No. 10-Aluminum Lake and FD&C Blue No. 1-Aluminum Lake).

CLINICAL PHARMACOLOGY

Cholesterol and triglycerides in the bloodstream circulate as part of lipoprotein complexes. These complexes can be separated by density ultracentrifugation into high (HDL), intermediate (IDL), low (LDL), and very low (VLDL) density lipoprotein fractions. Triglycerides (TG) and cholesterol synthesized in the liver are incorporated into very low density lipoproteins (VLDLs) and released into the plasma for delivery to peripheral tissues. In a series of subsequent steps, VLDLs are transformed into intermediate density lipoproteins (IDLs), and cholesterol-rich low density lipoproteins (LDLs). High density lipoproteins (HDLs), containing apolipoprotein A, are hypothesized to participate in the reverse transport of cholesterol from tissues back to the liver.

PRAVACHOL produces its lipid-lowering effect in two ways. First, as a consequence of its reversible inhibition of HMG-CoA reductase activity, it effects modest reductions in intracellular pools of cholesterol. This results in an increase in the number of LDL-receptors on cell surfaces and enhanced receptor-mediated catabolism and clearance of circulating LDL. Second, pravastatin inhibits LDL production by inhibiting hepatic synthesis of VLDL, the LDL precursor.

Clinical and pathologic studies have shown that elevated levels of total cholesterol (Total-C), low density lipoprotein cholesterol (LDL-C), and apolipoprotein B (Apo B - a membrane transport complex for LDL) promote human atherosclerosis. Similarly, decreased levels of HDL-cholesterol (HDL-C) and its transport complex, apolipoprotein A, are associated with the development of atherosclerosis. Epidemiologic investigations have established that cardiovascular morbidity and mortality vary directly with the level of Total-C and LDL-C and inversely with the level of HDL-C. Like LDL, cholesterol-enriched triglyceride-rich lipoproteins, including VLDL, IDL, and remnants, can also promote atherosclerosis. Elevated plasma TG are frequently found in a triad with low HDL-C levels and small LDL particles, as well as in association with non-lipid metabolic risk factors for coronary heart disease. As such, total plasma TG has not consistently been shown to be an independent risk factor for CHD. Furthermore, the independent effect of raising HDL or lowering TG on the risk of coronary and cardiovascular morbidity and mortality has not been determined. In both normal volunteers and patients with hypercholesterolemia, treatment with PRAVACHOL reduced Total-C, LDL-C, and apolipoprotein B. PRAVACHOL also reduced VLDL-C and TG and produced increases in HDL-C and apolipoprotein A. The effects of pravastatin on Lp (a), fibrinogen, and certain other independent biochemical risk markers for coronary heart disease are unknown. Although pravastatin is relatively more hydrophilic than other HMG-CoA reductase inhibitors, the effect of relative hydrophilicity, if any, on either efficacy or safety has not been established.

In one primary (West of Scotland Coronary Prevention Study – WOS)[1] and two secondary (Long-term Intervention with Pravastatin in Ischemic Disease – LIPID[2] and the Cholesterol and Recurrent Events – CARE[3]) prevention studies, PRAVACHOL has been shown to reduce cardiovascular morbidity and mortality across a wide range of cholesterol levels (see **Clinical Studies**).

Pharmacokinetics/Metabolism

PRAVACHOL (pravastatin sodium) is administered orally in the active form. In clinical pharmacology studies in man, pravastatin is rapidly absorbed, with peak plasma levels of parent compound attained 1 to 1.5 hours following ingestion. Based on urinary recovery of radiolabeled drug, the average oral absorption of pravastatin is 34% and absolute bioavailability is 17%. While the presence of food in the gastrointestinal tract reduces systemic bioavailability, the lipid-lowering effects of the drug are similar whether taken with, or 1 hour prior, to meals.

Pravastatin undergoes extensive first-pass extraction in the liver (extraction ratio 0.66), which is its primary site of action, and the primary site of cholesterol synthesis and of LDL-C clearance. In vitro studies demonstrated that pravastatin is transported into hepatocytes with substantially less uptake into other cells. In view of pravastatin's apparently extensive first-pass hepatic metabolism, plasma levels may not necessarily correlate perfectly with lipid-lowering efficacy. Pravastatin plasma concentrations [including: area under the concentration-time curve (AUC), peak (C_{max}), and steady-state minimum (C_{min})] are directly proportional to administered dose. Systemic bioavailability of pravastatin administered following a bedtime dose was decreased 60% compared to that following an AM dose. Despite this decrease in systemic bioavailability, the efficacy of pravastatin administered once daily in the evening, although not statistically significant, was marginally more effective than that after a morning dose. This finding of lower systemic bioavailability suggests greater hepatic extraction of the drug following the evening dose. Steady-state AUCs, C_{max} and C_{min} plasma concentrations showed no evidence of pravastatin accumulation following once or twice daily administration of PRAVACHOL (pravastatin sodium) tablets. Approximately 50% of the circulating drug is bound to plasma proteins. Following single dose administration of ^{14}C- pravastatin, the elimination half-life (t½) for total radioactivity (pravastatin plus metabolites) in humans is 77 hours.

Pravastatin, like other HMG-CoA reductase inhibitors, has variable bioavailability. The coefficient of variation, based on between-subject variability, was 50% to 60% for AUC.

Approximately 20% of a radiolabeled oral dose is excreted in urine and 70% in the feces. After intravenous administration of radiolabeled pravastatin to normal volunteers, approximately 47% of total body clearance was via renal excretion and 53% by non-renal routes (i.e., biliary excretion and biotransformation). Since there are dual routes of elimination, the potential exists both for compensatory excretion by the alternate route as well as for accumulation of drug and/or metabolites in patients with renal or hepatic insufficiency.

In a study comparing the kinetics of pravastatin in patients with biopsy confirmed cirrhosis (N=7) and normal subjects (N=7), the mean AUC varied 18-fold in cirrhotic patients and 5-fold in healthy subjects. Similarly, the peak pravastatin values varied 47-fold for cirrhotic patients compared to 6-fold for healthy subjects.

Biotransformation pathways elucidated for pravastatin include: (a) isomerization to 6-epi pravastatin and the 3α-hydroxyisomer of pravastatin (SQ 31,906), (b) enzymatic ring hydroxylation to SQ 31,945, (c) ω-1 oxidation of the ester side chain, (d) β-oxidation of the carboxy side chain, (e) ring oxidation followed by aromatization, (f) oxidation of a hydroxyl group to a keto group, and (g) conjugation. The major degradation product is the 3α-hydroxy isomeric metabolite, which has one-tenth to one-fortieth the HMG-CoA reductase inhibitory activity of the parent compound.

In a single oral dose study using pravastatin 20 mg, the mean AUC for pravastatin was approximately 27% greater and the mean cumulative urinary excretion (CUE) approximately 19% lower in elderly men (65 to 75 years old) compared with younger men (19 to 31 years old). In a similar study conducted in women, the mean AUC for pravastatin was approximately 46% higher and the mean CUE approximately 18% lower in elderly women (65 to 78 years old) compared with younger women (18 to 38 years old). In both studies, C_{max}, T_{max} and t½ values were similar in older and younger subjects.

Clinical Studies

Prevention of Coronary Heart Disease

In the Pravastatin Primary Prevention Study (West of Scotland Coronary Prevention Study – WOS),[1] the effect of PRAVACHOL (pravastatin sodium) on fatal and nonfatal coronary heart disease (CHD) was assessed in 6595 men 45–64 years of age, without a previous myocardial infarction (MI), and with LDL-C levels between 156–254 mg/dL (4–6.7 mmol/L). In this randomized, double-blind, placebo-controlled study, patients were treated with standard care, including dietary advice, and either PRAVACHOL 40 mg daily (N=3302) or placebo (N=3293) and followed for a median duration of 4.8 years. Median (25th, 75th percentile) percent changes from baseline after 6 months of pravastatin treatment in Total C, LDL-C, TG, and HDL were -20.3 (-26.9, -11.7), -27.7 (-36.0, -16.9), -9.1 (-27.6, 12.5), and 6.7 (-2.1, 15.6), respectively.

PRAVACHOL significantly reduced the rate of first coronary events (either coronary heart disease (CHD) death or nonfatal MI) by 31% [248 events in the placebo group (CHD death=44, nonfatal MI=204) vs 174 events in the PRAVACHOL group (CHD death=31, nonfatal MI=143), p=0.0001 (see figure below)]. The risk reduction with PRAVACHOL was similar and significant throughout the entire range of baseline LDL cholesterol levels. This reduction was also similar and significant across the age range studied with a 40% risk reduction for patients younger than 55 years and a 27% risk reduction for patients 55 years and older. The Pravastatin Primary Prevention Study included only men and therefore it is not clear to what extent these data can be extrapolated to a similar population of female patients.

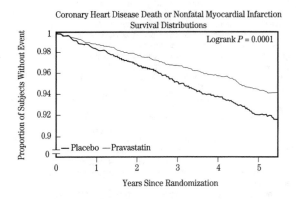

Coronary Heart Disease Death or Nonfatal Myocardial Infarction Survival Distributions

PRAVACHOL also significantly decreased the risk for undergoing myocardial revascularization procedures (coronary artery bypass graft [CABG] surgery or percutaneous transluminal coronary angioplasty [PTCA]) by 37% (80 vs 51 patients, p=0.009) and coronary angiography by 31% (128 vs 90, p=0.007). Cardiovascular deaths were decreased by 32% (73 vs 50, p=0.03) and there was no increase in death from non-cardiovascular causes.

Secondary Prevention of Cardiovascular Events

In the Long-term Intervention with Pravastatin in Ischemic Disease (LIPID)[2] study, the effect of PRAVACHOL, 40 mg daily, was assessed in 9014 patients (7498 men; 1516 women; 3514 elderly patients [age ≥65 years]; 782 diabetic patients) who had experienced either an MI (5754 patients) or had been hospitalized for unstable angina pectoris (3260 patients) in the preceding 3-36 months. In this multicenter, double-blind, placebo-controlled study participated for an average of 5.6 years (median of 5.9 years) and at randomization had total cholesterol between 114 and 563 mg/dL (mean 219 mg/dL), LDL-C between 46 and 274 mg/dL (mean 150 mg/dL), triglycerides between 35 and 2710 mg/dL (mean 160 mg/dL), and HDL-C between 1 and 103 mg/dL (mean 37 mg/dL). At baseline, 82% of patients were receiving aspirin and 76% were receiving antihypertensive medication. Treatment with PRAVACHOL significantly reduced the risk for total mortality by reducing coronary death (see Table 1). The risk reduction due to treatment with PRAVACHOL on CHD mortality was consistent regardless of age. PRAVACHOL significantly reduced the risk for total mortality (by reducing CHD death) and CHD events (CHD mortality or nonfatal MI) in patients who qualified with a history of either MI or hospitalization for unstable angina pectoris.

Table 1 LIPID – Primary and Secondary Endpoints

Event	Number (%) of Subjects		Risk Reduction	*P*-value
	Pravastatin (N = 4512)	Placebo (N = 4502)		
Primary Endpoint				
CHD mortality	287 (6.4)	373 (8.3)	24%	0.0004
Secondary Endpoints				
Total mortality	498 (11.0)	633 (14.1)	23%	<0.0001
CHD mortality or non-fatal MI	557 (12.3)	715 (15.9)	24%	<0.0001
Myocardial revascularization procedures (CABG or PTCA)	584 (12.9)	706 (15.7)	20%	<0.0001
Stroke				
All-cause	169 (3.7)	204 (4.5)	19%	0.0477
Non-hemorrhagic	154 (3.4)	196 (4.4)	23%	0.0154
Cardiovascular mortality	331 (7.3)	433 (9.6)	25%	<0.0001

In the Cholesterol and Recurrent Events (CARE)[3] study the effect of PRAVACHOL, 40 mg daily, on coronary heart disease death and nonfatal MI was assessed in 4159 patients (3583 men and 576 women) who had experienced a myocardial infarction in the preceding 3–20 months and who had normal (below the 75th percentile of the general population) plasma total cholesterol levels. Patients in this double-blind, placebo controlled study participated for an average of 4.9 years and had a mean baseline total cholesterol of 209 mg/dL. LDL cholesterol levels in this patient population ranged from 101 mg/dL – 180 mg/dL (mean = 139 mg/dL). At baseline, 84% of patients were receiving aspirin and 82% were taking antihypertensive medications. Median (25th, 75th percentile) percent changes from baseline after 6 months of pravastatin treatment in Total C, LDL-C, TG, and HDL were -22.0 (-28.4, -14.9), -32.4 (-39.9, -23.7), -11.0 (-26.5, 8.6), and 5.1 (-2.9, 12.7), respectively. Treatment with PRAVACHOL significantly reduced the rate of first recurrent coronary events (either CHD death or nonfatal MI), the risk of undergoing revascularization procedures (PTCA, CABG), and the risk for stroke or transient ischemic attack (TIA) (see Table 2).

Table 2 CARE – Primary and Secondary Endpoints

Event	Number (%) of Subjects		Risk Reduction	*P*-value
	Pravastatin (N = 2081)	Placebo (N = 2078)		
Primary Endpoint				
CHD mortality or nonfatal MI*	212 (10.2)	274 (13.2)	24%	0.003
Secondary Endpoints				
Myocardial revascularization procedures (CABG or PTCA)	294 (14.1)	391 (18.8)	27%	<0.001
Stroke or TIA	93 (4.5)	124 (6.0)	26%	0.029

* The risk reduction due to treatment with PRAVACHOL (pravastatin sodium) was consistent in both sexes.

In the Pravastatin Limitation of Atherosclerosis in the Coronary Arteries (PLAC I)[4] study, the effect of pravastatin therapy on coronary atherosclerosis was assessed by coronary angiography in patients with coronary disease and moderate hypercholesterolemia (baseline LDL-C range = 130-190 mg/dL). In this double-blind, multicenter, controlled clinical trial angiograms were evaluated at baseline and at three years in 264 patients. Although the difference between pravastatin and placebo for the primary endpoint (per-patient change in mean coronary artery diameter) and one of two secondary endpoints (change in percent lumen diameter stenosis) did not reach statistical significance, for the secondary endpoint of change in minimum lumen diameter, statistically significant slowing of disease was seen in the pravastatin treatment group (p = 0.02).

In the Regression Growth Evaluation Statin Study (REGRESS)[5], the effect of pravastatin on coronary atherosclerosis was assessed by coronary angiography in 885 patients with angina pectoris, angiographically documented coronary artery disease and hypercholesterolemia (baseline total cholesterol range = 160-310 mg/dL). In this double-blind, multicenter, controlled clinical trial, angiograms were evaluated at baseline and at two years in 653 patients (323 treated with pravastatin). Progression of coronary atherosclerosis was significantly slowed in the pravastatin group as assessed by changes in mean segment diameter (p=0.037) and minimum obstruction diameter (p=0.001).

Analysis of pooled events from PLAC I, the Pravastatin, Lipids and Atherosclerosis in the Carotids Study (PLAC II)[6], REGRESS, and the Kuopio Atherosclerosis Prevention Study (KAPS)[7] (combined N=1891) showed that treatment with pravastatin was associated with a statistically significant reduction in the composite event rate of fatal and nonfatal myocardial infarction (46 events or 6.4% for placebo versus 21 events or 2.4% for pravastatin, p=0.001). The predominant effect of pravastatin was to reduce the rate of nonfatal myocardial infarction.

Primary Hypercholesterolemia (Fredrickson Type IIa and IIb)
PRAVACHOL (pravastatin sodium) is highly effective in reducing Total-C, LDL-C and Triglycerides (TG) in patients with heterozygous familial, presumed familial combined and non-familial (non-FH) forms of primary hypercholesterolemia, and mixed dyslipidemia. A therapeutic response is seen within 1 week, and the maximum response usually is achieved within 4 weeks. This response is maintained during extended periods of therapy. In addition, PRAVACHOL is effective in reducing the risk of acute coronary events in hypercholesterolemic patients with and without previous myocardial infarction.

A single daily dose is as effective as the same total daily dose given twice a day. In multicenter, double-blind, placebo-controlled studies of patients with primary hypercholesterolemia, treatment with pravastatin in daily doses ranging from 10 mg to 40 mg consistently and significantly decreased Total-C, LDL-C, TG, and Total-C/HDL-C and LDL-C/HDL-C ratios; modestly decreased VLDL-C and produced variable increases in HDL-C.

Primary Hypercholesterolemia Study
Dose Response of PRAVACHOL*
Once Daily Administration At Bedtime

Dose	Total-C	LDL-C	HDL-C	TG
10 mg	-16%	-22%	+ 7%	-15%
20 mg	-24%	-32%	+ 2%	-11%
40 mg	-25%	-34%	+12%	-24%

*Mean percent change from baseline after 8 weeks

In another clinical trial, patients treated with pravastatin in combination with cholestyramine (70% of patients were taking cholestyramine 20 or 24 g per day) had reductions equal to or greater than 50% in LDL-C. Furthermore, pravastatin attenuated cholestyramine-induced increases in TG levels (which are themselves of uncertain clinical significance).

Hypertriglyceridemia (Fredrickson Type IV)
The response to pravastatin in patients with Type IV hyperlipidemia (baseline TG > 200 mg/dL and LDL-C < 160 mg/dL) was evaluated in a subset of 429 patients from the Cholesterol and Recurrent Events (CARE) study. For pravastatin-treated subjects, the median (min, max) baseline triglyceride level was 246.0 (200.5, 349.5) mg/dL.

Patients With Fredrickson Type IV Hyperlipidemia
Median (25th,75th percentile) Percent Change From Baseline

	Pravastatin 40 mg (N=429)	Placebo (N=430)
Triglycerides	-21.1 (-34.8, 1.3)	-6.3 (-23.1, 18.3)
Total-C	-22.1 (-27.1, -14.8)	0.2 (-6.9, 6.8)
LDL-C	-31.7 (-39.6, -21.5)	0.7 (-9.0, 10.0)
HDL-C	7.4 (-1.2, 17.7)	2.8 (-5.7, 11.7)
Non-HDL-C	-27.2 (-34.0, -18.5)	-0.8 (-8.2, 7.0)

Dysbetalipoproteinemia (Fredrickson Type III)
The response to pravastatin in two double-blind crossover studies of 46 patients with genotype E2/E2 and Fredrickson Type III dysbetalipoproteinemia is shown in the table below.

Patients With Fredrickson Type III Dysbetalipoproteinemia
Median (min, max) Percent Change From Baseline

	Median (min, max) at Baseline (mg/dL)	Median % Change (min, max) Pravastatin 40 mg (N=20)
Study 1		
Total-C	386.5 (245.0, 672.0)	-32.7 (-58.5, 4.6)
Triglycerides	443.0 (275.0, 1299.0)	-23.7 (-68.5, 44.7)
VLDL-C*	206.5 (110.0, 379.0)	-43.8 (-73.1, -14.3)
LDL-C*	117.5 (80.0, 170.0)	-40.8 (-63.7, 4.6)
HDL-C	30.0 (18.0, 88.0)	6.4 (-45.0, 105.6)
Non-HDL-C	344.5 (215.0, 646.0)	-36.7 (-66.3, 5.8)
*N=14		

	Median (min, max) at Baseline (mg/dL)	Median % Change (min, max) Pravastatin 40 mg (N=26)
Study 2		
Total-C	340.3 (230.1, 448.6)	-31.4 (-54.5, -13.0)
Triglycerides	343.2 (212.6, 845.9)	-11.9 (-56.5, 44.8)
VLDL-C	145.0 (71.5, 309.4)	-35.7 (-74.7, 19.1)
LDL-C	128.6 (63.8, 177.9)	-30.3 (-52.2, 13.5)
HDL-C	38.7 (27.1, 58.0)	5.0 (-17.7, 66.7)
Non-HDL-C	295.8 (195.3, 421.5)	-35.5 (-81.0, -13.5)

INDICATIONS AND USAGE

Therapy with PRAVACHOL (pravastatin sodium) should be considered in those individuals at increased risk for atherosclerosis-related clinical events as a function of cholesterol level, the presence or absence of coronary heart disease, and other risk factors.

Primary Prevention of Coronary Events
In hypercholesterolemic patients without clinically evident coronary heart disease, PRAVACHOL (pravastatin sodium) is indicated to:
 – Reduce the risk of myocardial infarction
 – Reduce the risk of undergoing myocardial revascularization procedures
 – Reduce the risk of cardiovascular mortality with no increase in death from non-cardiovascular causes

Secondary Prevention of Cardiovascular Events
In patients with clinically evident coronary heart disease, PRAVACHOL is indicated to:
 – Reduce the risk of total mortality by reducing coronary death
 – Reduce the risk of myocardial infarction
 – Reduce the risk of undergoing myocardial revascularization procedures
 – Reduce the risk of stroke and stroke/transient ischemic attack (TIA)
 – Slow the progression of coronary atherosclerosis

Hyperlipidemia
PRAVACHOL is indicated as an adjunct to diet to reduce elevated Total-C, LDL-C, Apo B, and TG levels and to increase HDL-C in patients with primary hypercholesterolemia and mixed dyslipidemia (Fredrickson Type IIa and IIb).[8]

PRAVACHOL is indicated as adjunctive therapy to diet for the treatment of patients with elevated serum triglyceride levels (Fredrickson Type IV).

PRAVACHOL is indicated for the treatment of patients with primary dysbetalipoproteinemia (Fredrickson Type III) who do not respond adequately to diet.

Lipid-altering agents should be used in addition to a diet restricted in saturated fat and cholesterol when the response to diet and other nonpharmacological measures alone has been inadequate (see NCEP Guidelines below).

Prior to initiating therapy with pravastatin, secondary causes for hypercholesterolemia (e.g., poorly controlled diabetes mellitus, hypothyroidism, nephrotic syndrome, dysproteinemias, obstructive liver disease, other drug therapy, alcoholism) should be excluded, and a lipid profile performed to measure Total-C, HDL-C, and TG. For patients with triglycerides (TG) <400 mg/dL (<4.5 mmol/L), LDL-C can be estimated using the following equation:

$$LDL\text{-}C = Total\text{-}C - HDL\text{-}C - \tfrac{1}{5}\,TG$$

For TG levels >400 mg/dL (>4.5 mmol/L), this equation is less accurate and LDL-C concentrations should be determined by ultracentrifugation. In many hypertriglyceridemic patients, LDL-C may be low or normal despite elevated Total-C. In such cases, HMG-CoA reductase inhibitors are not indicated.

Lipid determinations should be performed at intervals of no less than four weeks and dosage adjusted according to the patient's response to therapy.

The National Cholesterol Education Program's Treatment Guidelines are summarized below:

		LDL Cholesterol mg/dL (mmol/L)	
Definite Atherosclerotic Disease*	Two or more Other Risk Factors**	Initiation Level***	Goal
NO	NO	≥190 (>4.9)	<160 (<4.1)
NO	YES	≥160 (≥4.1)	<130 (<3.4)
YES	YES or NO	≥130 (≥3.4)	≤100 (≤2.6)

* Coronary heart disease or peripheral vascular disease (including symptomatic carotid artery disease).
** Other risk factors for coronary heart disease (CHD) include: age (males: ≥45 years; females: ≥55 years or premature menopause without estrogen replacement therapy); family history of premature CHD; current cigarette smoking; hypertension; confirmed HDL-C <35 mg/dL (<0.91 mmol/L); and diabetes mellitus. Subtract one risk factor if HDL-C is ≥60 mg/dL (≥1.6 mmol/L).
*** In CHD patients with LDL-C levels 100-129 mg/dL, the physician should exercise clinical judgement in deciding whether to initiate drug treatment.

At the time of hospitalization for an acute coronary event, consideration can be given to initiating drug therapy at discharge if the LDL-C is ≥130 mg/dL (see NCEP Guidelines, above).

Since the goal of treatment is to lower LDL-C, the NCEP recommends that LDL-C levels be used to initiate and assess treatment response. Only if LDL-C levels are not available, should the Total-C be used to monitor therapy.

As with other lipid-lowering therapy, PRAVACHOL (pravastatin sodium) is not indicated when hypercholesterolemia is due to hyperalphalipoproteinemia (elevated HDL-C).

CONTRAINDICATIONS

Hypersensitivity to any component of this medication.

Active liver disease or unexplained, persistent elevations in liver function tests (see **WARNINGS**).

Pregnancy and lactation. Atherosclerosis is a chronic process and discontinuation of lipid-lowering drugs during pregnancy should have little impact on the outcome of long-term therapy of primary hypercholesterolemia. Cholesterol and other products of cholesterol biosynthesis are essential components for fetal development (including synthesis of steroids and cell membranes). Since HMG-CoA reductase inhibitors decrease cholesterol synthesis and possibly the synthesis of other biologically active substances derived from cholesterol, they are contraindicated during pregnancy and in nursing mothers. **Pravastatin should be administered to women of childbearing age only when such patients are highly unlikely to conceive and have been informed of the potential hazards.** If the patient becomes pregnant while taking this class of drug, therapy should be discontinued immediately and the patient apprised of the potential hazard to the fetus (see **PRECAUTIONS: Pregnancy**).

WARNINGS

Liver Enzymes

HMG-CoA reductase inhibitors, like some other lipid-lowering therapies, have been associated with biochemical abnormalities of liver function. In three long-term (4.8-5.9 years), placebo-controlled clinical trials (WOS, LIPID, CARE; see **CLINICAL PHARMACOLOGY: Clinical Studies**), 19,592 subjects (19,768 randomized), were exposed to pravastatin or placebo. In an analysis of serum transaminase values (ALT, AST), incidences of marked abnormalities were compared between the pravastatin and placebo treatment groups; a marked abnormality was defined as a post-treatment test value greater than three times the upper limit of normal for subjects with pretreatment values less than or equal to the upper limit of normal, or four times the pretreatment value for subjects with pretreatment values greater than the upper limit of normal but less than 1.5 times the upper limit of normal. Marked abnormalities of ALT or AST occurred with similar low frequency (≤1.2%) in both treatment groups. Overall, clinical trial experience showed that liver function test abnormalities observed during pravastatin therapy were usually asymptomatic, not associated with cholestasis, and did not appear to be related to treatment duration.

It is recommended that liver function tests be performed prior to the initiation of therapy, prior to the elevation of the dose, and when otherwise clinically indicated.

Active liver disease or unexplained persistent transaminase elevations are contraindications to the use of pravastatin (see **CONTRAINDICATIONS**). Caution should be exercised when pravastatin is administered to patients who have a recent history of liver disease, have signs that may suggest liver disease (e.g., unexplained aminotransferase elevations, jaundice), or are heavy users of alcohol (see **CLINICAL PHARMACOLOGY: Pharmacokinetics/Metabolism**). Such patients should be closely monitored, started at the lower end of the recommended dosing range, and titrated to the desired therapeutic effect.

Patients who develop increased transaminase levels or signs and symptoms of liver disease should be monitored with a second liver function evaluation to confirm the finding and be followed thereafter with frequent liver function tests until the abnormality(ies) return to normal. Should an increase in AST or ALT of three times the upper limit of normal or greater persist, withdrawal of pravastatin therapy is recommended.

Skeletal Muscle

Rare cases of rhabdomyolysis with acute renal failure secondary to myoglobinuria have been reported with pravastatin and other drugs in this class. Uncomplicated myalgia has also been reported in pravastatin-treated patients (see **ADVERSE REACTIONS**). Myopathy, defined as muscle aching or muscle weakness in conjunction with increases in creatine phosphokinase (CPK) values to greater than 10 times the upper normal limit, was rare (<0.1%) in pravastatin clinical trials. Myopathy should be considered in any patient with diffuse myalgias, muscle tenderness or weakness, and/or marked elevation of CPK. Patients should be advised to report promptly unexplained muscle pain, tenderness or weakness, particularly if accompanied by malaise or fever. **Pravastatin therapy should be discontinued if markedly elevated CPK levels occur or myopathy is diagnosed or suspected. Pravastatin therapy should also be temporarily withheld in any patient experiencing an acute or serious condition predisposing to the development of renal failure secondary to rhabdomyolysis, e.g., sepsis; hypotension; major surgery; trauma; severe metabolic, endocrine, or electrolyte disorders; or uncontrolled epilepsy.**

The risk of myopathy during treatment with another HMG-CoA reductase inhibitor is increased with concurrent therapy with either erythromycin, cyclosporine, niacin, or fibrates. However, neither myopathy nor significant increases in CPK levels have been observed in three reports involving a total of 100 post-transplant patients (24 renal and 76 cardiac) treated for up to two years concurrently with pravastatin 10-40 mg and cyclosporine. Some of these patients also received other concomitant immunosuppressive therapies. Further, in clinical trials involving small numbers of patients who were treated concurrently with pravastatin and niacin, there were no reports of myopathy. Also, myopathy was not reported in a trial of combination pravastatin (40 mg/day) and gemfibrozil (1200 mg/day), although 4 of 75 patients on the combination showed marked CPK elevations versus one of 73 patients receiving placebo. There was a trend toward more frequent CPK elevations and patient withdrawals due to musculoskeletal symptoms in the group receiving combined treatment as compared with the groups receiving placebo, gemfibrozil, or pravastatin monotherapy (see **PRECAUTIONS: Drug Interactions**). The use of fibrates alone may occasionally be associated with myopathy. The combined use of pravastatin and fibrates should be avoided unless the benefit of further alterations in lipid levels is likely to outweigh the increased risk of this drug combination.

PRECAUTIONS

General

PRAVACHOL (pravastatin sodium) may elevate creatine phosphokinase and transaminase levels (see **ADVERSE REACTIONS**). This should be considered in the differential diagnosis of chest pain in a patient on therapy with pravastatin.

Homozygous Familial Hypercholesterolemia. Pravastatin has not been evaluated in patients with rare homozygous familial hypercholesterolemia. In this group of patients, it has been reported that HMG-CoA reductase inhibitors are less effective because the patients lack functional LDL receptors.

Renal Insufficiency. A single 20 mg oral dose of pravastatin was administered to 24 patients with varying degrees of renal impairment (as determined by creatinine clearance). No effect was observed on the pharmacokinetics of pravastatin or its 3α-hydroxy isomeric metabolite (SQ 31,906). A small increase was seen in mean AUC values and half-life ($t\frac{1}{2}$) for the inactive enzymatic ring hydroxylation metabolite (SQ 31,945). Given this small sample size, the dosage administered, and the degree of individual variability, patients with renal impairment who are receiving pravastatin should be closely monitored.

Information for Patients

Patients should be advised to report promptly unexplained muscle pain, tenderness or weakness, particularly if accompanied by malaise or fever (see **WARNINGS: Skeletal Muscle**).

Drug Interactions

Immunosuppressive Drugs, Gemfibrozil, Niacin (Nicotinic Acid), Erythromycin: See **WARNINGS: Skeletal Muscle.**

Cytochrome P450 3A4 Inhibitors: In vitro and in vivo data indicate that pravastatin is not metabolized by cytochrome P450 3A4 to a clinically significant extent. This has been shown in studies with known cytochrome P450 3A4 inhibitors (see diltiazem and itraconazole below). Other examples of cytochrome P450 3A4 inhibitors include ketoconazole, mibefradil, and erythromycin.

Diltiazem – Steady-state levels of diltiazem (a known, weak inhibitor of P450 3A4) had no effect on the pharmacokinetics of pravastatin. In this study, the AUC and C_{max} of another HMG-CoA reductase inhibitor which is known to be metabolized by cytochrome P450 3A4 increased by factors of 3.6 and 4.3, respectively.

Itraconazole – The mean AUC and C_{max} for pravastatin were increased by factors of 1.7 and 2.5, respectively, when given with itraconazole (a potent P450 3A4 inhibitor which also inhibits p-glycoprotein transport) as compared to placebo. The mean $t\frac{1}{2}$ was not affected by itraconazole, suggesting that the relatively small increases in C_{max} and AUC were due solely to increased bioavailability rather than a decrease in clearance, consistent with inhibition of p-glycoprotein transport by itraconazole. This drug transport system is thought to affect bioavailability and excretion of HMG-CoA reductase inhibitors, including pravastatin. The AUC and C_{max} of another HMG-CoA reductase inhibitor which is known to be metabolized by cytochrome P450 3A4 increased by factors of 19 and 17, respectively, when given with itraconazole.

Antipyrine: Since concomitant administration of pravastatin had no effect on the clearance of antipyrine, interactions with other drugs metabolized via the same hepatic cytochrome isozymes are not expected.

Cholestyramine/Colestipol: Concomitant administration resulted in an approximately 40 to 50% decrease in the mean AUC of pravastatin. However, when pravastatin was administered 1 hour before or 4 hours after cholestyramine or 1 hour before colestipol and a standard meal, there was no clinically significant decrease in bioavailability or therapeutic effect. (See **DOSAGE AND ADMINISTRATION: Concomitant Therapy.**)

Warfarin: Pravastatin had no clinically significant effect on prothrombin time when administered in a study to normal elderly subjects who were stabilized on warfarin.

Cimetidine: The $AUC_{0-12\,hr}$ for pravastatin when given with cimetidine was not significantly different from the AUC for pravastatin when given alone. A significant difference was observed between the AUC's for pravastatin when given with cimetidine compared to when administered with antacid.

Digoxin: In a crossover trial involving 18 healthy male subjects given pravastatin and digoxin concurrently for 9 days, the bioavailability parameters of digoxin were not affected. The AUC of pravastatin tended to increase, but the overall bioavailability of pravastatin plus its metabolites SQ 31,906 and SQ 31,945 was not altered.

Cyclosporine: Some investigators have measured cyclosporine levels in patients on pravastatin, and to date, these results indicate no clinically meaningful elevations in cyclosporine levels. In one single-dose study, pravastatin levels were found to be increased in cardiac transplant patients receiving cyclosporine.

Gemfibrozil: In a crossover study in 20 healthy male volunteers given concomitant single doses of pravastatin and gemfibrozil, there was a significant decrease in urinary excretion and protein binding of pravastatin. In addition, there was a significant increase in AUC, C_{max}, and T_{max} for the pravastatin metabolite SQ 31,906. Combination therapy with pravastatin and gemfibrozil is generally not recommended.

In interaction studies with *aspirin, antacids* (1 hour prior to PRAVACHOL), *cimetidine, nicotinic acid,* or *probucol*, no statistically significant differences in bioavailability were seen when PRAVACHOL (pravastatin sodium) was administered.

Endocrine Function
HMG-CoA reductase inhibitors interfere with cholesterol synthesis and lower circulating cholesterol levels and, as such, might theoretically blunt adrenal or gonadal steroid hormone production. Results of clinical trials with pravastatin in males and post-menopausal females were inconsistent with regard to possible effects of the drug on basal steroid hormone levels. In a study of 21 males, the mean testosterone response to human chorionic gonadotropin was significantly reduced (p<0.004) after 16 weeks of treatment with 40 mg of pravastatin. However, the percentage of patients showing a ≥50% rise in plasma testosterone after human chorionic gonadotropin stimulation did not change significantly after therapy in these patients. The effects of HMG-CoA reductase inhibitors on spermatogenesis and fertility have not been studied in adequate numbers of patients. The effects, if any, of pravastatin on the pituitary-gonadal axis in pre-menopausal females are unknown. Patients treated with pravastatin who display clinical evidence of endocrine dysfunction should be evaluated appropriately. Caution should also be exercised if an HMG-CoA reductase inhibitor or other agent used to lower cholesterol levels is administered to patients also receiving other drugs (e.g., ketoconazole, spironolactone, cimetidine) that may diminish the levels or activity of steroid hormones.

CNS Toxicity
CNS vascular lesions, characterized by perivascular hemorrhage and edema and mononuclear cell infiltration of perivascular spaces, were seen in dogs treated with pravastatin at a dose of 25 mg/kg/day, a dose that produced a plasma drug level about 50 times higher than the mean drug level in humans taking 40 mg/day. Similar CNS vascular lesions have been observed with several other drugs in this class.

A chemically similar drug in this class produced optic nerve degeneration (Wallerian degeneration of retinogeniculate fibers) in clinically normal dogs in a dose-dependent fashion starting at 60 mg/kg/day, a dose that produced mean plasma drug levels about 30 times higher than the mean drug level in humans taking the highest recommended dose (as measured by total enzyme inhibitory activity). This same drug also produced vestibulocochlear Wallerian-like degeneration and retinal ganglion cell chromatolysis in dogs treated for 14 weeks at 180 mg/kg/day, a dose which resulted in a mean plasma drug level similar to that seen with the 60 mg/kg/day dose.

Carcinogenesis, Mutagenesis, Impairment of Fertility
In a 2-year study in rats fed pravastatin at doses of 10, 30, or 100 mg/kg body weight, there was an increased incidence of hepatocellular carcinomas in males at the highest dose (p <0.01). Although rats were given up to 125 times the human dose (HD) on a mg/kg body weight basis, serum drug levels were only 6 to 10 times higher than those measured in humans given 40 mg pravastatin as measured by AUC.

In a 2-year study in mice fed pravastatin at doses of 250 and 500 mg/kg/day, there was an increased incidence of hepatocellular carcinomas in males and females at both 250 and 500 mg/kg/day (p<0.0001). At these doses, lung adenomas in females were increased (p=0.013). Serum drug levels were 30 to 40 times (250 mg/kg/day) and 50 times (500 mg/kg/day) that of humans given 40 mg pravastatin, as measured by AUC. In another 2-year study in mice with doses at up to 100 mg/kg/day (producing plasma drug levels up to 5 times human drug levels at 40 mg), there were no drug-induced tumors.

No evidence of mutagenicity was observed *in vitro*, with or without rat-liver metabolic activation, in the following studies: microbial mutagen tests, using mutant strains of *Salmonella typhimurium* or *Escherichia coli*; a forward mutation assay in L5178Y TK +/- mouse lymphoma cells; a chromosomal aberration test in hamster cells; and a gene conversion assay using *Saccharomyces cerevisiae*. In addition, there was no evidence of mutagenicity in either a dominant lethal test in mice or a micronucleus test in mice.

In a study in rats, with daily doses up to 500 mg/kg, pravastatin did not produce any adverse effects on fertility or general reproductive performance. However, in a study with another HMG-CoA reductase inhibitor, there was decreased fertility in male rats treated for 34 weeks at 25 mg/kg body weight, although this effect was not observed in a subsequent fertility study when this same dose was administered for 11 weeks (the entire cycle of spermatogenesis, including epididymal maturation). In rats treated with this same reductase inhibitor at 180 mg/kg/day, seminiferous tubule degeneration (necrosis and loss of spermatogenic epithelium) was observed. Although not seen with pravastatin, two similar drugs in this class caused drug-related testicular atrophy, decreased spermatogenesis, spermatocytic degeneration, and giant cell formation in dogs. The clinical significance of these findings is unclear.

Pregnancy
Pregnancy Category X.
See **CONTRAINDICATIONS**.

Safety in pregnant women has not been established. Pravastatin was not teratogenic in rats at doses up to 1000 mg/kg daily or in rabbits at doses of up to 50 mg/kg daily. These doses resulted in 20x (rabbit) or 240x (rat) the human exposure based on surface area (mg/meter[2]). Rare reports of congenital anomalies have been received following intrauterine exposure to other HMG-CoA reductase inhibitors. In a review[9] of approximately 100 prospectively followed pregnancies in women exposed to simvastatin or lovastatin, the incidences of congenital anomalies, spontaneous abortions and fetal deaths/stillbirths did not exceed what would be expected in the general population. The number of cases is adequate only to exclude a three-to-four-fold increase in congenital anomalies over the background incidence. In 89% of the prospectively followed pregnancies, drug treatment was initiated prior to pregnancy and was discontinued at some point in the first trimester when pregnancy was identified. As safety in pregnant women has not been established and there is no apparent benefit to therapy with PRAVACHOL during pregnancy (see **CONTRAINDICATIONS**), treatment should be immediately discontinued as soon as pregnancy is recognized. PRAVACHOL (pravastatin sodium) should be administered to women of child-bearing potential only when such patients are highly unlikely to conceive and have been informed of the potential hazards.

Nursing Mothers
A small amount of pravastatin is excreted in human breast milk. Because of the potential for serious adverse reactions in nursing infants, women taking PRAVACHOL should not nurse (see **CONTRAINDICATIONS**).

Pediatric Use

Safety and effectiveness in individuals less than 18 years old have not been established. Hence, treatment in patients less than 18 years old is not recommended at this time.

Geriatric Use

Two secondary prevention trials with pravastatin (CARE and LIPID) included a total of 6,593 subjects treated with pravastatin 40 mg for periods ranging up to 6 years. Across these two studies, 36.1% of pravastatin subjects were aged 65 and older and 0.8% were aged 75 and older. The beneficial effect of pravastatin in elderly subjects in reducing cardiovascular events and in modifying lipid profiles was similar to that seen in younger subjects. The adverse event profile in the elderly was similar to that in the overall population. Other reported clinical experience has not identified differences in responses to pravastatin between elderly and younger patients.

Mean pravastatin AUCs are slightly (25-50%) higher in elderly subjects than in healthy young subjects, but mean C_{max}, T_{max} and $t½$ values are similar in both age groups and substantial accumulation of pravastatin would not be expected in the elderly (see **CLINICAL PHARMACOLOGY: Pharmacokinetics/ Metabolism**).

ADVERSE REACTIONS

Pravastatin is generally well tolerated; adverse reactions have usually been mild and transient. In 4-month long placebo-controlled trials, 1.7% of pravastatin-treated patients and 1.2% of placebo-treated patients were discontinued from treatment because of adverse experiences attributed to study drug therapy; this difference was not statistically significant. (See also **PRECAUTIONS: Geriatric Use** section).

Adverse Clinical Events

All adverse clinical events (regardless of attribution) reported in more than 2% of pravastatin-treated patients in the placebo-controlled trials are identified in the table below; also shown are the percentages of patients in whom these medical events were believed to be related or possibly related to the drug:

Body System/Event	All Events		Events Attributed to Study Drug	
	Pravastatin (N = 900) %	Placebo (N = 411) %	Pravastatin (N = 900) %	Placebo (N = 411) %
Cardiovascular				
Cardiac Chest Pain	4.0	3.4	0.1	0.0
Dermatologic Rash	4.0*	1.1	1.3	0.9
Gastrointestinal				
Nausea/Vomiting	7.3	7.1	2.9	3.4
Diarrhea	6.2	5.6	2.0	1.9
Abdominal Pain	5.4	6.9	2.0	3.9
Constipation	4.0	7.1	2.4	5.1
Flatulence	3.3	3.6	2.7	3.4
Heartburn	2.9	1.9	2.0	0.7
General				
Fatigue	3.8	3.4	1.9	1.0
Chest Pain	3.7	1.9	0.3	0.2
Influenza	2.4*	0.7	0.0	0.0
Musculoskeletal				
Localized Pain	10.0	9.0	1.4	1.5
Myalgia	2.7	1.0	0.6	0.0
Nervous System				
Headache	6.2	3.9	1.7*	0.2
Dizziness	3.3	3.2	1.0	0.5
Renal/Genitourinary				
Urinary Abnormality	2.4	2.9	0.7	1.2
Respiratory				
Common Cold	7.0	6.3	0.0	0.0
Rhinitis	4.0	4.1	0.1	0.0
Cough	2.6	1.7	0.1	0.0

*Statistically significantly different from placebo.

In three large, placebo-controlled trials (West of Scotland Coronary Prevention study [WOS], Cholesterol and Recurrent Events study [CARE], and Long-term Intervention with Pravastatin in Ischemic Disease study [LIPID]) involving a total of 19,768 patients treated with PRAVACHOL (pravastatin sodium) (N=9895) or placebo (N=9873), the safety and tolerability profile in the pravastatin group was comparable to that of the placebo group over the median 4.8 to 5.9 years of follow-up. In these long-term trials, the most common reasons for discontinuation were mild, non-specific gastrointestinal complaints.

The following effects have been reported with drugs in this class; not all the effects listed below have necessarily been associated with pravastatin therapy:

Skeletal: myopathy, rhabdomyolysis, arthralgia.

Neurological: dysfunction of certain cranial nerves (including alteration of taste, impairment of extra-ocular movement, facial paresis), tremor, vertigo, memory loss, paresthesia, peripheral neuropathy, peripheral nerve palsy, anxiety, insomnia, depression.

Hypersensitivity Reactions: An apparent hypersensitivity syndrome has been reported rarely which has included one or more of the following features: anaphylaxis, angioedema, lupus erythematous-like syndrome, polymyalgia rheumatica, dermatomyositis, vasculitis, purpura, thrombocytopenia, leukopenia, hemolytic anemia, positive ANA, ESR increase, eosinophilia, arthritis, arthralgia, urticaria, asthenia, photosensitivity, fever, chills, flushing, malaise, dyspnea, toxic epidermal necrolysis, erythema multiforme, including Stevens-Johnson syndrome.

Gastrointestinal: pancreatitis, hepatitis, including chronic active hepatitis, cholestatic jaundice, fatty change in liver, and, rarely, cirrhosis, fulminant hepatic necrosis, and hepatoma; anorexia, vomiting.

Skin: alopecia, pruritus. A variety of skin changes (e.g., nodules, discoloration, dryness of skin/mucous membranes, changes to hair/nails) have been reported.

Reproductive: gynecomastia, loss of libido, erectile dysfunction.

Eye: progression of cataracts (lens opacities), ophthalmoplegia.

Laboratory Abnormalities: elevated transaminases, alkaline phosphatase, and bilirubin; thyroid function abnormalities.

Laboratory Test Abnormalities

Increases in serum transaminase (ALT, AST) values and CPK have been observed (see **WARNINGS**).

Transient, asymptomatic eosinophilia has been reported. Eosinophil counts usually returned to normal despite continued therapy. Anemia, thrombocytopenia, and leukopenia have been reported with HMG-CoA reductase inhibitors.

Concomitant Therapy

Pravastatin has been administered concurrently with cholestyramine, colestipol, nicotinic acid, probucol and gemfibrozil. Preliminary data suggest that the addition of either probucol or gemfibrozil to therapy with lovastatin or pravastatin is **not** associated with greater reduction in LDL-cholesterol than that achieved with lovastatin or pravastatin alone. No adverse reactions unique to the combination or in addition to those previously reported for each drug alone have been reported. Myopathy and rhabdomyolysis (with or without acute renal failure) have been reported when another HMG-CoA reductase inhibitor was used in combination with immunosuppressive drugs, gemfibrozil, erythromycin, or lipid-lowering doses of nicotinic acid. Concomitant therapy with HMG-CoA reductase inhibitors and these agents is generally not recommended. (See **WARNINGS: Skeletal Muscle** and **PRECAUTIONS: Drug Interactions**.)

OVERDOSAGE

To date, there are two reported cases of overdosage with pravastatin, both of which were asymptomatic and not associated with clinical laboratory abnormalities. If an overdose occurs, it should be treated symptomatically and supportive measures should be instituted as required.

DOSAGE AND ADMINISTRATION

The patient should be placed on a standard cholesterol-lowering diet before receiving PRAVACHOL (pravastatin sodium) and should continue on this diet during treatment with PRAVACHOL (see NCEP Treatment Guidelines for details on dietary therapy).

The recommended starting dose is 10, 20 or 40 mg once daily. PRAVACHOL can be administered as a single dose at any time of the day, with or without food. In patients with a history of significant renal or hepatic dysfunction, a starting dose of 10 mg daily is recommended.

Since the maximal effect of a given dose is seen within 4 weeks, periodic lipid determinations should be performed at this time and dosage adjusted according to the patient's response to therapy and established treatment guidelines.

In patients taking immunosuppressive drugs such as cyclosporine (see **WARNINGS: Skeletal Muscle**) concomitantly with pravastatin, therapy should begin with 10 mg of pravastatin once-a-day at bedtime and titration to higher doses should be done with caution. Most patients treated with this combination received a maximum pravastatin dose of 20 mg/day.

Concomitant Therapy

The lipid-lowering effects of PRAVACHOL (pravastatin sodium) on total and LDL cholesterol are enhanced when combined with a bile-acid-binding resin. When administering a bile-acid-binding resin (e.g., cholestyramine, colestipol) and pravastatin, PRAVACHOL should be given either 1 hour or more before or at least 4 hours following the resin. See also **ADVERSE REACTIONS: Concomitant Therapy**.

HOW SUPPLIED

PRAVACHOL® (pravastatin sodium) Tablets are supplied as:

10 mg tablets: Pink to peach, rounded, rectangular-shaped, biconvex with a P embossed on one side and PRAVACHOL 10 engraved on the opposite side. They are supplied in bottles of 90 (NDC 0003-5154-05). Bottles contain a desiccant canister.

20 mg tablets: Yellow, rounded, rectangular-shaped, biconvex with a P embossed on one side and PRAVACHOL 20 engraved on the opposite side. They are supplied in bottles of 90 (NDC 0003-5178-05) and bottles of 1000 (NDC 0003-5178-75). Bottles contain a desiccant canister.

40 mg tablets: Green, rounded, rectangular-shaped, biconvex with a P embossed on one side and PRAVACHOL 40 engraved on the opposite side. They are supplied in bottles of 90 (NDC 0003-5194-10). Bottles contain a desiccant canister.

Unimatic® unit-dose packs containing 100 tablets are also available for the **20 mg** (NDC 0003-5178-06) potency.

Storage

Do not store above 86° F (30° C). Keep tightly closed (protect from moisture). Protect from light.

REFERENCES

[1] Shepherd J, et al. Prevention of coronary heart disease with pravastatin in men with hypercholesterolemia (WOS). *N Engl J Med* 1995;333:1301–7.

[2] The Long-term Intervention with Pravastatin in Ischemic Disease Group. Prevention of cardiovascular events and death with pravastatin in patients with coronary heart disease and a broad range of initial cholesterol levels (LIPID). *N Engl J Med* 1998;339:1349–1357.

[3] Sacks FM, et al. The effect of pravastatin on coronary events after myocardial infarction in patients with average cholesterol levels (CARE). *N Engl J Med.* 1996;335:1001-9.

[4] Pitt B, et al. Pravastatin Limitation of Atherosclerosis in the Coronary Arteries (PLAC I): Reduction in Atherosclerosis Progression and Clinical Events. *J Am Coll Cardiol* 1995;26:1133-9.

[5] Jukema JW, et al. Effects of Lipid Lowering by Pravastatin on Progression and Regression of Coronary Artery Disease in Symptomatic Man With Normal to Moderately Elevated Serum Cholesterol Levels. The Regression Growth Evaluation Statin Study (REGRESS). *Circulation* 1995;91:2528–2540.

[6] Crouse JR, et al. Pravastatin, lipids, and atherosclerosis in the carotid arteries: design features of a clinical trial with carotid atherosclerosis outcome (PLAC II).*Controlled Clinical Trials* 13:495, 1992.

[7] Salonen R, et al. Kuopio Atherosclerosis Prevention Study (KAPS). A population-based primary preventive trial of the effect of LDL lowering on atherosclerotic progression in carotid and femoral arteries. Research Institute of Public Health, University of Kuopio, Finland. *Circulation* 92:1758, 1995.

[8] Fredrickson DS, et, al. Fat transport in lipoproteins-an integrated approach to mechanisms and disorders. *N Engl J Med* 1967; 276:34-42, 94-102, 148-156, 215-224, 273-281.

[9] Manson JM, Freyssinges C, Ducrocq MB, Stephenson WP. Postmarketing Surveillance of Lovastatin and Simvastatin Exposure During Pregnancy. *Reproductive Toxicology* 10(6):439-446, 1996.

U.S. Patent Nos.: 4,346,227; 5,030,447; 5,180,589; 5,622,985

D3-B001-07-01
Revised July 2001

5154DIM-16

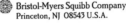

Bristol-Myers Squibb Company
Princeton, NJ 08543 U.S.A.